Cancer Consult

Cancer Consult

Expertise in Clinical Practice, Second Edition.

Volume 1: Solid Tumors & Supportive Care

Edited by

Syed A. Abutalib, Maurie Markman, Al B. Benson III, and Hope S. Rugo

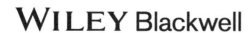

This second edition first published 2024
© 2024 John Wiley & Sons Ltd

Edition History
Cancer Consult: Expertise for Clinical Practice, John Wiley and Sons, Inc. (2014)

All rights reserved. No part of this publication may be reproduced, stored in a retrieval system, or transmitted, in any form or by any means, electronic, mechanical, photocopying, recording or otherwise, except as permitted by law. Advice on how to obtain permission to reuse material from this title is available at http://www.wiley.com/go/permissions.

The right of Syed A. Abutalib, Maurie Markman, Al B. Benson III and Hope S. Rugo to be identified as the authors of the editorial material in this work has been asserted in accordance with law.

Registered Offices
John Wiley & Sons, Inc., 111 River Street, Hoboken, NJ 07030, USA
John Wiley & Sons Ltd, The Atrium, Southern Gate, Chichester, West Sussex, PO19 8SQ, UK

Editorial Office
The Atrium, Southern Gate, Chichester, West Sussex, PO19 8SQ, UK

For details of our global editorial offices, customer services, and more information about Wiley products visit us at www.wiley.com.

Wiley also publishes its books in a variety of electronic formats and by print-on-demand. Some content that appears in standard print versions of this book may not be available in other formats.

Trademarks: Wiley and the Wiley logo are trademarks or registered trademarks of John Wiley & Sons, Inc. and/or its affiliates in the United States and other countries and may not be used without written permission. All other trademarks are the property of their respective owners. John Wiley & Sons, Inc. is not associated with any product or vendor mentioned in this book.

Limit of Liability/Disclaimer of Warranty
The contents of this work are intended to further general scientific research, understanding, and discussion only and are not intended and should not be relied upon as recommending or promoting scientific method, diagnosis, or treatment by physicians for any particular patient. In view of ongoing research, equipment modifications, changes in governmental regulations, and the constant flow of information relating to the use of medicines, equipment, and devices, the reader is urged to review and evaluate the information provided in the package insert or instructions for each medicine, equipment, or device for, among other things, any changes in the instructions or indication of usage and for added warnings and precautions. While the publisher and authors have used their best efforts in preparing this work, they make no representations or warranties with respect to the accuracy or completeness of the contents of this work and specifically disclaim all warranties, including without limitation any implied warranties of merchantability or fitness for a particular purpose. No warranty may be created or extended by sales representatives, written sales materials or promotional statements for this work. The fact that an organization, website, or product is referred to in this work as a citation and/or potential source of further information does not mean that the publisher and authors endorse the information or services the organization, website, or product may provide or recommendations it may make. This work is sold with the understanding that the publisher is not engaged in rendering professional services. The advice and strategies contained herein may not be suitable for your situation. You should consult with a specialist where appropriate. Further, readers should be aware that websites listed in this work may have changed or disappeared between when this work was written and when it is read. Neither the publisher nor authors shall be liable for any loss of profit or any other commercial damages, including but not limited to special, incidental, consequential, or other damages.

Library of Congress Cataloging-in-Publication Data
Names: Abutalib, Syed A., editor. | Markman, Maurie, editor.
Title: Cancer consult : expertise in clinical practice. Volume 1, Solid tumors & supportive care / edited by Syed A. Abutalib, Maurie Markman, Al B. Benson and Hope S. Rugo.
Description: Second edition. | Hokoben, NJ : John Wiley & Sons Ltd., 2023. | Includes bibliographical references.
Identifiers: LCCN 2023024465 | ISBN 9781119823735 (paperback) | ISBN 9781119823742 (pdf) | ISBN 9781119823759 (epub) | ISBN 9781119823766 (ebook)
Subjects: LCSH: Tumors--Treatment--Examinations, questions, etc.
Classification: LCC RC256 .C36 2023 | DDC 616.99/40076--dc23/eng/20230623
LC record available at https://lccn.loc.gov/2023024465

Cover image: © Kotkoa/Shutterstock
Cover design by Wiley

Set in 9.5/12.5pt STIXTwoText by Integra Software Services Pvt. Ltd, Pondicherry, India

Contents

Editors Volume 1 *xi*
**Volume 2: Neoplastic Hematology & Cellular Therapy
Editors** *xii*
Editor's Biography *xiii*
Preface *xv*
Acknowledgment *xvii*

Part 1   Central Nervous System   *1*

1 **Central Nervous System Tumors**   *3*
    Mark R. Gilbert and Edina Komlodi-Pasztor

Part 2   Head and Neck and Thoracic Cancers   *13*

2 **Localized Head and Neck Cancer**   *15*
    Emrullah Yilmaz and Jessica L. Geiger

3 **Recurrent and Metastatic Head and Neck Cancer**   *31*
    Chloe Weidenbaum and Mike Gibson

4 **Thyroid Cancers**   *39*
    Kartik Sehgal and Jochen H. Lorch

5 **Non-Small Cell Lung Cancer: Screening, Staging, and Stage I**   *51*
    Ryan D. Gentzler and Linda W. Martin

6 **Non-Small Cell Lung Cancer: Stages II and III**   *63*
    Gregory Peter Kalemkerian, Kamya Sankar, and Angel Qin

7 **Recurrent and Metastatic Non-Small Cell Lung Cancer**   *79*
    Julia Judd, J. Nicholas Bodor, and Hossein Borghaei

8 **Small Cell Lung Cancer**   *97*
    Jyoti D. Patel and Husam Hafzah

9 **Mesothelioma** *105*
Harvey I. Pass, David Chen, and Jack Donaghue

Part 3 Breast Cancer *115*

10 **DCIS and LCIS** *117*
Amanda Nash, Rita Mukhtar, and Shelley Hwang

11 **Early-Stage ER/PR–Positive, HER2-Negative Breast Cancer** *129*
William J. Gradishar

12 **ER/PR-Positive, HER2-Negative Metastatic Breast Cancer** *139*
Sara Nunnery, Laura Kennedy, and Sonya Reid

13 **Early-Stage HER2-Positive Breast Cancer** *151*
Erin Roesch and Jame Abraham

14 **HER2-Positive Metastatic Breast Cancer** *163*
Reshma L. Mahtani, Naomi G. Dempsey, and Ana Sandoval

15 **Early-Stage Triple-Negative Breast Cancer** *179*
Tiffany A. Traina, Carlos dos Anjos, and Elaine Walsh

16 **Triple-Negative Metastatic Breast Cancer** *191*
Azadeh Nasrazadani, Juan Gomez, and Adam Brufsky

17 **Inflammatory Breast Cancer – A Distinct Entity** *201*
Massimo Cristofanilli and Elena Vagia

18 **Male Breast Cancer** *213*
Laura A. Huppert, Ozge Gumusay, Shreya Desai, and Hope S. Rugo

19 **Breast Cancer in Pregnancy and Fertility Preservation** *225*
Fedro A. Peccatori, Hatem Azim, and Matteo Lambertini

Part 4 Gastrointestinal Cancers *233*

20 **Early-Stage Gastroesophageal Cancer and Precursor Lesions** *235*
Yixing Jiang and Aaron Ciner

21 **Metastatic Esophagogastric Cancer** *249*
Geoffrey Y. Ku and David H. Ilson

22 **Early-Stage Colon Cancer** *255*
    John Krauss, Vaibhav Sahai, and Al B. Benson III

23 **Early-Stage Rectal Cancer** *267*
    Hannah J. Roberts, Theodore Hong, and Aparna Parikh

24 **Recurrent and Metastatic Colorectal Cancer** *283*
    Joseph Heng and Blase Polite

25 **Pancreatic Adenocarcinoma** *291*
    Evan Walker, Andrew Ko, and Margaret Tempero

26 **Hepatocellular Cancer** *309*
    Pedro Luiz Serrano Uson Junior and Mitesh Borad

27 **Biliary Tract Cancers** *319*
    David B. Zhen and Vaibhav Sahai

28 **Carcinoid and Neuroendocrine Tumors** *327*
    Mintallah Haider and Jonathan Strosberg

29 **Anal Cancer** *343*
    Asad Mahmood and Rob Glynne-Jones

Part 5   Genitourinary Cancers *359*

30 **Renal Cancer** *361*
    James L. Coggan, Alan Tan, and Timothy M. Kuzel

31 **Bladder Cancer** *375*
    Revathi Kollipara, Alan Tan, and Timothy M. Kuzel

32 **Prostate Cancer: Screening, Surveillance, Prognostic Algorithms, and Independent Pathologic Predictive Parameters** *389*
    Eduardo Benzi and Thomas M. Wheeler

33 **Early and Locally Advanced Prostate Cancer** *399*
    James Randall, Mohammad R. Siddiqui, Ashley Ross, and Sean Sachdev

34 **Metastatic Prostate Cancer** *421*
    Priyanka Chablani, Natalie Reizine, and Walter Stadler

35 **Germ Cell Tumors** *437*
    Hamid Emamekhoo, Syed A. Abutalib, and Timothy Gilligan

Part 6 Skin Malignancies 453

36 Melanoma *455*
Ana M. Ciurea and Kim Margolin

37 Nonmelanoma Skin Cancers *477*
Chrysalyne D. Schmults and Danielle A. Parker

Part 7 Gynecological Cancers 497

38 Ovarian Cancer: Primary Treatment and Approach to Recurrent Disease *499*
Rani Bansal, Don Dizon, and Martina Murphy

39 Ovarian Cancer: Second-line Treatment Strategies *511*
Maurie Markman

40 Endometrial Cancer *523*
Maurie Markman

41 Cancer of the Cervix, Vulva, and Vagina *533*
Sabrina M. Bedell and Peter G. Rose

42 Uncommon Gynecologic Cancers *549*
Michael Frumovitz, Shannon Westin, and David M. Gershenson

Part 8 Sarcomas 565

43 Bone Sarcomas *567*
Nicole Larrier, William Eward, and Richard F. Riedel

44 Soft Tissue Sarcomas *579*
Jeffrey Farma, Krisha Howell, and Margaret von Mehren

Part 9 Hereditary Cancer Syndromes and Genetic Testing 595

45 Hereditary Cancer Syndromes *597*
Mary B. Daly

46 Hereditary Breast and Ovarian Cancer Syndromes *611*
Kristen Whitaker and Elias Obeid

47 Hereditary Gastrointestinal and Pancreatic Cancer Syndromes *625*
Kristen M. Shannon, Linda H. Rodgers-Fouche, and Daniel C. Chung

Part 10 Special Issues in Oncology *637*

48 Cancer of Unknown Primary *639*
Tony Greco

49 Anticoagulation in Cancer *651*
Jean Marie Connors

50 Identification and Management of Immunotherapy-Related Adverse Events in Oncology *663*
Ozge Gumusay, Laura A. Huppert, Dame Idossa, and Hope S. Rugo

51 Geriatric Oncology *677*
Sukeshi Patel Arora and Efrat Dotan

52 Palliative Medicine for Curable and Terminal Cancers *693*
Isabelle Blanchard, Kavitha Jennifer Ramachandran, and Divya Gupta

Index *709*

Editors Volume 1

Syed Ali Abutalib, MD
Medical Director
Hematologic Malignancies and
Transplantation and Cellular Therapy
Aurora St. Luke's Medical Center
Advocate Aurora Health Care
Milwaukee, Wisconsin

Maurie Markman, MD
Professor, Department of Medical
Oncology and Therapeutics Research
City of Hope

President, Medicine & Science
City of Hope, Atlanta,
Chicago and Phoenix

Al B. Benson III, MD, FACP, FASCO
Professor of Medicine
Associate Director for Cooperative Groups
Robert H. Lurie Comprehensive Cancer
Center of Northwestern University
Chicago, IL

Hope S. Rugo, MD, FASCO
Professor of Medicine
Director, Breast Oncology and Clinical
Trials Education
University of California San Francisco
Helen Diller Family Comprehensive
Cancer Center, San Francisco, CA

Volume 2: Neoplastic Hematology & Cellular Therapy

Editors

Syed Ali Abutalib, MD
Medical Director
Hematologic Malignancies and
Transplantation and Cellular Therapy
Aurora St. Luke's Medical Center
Advocate Aurora Health Care
Milwaukee, Wisconsin

Maurie Markman, MD
Professor, Department of Medical
Oncology and Therapeutics Research
City of Hope

President, Medicine & Science, City of
Hope, Atlanta, Chicago, and Phoenix

Kenneth C. Anderson, MD
Program Director, Jerome Lipper Multiple
Myeloma Center and LeBow Institute for
Myeloma Therapeutics
Kraft Family Professor of Medicine
Harvard Medical School
Dana Farber Cancer Institute, Boston, MA

James O. Armitage, MD
Joe Shapiro Professor of Medicine,
University of Nebraska Medical Center
Omaha, NE

Editor's Biography

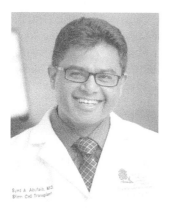

Syed Ali Abutalib, MD, is Medical Director, Hematologic Malignancies and Transplantation and Cellular Therapy, Aurora St. Luke's Medical Center. He also served as active member of Executive Committee on Education for American Society of Transplantation and Cellular therapy (ASTCT®) and is one of the Associate Editors for The ASCO Post®. Dr. Abutalib is the Founding Editor of Advances in Cell and Gene Therapy, a Wiley Journal. In addition, he is Associate Professor of Medicine at Rosalind Franklin University of Medicine and Science. Dr. Abutalib has co-edited 16 Hematology/Oncology and Cellular/Gene therapy books over a short span of 10 years and has published in a number of cancer magazines, journals, and textbooks. He continues to collaborate with most cancer experts worldwide in the area of Hematology/Oncology and stem cell transplantation to explore and develop innovative ideas and breakthroughs in Medical Education with a prime focus to improve patient care.

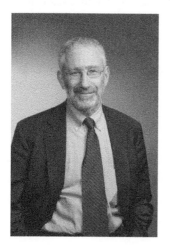

Maurie Markman, MD, is Professor of Oncology and Therapeutics Research, City of Hope and President of Medicine & Science, City of Hope Atlanta, Chicago, Phoenix. A nationally renowned oncologist, Dr. Markman has more than 20 years of experience in cancer treatment and gynecologic research at some of the country's most recognized facilities. Dr. Markman has served as the Vice President for Clinical Research and Chairman of the Department of Gynecologic Medical Oncology at M.D. Anderson Cancer Center in Houston, Texas. Prior to that, Dr. Markman spent 11 years as Chairman of the Department of Hematology/Oncology and Director of the Taussig Cancer Center at the Cleveland Clinic Foundation. He also spent five years as Vice Chairman of the Department of Medicine at Memorial Sloan-Kettering Cancer Center in New York.

Editor's Biography

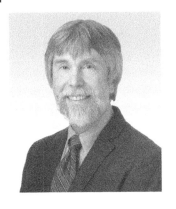

Al B. Benson III, M.D FACP FASCO is a Professor of Medicine in the Division of Hematology/Oncology at Northwestern University's Feinberg School of Medicine in Chicago, Illinois, and the Associate Director for Cooperative Groups at the Robert H. Lurie Comprehensive Cancer Center. He is a recipient of the American Society of Clinical Oncology (ASCO) Statesman Award (Fellow of ASCO) and has served on a number of ASCO committees, often as chair or co-chair. Dr Benson is currently Vice-Chair of the ECOG-ACRIN Cancer Research Group, past Chair of the ECOG-ACRIN Gastrointestinal Committee, Co-Chair of Cancer Care Delivery Research Committee, a member of the NCI Rectal/Anal Task Force and Co-Chair of the International Rare Cancers Initiative (IRCI), Anal Cancers Committee. In addition, he is a Past President of the Illinois Medical Oncology Society, Past President of the Association of Community Cancer Centers (ACCC), a board member and past-Chair of the Board of Directors of the National Comprehensive Cancer Network (NCCN) and the past President of the National Patient Advocate Foundation. Dr. Benson has published extensively in the areas of gastrointestinal cancer clinical trials, health services research and cancer treatment guidelines.

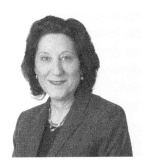

Hope S. Rugo, MD, FASCO, is Director of Breast Oncology and Clinical Trials Education and a Professor of Medicine at the University of California San Francisco Comprehensive Cancer Center. Dr. Rugo is an internationally well-known medical oncologist specializing in breast cancer research and treatment. She entered the field of breast cancer in order to incorporate novel therapies with excellent quality of care into the treatment of breast cancer and is a principal investigator of multiple clinical trials focusing on novel targeted therapeutics to improve the treatment of breast cancer. Her research interests include immunotherapy and combinations of targeted agents to treat breast cancer, and management of toxicity. She is co-chair of the Safety Committee for the multicenter adaptively randomized phase II I-SPY2 trial, co-chair of the Triple Negative Working Group of the Translational Breast Cancer Research Consortium (TBCRC) and a member of the Alliance breast committee. Dr. Rugo is an active clinician committed to education.

Preface

Over the past decade there have been tremendous advances in the oncology arena resulting in both improved survival and quality of life for individuals requiring management of a malignant disease. However, this surge in available therapeutic options has quite often resulted in increased complexity of care. As a result, patients frequently request a "second opinion."

It is also commonplace for oncologists to discuss with a colleague a difficult or unusual case, or the management of a patient who presents with serious comorbidities, to insure that the individual is given the greatest opportunity to experience the benefits of therapy while minimizing the risks of possible treatment- related harm. Such discussions occur both within a particular specialty (e.g., surgery, radiation, or medical oncology) and between various specialties.

Further, as cancer management becomes more multimodal in nature, with an increasing focus on maximizing the opportunity for extended survival and at the same time optimizing quality of life, the requirement for essential communication between individual specialists with their own unique knowledge and experience of critically relevant components of care becomes ever more important.

It is with these thoughts in mind that the editors conceived of an oncology text that would focus on the "Expert Perspectives" of oncology professionals. The intent of this distinctive effort is to have each individual chapter be viewed as a "miniconsultation" provided by a specialist regarding a specific, highly clinically relevant issue in cancer management.

Considering the specific purpose and focus of the material presented, the book is written without detailed references (although "Recommended Readings" are included at the end of each chapter). However, many of the authors have prepared a more extensive reference list, and the editors will be happy to email any reader the more detailed reference lists for individual book chapters, if so requested.

The chapters that follow have been written by clinicians selected for their recognized clinical expertise and experience. It is hoped that those reading this book will find the material of value in their own interactions with their patients.

Syed A. Abutalib, Maurie Markman, Al B. Benson III, and Hope S. Rugo

Acknowledgment

Syed Ali Abutalib: I am immensely grateful to God for providing me with the inspiration, and strength throughout this endeavour. I would like to extend my heartfelt acknowledgment to the timeless wisdom of Ali Ibne Abutalib (PBUH), who once said, "Knowledge is a companion that will never betray you, an ornament that will enhance your worth, a friend that will be with you in solitude, and a guide that will lead you to righteousness." Inspired by these profound words, I express my gratitude to the co-editors, and esteem contributors of this text. Their expertise, and dedication have significantly enhanced the breadth and depth of the content. Also, I would like to acknowledge my grandparents, Hamid, and Laila Jafry for their unwavering support, and my daughter, Sakeena Ali Abutalib. Lastly, I would like to extend my appreciation to the courageous cancer patients and their families for making me a better physician and a person.

Maurie Markman: To my grandsons, James, William, and Conrad.

Al B. Benson III: This text is dedicated to our patients who deserve the best we can offer and to the entire health care team that works tirelessly to help provide our patients the comprehensive cancer care that is so essential during the course of their illness.

Hope S. Rugo: To our dedicated colleagues who worked so hard to contribute excellent and updated manuscripts and who responded to revision requests and proof reviews with enthusiasm. To the editor, Dr. Abutalib, who has worked tirelessly and for untold hours to put this remarkable collection together, and of course to my co-editors and colleagues at Wiley as well. And of course, to my family, for your unwavering support and enthusiasm. This work is truly a tribute to the passion of oncologists to educate broadly, with the goal of improving patient care.

Part 1

Central Nervous System

1

Central Nervous System Tumors

Mark R. Gilbert and Edina Komlodi-Pasztor

Introduction

Central nervous system tumors can be divided into primary brain tumors and metastatic lesions. This chapter will focus on the most frequently occurring questions related to tumors originating from the brain, spinal cord, or associated tissue. Primary central nervous system lymphoma is discussed in a separate chapter. We will review practical questions related to epidemiology, classification, and treatment of primary brain tumors. We will discuss the incidence rates and the genetic and environmental predisposing factors related to brain cancers. A brief overview of the new fifth edition of the World Health Organization (WHO) classification system will be provided. We will summarize treatment recommendations of the most commonly occurring benign and malignant primary brain tumors, such as meningioma, oligodendroglioma, astrocytoma, and glioblastoma.

1. How do we classify brain tumors?

Expert Perspective: Brain tumors can be divided into two main groups: benign tumors and malignant cancers. Malignant cancers can be further subdivided into metastatic lesions and primary central nervous system cancers (PCNSC).

Instead of using the tumor, node, and metastasis (TNM) staging system as in systemic solid tumors and hematologic malignancies, central nervous system (CNS) cancers are classified based on the World Health Organization (WHO) grading system. This grading system has been undergoing dynamic changes in the setting of new advances in molecular genetics. Although traditionally this grading system was based on histological features, the revised WHO classification published in 2016 used molecular parameters for the first time in addition to histology to categorize tumor tissues. The role of molecular diagnostics in CNS tumor classification is being further solidified in the 2021 WHO classification, which follows the recommendations of the 2019 cIMPACT-NOW Utrecht meeting (Louis et al. 2021).

As described in the new fifth edition of the WHO classification system, using a layered reporting structure, including integrated diagnosis, histological diagnosis, CNS grading, followed by molecular information, is recommended. The integrated diagnosis incorporates important molecular features in addition to tissue-based histological findings, highlighting the importance of different diagnostic modalities in the accurate diagnosis in CNS tumors.

Brain and spinal cord tumors are graded from 1 to 4, where the higher numbers indicate faster growth and/or greater aggressiveness. Each tumor type has its own grading that represents its historically determined natural history but does not necessarily correlate with prognosis in this current era. For example, the five-year survival of a grade 3 meningioma is 64%, whereas almost all patients with a grade 4 WNT-activated medulloblastoma have long-term survival if treatment is provided. In recent years, molecular biomarkers became an important part of clinical care in neuro-oncology because they have promoted better categorization of CNS tumors. Consequently, the 2021 WHO classification enhances the use of molecular biomarkers to influence grading in many tumor types due to their powerful prognostic value. In addition, molecular biomarkers also have the potential to influence treatment in some cases. Imminent advances in molecular diagnostics are expected to further evolve the landscape of neuro-oncology soon.

2. What is the incidence of primary brain cancers?

Expert Perspective: Although CNS tumors (including malignant and non-malignant etiology) are the most common solid tumor types in children below age 14, they are less frequent in adults. Brain tumors are the 3rd most common tumor types in people between the ages of 15 and 39 with an average annual age-adjusted incidence rate of 11.54 per 100,000 population, and the 8th most common tumor type above age 40 with an average annual age-adjusted incidence rate of 42.85 per 100,000 population. In adults, 70.3% of brain tumors are non-malignant, and among them, meningioma is the most common tumor type (Table 1.1). Regarding adult malignant tumors, glioblastoma leads in frequency because it represents 14.5% of all brain tumors and 48.6% of malignant brain cancers. Malignant brain cancers are more prevalent in males than females (56% vs 44%, respectively). Gender differences are reversed in non-malignant cancers, where 36% of the cases occurred in males and 64% in females. Incidence rates for malignant primary brain tumors are highest in Whites (7.58 per 100,000), but non-malignant primary brain tumors are more common in Blacks (19.45 per 100,000) (Ostrom et al. 2020).

3. Do primary brain cancers have genetic predisposition?

Expert Perspective: Most adult primary brain tumors occur sporadically without an identifiable genetic predisposition. However, genetic susceptibility to brain cancers is suggested by tumor aggregation in families, genetic cancer syndromes, linkage analyses, and lymphocyte

Table 1.1 Molecular characteristics and grading of the most frequently occurring CNS tumors in adults.

Name	Molecular characteristics	Grading	Frequency (% of all primary brain tumors)
Meningioma	N/A	1,2,3	38
Oligodendroglioma	IDH-mutant, 1p/19q-codeleted	2,3	4
Astrocytoma	IDH-mutant	2,3,4	5–8
Glioblastoma	IDH-wildtype	4	14

mutagen sensitivity. Thorough medical history taking with close attention to the family cancer history can reveal family cancer clusters and/or raise suspicion for a genetic syndrome associated with brain cancers. The most common genetic conditions associated with primary CNS tumors include Lynch syndrome, neurofibromatosis type 1, Li-Fraumeni syndrome, tuberous sclerosis (Table 1.2). In addition to colorectal cancer, endometrial cancer, upper urinary tract cancer, and ovarian cancer, patients with Lynch syndrome are at high risk of developing gliomas in their fifth decade. Patients with neurofibromatosis type 1 can develop optic pathway tumors in childhood and/or glioblastoma, as well as malignant peripheral nerve sheath tumors in early adulthood. They are also more prone to be diagnosed with breast cancer, endocrine cancers, sarcoma, melanoma, ovarian cancer, and prostate cancer. Patients with Li-Fraumeni syndrome can also develop multiple cancers, including solid tumors (breast cancer, osteosarcoma, sarcoma, and adrenocortical cancer), hematologic malignancies (leukemia), and CNS tumors (choroid plexus tumor in infancy, medulloblastoma in childhood, and high-grade glioma in early adulthood). Patients with tuberous sclerosis may develop subependymal giant-cell astrocytomas before age 25 in addition to other solid tumors (like rhabdomyoma and kidney cancer). Recognizing a genetic syndrome based on clinical signs and genetic markers is crucial to provide appropriate medical management. The identification of a genetic syndrome may influence the treatment plan because targeted therapy has been increasingly accessible for specific mutations. In addition to that, it may also guide future cancer surveillance and the need for family cancer screening. (See Chapters 45–47.)

Table 1.2 Characteristics of the most common genetic conditions associated with primary central nervous system tumors.

Name	Frequency	Mutation	Gene/protein	Common CNS tumors	Other tumors
Lynch syndrome	Estimated 1 in 279	Multiple chromosomes, including chromosomes 2, 3, and 7	*MLH1*, *MSH2*, *MSH6*, *PMS2*, *EPCAM*	Glioblastoma, astrocytoma, oligodendroglioma, medulloblastoma	Colon, endometrial, upper urinary tract, ovarian
Neurofibromatosis type 1	1 in 3,000–4,000	Chromosome 17	*NF1*/neurofibromin	Plexiform neurofibroma, optic pathway tumors, glioblastoma, malignant peripheral nerve sheath tumors	Breast, endocrine, sarcoma, melanoma, ovarian, prostate
Li-Fraumeni syndrome	1 in 5,000–20,000	Chromosome 17	*TP53*/p53	Choroid plexus tumor, medulloblastoma, high-grade glioma	Breast, osteosarcoma, sarcoma, leukemia, adrenocortical
Tuberous sclerosis	Estimated 1 in 6,000–18,000	Chromosomes 9 and 16	*TS1*, *TS2*	Subependymal giant-cell astrocytoma	Rhabdomyomas, kidney

4. Do environment factors cause brain tumors?

Expert Perspective: The question of environmental factors leading to brain tumors has been extensively investigated, but there are only a few environmental factors that have been confidently linked to tumorigenesis in the CNS. Among these, therapeutic ionizing radiation has been uniformly accepted as a risk factor for brain cancers including meningiomas, gliomas, and nerve sheath tumors. This risk is even higher when radiation exposure occurs at young age. Although the significance of diagnostic radiation exposure has not been fully clarified, some studies suggest increased risk of brain cancers in patients who receive head CT scans in childhood. In contrast, allergic and ectopic conditions seem to reduce the risk of developing CNS tumors (such as glioma and meningioma) based on large epidemiologic studies. The role of hormones and hormonal therapy in brain cancer development has been thoroughly investigated without firm conclusion. The fact that meningioma is three to six times more common in females than males provided the biological basis of this hypothesis. So far, there is no clear evidence that hormone treatment would increase the risk of brain cancers, including meningioma and glioma. Another area of active investigation aims to explore the possible connection between cell-phone use and brain tumors. Although no consensus has yet been reached on this issue, some studies suggest that long-term use of or childhood exposure to cell phones is potentially carcinogenic. Occupational exposures and environmental factors, including but not limited to pesticides, lead, dust, formaldehyde, and sulfur dioxide, have been also explored without finding a significant relationship to brain cancers.

5. Does a grade 1 meningioma require treatment?

Expert Perspective: Meningiomas are the most common primary brain tumors, with an incidence rate of 8.81 per 100,000 population. They represent 38.3% of all tumors and 53.9% of all non-malignant brain tumors. Meningiomas are usually slow-growing, extra-axial tumors. Most often they are located along the parasagittal line, and less frequently they are in the spinal region. Usually they are found incidentally in asymptomatic patients, but they can cause progressive focal neurologic symptoms relevant to their location. Their incidence increases with age. They are more common in women, in Blacks, and in people with a remote history of radiation therapy to the CNS, especially if the exposure occurred in childhood. Some genetic disorders, such as neurofibromatosis type 2 and MEN1 syndrome, have been associated with an increased risk of developing meningiomas (Table 1.2).

Unlike most brain tumors, meningiomas are graded from 1 to 3 by the 2021 WHO classification system. Within the grades, 15 subtypes are distinguished histologically. Grade 1 benign tumors represent about 80% of meningiomas. Grade 2 is found in approximately 15–20% of the cases. Grades 1 and 2 are also referred to as non-malignant meningiomas, although both can undergo malignant transformation to higher grade, which is more likely with the grade 2 tumors. Grade 3 meningiomas are malignant tumors that represent 2% of meningiomas. The 10-year relative survival is 87.4% for non-malignant meningiomas and 59.6% for malignant meningiomas.

Due to the heterogeneous nature of meningioma cases (including patient factors and histological features of the specific tumor), individualized treatment should be offered for patients after careful evaluation of the risk and benefits of available therapeutic options.

Slow-growing asymptomatic tumors that do not invade or compromise healthy tissue can be monitored with periodic MRIs. Imaging should be repeated at three, six and twelve months after the diagnosis, then every 6–12 months for five years, followed by every one to three years thereafter. To determine tumor growth rate, imaging should be always compared to the first MRI. For large and symptomatic meningiomas, surgery is preferred if the location is accessible. For patients with unresectable meningioma, radiation treatment can be an effective alternative. Surgery followed by radiation therapy can be considered for grade 2 meningiomas, but prospective randomized trials comparing observation with radiation after resection are not yet completed. In contrast, radiation treatment is required for grade 3 meningiomas due to their high recurrence rates.

Increasing evidence supports the value of molecular sequencing of meningiomas, too. In addition to the undebatable role of the *NF2* gene mutation in the development of meningiomas, the prognostic significance of other genetic alternations has been recognized in recent years. Based on the new 2021 WHO classification, a histologically grade 1 meningioma can be upgraded to grade 3 in the integrated reporting system if it harbors a *TERT* promoter mutation and/or homozygous deletion of *CDKN2A/B*. Therefore, molecular characterization of a meningioma is critical for the accurate tissue diagnosis and for the selection of appropriate treatment. In addition, molecular advances not only contribute to better characterization of specific tumor samples but may also contribute to the development of targeted therapy and better patient outcome in the near future.

6. What is the standard of care treatment of oligodendroglioma?

Expert Perspective: The diagnostic criteria have changed in the last few decades, and the 2021 WHO classification guideline categorizes tumors with mutation in the isocitrate dehydrogenase gene (*IDH* mutation) and combined whole-arm losses of 1p and 19q (1p/19q codeletion) as oligodendroglioma. This clear separation from other gliomas were needed due to the distinct pathology, molecular pathogenesis, treatment response, and prognosis of oligodendrogliomas. They are grouped into two grades based on their histological and molecular characteristics.

Grade 2 oligodendrogliomas are low-grade tumors. They have low mitotic activity and grow slowly, often for years prior to diagnosis. Molecular sequencing reveals no *ATRX* mutation but shows *TERT* promoter mutations. Grade 3 oligodendrogliomas, used to be called anaplastic oligodendrogliomas, are malignant tumors with atypical features including high cell density, increased mitotic rate, nuclear atypia, microvascular proliferation, and necrosis, but they also lack *ATRX* mutation and they harbor *TERT* promoter mutations. Patients with grade 3 oligodendroglioma have worse prognosis compared with patients with grade 2 tumors. There is some evidence that oligodendrogliomas start at low grade and ultimately evolve into more aggressive tumors, although this progression can't always be detected because some patients are diagnosed with high-grade tumors at presentation.

Oligodendroglioma treatment should include maximal safe resection followed by additional treatment, which can include radiotherapy and chemotherapy at some point in the course of disease. Because the clear classification of oligodendroglioma is recent, prior clinical studies provide data on the treatment of oligodendroglioma mixed with other tumor types, like astrocytoma (per current classification). The most notable studies include RTOG 9802 for grade 2 tumors and RTOG 9402 and EORTC 269521 for grade 3 tumors. In general, it is accepted that patients under 40 years old who underwent complete resection of a grade 2 oligodendroglioma and with no evidence of *CDNK2A/B* homozygous deletion may be followed by regular imaging. MRI with and without contrast is recommended every three to six months in the first five years, followed by every six to nine months or as clinically indicated, before transitioning to annual imaging. In this age group, the delay of treatment may improve quality of life without worsening the disease outcome. For grade 2 oligodendrogliomas diagnosed above age 40 or with incomplete resection, and for grade 3 tumors, fractionated external beam radiation treatment followed by chemotherapy is recommended. Beside the acute toxicities (including fatigue, headaches, and hair loss), long-term side effects of radiation treatment include cognitive impairment, hearing loss, meningioma, and overt brain injury called radiation-induced necrosis. The choice of post-radiation chemotherapy remains controversial. Most data support the use of procarbazine, lomustine, and vincristine (PCV) as a choice of chemotherapy, although some centers avoid the use of vincristine due to lack of evidence of blood-brain barrier penetration and the universal development of peripheral neuropathy. Furthermore, the inclusion of a nitrosourea raises concerns about prolonged hematologic toxicity. Temozolomide, commonly used for astrocytoma and glioblastoma, has not been compared prospectively with PCV in the post-radiation setting but has a much better toxicity profile. However, clinical trials are underway to assess the utility of temozolomide in the treatment of oligodendroglioma. The initial study reported inferiority of temozolomide compared to radiation treatment. The current phase of the study compares radiotherapy with temozolomide to radiotherapy with PCV treatment.

Key Clinical Trials: RTOG 9802, RTOG 9402, EORTC 269521, CODEL.

7. How does one treat a WHO grade 3 *IDH* mutant astrocytoma?

Expert Perspective: Traditionally, an anaplastic astrocytoma was classified as a grade 3 astrocytoma. With the current 2021 WHO grading system, all astrocytomas are *IDH* mutant by definition and range from grade 2 to grade 4. Because clinical studies were designed based on prior classification systems or even before some of the currently used biomarkers were identified, data interpretation can be challenging at times.

In case of a WHO grade 3 *IDH* mutant astrocytoma, the CATNON study can be used for treatment guidance. The CATNON study is a randomized, open-labeled, phase III study that, using an innovative 2 × 2 factorial design, randomized 751 patients into four groups: radiation treatment alone, radiation treatment with concomitant temozolomide, radiation with adjuvant temozolomide, and radiation treatment with concomitant as well as adjuvant temozolomide (1:1:1:1). During data analysis, patients were divided based on *IDH* mutations status. Ultimately, data from 660 patients (444 with *IDH* mutation) were used to determine whether concomitant temozolomide or adjuvant temozolomide improve survival. The study revealed clinical benefit from adjuvant temozolomide (for 12 months) in patients with *IDH1* or *IDH2* mutant tumors. The five-year overall survival was 64.8% in the patients who did not receive adjuvant temozolomide compared to 82.8% who did. On the other hand, no benefit was found from daily concomitant temozolomide during radiation treatment in this patient population. The five-year survival was 80.5% without concomitant chemotherapy compared with 82.8% with concomitant temozolomide (van den Bent et al. 2021).

Mutations in the *IDH1* or *IDH2* gene provides an exciting opportunity for molecularly targeted treatment. Multiple studies are investigating the utility of IDH targeting treatment in different cancers, including glioma. For example, *IDH*-mutant inhibitors, ivosidenib and vorasidenib, have been approved by the Food and Drug Administration as a therapeutic option for *IDH*-mutated AML. In gliomas, the efficacy of ivosidenib has been assessed in a multicenter, open-label, phase I, dose escalation and expansion study. This study revealed median progression free survival benefit from ivosidenib in non-enhancing gliomas (considered to be low grade gliomas) but not in enhancing gliomas (considered to be high grade gliomas). Vorasidenib, an oral dual inhibitor of mutant *IDH1/2* enzymes, significantly improved progression-free survival in patients with residual or recurrent grade 2 gliomas. This treatment delayed disease progression. These findings from the INDIGO trial represent a significant step forward in the treatment of patients with grade 2 glioma with *IDH* mutations. Moreover, there is increasing evidence that poly(ADP-ribose) polymerase (PARP) inhibition may be another treatment option; clinical trials are undergoing to assess the benefit of pamiparib with temozolomide. Also, vorasidenib is under evaluation in combination with pembrolizumab in an ongoing phase I study in grade 2/3 glioma.

Key clinical trial: CATNON, INDIGO.

8. Does age matter for glioblastoma treatment?

Expert Perspective: In 2005, a paper reported survival benefit from adding concomitant and adjuvant temozolomide to radiotherapy in glioblastoma patients. Since then, the Stupp protocol described in this paper became the standard of care in the treatment of this aggressive brain tumor. The regimen includes irradiation for a total of 60 Gy, 5 days per week for 6 weeks along with daily temozolomide (7 days a week) at 75 mg/m^2, followed by 6 cycles of adjuvant temozolomide for 5 days in a 28-day cycle at 150–200 mg/m^2. The median age of patients participating in the original study and who received the combination treatment with temozolomide with radiotherapy was 56 (ranged between 19 and 70 years old). The most common side effects include fatigue, thrombocytopenia, neutropenia, leukopenia, and constipation. The median survival benefit of this regimen was an additional 2.5 months for a total of 14.6 months, significantly longer than the 12.1 months in the "radiotherapy alone" arm.

The incidence of glioblastoma is increasing with age, and the median age at diagnosis is 65 years (Figure 1.1). At the same time, older patients are usually underrepresented in clinical studies aimed to treat glioblastoma. In addition to limited data on optimal treatment in this age group, clinicians need to consider other factors associated with age, such as poor performance status, additional medical conditions, increased risk of toxicity, and social support system. A small number of studies were specifically designed to address these issues. Among them, a phase III clinical study assessed the benefit of a short-course radiation treatment along with temozolomide in patients ≥ 65 years of age. Patients were randomized to receive either radiotherapy alone or concomitant chemoradiation. A total of 40.5 Gy radiation treatment was administered in 15 fractions over three weeks. Concomitant temozolomide was given at 75 mg/m^2 for 21 days followed by adjuvant temozolomide at 150–200 mg/m^2 dose for 5 days in a 28-day long cycle, for up to 12 cycles. The results showed that this short course of radiation treatment with or without temozolomide was well tolerated in this age group. The median number of adjuvant cycles was 5. The overall survival rate increased from 7.6 months (of the radiation treatment alone arm) to 9.3

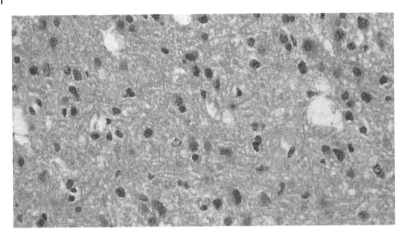

Figure 1.1 Histologic features of grade II astrocytoma, including increased astrocytic cellularity ("hypercellularity"). (Color Plate 1.1)

months with the combination treatment. The benefit of chemotherapy was even greater in patients with MGMT methylated glioblastoma. This study provided evidence that it is reasonable to consider a shorter course, hypofractionated radiation therapy with temozolomide for the treatment of older patients (based on chronological or biological age).

Key Clinical Trial: Perry et al. 2017.

9. How does one diagnose pseudo-progression and necrosis?

Expert Perspective: Clinicians are often puzzled by the etiology of the non-specific post-treatment changes seen on brain MRI following completion of treatment for CNS tumors. These changes may represent tumor progression, pseudo-progression, or necrosis. Radiologically, they all present with new or enlarging contrast enhancement at the area of radiation exposure.

Even with additional imaging techniques, the exact diagnosis can be rarely given with confidence. Special MRI sequences, such as perfusion and diffusion weighted imaging, are frequently used even though they provide suboptimal sensitivity and specificity to distinguish tumor progression from tumor necrosis. MR spectroscopy may increase accuracy of the assessment; however, the imaging data may misrepresent the true etiology of the changes. Needless to say, that the proper diagnosis is crucial in order to provide appropriate management for the patient.

Pseudo-progression typically presents within three months of completing radiation treatment. The hypothesis is that radiation treatment damages all cells in the exposure field and leads to cell death of the tumor cells as well as healthy cells, including neurons and vascular cells. This cell death will initiate inflammatory changes and some local edema, which ultimately leads to blood brain barrier impairment. As a result, post-radiation scans are always used as a new baseline scan but not for treatment decisions. In cases of suspected pseudo-progression, it is advised to continue treatment and reimage the patient in 2–3 months, or sooner if needed. Pseudo-progression is usually asymptomatic, but if symptoms arise, a course of steroid treatment may lead to clinical and radiological improvement. Eventually, the contrast enhancing area on the MRI is expected to stabilize or regress if the changes are due to pseudo-progression. In questionable cases, surgery may be necessary for the proper diagnosis.

Treatment-related (radiation) necrosis presents as a delayed, severe degree of local tissue and vascular injury. It typically occurs 12–24 months following chemoradiation, but it may evolve several years later. There are multiple factors that play a role in the development of radiation necrosis, including the cumulative dose and fractionation of radiation treatment. Unlike pseudo-progression, which is often asymptomatic, radiation necrosis is often symptomatic and irreversible. It may even result in slowly progressive neurologic dysfunction. The risk of radiation necrosis needs to be discussed with patients who are expected to have a longer clinical course.

In many cases, time will help distinguish between progression, pseudo-progression, and necrosis. Yet time is of the essence when treatment is needed for true tumor progression. Until novel innovative methods become available for the precise diagnosis of these changes, clinicians need to exercise careful consideration when deciding between conservative management and active intervention.

10. What is the role of bevacizumab in neuro-oncology?

Expert Perspective: In solid tumors (such as renal cell carcinoma, metastatic colon cancer, and ovarian cancer), bevacizumab is used for its antitumor effect. In neuro-oncology, bevacizumab is used for its anti-angiogenic effect and often leads to clinical improvement as well as radiologic response evident by decreased contrast enhancement on MRI. Indeed, single-agent bevacizumab received accelerated FDA approval in 2009 followed by full approval in 2017 for the treatment of recurrent glioblastoma, based on demonstration of significantly increased progression-free survival based on the EORTC 26101 study, although there was no improvement in overall survival or time to neurologic deterioration. Subsequent studies also demonstrated no benefit on overall survival in patients with newly diagnosed or recurrent glioblastoma (AVAglio and RTOG 0825, EORTC 26101). In addition, some evidence suggests that patients who progress while undergoing treatment with bevacizumab do not respond well to further salvage therapy and, as a result, have limited eligibility for clinical trials. Therefore, it may be prudent to reserve bevacizumab as the final salvage option.

Bevacizumab is frequently used as a steroid-spearing agent. Dexamethasone is the drug of choice in patients who are symptomatic from brain edema. Some patients require short-term use of steroids, whereas others need it for longer time and may even become dependent on it. Long-term steroid use may significantly decrease patients' quality of life and lead to multiple medical problems, especially in elderly patients or those who already have multiple comorbidities. Steroid-induced myopathy, insomnia, diabetes, weight gain, decrease in physical activity, mood changes, change in physical appearance, and fluid retention are among the most commonly experienced side effects. To avoid these problems, it is reasonable to consider bevacizumab after assessing the risks and benefits of this medications. The common side effects of bevacizumab include hypertension, headaches, epistaxis, and delayed would healing. The dangerous side effects include hemorrhage, thromboembolism, and spontaneous bowel perforation.

Bevacizumab has been shown in a randomized, placebo-controlled clinical trial to improve radiation-induced necrosis. A low dose and short course of treatment of bevacizumab is used for this purpose.

Key Clinical Trials: EORTC 26101, AVAglio, RTOG 0825, Levin et al. 2011.

Recommended Readings

Louis, D.N., Perry, A., Wesseling, P. et al. (2021). The 2021 WHO classification of tumors of the central nervous system: A summary. *Neuro Oncol* 23 (8):1231–1251. doi: 10.1093/neuonc/noab106. PMID: 34185076; PMCID: PMC8328013.

Mellinghoff, I.K., van den Bent, M.J., Blumenthal, D.T. et al. (2023 June 4). Vorasidenib in IDH1- or IDH2-mutant low-grade Glioma. *N Engl J Med*. doi: 10.1056/NEJMoa2304194. Epub ahead of print. PMID: 37272516.

Ostrom, Q.T., Patil, N., Cioffi, G. et al. (2022). Corrigendum to: CBTRUS statistical report: Primary brain and other central nervous system tumors diagnosed in the United States in 2013–2017. *Neuro Oncol* 24 (7):1214. doi:10.1093/neuonc/noaa269. Erratum for: *Neuro Oncol* 22 (12 Suppl 2): iv1–iv96. PMID: 33340329; PMCID: PMC9248396.

Perry, J.R., Laperriere, N., O'Callaghan, C.J. et al. (2017). Trial investigators. Short-course radiation plus temozolomide in elderly patients with glioblastoma. *N Engl J Med* 376 (11): 1027–1037. doi:10.1056/NEJMoa1611977. PMID: 28296618.

van den Bent, M.J., Brandes, A.A., Taphoorn, M.J. et al. (2013). Adjuvant procarbazine, lomustine, and vincristine chemotherapy in newly diagnosed anaplastic oligodendroglioma: Long-term follow-up of EORTC brain tumor group study 26951. *J Clin Oncol* 31 (3): 344–50. doi:10.1200/JCO.2012.43.2229. Epub 2012 Oct 15. PMID: 23071237.

van den Bent, M.J., Tesileanu, C.M.S., Wick, W. et al. (2021). Adjuvant and concurrent temozolomide for 1p/19q non-co-deleted anaplastic glioma (CATNON; EORTC study 26053–22054): Second interim analysis of a randomised, open-label, phase 3 study. *Lancet Oncol* 22 (6): 813–823. doi:10.1016/S1470-2045(21)00090-5. Epub 2021 May 14. PMID: 34000245; PMCID: PMC8191233.

Wick, W., Gorlia, T., Bendszus, M. et al. (2017). Lomustine and bevacizumab in progressive glioblastoma. *N Engl J Med* 377 (20): 1954–1963. doi:10.1056/NEJMoa1707358. PMID: 29141164.

Part 2

Head and Neck and Thoracic Cancers

2

Localized Head and Neck Cancer

Emrullah Yilmaz and Jessica L. Geiger

Taussig Cancer Institute, Cleveland Clinic, Cleveland, OH, USA

Introduction

Head and neck cancer is the seventh most common type of cancer worldwide and comprises a diverse group of cancers affecting the upper aerodigestive tract (including the oral cavity (Table 2.1), nasopharynx, oropharynx (Tables 2.2–3), hypopharynx (Table 2.4), and larynx), the paranasal sinuses, and the salivary glands. Although many different histologies exist, the most common is squamous cell carcinoma. In general, men are at twofold to fourfold higher risk than women for developing Head and Neck squamous cell carcinoma (HNSCC). Predominant risk factors include tobacco use, alcohol abuse, and oncogenic viruses, including human papillomavirus and Epstein-Barr virus. Most head and neck cancers (73% in the United States) are now related to human papillomavirus infection rather than tobacco and alcohol. Head and neck malignancies remain challenging to treat, requiring a multidisciplinary approach, with surgery, radiotherapy, and systemic therapy serving as key components of the treatment of locally advanced disease. Although many treatment principles overlap, treatment is generally site-specific and histology-specific. Recurrent and metastatic Head and Neck Cancers are discussed in the next chapter.

Case Study 1

A 56-year-old male presented with a left neck lump enlarging for four months. He denied any swallowing difficulty or sore throat. He never smoked cigarettes and denied alcohol drinking as well. He works as an engineer. His father had lung cancer and prostate cancer. He was seen by his primary care physician and referred to an ear, nose, and throat (ENT) doctor. A flexible laryngoscopy was performed during the clinic visit, which showed a small left tonsil mass (Table 2.2).

1) What is the possible cause of his mass?
    A) EBV
    B) HPV

Cancer Consult: Expertise in Clinical Practice, Volume 1: Solid Tumors & Supportive Care,
Second Edition. Edited by Syed A. Abutalib, Maurie Markman, Al B. Benson III, and Hope S. Rugo.
© 2024 John Wiley & Sons Ltd. Published 2024 by John Wiley & Sons Ltd.

C) Hereditary
D) Occupational exposure

Expert Perspective: Human papillomavirus (HPV) can lead to oropharyngeal squamous cell carcinomas. It has been reported that more than 70% of oropharyngeal cancers are caused by HPV, and HPV type 16 (HPV-16) accounts for almost 90% of the HPV-positive oropharyngeal cancers in the United States. The incidence of HPV-related head and neck squamous cell carcinomas (HNSCC) has increased in recent decades. As the most common oncogenic HPVs, HPV-16 and HPV-18 are covered by FDA-approved HPV vaccines. It is feasible that HPV-positive HNSCC could be prevented by successful vaccination campaigns worldwide. Once the cancer develops, high-risk HPV testing is recommended for all oropharyngeal (soft palate, tonsil, posterior and lateral pharyngeal walls, and base of the tongue) squamous cell carcinomas. HPV-related oropharyngeal squamous cell carcinomas have a favorable outcome compared with HPV-negative squamous cell carcinomas. The College of American Pathologists recommends p16 immunohistochemistry testing as a surrogate marker of high-risk HPV. (See chapters on cervical and anal cancers.)

Correct Answer: B

Table 2.1 Cancer of the mucosal lip and oral cavity† TNM staging (AJCC UICC 8th edition).

Staging	Description
T1	Tumor ≤2 cm with depth of invasion ≤5 mm
T2	Tumor ≤2 cm, with depth of invasion ≤5 mm and ≤10 mm; or Tumor >2 cm and ≤4 cm, with depth of invasion ≤10 mm
T3	Tumor >2 cm and ≤4 cm with depth of invasion >10 mm; or Tumor >4 cm with depth of invasion ≤10 mm
T4a	Moderately advanced local diseaseTumor >4 cm with depth of invasion >10 mm; or Tumor invades adjacent structures only (e.g. through cortical bone of the mandible or maxilla, or involves the maxillary sinus or skin of the face)*
T4b	Very advanced local diseaseTumor invades masticator space, pterygoid plates, or skull base and/or encases the internal carotid artery
N1	Metastasis in a single ipsilateral lymph node, ≤3 cm in greatest negative for dimension extranodal extension
N2a	Metastasis in a single ipsilateral node larger than 3 cm but not larger than 6 cm in greatest dimension, and negative for extranodal extension
N2b	Metastases in multiple ipsilateral nodes, none larger than 6 cm in greatest dimension, and negative for dimension extranodal extension
Nc	Metastases in bilateral or contralateral lymph nodes, none larger than 6 cm in greatest dimension, and negative for dimension extranodal extension
N3a	Metastasis in a lymph node >6 cm in greatest dimension and negative for dimension extranodal extension

Table 2.1 (Continued)

Staging	Description
N3b	Metastasis in any node(s) and clinically overt positive for dimension extranodal extension
M1	Distant metastasis

† Oral cavity tumors include the mucosa of the lip (not the external, dry lip), floor of the mouth, oral tongue, alveolar ridge, retromolar trigone, hard palate, and buccal mucosa.
* Superficial erosion of bone/tooth socket (alone) by a gingival primary is not sufficient to classify a tumor as T4.
Source: Adapted from *AJCC Cancer Staging Manual, Eighth Edition* (2017).

Table 2.2 HPV-related oropharyngeal cancer† TNM clinical staging (AJCC UICC 8th edition).

Staging	Description
T1	Tumor 2 cm or smaller in greatest dimension
T2	Tumor larger than 2 cm but not larger than 4 cm in greatest dimension
T3	Tumor larger than 4 cm in greatest dimension or extension to lingual surface of epiglottis
T4	Moderately advanced local diseaseTumor invades the larynx, extrinsic muscle of tongue, medial pterygoid, hard palate, or mandible; mucosal extension to lingual surface of epiglottis from primary tumors of the base of the tongue and vallecula does not constitute invasion of the larynx
N1	One or more ipsilateral lymph nodes, none larger than 6 cm
N2	Contralateral or bilateral lymph nodes, none larger than 6 cm
N3	Lymph node(s) larger than 6 cm
M1	Distant metastasis

† Oropharyngeal carcinoma includes the soft palate, tonsil, posterior and lateral pharyngeal walls, and base of the tongue.
Source: Adapted from *AJCC Cancer Staging Manual, Eighth Edition* (2017).

Table 2.3 Oropharyngeal (p16 negative) cancer† TNM clinical staging (AJCC UICC 8th edition).

Staging	Description
T1	Tumor 2 cm or smaller in greatest dimension
T2	Tumor larger than 2 cm but not larger than 4 cm in greatest dimension
T3	Tumor larger than 4 cm in greatest dimension or extension to lingual surface of epiglottis
T4a	Moderately advanced local disease Tumor invades the larynx, extrinsic muscle of tongue, medial pterygoid, hard palate, mandible, mucosal extension to lingual surface of epiglottis from primary tumors of the base of the tongue and vallecula does not constitute invasion of the larynx

(Continued)

Table 2.3 (Continued)

Staging	Description
T4b	Very advanced local disease
	Tumor invades lateral pterygoid muscle, pterygoid plates, lateral nasopharynx, or skull base or encases carotid artery.
N	Same as Table 2.1
M1	Distant metastasis

[†] Oropharyngeal carcinoma includes the soft palate, tonsil, posterior and lateral pharyngeal walls, and base of the tongue.
Source: Adapted from *AJCC Cancer Staging Manual, Eighth Edition* (2017).

Table 2.4 Hypopharyngeal cancer[†] TNM clinical staging AJCC UICC 8th edition.

Staging	Description
T1	Tumor limited to one subsite of hypopharynx and/or 2 cm or smaller in greatest dimension
T2	Tumor invades more than one subsite of hypopharynx or an adjacent site, or measures larger than 2 cm but not larger than 4 cm in greatest dimension without fixation of hemilarynx
T3	Tumor larger than 4 cm in greatest dimension or with fixation of hemilarynx or extension to esophageal mucosa
T4a	Moderately advanced local disease
	Tumor invades thyroid/cricoid cartilage, hyoid bone, thyroid gland, esophageal muscle, or central compartment soft tissue; central compartment soft tissue includes prelaryngeal strap muscles and subcutaneous fat
T4b	Very advanced local disease
	Tumor invades prevertebral fascia or encases carotid artery, or involves mediastinal structures
N	Same as Table 2.1
M1	Distant metastasis

[†] Hypopharyngeal cancer includes the pyriform fossa, lateral and posterior hypopharyngeal walls, and postcricoid region.
Source: Adapted from *AJCC Cancer Staging Manual, Eighth Edition* (2017).

Case Study 2

A 67-year-old male went to the dentist for routine follow-up and was found to have a 1.5 cm right anterior tongue lesion. He was then referred to ENT, and a biopsy from the tongue lesion showed squamous cell carcinoma; immunohistochemistry for p16 staining was positive. A PET-CT was done showing a 1.5 cm right tongue lesion, bilateral cervical lymph nodes (largest 2 cm), and no evidence of distant metastasis. He has no history of tobacco smoking, but he has been chewing betel nut for 30 years. His mother died of breast cancer at age 65.

2) Which of the following statements regarding the patient's diagnosis is correct?
    A) He has a good prognosis due to no history of tobacco smoking
    B) He has a good prognosis due to p16 positivity
    C) His cancer is associated with betel nut chewing
    D) His family needs genetics counseling.

Expert Perspective: The prognostic effect of HPV is limited to oropharyngeal squamous cell carcinomas and is not observed in non-oropharyngeal squamous cell carcinomas. Therefore, routine high-risk HPV testing for non-oropharyngeal cancers is not recommended by the College of American Pathologists. A positive p16 test is not associated with a good prognosis in this patient. Betel nut chewing is among the risk factors for oral cavity squamous cell carcinoma. Betel nut chewing is shown to be associated with poor prognosis as well. Oral cavity tumors include the mucosa of the lip (not the external, dry lip), floor of the mouth, oral tongue, alveolar ridge, retromolar trigone, hard palate, and buccal mucosa.

Correct Answer: C

Case Study 3

A 58-year-old male with a smoking history of 35 packs per year presented with hoarseness for three months. He was referred to an ENT, and a direct laryngoscopy was done, showing right true vocal cord mass with vocal cord fixation. Biopsy showed moderately differentiated squamous cell carcinoma. PET-CT showed the true vocal cord mass with no cervical lymph node involvement or distant metastasis. The patient was diagnosed with Stage III larynx cancer due to vocal cord fixation.

3) What is the best treatment option for the patient?
    A) Radiation therapy
    B) Radiation therapy with concurrent chemotherapy
    C) Endoscopic resection
    D) Total laryngectomy with bilateral neck dissection

Expert Perspective: Stage I and II larynx cancers are considered as early stage, and radiation therapy alone is an effective treatment for early stage larynx cancers. However, the patient has T3 tumor stage due to the vocal cord fixation. Therefore, he has stage III disease.

Concurrent chemoradiation with cisplatin is an effective treatment for stages III and IVA laryngeal squamous cell carcinomas. A Veteran Affairs Laryngeal Cancer Study Group compared induction chemotherapy plus radiation to surgery plus radiation for stage III and IV laryngeal cancers. The patients were randomized to receive three cycles of cisplatin and fluorouracil and then radiation therapy or surgery and postoperative radiation therapy. Larynx preservation was observed in 64% of the patients. Given the results with laryngeal preservation, RTOG 91–11 trial was designed to determine the optimal treatment for larynx preservation. The trial excluded T4a larynx cancer patients with bulky disease. Patients were randomized to receive induction chemotherapy with cisplatin and fluorouracil followed by radiation therapy, concurrent chemoradiotherapy (CCRT) with cisplatin, and radiation therapy alone. The study results showed that CCRT improved laryngeal preservation compared to induction chemotherapy followed by radiation therapy and radiation therapy alone.

Because this patient has stage III larynx cancer, he would be a good candidate for laryngeal preservation with concurrent chemoradiation.

Correct Answer: B

Case Study continued: The patient completed chemoradiation with cisplatin. During his follow-up after treatment completion, he was found to have a left neck mass. A biopsy of the mass showed moderately differentiated squamous cell carcinoma consistent with residual disease from laryngeal cancer. Direct laryngoscopy showed residual disease in the larynx as well. CT chest did not show any distant metastasis.

4) What is the treatment option that you would recommend?
   A) Carboplatin/paclitaxel
   B) Pembrolizumab
   C) Re-irradiation
   D) Total laryngectomy with bilateral neck dissection

Expert Perspective: Patients who fail treatment with organ preservation strategy are treated with salvage laryngectomy. RTOG 91–11 trial reported 16% of the patients on the concurrent chemoradiation arm required total laryngectomy. Furthermore, the local-regional control following salvage total laryngectomy with bilateral neck dissection was 74% in this arm. So, salvage total laryngectomy with bilateral neck dissection is an effective treatment for patients with residual disease or local recurrence following the chemoradiation.

Correct Answer: D

Case Study 4

A-63-year-old male with a smoking history of 30 packs per year presented with hoarseness and swallowing difficulty for one month. He was then referred to an ENT. Direct laryngoscopy was done, showing a glottis mass with vocal cord fixation. PET-CT showed thyroid cartilage and prevertebral space invasion, no lymphadenopathy, and no distant metastasis. He had no other significant health problem.

5) What is the best treatment option for the patient?
   A) Laryngectomy without neck dissection followed with adjuvant radiation
   B) Laryngectomy and bilateral neck dissection followed with adjuvant radiation
   C) Laryngectomy and bilateral neck dissection followed with adjuvant chemoradiation
   D) Chemoradiation with cisplatin 100 mg/m^2 every three weeks
   E) Chemoradiation with cisplatin 100 mg/m^2 every three weeks and avelumab every three weeks

Expert Perspective: The patient presents with T4bN0M0 laryngeal squamous cell carcinomas. Because the patient doesn't have distant metastasis, treatment should be curative intent.

The patients with locally advanced laryngeal cancers require multidisciplinary evaluation. Although surgery with laryngectomy is preferred treatment for large T3 or T4a lesions, T4b lesions are treated with concurrent chemoradiation. Due to the prevertebral space invasion, the patient has T4b disease. Therefore, he is not a good surgical candidate. Encasement of the carotid artery and invasion of mediastinal structures are other criteria for T4b stage laryngeal cancer.

Cisplatin is the standard chemotherapy for concurrent chemoradiation for HNSCC. High-dose cisplatin 100 mg/m^2 administered with radiation therapy every three weeks is the chemotherapy regimen used in most clinical trials. Although weekly cisplatin 40 mg/m^2 is used in practice, there isn't a large trial comparing the effectiveness of weekly chemotherapy with high-dose cisplatin in definitive treatment.

A recent phase III clinical trial evaluated the role of immunotherapy with chemoradiation. The addition of PD-L1 inhibitor avelumab did not prolong the survival of the patients undergoing concurrent chemoradiation. Therefore, chemoradiation with cisplatin remains the standard of care for cisplatin-eligible patients.

Correct Answer: D

Case Study 5

A 78-year-old male presented with swallowing difficulty for three months. He was seen by gastroenterology, and esophagogastroduodenoscopy (EGD) was done showing no esophageal mass. He then had a CT neck showing a 3 cm right base of tongue mass and multiple right cervical lymph nodes, largest 4 cm with clinical extranodal extension. He was referred to an ENT, and an fine-needle aspiration (FNA) from the right cervical node showed squamous cell carcinoma; p16 immunohistochemistry was negative. He has a history of coronary artery disease, congestive heart failure, hypertension, and chronic kidney disease. He was not found by the ENT to be a candidate for surgery due to the location of the base of tongue mass. He is still able to continue his daily activities. He was referred to medical oncology and radiation oncology for evaluation of treatment options.

6) What is the best treatment for the patient?
   A) Radiation and concurrent cisplatin
   B) Radiation and concurrent cetuximab
   C) Radiation alone
   D) Carboplatin and paclitaxel
   E) Cetuximab

Expert Perspective: The patient is presenting with T2N3bM0 oropharyngeal squamous cell carcinomas, HPV-unrelated. The most recent AJCC staging (8th edition) included the extranodal extension to the staging of p16-negative HNSCC. The presence of the clinically overt extranodal extension in imaging is staged as N3b; therefore, this patient has N3b disease.

Chemoradiation with cisplatin is the standard of care for nonsurgical treatment of HNSCC. However, due to several factors, patients may not be eligible for cisplatin. This patient wouldn't be able to get cisplatin due to chronic kidney disease. However, given his good performance, he would still be a candidate for curative-intent treatment. Therefore chemotherapy or cetuximab without radiation shouldn't be considered.

A large, randomized phase III trial compared radiotherapy with radiation therapy with concurrent cetuximab for locally advanced stage III and IV HNSCC patients. Cetuximab is a monoclonal antibody against epidermal growth factor receptor (EGFR), and it was administered weekly with radiation therapy, starting with the week before radiation with a loading dose. The study results showed increased locoregional control and improved progression-free survival with cetuximab and radiation therapy. Therefore, cetuximab can be considered for the cisplatin-ineligible patients concurrent with radiation therapy for locally advanced HNSCC.

Correct Answer: B

7) **What is the next best step following completion of therapy?**
    A) Observation
    B) Direct laryngoscopy with biopsy from vocal cord
    C) Bilateral neck dissection
    D) PET-CT within 12 weeks of treatment completion

Expert Perspective: Historically, neck dissection was performed following chemoradiation for nodal disease. PET-NECK trial Management Group designed a randomized clinical trial to evaluate the role of post-treatment PET-CT to evaluate response to chemoradiation in the United Kingdom. HNSCC patients with N2 and N3 disease treated with chemoradiation were randomly assigned to undergo planned neck dissection or PET-CT 12 weeks after chemoradiation and neck dissection if they didn't respond. Fewer neck dissections were done in the PET-CT surveillance group (54 vs. 224), and overall survival was similar.

Correct Answer: D

Case Study 6

A 52-year-old female was found to have right cervical lymphadenopathy during her routine annual primary care follow-up. An ultrasound of the neck showed a 4 cm right cervical lymph node. An FNA of the lymph node showed keratinizing squamous cell carcinoma, p16-positive. She was referred to an ENT, and a flexible laryngoscopy showed a small right tonsil mass. The patient wanted nonsurgical treatment and was referred to medical oncology and radiation oncology. PET-CT showed a 1 cm right tonsil mass and four cervical lymph nodes (largest 4.5 cm). She has no other medical problem and denied tobacco smoking and alcohol consumption.

8) **Which is the best treatment option for the patient?**
    A) Radiation alone
    B) Radiation with concurrent cisplatin
    C) Radiation with concurrent cetuximab
    D) Carboplatin/5-FU/pembrolizumab
    E) Pembrolizumab

Expert Perspective: The patient has T1N1M0 oropharyngeal squamous cell carcinomas, p16-positive. Trans-oral robotic surgery with risk stratified adjuvant treatment is an effective treatment for HPV-related HNSCC. However, definitive chemoradiation has comparable responses, although there is not a large, randomized study comparing surgery to chemoradiation.

Chemoradiation with cisplatin is the standard of care for patients who are not undergoing surgery. Given the good response rates to the treatment of HPV-related HNSCC, treatment de-intensification strategies are being evaluated. A randomized phase III RTOG 1016 trial compared cisplatin to cetuximab with concurrent radiation therapy to see whether cisplatin can be replaced with cetuximab for HPV-related HNSCC. This study included stages III and IV (AJCC 7th edition) HPV-positive oropharyngeal cancers. Radiation therapy with cetuximab showed inferior overall survival and progression-free survival.

Therefore, cisplatin remains the standard systemic treatment with concurrent radiation therapy for HPV-related oropharyngeal squamous cell carcinomas, and cetuximab shouldn't be recommended unless the patient is cisplatin-ineligible.

Correct Answer: B

Case Study 7

A 62-year-old male with a smoking history of 50 packs per year presented with nonhealing tongue ulcer. He was found to have a 1 cm right tongue lesion and right cervical lymph nodes.

9) What treatment do you recommend?
   A) Partial glossectomy with selective neck dissection
   B) Induction chemotherapy followed by partial glossectomy and selective neck dissection
   C) Induction chemotherapy followed by concurrent chemoradiation
   D) Chemoradiation

Expert Perspective: Surgery is preferred treatment for locally advanced oral cavity squamous cell carcinomas even though there isn't a large trial comparing surgery with radiation-based treatment. However, chemoradiation with cisplatin can be considered for the patients with unresectable tumors. The role of the induction chemotherapy before surgery is not well established. Although for select patients undergoing chemoradiation, induction chemotherapy with TPF regimen (docetaxel, platinum agent, and fluorouracil) can be considered, there is no survival benefit shown with induction chemotherapy. Given the small size of the tumor, partial glossectomy with selective right neck dissection is the best initial treatment for this patient.

Correct Answer: A

Case Study continued: The patient underwent partial glossectomy with right neck dissection. Pathology revealed a 1.5 cm right tongue squamous cell carcinoma with depth of invasion of 6 mm, negative margins, and positive perineural invasion, and 1 out of 43 lymph nodes were positive with extranodal extension, with 2 cm size.

10) Which do you recommend?
   A) Observation
   B) Radiation therapy

C) Radiation therapy with concurrent cisplatin
D) Total glossectomy with left neck dissection.

Expert Perspective: The patient's pathologic stage is T2N1. Depth of invasion was added to T stage in AJCC 8th edition. The tumor size is less than 2 cm; however, the depth of invasion is more than 5 mm. Therefore, the tumor stage is T2.

The patients with positive margin and/or extranodal extension show benefit from adjuvant chemoradiation with cisplatin. Two large cooperative group trials, EORTC 22931 and RTOG 0501, compared postoperative radiation therapy to chemoradiation. The subgroup analysis observed the benefit of chemoradiation in patients with positive margin and extranodal extension.

Because the patient had extranodal extension, adjuvant radiation therapy with concurrent cisplatin is recommended.

Correct Answer: C

Case Study 8

A 54-year-old male with no smoking history presented with a sore throat and a left neck lump. He underwent direct laryngoscopy showing a left oropharyngeal mass, and a biopsy was done showing squamous cell carcinoma, p16-positive. Trans-oral robotic surgery and left neck dissection was done. Pathology showed 2.5 cm oropharyngeal mass with positive margin, and 4 out of 31 lymph nodes were positive with 3 mm extranodal extension.

11) **Which treatment would you recommend?**
    A) Observation
    B) Radiation therapy
    C) Radiation with concurrent cetuximab
    D) Radiation with concurrent cisplatin

Expert Perspective: The patient has high-risk features including positive margin and extranodal extension. Adjuvant chemoradiation is recommended for HPV-related HNSCC positive margin and extranodal extension. ECOG E3311 was designed to evaluate reduced postoperative radiation therapy for p16-positive oropharyngeal squamous cell carcinomas in patients with intermediate risk factors including clear/close margins, two to four nodes, and extranodal extension of ⩽1 mm. The two-year progression-free survival shows no difference with reduced-dose postoperative radiation therapy in intermediate risk group. However, the patients in the high-risk group received chemoradiation with cisplatin in this study as well. Therefore, this patient with positive margin and extranodal extension should receive adjuvant chemoradiation with cisplatin.

Correct Answer: D

Case Study 9

A 45-year-old Asian female presented with left ear pain for three months. She was given antibiotics, which didn't help her pain. She was seen by an ENT, and a flexible laryngoscopy showed left nasopharyngeal mass. A CT neck was done showing a 3 cm nasopharyngeal mass with parapharyngeal space extension and left cervical lymph nodes (largest 4 cm). A CT of the chest didn't show any evidence of distant metastasis. The biopsy from the cervical node was consistent with undifferentiated carcinoma, EBV-positive.

12) What treatment would you recommend?
   A) Radiation therapy
   B) Resection of the mass with bilateral neck dissection.
   C) Systemic treatment alone with cisplatin and 5-fluorouracil
   D) Induction chemotherapy with cisplatin and gemcitabine followed by chemoradiation with cisplatin

Expert Perspective: The patient has locally advanced nasopharyngeal carcinoma. Nasopharyngeal carcinoma is a different group of head and neck cancers, and the treatment algorithm is not the same as non-nasopharyngeal HNSCC.

Epstein-Barr virus (EBV) has a strong association with nasopharyngeal carcinoma. There are three different histopathologic subtypes of nasopharyngeal carcinoma: keratinizing squamous cell carcinomas (WHO type I), and non-keratinizing carcinoma differentiated (WHO type II) and undifferentiated (WHO type III) basaloid squamous cell carcinomas. Undifferentiated carcinoma is seen in the majority of cases in Southern China, where nasopharyngeal carcinoma is endemic.

Most of the patients with nasopharyngeal carcinoma present with locally advanced disease with lymph node involvement. Due to the location of the nasopharyngeal carcinoma, surgical treatment is usually not considered. Therefore, locally advanced nasopharyngeal carcinoma patients are treated with nonsurgical treatment.

Early stage nasopharyngeal carcinoma patients can be treated with radiation alone, but patients usually present with locally advanced disease. Chemoradiation followed by adjuvant chemotherapy has been standard of care for several years. Intergroup 0099 trial randomized nasopharyngeal carcinoma patients to receive radiation therapy alone versus chemoradiation with cisplatin followed by chemotherapy with cisplatin and fluorouracil for three cycles. The patients on the chemotherapy arm had better overall survival and progression-free survival.

Cisplatin and gemcitabine combination was found have better response rates when compared with cisplatin and fluorouracil in metastatic nasopharyngeal carcinoma. Given the effectiveness of this combination, a phase III trial was designed to evaluate role of cisplatin and gemcitabine induction chemotherapy in China. Locally advanced nasopharyngeal carcinoma patients were randomized to receive three cycles of cisplatin gemcitabine followed by chemoradiation with cisplatin versus chemoradiation alone. Induction chemotherapy improved recurrence-free survival and overall survival. However, there isn't a current data comparing induction chemotherapy with adjuvant chemotherapy following chemoradiation.

Correct Answer: D

Case Study 10

A 71-year-old male with no smoking history presented with swallowing difficulty and neck pain. He was found to have a base of tongue mass, and a biopsy showed squamous cell carcinoma with positive p16. A PET-CT was done showing base of tongue mass, bilateral cervical lymph nodes, and five lung nodules (largest 3 cm). A biopsy from one of the lung nodules showed squamous cell carcinoma. Immunhistochemistry showed positive p16, and PDL-1 CPS score was 75. He has hypertension that is controlled well, and he is able to continue daily activities without difficulty.

13) **What is the best next step for the treatment?**
    A) Hospice care
    B) Radiation therapy with concurrent cisplatin
    C) Carboplatin/5-Fluorouracil/cetuximab
    D) Cetuximab
    E) Pembrolizumab

Expert Perspective: The patient has distant metastasis, and he has good performance status. Therefore, systemic treatment can be considered.

EXTREME regimen with platinum, fluorouracol, and cetuximab was prior standard treatment for first-line treatment of recurrent/metastatic HNSCC. KEYNOTE-048 trial randomized recurrent/metastatic HNSCC patients to EXTREME regimen, pembrolizumab and chemotherapy (platinum/fluorouracil), and pembrolizumab alone. Pembrolizumab alone improved overall survival in patients with a PDL1 CPS score of 20 or more when compared to EXTREME. Pembrolizumab and chemotherapy improved overall survival regardless of the PDL1 status.

Because this patient has a high PDL1 CPS score, pembrolizumab would be the choice of treatment.

Correct Answer: E

Case Study 11

A 52-year-old female with p16-positive squamous cell carcinoma of base of tongue completed chemoradiation with cisplatin. Post-treatment PET-CT showed complete response. She presented with fever and cough seven years after completing treatment. A CT of the chest showed right lower lung infiltrate.

14) **What would you recommend?**
    A) Biopsy from the infiltrate
    B) Radiation to right lower lobe
    C) Pembrolizumab
    D) Antibiotics and swallow study

Expert Perspective: Chemoradiation is an effective treatment for HPV-related oropharyngeal cancer patients. However, patients may have late toxicities due to the treatment. Osteoradionecrosis, xerostomia, trismus, carotid artery injury, and dysphagia are among the late complications seen in long-term survivors.

Dysphagia can be seen due to late esophageal toxicity from radiation induced fibrosis. Patients may present with aspiration pneumonia. A swallow study is needed to evaluate the dysphagia. Patients with esophageal stricture can be treated with dilatation.

Correct Answer: D

Case Study 12

A 62-year-old male with squamous cell carcinoma of hypopharynx completed chemoradiation with cisplatin. He has a smoking history of 30 packs per year. His post-treatment PET-CT three months after completing the treatment showed no evidence of recurrence. He presents for routine follow-up two years after completing treatment. He denied any neck pain, swallowing difficulty, or fatigue. His recent flexible laryngoscopy done by an ENT shows no evidence of recurrence.

15) Which of the below would you not recommend to the patient?
   A) Tobacco cessation
   B) Low-dose CT chest
   C) Dental exam at least twice a year
   D) PET-CT
   E) TSH (thyroid stimulating hormone)

Expert Perspective: Due to multimodality of the treatment of head and neck cancers including chemotherapy, radiation therapy, or surgery, patients who survive HNSCC may experience several short-term and long-term adverse events. The patients need close follow-up following the completion of the treatment not only for cancer surveillance but also for evaluation of toxicities.

Tobacco cessation is proven to improve outcome from the treatment. It also helps prevent dental problems that may be seen following chemoradiation. The patients should continue screening for other cancers, and a low-dose CT of the chest should be considered for the lung cancer screening for patient with smoking history. Due to several factors including xerostomia, the patients are prone to increased risk for dental problems, so close dental follow-up is recommended. Radiation therapy can increase risk of hypothyroidism, and TSH evaluation is recommended every 6–12 months following radiation to neck. Once a post-treatment PET-CT shows complete response, there is no role for surveillance with PET-CT imaging.

The American Society of Oncology established survivorship guidelines that may help the providers following the patients after their treatment.

Correct Answer: D

Case Study 13

A 76-year-old male presented with a left neck mass enlarging for six months. A CT of the neck showed a left parotid mass. The biopsy was consistent with high-grade salivary duct carcinoma. A CT of the chest didn't show any metastasis.

2 Localized Head and Neck Cancer

16) **What would you recommend for the treatment?**
    A) Radiation therapy alone
    B) Concurrent chemoradiation
    C) Parotidectomy followed by postoperative radiation therapy
    D) Chemotherapy with carboplatin and paclitaxel

Expert Perspective: Surgical resection is the preferred treatment for locally advanced salivary gland cancers. Low-grade tumors can be treated with surgery alone. Postoperative radiation therapy is considered for the high risk patients with high-grade histopathology. There isn't enough evidence of adjuvant chemoradiation for salivary gland cancers. RTOG 1008 recently completed enrollment, and it randomized high-risk salivary gland cancer patients to receive postoperative radiation therapy or chemoradiation.

Definitive radiation therapy can be considered for the patients presenting with unresectable disease. The role of the concurrent chemoradiation is not established for salivary gland carcinomas in definitive setting.

Correct Answer: A

Case Study continued: The patient underwent parotidectomy and adjuvant radiation therapy due to high-risk features. A CT of the chest was done two years after completing treatment for shortness of breath showing multiple lung nodules. Biopsy from one of the lung nodules was consistent with metastasis from salivary duct carcinoma.

17) **Which is not among the molecular markers that can help selecting best treatment for the patient?**
    A) p16
    B) Androgen receptor
    C) HER2
    D) Tumor mutational burden

Expert Perspective: Low-grade salivary gland cancers with metastasis have an indolent course with slow progression over time, and they can be observed closely. However, patients with high-grade carcinomas can present with rapidly progressing disease, and systemic treatment can be offered.

Given the rarity of the salivary gland carcinomas, the chemotherapy regimens are selected from the results of small phase I or II clinical trials. Platinum-, taxane-, and doxorubicin-based chemotherapies can be used depending on the patient's performance status. However, biomarker-driven treatment has been emerging as the preferred treatment for metastatic salivary gland carcinomas. In metastatic BRAF V600E mutated salivary duct carcinomas of any histology and no other actionable molecular alterations, combination of dabrafenib and trametinib is reasonable consideration.

HER2 overexpression is common in salivary duct carcinomas and mucoepidermoid carcinomas. Combination of chemotherapy and trastuzumab can be considered for HER2-positive salivary gland carcinomas. Trastuzumab plus pertuzumab can be considered as initial therapy in patients who wish to avoid or have contraindications to chemotherapy. T-DM1 can be considered for the patients who progress after trastuzumab.

More than 80% of salivary duct carcinoma patients have androgen receptor positivity. A leuprolide and bicalutamide combination can be offered to salivary gland cancer patients with androgen receptor expression.

Tumor mutational burden (TMB) is an emerging biomarker for immunotherapy response, and pembrolizmab is FDA approved for solid tumors with TMB more than 10 muts/Mb (mutations/megabase).

Given the lack of effective systemic chemotherapy for salivary gland cancer patients, checking biomarkers for treatment selection is crucial for patient with metastatic disease.

Correct Answer: A

Recommended Readings

Bonner, J.A., Harari, P.M., Giralt, J. et al. (2006). Radiotherapy plus cetuximab for squamous-cell carcinoma of the head and neck. *N Engl J of Med* 354 (6): 567–578.

Burtness, B., Harrington, K.J., Greil, R. et al. (2019). Pembrolizumab alone or with chemotherapy versus cetuximab with chemotherapy for recurrent or metastatic squamous cell carcinoma of the head and neck (KEYNOTE-048): a randomised, open-label, phase 3 study. *Lancet (London, England)* 394 (10212): 1915–1928.

Chaturvedi, A.K., Engels, E.A., Pfeiffer, R.M. et al. (2011). Human papillomavirus and rising oropharyngeal cancer incidence in the United States. *J Clin Oncol Am J Clin Oncol* 29 (32): 4294–4301.

Cooper, J.S., Zhang, Q., Pajak, T.F. et al. (2012). Long-term follow-up of the RTOG 9501/intergroup phase III trial: postoperative concurrent radiation therapy and chemotherapy in high-risk squamous cell carcinoma of the head and neck. *Int J Radiat Oncol Biol Phys* 84 (5): 1198–1205.

Forastiere, A.A., Zhang, Q., Weber, R.S. et al. (2013). Long-term results of RTOG 91-11: a comparison of three nonsurgical treatment strategies to preserve the larynx in patients with locally advanced larynx cancer. *J Clin Oncol Am J Clin Oncol* 31 (7): 845–852.

Gillison, M.L., Trotti, A.M., Harris, J. et al. (2019). Radiotherapy plus cetuximab or cisplatin in human papillomavirus-positive oropharyngeal cancer (NRG Oncology RTOG 1016): a randomised, multicentre, non-inferiority trial. *Lancet (London, England)* 393 (10166): 40–50.

Huang, S.H. and O'Sullivan, B. (2017). Overview of the 8th edition TNM classification for head and neck cancer. *Curr Treat Options Oncol* 18 (7): 40.

Lee, N.Y., Ferris, R.L., Psyrri, A. et al. (2021). Avelumab plus standard-of-care chemoradiotherapy versus chemoradiotherapy alone in patients with locally advanced squamous cell carcinoma of the head and neck: a randomised, double-blind, placebo-controlled, multicentre, phase 3 trial. *Lancet Oncol* 22 (4): 450–462.

Mehanna, H., Wong, W.-L., McConkey, C.C. et al. (2016). PET-CT surveillance versus neck dissection in advanced head and neck cancer. *N Engl J Med* 374 (15): 1444–1454.

Zhang, Y., Chen, L., Hu, G.-Q. et al. (2019). Gemcitabine and cisplatin induction chemotherapy in nasopharyngeal carcinoma. *N Engl J Med* 381 (12): 1124–1135.

3

Recurrent and Metastatic Head and Neck Cancer

Chloe Weidenbaum and Mike Gibson

Vanderbilt University Medical Center, Nashville, TN, USA

Introduction

Head and neck cancers constitute a heterogenous group of malignancies that are predominantly squamous cell carcinoma. The highest rates of head and neck cancers are seen in older males, with low- and middle-income countries being disproportionately affected. Treatment is challenging, and 15–50% of patients develop recurrent disease. Prognosis remains generally poor despite advances in treatment, with a median survival of 6–15 months depending on patient- and disease-related factors. This highlights the need for more effective treatment options as well as the importance of multidisciplinary care with options aimed at both symptomatic and curative treatment. Here, we review several cases discussing the epidemiology, diagnosis, and treatment of recurrent and metastatic head and neck cancers.

Case Study 1

A 62-year-old male is referred to you for recurrent oropharyngeal squamous cell carcinoma (SCC). He was treated with a combination of chemotherapy and radiation five years ago. He drinks alcohol occasionally and has a 25-pack-year history of tobacco use. He works in a grocery store and has no history of exposure to toxic fumes. His mother had breast cancer, and his father had lung cancer. He asks why he developed oropharyngeal cancer.

1) **What do you tell him is the most likely etiology of his cancer?**
    A) Alcohol use
    B) HPV infection
    C) Family history of cancer
    D) Tobacco use
    E) Occupational exposure
    F) EBV infection

Cancer Consult: Expertise in Clinical Practice, Volume 1: Solid Tumors & Supportive Care,
Second Edition. Edited by Syed A. Abutalib, Maurie Markman, Al B. Benson III, and Hope S. Rugo.
© 2024 John Wiley & Sons Ltd. Published 2024 by John Wiley & Sons Ltd.

Expert Perspective: The single most important known risk factor for head and neck squamous cell carcinoma (HNSCC) is tobacco use. This includes both smoked and smokeless forms of tobacco products. Alcohol is also an important risk factor for HNSCC. Interestingly, alcohol and tobacco use have been shown to have a synergistic effect on the development of HNSCC through repeated exposure to local mucosa; this is known as field cancerization. Human papillomavirus (HPV), primarily type 16, infection is another risk factor for HNSCC. HPV-associated HNSCC is most commonly oropharyngeal and is primarily found in male patients. It has a predilection for the base of the tongue and tonsils and is seen more often in younger patients, although HPV associated oropharyngeal cancer has a biphasic distribution with peaks around 30 and 55 years of age. Recent studies suggest that HPV accounts for 70–80% of oropharyngeal cancer cases in North America. Thus, it is also plausible HPV is the etiology of this patient's cancer. Other risk factors for HNSCC include radiation and other environmental/occupational exposures, periodontal disease, and immunosuppression. Epstein-Barr virus (EBV) is associated with nasopharyngeal carcinoma. HIV infection is also associated with HNSCC.

Correct Answer: B or D

Case Study 2

A 75-year-old male presented to his primary care physician with hoarseness and dysphagia of eight months' duration. He has a remote history of tobacco use. He was referred to an ear, nose, and throat (ENT) doctor, and direct laryngoscopy showed a vocal cord mass (larynx). Biopsy shows poorly differentiated squamous cell carcinoma, and PET-CT shows local lymph node involvement with metastasis to the liver. He has a remote history of HNSCC, which was treated with definitive chemotherapy and radiation.

2) **Which of the following is associated with a poor prognosis?**
   A) HPV positivity
   B) Increased tumor PD-L1 expression status
   C) History of tobacco use
   D) Prior chemotherapy for HNSCC
   E) Prior radiation therapy at the disease site

Expert Perspective: In patients with recurrent or metastatic HNSCC, there are many factors influencing prognosis. This is important to consider when developing an individualized treatment approach. Factors associated with a better prognosis (i.e. longer survival) include HPV positivity, prior response to chemotherapy, time since completion of prior definitive therapy, higher performance status, and tumor programmed death-ligand 1 (PD-L1) expression. In particular, PD-L1 expression predicts positive response to PD-1 therapy. Conversely, factors associated with a poor prognosis in HNSCC include prior radiation therapy, poor performance status, weight loss, significant comorbidity, and active (but not solely a history of) smoking.

Correct Answer: E

Case Study 3

A 58-year-old female presents to you with a right-sided neck lump that has been enlarging for six weeks. She has a history of localized soft palate (oropharyngeal) squamous cell carcinoma, which was diagnosed three years ago and was treated with definitive concurrent chemoradiation therapy. Her symptoms resolved following treatment, and imaging last year did not show any residual disease. She denies any recent dysphagia or odynophagia and does not have history of tobacco or alcohol use. Physical exam reveals a right-sided 5 cm cervical lymph node. Chest X-ray is unremarkable.

3) **What is the next best management strategy?**
   A) MRI
   B) CT
   C) PET scan
   D) Endoscopy
   E) Fine-needle aspiration

Expert Perspective: Initial assessment for primary HNSCC involves history and physical examination, often including inspection, palpation, and direct endoscopy. Some patients present with a neck mass as their primary complaint and no clear primary site of the tumor, making a fine-needle aspiration (FNA) biopsy useful for diagnosis. Assessment of local infiltration, lymph node involvement, and distant metastases is also important and can involve CT, MRI, PET scan, and PET-CT imaging modalities. Staging involves the use of CT or MRI of the head and neck. PET-CT may be particularly useful in staging recurrent HNSCC.

Correct Answer: E

Case Study 4

A 67-year-old male is seeing you for recently diagnosed metastatic squamous cell carcinoma of the right maxillary sinus (paranasal sinus). He has not undergone any treatment. His comorbidities are coronary artery disease, hypertension, and hyperlipidemia. He has an Eastern Cooperative Oncology Group (ECOG) score of 1.

4) **What is the role of biomarkers in the management and prognosis of metastatic paranasal sinus (maxillary, ethmoid, sphenoid, frontal) squamous cell carcinoma?**
   A) PD-L1 combined positive score
   B) Pre- and posttreatment HPV DNA
   C) Pre- and posttreatment Epstein-Barr virus (EBV) DNA
   D) Circulating tumor DNA (ctDNA)
   E) None of the above

Expert Perspective: Research in HNSCC over the past few years has led to the landmark development of the PD-L1 combined positive score (CPS). This is a clinically relevant scoring method created to identify patients who will respond effectively to anti-PD-1 therapy. It is based on the number of PD-L1-staining cells (including tumor cells, lymphocytes, and macrophages) relative to the total number of tumor cells. In recent years, its expression has become associated with a better prognosis in recurrent/metastatic HNSCC, with increasing use of CPS in risk stratification for the treatment of HNSCC.

The KEYNOTE-048 trial established use of pembrolizumab (a PD-1 inhibitor) as first-line treatment in recurrent/metastatic HNSCC, with or without the use of chemotherapy. Pembrolizumab improved overall survival (OS) when added to a platinum and fluorouracil regimen as compared to cetuximab with platinum and fluorouracil regardless of CPS. In patients with a CPS of >1, pembrolizumab alone improved OS. HPV, EBV, and ctDNA are being studied for use as biomarkers in HNSCC but do not yet have an established role in the clinical setting.

The recommended dosing of pembrolizumab is 200 mg once every three weeks or 400 mg once every six weeks. This would be continued until disease progression or unacceptable toxicity, or up to 24 months in the absence of disease progression.

Correct Answer: A

Case Study 5

A 65-year-old male with a history of hypertension and tobacco use was referred to you for oropharyngeal squamous cell carcinoma that has metastasized to the liver and lung. He has not undergone any treatment. He complains of worsening dysphagia and cough. He has a 30-pack-per-year history of cigarette smoking and continues to smoke tobacco. He has good performance status. The PD-L1 CPS is 2.

5) What treatment do you recommend?
   A) Radiation therapy followed by chemoimmunotherapy
   B) Surgical resection followed by chemoimmunotherapy
   C) Radiation therapy alone
   D) Chemotherapy alone
   E) Immunotherapy alone

Expert Perspective: Based on the KEYNOTE-048 trial discussed above, given his CPS of >1 systemic therapy with pembrolizumab alone would be indicated in this patient with gwood performance status and relatively limited comorbidities. Radiation can be considered for controlling the primary tumor or providing symptomatic relief; however, the goal of treatment for his metastatic cancer is palliative.

Correct Answer: E

Case Study 6

A 60-year-old female whom you previously saw one year ago for localized laryngeal carcinoma and who was treated with cisplatin and fluorouracil followed by radiation presents with recurrent hoarseness and cough. She otherwise feels well, has no significant past medical history, and walks two miles daily without difficulty. The PET scan shows hypermetabolic activity in the larynx, and FNA biopsy reveals recurrent squamous cell carcinoma.

6) Which of the following would be the preferred management strategy?
   A) Radiation therapy and/or chemotherapy
   B) Surgery and/or radiation
   C) Chemotherapy alone
   D) Radiation therapy alone
   E) Supportive care alone

Expert Perspective: This patient has localized recurrent laryngeal SCC with favorable features. She has several options, including salvage surgery, re-irradiation, or palliative chemoimmunotherapy. If she is a surgical candidate, it would be reasonable to offer the patient the option of curative intent with salvage surgery. If high-risk pathologic features are seen after surgical resection, postoperative reirradiation should also be considered. If the patient is not a surgical candidate or the tumor is not amenable to resection, reir-radiation and/or chemotherapy should be considered. However, there are significant complications associated with re-irradiation, including infection, bleeding, and tissue necrosis. In choosing a treatment option, it is important to consider the initial treatment regimen type and response, interval between initial treatment and disease progression, and patient comorbidities and performance status. Depending on her CPS, options also include combination chemotherapy, single-agent immunotherapy, or combination chemoimmunotherapy.

Correct Answer: B

Case Study 7

A 71-year-old male is referred to you with an enlarging left-sided neck mass. Further questioning reveals he has a remote history of locally advanced oropharyngeal squamous cell carcinoma, successfully treated with a combination of radiation and platinum-based chemotherapy. He does not smoke and denies weight loss. He has excellent performance status. The PD-L1 CPS is 0.

7) What systemic treatment do you recommend for the most likely diagnosis?
   A) Platinum plus fluorouracil with pembrolizumab
   B) Platinum plus fluorouracil with concurrent or sequential cetuximab
   C) Platinum plus taxane with concurrent or sequential cetuximab
   D) Platinum plus taxane
   E) Any of the above

Expert Perspective: For patients with recurrent HNSCC (the most likely diagnosis in this patient), the choice of subsequent treatment regimen depends on timing of relapsed disease, prior systemic treatment, PD-L1 CPS, performance status, and comorbidities. For those with progressive or recurrent disease within six months of receiving platinum-based chemotherapy (with or without cetuximab), options include single-agent PD-1 targeted therapy using either pembrolizumab or nivolumab. Single-agent pembrolizumab or nivolumab would not be an ideal choice for this patient due to the timing of his initial disease being greater than six months prior.

Because of this, the next step would be to calculate the CPS for further stratification. If the CPS was ≥1, he would be eligible for single-agent pembrolizumab. With a CPS of <1 (or unavailable) and good performance status, treatment is chemotherapy with pembrolizumab.

In the EXTREME trial, cetuximab with a combination regimen of platinum plus fluorouracil showed significantly increased OS (10.1 versus 7.4 months), progression-free survival (5.6 versus 3.3 months), and objective response rate (36 versus 20%) compared with chemotherapy alone. Similar efficacy but less toxicity was seen when taxane was used in place of fluorouracil.

Single-agent chemotherapy has been studied in recurrent HNSCC, although several have shown limited survival impact and treatment-related toxicities are a substantial concern. If the patient had poor performance status with a CPS of 0 or unavailable, options would be further limited to single-agent chemotherapy such as carboplatin, taxane, cetuximab, fluorouracil, and/or palliative care, or hospice care would be recommended.

Correct Answer: A

Case Study 8

The patient in the previous question chooses treatment with carboplatin, fluorouracil, and cetuximab. He tolerates treatment well with subsequent imaging showing no residual disease. However, six months later, he again relapses. His performance status remains good.

8) What would be the next step in managing his recurrent oropharyngeal squamous cell carcinoma?
   A) Repeat same treatment as prior due to his previous positive response
   B) Immunotherapy with a PD-1 antibody
   C) Cetuximab only at higher dosing
   D) Taxane followed by cetuximab
   E) Palliative treatment only

Expert Perspective: Many patients with HNSCC find themselves in this situation of multiple recurrences; there is currently no universally accepted standard of care. Additionally, in this and many of the above scenarios, patients can consider enrollment in a clinical trial. All patients should be comanaged with a supportive care team (see chapter on palliative care).

In this case, the patient progressed following treatment with systemic platinum-based chemotherapy. Based on his good performance status and lack of advanced comorbidities, he would be eligible for immunotherapy with nivolumab or pembrolizumab despite a CPS of 0. The CheckMate 141 trial demonstrated that in patients with recurrent HNSCC who had progressed within six months after platinum-based chemotherapy without prior immunotherapy exposure, the PD-1 inhibitor nivolumab showed improved survival and less toxicity versus single-agent systemic chemotherapy regardless of PD-L1 expression.

The combination of pembrolizumab and cetuximab is currently being investigated. A recent phase II trial in patients with platinum-based chemotherapy refractory recurrent/metastatic HNSCC without prior immunotherapy or cetuximab exposure showed that by a median follow-up of seven months, overall responses were seen in 45% of patients.

Neither the panitumumab (a monoclonal antibody to epidermal growth factor receptor) nor bevacizumab (a monoclonal antibody to anti-vascular endothelial growth factor) has an established role in the treatment of metastatic or recurrent HNSCC due to their limited effects on survival and increased grade ≥3 toxicities.

Correct Answer: B

Case Study 9

An 82-year-old male with a history of end-stage renal disease, chronic obstructive pulmonary disease on home supplemental oxygen, and uncontrolled type 2 diabetes mellitus, is referred to you for evaluation of a 2 cm tongue lesion that he noticed three months ago. His performance status is limited, with an ECOG score of 3 (capable of only limited self-care; confined to bed or chair more than 50% of waking hours). He lives with family and does not leave the house due to physical limitations. FNA reveals squamous cell carcinoma. PET scan shows multiple hypermetabolic lung nodules, with CT-guided biopsy of one lesion revealing metastatic squamous cell carcinoma. The PD-L1 CPS is 8.

9) What would be the best treatment approach?
   A) Chemoradiotherapy
   B) Single-agent chemotherapy
   C) Palliative/hospice treatment only
   D) Surgical resection of the tongue lesion only
   E) Surgical resection of the tongue lesion and lung nodules
   F) Immunotherapy

Expert Perspective: This patient has multiple advanced comorbidities and poor performance status (ECOG score of 3). In such patients, the benefits of pursuing systemic treatment generally do not outweigh the risks. This includes immunotherapy treatment options. This patient's poor performance status and high burden of advanced comorbidities are indicative of a poor prognosis, and it is unlikely he would be able to tolerate the potential adverse effects of treatment, which are less with pembrolizumab than with chemotherapy but still notable. Symptomatic treatment focused on the patient's comfort may be the best option, provided that the patient feels likewise. A multidisciplinary approach to care is particularly important in this type of case.

Correct Answer: C

Recommended Readings

Burtness, B., Harrington, K., Greil, R. et al. (2019). Pembrolizumab alone or with chemotherapy versus cetuximab with chemotherapy for recurrent or metastatic squamous cell carcinoma of the head and neck (KEYNOTE-048): a randomized, open-label, phase 3 study. *Lancet* 394 (10212): 1915–1928.

Cogliano, V.J., Baan, R., Straif, K. et al. (2011). Preventable exposures associated with human cancers. *J Natl Cancer Inst* 103 (24): 1827–1839.

Craig, D.J., Nanavaty, N.S., Devanaboyina, M. et al. (2021). The abscopal effect of radiation therapy. *Future Onc* 17 (13): 1683–1694.

Dhull, A.K., Atri, R., Dhankhar, R. et al. (2018). Major risk factors in head and neck cancer: a retrospective analysis of 12-year experiences. *World J Oncol* 9 (3): 80–84.

Ferris, R.L., Blumenschein, G., Jr, Fayette, J. et al. (2016). Nivolumab for recurrent squamous-cell carcinoma of the head and neck. *N Engl J Med* 375 (19): 1856–1867.

Gillison, M.L., D'Souza, G., Westra, W. et al. (2008). Distinct risk factor profiles for human papillomavirus type 16-positive and human papillomavirus type 16-negative head and neck cancers. *J Natl Cancer Inst* 100 (6): 407.

Goodwin Jr, W.J. (2000). Salvage surgery for patients with recurrent squamous cell carcinoma of the upper aerodigestive tract: when do the ends justify the means? *Laryngoscope* 110 (Issue 3, Part 2, Suppl. 93): 1–18.

Guigay, J., Aupérin, A., Fayette, J. et al. (2021). Cetuximab, docetaxel, and cisplatin versus platinum, fluorouracil, and cetuximab as first-line treatment in patients with recurrent or metastatic head and neck squamous-cell carcinoma (GORTEC 2014-01 TPExtreme): a multicentre, open-label, randomised, phase 2 trial. *Lancet Oncol* 22 (4): 463–475.

Ionna, F., Bossi, P., Guida, A. et al. (2021). Recurrent/metastatic squamous cell carcinoma of the head and neck: a big and intriguing challenge which may be resolved by integrated treatments combining locoregional and systemic therapies. *Cancers* 13 (10): 2371.

Kulangara, K., Hanks, D.A., Waldroup, S. et al. (2017). Development of the combined positive score (CPS) for the evaluation of PD-L1 in solid tumors with the immunohistochemistry assay PD-L1 IHC 22C3 pharmDx. *J Clin Oncol* 35 (15 Suppl.): e14589–e14589.

National Comprehensive Cancer Network. Head and Neck Cancers (Version 3.2021). http://www.nccn.org/professionals/physician_gls/pdf/head-and-neck.pdf (accessed 12 November 2021).

Sacco, A.G., Chen, R., Worden, F.P. et al. (2021). Pembrolizumab plus cetuximab in patients with recurrent or metastatic head and neck squamous cell carcinoma: an open-label, multi-arm, non-randomised, multicentre phase 2 trial. *Lancet Oncol* 22 (6): 883–892.

Wheless, S.A., McKinney, K.A., and Zanation, A.M. (2010). A prospective study of the clinical impact of a multidisciplinary head and neck tumor board. *Otolaryngol Head Neck Surg* 143 (5): 650–654.

4

Thyroid Cancers

Kartik Sehgal[1] and Jochen H. Lorch[2]

[1] *Director, Thyroid Cancer Center, Dana-Farber Cancer Institute, Boston, USA*
[2] *Medical Director, Head and Neck/Thyroid Program, Robert H. Lurie Cancer Center of Northwestern University, Chicago, USA*

Introduction

Thyroid cancer is among the top-15 most common cancer types in the United States of America (USA) and the most common endocrine malignancy. Current estimates suggest that there will be 43,800 new cases of thyroid cancer and 2,230 deaths attributed to this cancer in 2022. Age-adjusted annual incidence rate has been reported at 14.1 per 100,000 in the 2014–2018 period. Females have a higher preponderance than males for development of these cancers, with an estimated ratio of approximately 2.7:1. The only well-documented etiologic factor for differentiated thyroid cancer is radiation exposure; however, more than 90% of these cancers are unrelated to radiation exposure. Approximately 915,664 people were living with thyroid cancer in the USA in 2019. Most patients with thyroid cancer carry a good prognosis with standard of care treatment. In the 2011–2017 reporting period, five-year overall survival rates for all stages combined were high at 98.4%. Similar rates were seen in those with locoregional disease. However, those with distant metastases had five-year survival rates of approximately 53.3%. Age-adjusted annual death rate in the 2015–2019 period was reported at 0.5 per 100,000.

Thyroid cancer is divided into the following histologic types: differentiated thyroid cancer (95–96%), anaplastic thyroid cancer (1–2%), and medullary thyroid cancer (1–2%). Differentiated thyroid cancer originates from thyroid follicular cells and is further subdivided into histologic subtypes: papillary (most frequent subtype and further histologically subdivided into classic and other variants), follicular, Hurthle cell, and poorly differentiated. Poorly differentiated and Hurthle cell thyroid cancer generally follow a more aggressive clinical course compared with papillary thyroid cancers. Anaplastic thyroid cancer is a rare but extremely aggressive undifferentiated malignancy, with median survival of three to seven months from diagnosis and disease-specific mortality approaching 100%. Medullary thyroid cancer is an uncommon thyroid carcinoma that arises from parafollicular or C cells of the thyroid gland. Thyroid cancers can exhibit a range of clinical patterns and growth behavior, ranging from slow-growing tumors with low mortality (most differentiated thyroid cancer) to aggressive clinical course (anaplastic thyroid cancer). Familial syndromes should be suspected when there is a family history of thyroid cancer or a history of a familial

Cancer Consult: Expertise in Clinical Practice, Volume 1: Solid Tumors & Supportive Care,
Second Edition. Edited by Syed A. Abutalib, Maurie Markman, Al B. Benson III, and Hope S. Rugo.
© 2024 John Wiley & Sons Ltd. Published 2024 by John Wiley & Sons Ltd.

syndrome associated with thyroid cancer. Approximately 5% of the differentiated thyroid cancers are associated with hereditary syndromes such as Gardner syndrome, familial adenomatous polyposis, Cowden syndrome, multiple endocrine neoplasia type 2A, familial medullary thyroid carcinoma, and Carney complex (see Chapters 45–47).

Case Study 1

Differentiated Thyroid Carcinoma

A 47-year-old woman, never smoker and otherwise healthy, was noted to have a lump in neck on routine physical examination by her primary care doctor. Evaluation with an ultrasound of the neck showed a 4.2 cm solid nodule with microcalcifications in the right upper lobe of thyroid and multiple borderline pathologically enlarged lymph nodes in the central and lateral neck. Fine needle aspiration (FNA) of right upper lobe nodule was suspicious for differentiated thyroid carcinoma.

1) **Should everyone with a diagnosis of differentiated thyroid cancer undergo total thyroidectomy?**

Expert Perspective: Surgery is the primary modality of treatment for most cases with a new diagnosis of differentiated thyroid cancer. The surgical options include thyroid lobectomy and total thyroidectomy with or without neck dissection. Total thyroidectomy is recommended for a new case of differentiated thyroid cancer in the presence of any of the following indications: (a) primary tumor greater than or equal to 4 cm in diameter, (b) presence of extrathyroidal extension of tumor, (c) presence of lymph node metastases, (d) presence of distant metastases, (e) history of radiation to head and neck region during childhood, (f) more than five foci of multifocal papillary microcarcinoma, particularly in the 8–9 mm range, and (g) a primary tumor 1–4 cm in size with abnormal imaging findings in the contralateral thyroid lobe, or a multidisciplinary team preference for treatment with adjuvant radioactive iodine therapy. These indications are supported by the benefit seen in the large, multicenter observational analyses performed by the National Thyroid Cancer Treatment Cooperative Study Group. In contrast, thyroid lobectomy is generally reserved for those with primary thyroid tumors less than 1 cm without presence of extrathyroidal extension, abnormal lymph nodes, or additional risk factors. For patients with 1–4 cm intrathyroidal tumors without the risk factors indicated earlier, the choice between thyroid lobectomy and total thyroidectomy is made on an individual patient level after considering patient preference and multidisciplinary team discussion. With proper selection of patients, outcomes have been shown to be equivalent in studies from analysis of the National Cancer Institute (NCI) Surveillance, Epidemiology, and End Results (SEER) Program database, leading to acceptance of thyroid lobectomy as an option in both National Comprehensive Cancer Network (NCCN) and American Thyroid Association (ATA) guidelines.

2) **Is total thyroidectomy followed by radioactive iodine therapy in every case?**

Expert Perspective: The practice to use radioactive iodine (RAI) in all versus selected patients with differentiated thyroid cancer is controversial. RAI therapy utilizes the principal of preferential uptake and concentration of iodine by thyroid follicular cells to cause acute cell death. The goals of RAI administration are to ablate any remaining normal thyroid tissue (to facilitate postsurgery surveillance by imaging or serum tumor markers) as well as destroy any microscopic or macroscopic disease that was not resected by surgery. The recommendations for RAI after surgery mostly rely on the ATA risk stratification system to estimate the risk of persistent disease or recurrence of cancer. It should be emphasized that recent use of iodinated contrast medium, an iodine-rich diet, and inadequate elevation of the level of thyroid-stimulating hormone (thyrotropin) can all undermine the effectiveness of RAI treatment. Human recombinant thyrotropin has replaced the need for a patient to be put into a hypothyroid state.

All differentiated thyroid cancer patients are stratified into low risk, intermediate risk, or high risk according to ATA classification, which utilizes clinicopathologic features of differentiated thyroid cancer (including but not limited to adequacy of surgical resection, histology of primary tumor, extent and involvement of lymph nodes, presence or absence of distant metastases, and presence or absence of high-risk activating mutations such as *BRAF* and *TERT* promotor) that predict persistent and recurrent disease risks of ≤5%, 5–20%, and ≥20% in low-, intermediate-, and high-risk ATA categories, respectively. Dosing strategies for RAI (ablative compared with higher therapeutic doses) are determined by the patient's prognostic risk, and they range from 50 to 75 mCi for ablation of remnants after total thyroidectomy for low-risk patients, from 100 to 150 mCi for the treatment of locoregional lymph nodes, and from 150 to 250 mCi for the treatment of lung and bone metastases.

RAI is recommended for those with high risk for persistent or recurrent disease (i.e. those with macroscopic tumor invasion, gross residual disease after surgery, presence of distant metastases). Those with low risk for persistent or recurrent disease (i.e. tumor <4 cm without any high-risk histologic features) are generally not treated with RAI. For those with intermediate risk for persistent or recurrent disease, RAI may be recommended after multidisciplinary team discussion in presence of high-risk characteristics such as aggressive histologic subtypes (poorly differentiated, insular, and tall cell), substantial lymph node involvement, and microscopic invasion into the perithyroidal soft tissues.

Our Patient: We would recommend total thyroidectomy along with central and lateral neck dissection. The ultimate decision for radioiodine therapy would depend upon ATA risk stratification, but with a tumor greater than 4 cm and age at diagnosis >45 years, we would strongly consider adjuvant RAI therapy.

3) How are the patients with differentiated thyroid cancer followed after surgery and/or radioiodine therapy? Are there any biomarkers for disease?

Expert Perspective: Dynamic risk stratification is recommended after initial management and subsequently at each follow-up visit. It considers clinical characteristics, course, surgical pathologic results, and serum tumor markers at each stratification. Based upon biochemical and structural evidence of disease, patients are categorized into the following risk categories: (a) excellent response (1–4% risk of recurrence), (b) biochemical incomplete response (approximately 20% risk of recurrence), (c) structural incomplete response (50–85% risk of recurrence), and (d) indeterminate response (15–20% risk of recurrence). Serum thyroglobulin is an established tumor marker for differentiated thyroid cancer and is synthesized only by thyroid follicular cells. It is measured along with antithyroglobulin antibodies preferentially using the same laboratory facility.

Thyroid-stimulating hormone (TSH) suppressive therapy with supratherapeutic doses of thyroid hormone supplementation is recommended in most cases after initial surgical management. The recommendations for goal serum TSH suppression and frequency of surveillance/monitoring with serum biomarkers, ultrasonography of neck, and/or additional imaging studies for recurrent/persistent disease are initially determined and subsequently adjusted based upon the dynamic risk stratification at each follow-up visit. Timing of follow-up visits can vary depending on risk assessment and may range from every three to six months in high-risk cases to once every year or longer. The suggested follow-up plan, including goals for TSH suppression for patients in the first year following thyroid surgery, is included in Table 4.1. The serum TSH goal is adjusted based upon dynamic risk stratification: 0.5–2.0 mU/L for those with excellent response, 0.1–0.5 mU/L for those with indeterminate response or biochemical incomplete response, and <0.1 mU/L for those with structural incomplete response.

4) Is there any role for radiation therapy to thyroid bed or other areas in management of differentiated thyroid cancer?

Expert Perspective: External beam radiation therapy (EBRT) to thyroid bed and known disease sites is considered only in select cases: patients with gross unresectable disease, those with high likelihood of microscopic disease of a histologic subtype (such as poorly differentiated and insular) that is known or strongly suspected to be refractory to RAI, and those with multiple locoregional recurrences despite repeat surgery and RAI courses and/or with unacceptable morbidity expected with additional surgical interventions. EBRT is more widely utilized in the poor prognostic subgroup of patients aged 45 years or older. The recommendation for EBRT is made after multidisciplinary discussion between surgery, radiation oncology, endocrinology, and medical oncology teams because high level evidence from randomized trials showing improvement of survival outcomes is not available. Radiation therapy with palliative intent using either EBRT or stereotactic body radiation therapy is recommended for symptomatic and/or progressive oligometastatic or for "oligoprogressive" disease not amenable for surgical resection and refractory to RAI (e.g. oligometastatic lung lesions, brain metastases, and painful bone lesions).

Table 4.1 Management during first year after thyroid surgery for differentiated thyroid cancer.

ATA risk stratification	Serum TSH goal	Unstimulated serum Tg	Surveillance US neck imaging
Low risk	• Nonstimulated serum Tg Detectable: 0.1–0.5 mU/L • Nondetectable 0.5–2 mU/L	• 4–6 weeks • 3–6 months • 9–12 months	6–12 months
Intermediate risk	0.1–0.5 mU/L		6–12 months
High risk	<0.1 mU/L		Every 6 months

ATA, American Thyroid Association; Tg, Thyroglobulin; US, ultrasonography.

5) In cases of locoregional recurrence of differentiated thyroid cancer, should patients undergo interventions such as surgery and/or radioiodine therapy immediately after detection?

Expert Perspective: No. Locoregional recurrence of differentiated thyroid cancer can be biochemical (rising serum thyroglobulin levels) and/or structural (e.g. on ultrasonography of neck). The recurrent disease can often be slow growing and asymptomatic and can often be monitored without need for immediate interventions. Surgery (of head and neck region) and other locally directed therapies may be recommended for clinically significant disease, which is symptomatic, increasing in size, or has the potential to cause symptoms in the near future or affect critical structures in the neck by virtue of their location. Asymptomatic, low-volume disease not close to critical structures in neck can be monitored clinically along with ultrasonography of neck. For unresectable recurrent disease, we recommend evaluation with diagnostic radioiodine scanning to consider repeat course of RAI therapy. If there is high suspicion for or proven RAI refractory disease, other local therapies such as EBRT, percutaneous ethanol injection, and radiofrequency ablation can be utilized after multidisciplinary team discussion.

Those who undergo second surgery (or other local interventions) for locoregional recurrence should be evaluated in follow-up with serum thyroglobulin levels and often diagnostic radioiodine scanning. A repeat course of radioiodine therapy should be considered based upon surgical histopathologic features and change or decline in serum thyroglobulin levels postsurgery. If presurgical PET-CT is available and showed fluorodeoxyglucose (FDG) avidity of recurrent disease, RAI therapy is unlikely to be effective; however, this information is not available for all cases with recurrent disease.

6) How is differentiated thyroid cancer managed if there are suspicious or confirmed distant metastases at the time of diagnosis?

Expert Perspective: The common sites of distant metastatic spread from thyroid cancer are lung (most common) and bone. Brain, kidney, adrenal glands, and liver are other less common sites of metastases. Unlike most other cancer types, surgical resection of thyroid and lymph nodes is recommended in most cases for management of differentiated thyroid cancer with presence of suspicious or pathologically confirmed distant metastases. Total thyroidectomy in these cases has two predominant purposes even in patients who present with metastatic disease; (a) administration of radioactive iodine therapy with curative intent (presence of distant metastases is one of the criteria for stratification into the ATA-based high-risk category), and (b) utilization of TSH suppressive therapy to slow the rate of growth of distant metastases and prolong the time to need for start of systemic therapy with tyrosine kinase inhibitors (TKI).

Our Patient: We would recommend proceeding with total thyroidectomy along with neck dissection, followed by radioiodine therapy. A post-treatment scan should be done to evaluate whether lung nodules or other areas showed uptake of radioiodine therapy.

She underwent total thyroidectomy and central and bilateral modified radical neck dissection, which confirmed the presence of papillary thyroid carcinoma, classic type. She was started on thyroid hormone suppression therapy with levothyroxine and received adjuvant RAI therapy. A post-treatment radioiodine scan did not show uptake in the lung lesions. She was referred to medical oncology for further management.

7) When should patients with metastatic radioactive iodine refractory differentiated thyroid cancer start systemic therapy?

Expert Perspective: RAI refractory differentiated thyroid cancer is defined by lack of iodine uptake on radioiodine scanning, progression of disease within 12 months of radioiodine treatment, and after a cumulative dose of 600 mCi. The majority of patients with RAI refractory disease do not need to start systemic therapy immediately. The ATA guidelines state that treatment should be started upon development of symptomatic disease, but treatment is often initiated prior to this. We recommend start of systemic treatment based upon presence of symptoms, disease burden, and rate of progression of disease. Those with asymptomatic metastatic disease not close to critical structures growing in diameter less than 20% per year and doubling time greater than 12 months can be monitored as active surveillance. There are no universally accepted cutoffs for size of metastatic lesions that warrant start of systemic therapy, but lesions greater than 2 cm require closer monitoring. Locally directed therapies such as palliative radiation therapy, metastasectomy, and radiofrequency ablation could be considered for oligometastatic or oligoprogressive disease before starting systemic therapy. This approach is preferred given potential for adverse events and change in quality of life with most systemic therapy agents, with likely no impact on survival. As phase III studies have shown, there seems to be no survival advantage to starting treatment earlier versus later, particularly in slow growing disease.

8) What systemic therapy options are available for radioactive iodine refractory differentiated thyroid cancer?

Expert Perspective: Systemic therapy is recommended for patients with extensive burden of metastatic disease that is symptomatic or expected to be symptomatic in the near future and/or with rapidly progressive lesions, as discussed previously. We recommend obtaining somatic genomic profiling of tumor in all patients with radioactive iodine refractory differentiated thyroid cancer. In absence of alterations targetable with the FDA-approved therapies or nonavailability of molecular results, we recommend treatment with either oral anti-angiogenic therapy, lenvatinib, or participation in available clinical trials. Lenvatinib was approved based upon improvement of median progression-free survival from 3.6 to 18.3 months in the phase III randomized placebo-controlled SELECT trial. Sorafenib is another FDA-approved therapy in this setting based upon improvement in progression free survival seen in the phase III DECISION trial. However, it is generally associated with substantial adverse events and is not routinely utilized by us. After progression of disease on lenvatinib, we recommend treatment with either cabozantinib or participation in available clinical trials. Cabozantinib has been approved by the FDA based upon improvement in progression-free survival in the phase III randomized placebo-controlled COSMIC trial.

If the molecular profiling of tumor identifies rearrangements in the *RET* gene, we recommend treatment with FDA-approved *RET* selective inhibitors (selpercatinib or pralsetinib) as first-line treatment. This recommendation is supported by high objective response rates of approximately 80–90% and an overall more favorable safety profile compared with multitargeted tyrosine kinase inhibitor, which was seen in LIBRETTO-001 (selpercatinib) and ARROW (pralsetinib) trials. If the tumor harbors rearrangements in the *NTRK1* gene, we recommend treatment with FDA-approved, mutation-specific inhibitor larotrectinib or entrectinib. For patients with tumors harboring the *BRAF V600E* mutation, *BRAF/MEK* inhibitors are currently approved for management in differentiated thyroid cancers refractory to standard of care. Phase II data supports efficacy in this population; use of a *BRAF* inhibitor alone or in combination with a MEK inhibitors could be considered as first-line treatment, particularly in patients with contraindications to use of multitargeted TKI therapy or as second- or third-line therapy after progression of disease on lenvatinib and/or cabozantinib. First-generation mammalian target of rapamycin (mTOR) inhibitors such as everolimus also have considerable activity in this disease and should be considered in cases with resistance or contraindications to multitargeted tyrosine kinase inhibitor or in those who are unsuitable for other treatments. Drugs in development include second-generation mTOR inhibitors and MEK inhibitors. Immunotherapy with immune checkpoint inhibitors appears to be effective in anaplastic and certain subtypes of differentiated thyroid cancer such as Hurthle cell thyroid cancer, but it generally appears to have low activity in differentiated thyroid cancer. Figure 4.1 describes a suggested algorithm for management of these patients.

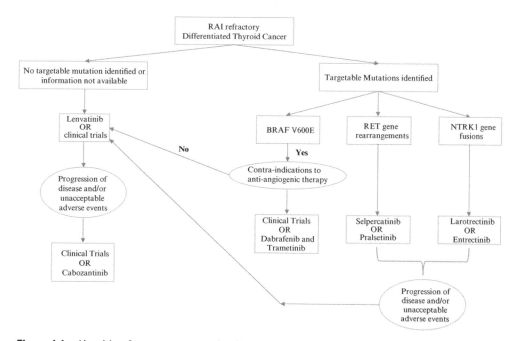

Figure 4.1 Algorithm for management of radioactive iodine (RAI) refractory differentiated thyroid cancer.

9) Should patients with *BRAF V600E* mutated differentiated thyroid cancer be treated with upfront *BRAF/MEK* inhibitors when it is time for systemic therapy?

Expert Perspective: *BRAF V600E* mutation is seen in approximately 40–45% of patients with papillary thyroid cancer. Both vemurafenib and dabrafenib (with or without trametinib) have shown efficacy as monotherapy in differentiated thyroid cancers harboring *BRAF V600E* mutation in phase II studies; results from an ongoing phase III study (NCT04940052) are not available. We consider use of dabrafenib and trametinib in the presence of contraindications to antiangiogenic therapy such as uncontrolled hypertension, recent history of stroke or myocardial infarction, recent history of major bleeding, disease with concern for invasion of airway or upper gastrointestinal tract, and older patients with multiple comorbidities.

10) Are patients with poorly differentiated thyroid cancer managed differently than other common types of differentiated thyroid cancer?

Expert Perspective: Poorly differentiated cancer is an uncommon subtype of differentiated thyroid cancer (2–15%); however, it accounts for most deaths among (non-anaplastic) differentiated thyroid cancers. Turin criteria are the currently accepted definition for poorly differentiated cancer. We additionally consider MSKCC criteria (presence of five or more mitoses per 10 high-power microscopic fields and/or fresh tumor necrosis) to define differentiated thyroid cancers with high-grade features and manage them similarly to poorly differentiated thyroid cancers. These cancers tend to present with adverse features at diagnosis (older age, male predominance, advanced locoregional disease, and distant metastases).

Surgery remains the mainstay of treatment, and despite variable radioiodine avidity expected with this histology, we do generally recommend a one-time dose of RAI if indicated according to the ATA-based risk stratification. EBRT is strongly considered in adjuvant setting with this histology with large primary tumors (T3 or T4) and with extensive node involvement and extranodal extension. Of note, serum thyroglobulin level may not be a reliable tumor marker in these patients. We generally do not recommend repeat doses of RAI in cases of recurrence with this histology.

Patients with poorly differentiated thyroid cancer were included in the clinical trials of systemic therapy with lenvatinib and sorafenib, and similar benefits were seen in subgroup analyses. However, due to poor prognosis of these patients, participation in clinical trials is strongly recommended. Response to combination immunotherapy (nivolumab and ipilimumab) as well as combination of immunotherapy and antiangiogenic therapy have been described in small studies. Results are awaited from clinical trials evaluating a combination of lenvatinib with pembrolizumab (NCT02973997) and of cabozantinib with nivolumab and ipilimumab (NCT03914300).

Case Study 2

Anaplastic Thyroid Cancer

A 65-year-old man with a past medical history of hypertension presented with a rapidly enlarging mass in the neck and difficulty swallowing. Imaging of neck revealed a heterogenous, 4.6 cm mass arising from the right thyroid lobe with bilateral cervical lymphadenopathy. Systemic imaging showed two <5 mm lung nodules in the lower lobe of the left lung. A core needle biopsy of both thyroid mass and left enlarged cervical lymph node showed anaplastic thyroid cancer.

11) How are patients with anaplastic thyroid cancer without distant metastases managed?

Expert Perspective: All patients with anaplastic thyroid cancer are classified as stage IV, with stage IVA (tumor confined to thyroid and no regional lymph node involvement), stage IVB (tumor with extrathyroidal extension and/or regional lymph node involvement), or stage IVC (presence of distant metastases). For stage IVA disease and resectable stage IVB disease, we recommend definitive surgical resection followed by adjuvant concurrent chemoradiation therapy with carboplatin and paclitaxel as radiation sensitizers. For patients with unresectable stage IVB disease, we recommend immediate assessment of tumor for *BRAF V600E* mutation (immunohistochemistry and/or molecular analysis). In the presence of *BRAF V600E* mutated disease, we recommend treatment with upfront dabrafenib and trametinib; for non–*BRAF V600E* mutated disease, we recommend upfront treatment with combination immunotherapy with nivolumab and ipilimumab based upon our institutional experience from a phase II study in metastatic disease. Immune checkpoint inhibitors with a PD-1 inhibitor such as pembrolizumab are also recommended in the absence of a clinical trial. The role of surgery in this setting is unclear. We advocate continual assessment for candidacy for surgical resection starting from approximately after four to six weeks of systemic therapy. If these patients become candidate for surgical resection, surgery followed by adjuvant concurrent chemoradiation therapy with carboplatin and paclitaxel could be considered. It is important to note, however, that the possible impact on outcomes is unclear. Participation in clinical trials, whenever available, is always encouraged for these patients given overall poor prognosis of anaplastic thyroid cancer. Figure 4.2 describes a suggested algorithm for management of these patients.

12) Are any systemic therapies available for metastatic anaplastic thyroid cancer?

Expert Perspective: Similar to management for unresectable stage IVB disease, we perform rapid assessment of tumor for *BRAF V600E* mutation in patients with metastatic disease. In the presence of *BRAF V600E* mutated disease, we recommend treatment with FDA-approved *BRAF/MEK* inhibitor therapy with dabrafenib and trametinib. For non–*BRAF V600E* mutated disease, we recommend upfront treatment with combination immunotherapy with nivolumab and ipilimumab. This is based on a phase II study that reported an objective response rate of 30% with this combination therapy in 10 patients with anaplastic thyroid cancer. Based upon response to initial systemic therapy, consolidative therapy with surgery and/or external beam radiation therapy is considered in select cases. Immune checkpoint inhibitors with a PD-1 inhibitor such as pembrolizumab are also recommended in the absence of a clinical trial based on results from a phase II study using a likely comparable, but not FDA-approved, PD-1 inhibitor, spartalizumab, which showed a radiographic response rate of 19%.

We also recommend obtaining somatic molecular profiling of the tumor to evaluate for actionable alterations in *RET* and *NTRK1* genes as well as other targets for clinical trials.

48 | *4 Thyroid Cancers*

Because it usually takes time to carry out the analysis, we generally utilize *RET* and *TRK* inhibitors in second-line setting after progression of disease on immunotherapy in the presence of these mutations or when molecular results become available. For patients who progress beyond first- or second-line treatment, we often utilize off-label combinations of immunotherapy with antiangiogenic therapy (lenvatinib or cabozantinib), based on data from small studies of this combination from Germany, or mTOR inhibitor (everolimus) after informed discussion with patients. Participation in clinical trials and early discussions about goals of treatment and patient preferences regarding interventions are always recommended. Figure 4.2 describes a suggested algorithm for management of these patients.

Case Study 3

Medullary Thyroid Carcinoma

A 55-year-old woman presented with a slowly growing neck mass for four months and facial flushing for two weeks. Imaging of the neck revealed a heterogeneous mass in the left thyroid lobe and numerous bilateral cervical lymph nodes. FNA of cervical lymph node showed neuroendocrine malignant cells with tumor cells positive for calcitonin, consistent with a diagnosis of medullary thyroid carcinoma. Systemic imaging was notable for a solitary 1.5 cm lesion in liver, which confirmed the presence of medullary thyroid carcinoma on biopsy.

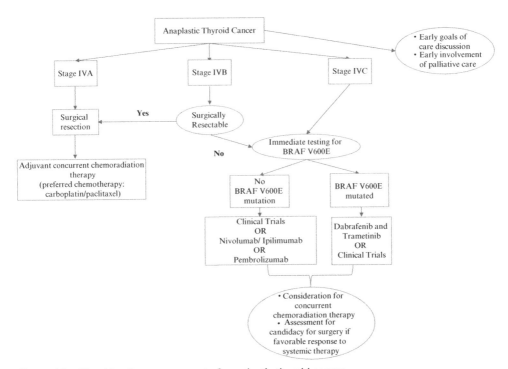

Figure 4.2 Algorithm for management of anaplastic thyroid cancer.

13) Should patients with metastatic medullary thyroid cancer immediately start systemic therapy?

Expert Perspective: Medullary thyroid cancer secretes calcitonin and carcinoembryonic antigen (CEA), both of which are obtained as serum tumor markers at the time of diagnosis. About 75% of medullary thyroid cancer cases are sporadic (with 65% of those harboring somatic *RET* mutation), whereas the remaining 25% cases are hereditary with germline *RET* mutation. Germline testing for *RET* mutation is recommended in all cases with new diagnoses of medullary thyroid cancer because it helps determine the need for biochemical screening for presence of coexisting endocrine tumors (especially pheochromocytoma and hyperparathyroidism, components of multiple endocrine neoplasia syndromes) preoperatively. Systemic imaging with CT of neck and chest, MRI of the abdomen, and an NM bone scan is recommended in patients with locoregional lymph nodes in neck and/or preoperative serum calcitonin > 500 pg/mL. PET-CT imaging is not recommended except with high calcitonin levels, due to lower sensitivity.

Total thyroidectomy along with neck dissection is recommended as the preferred step in most patients with or without distant metastatic disease. The exception would be cases with rapidly progressive (accelerated phase) and symptomatic disease with high tumor burden. Oligometastatic disease at diagnosis or "oligoprogressive" disease should be managed with local interventions such as metastasectomy, radiofrequency ablation, cryoablation, EBRT, and transarterial chemoembolization. Small-volume distant metastatic disease not amenable to local therapies may grow slowly and can be monitored without the need for systemic therapy for years.

The recommendations for the start of systemic therapy in medullary thyroid cancer are similar to those discussed earlier for differentiated thyroid cancer-symptomatic disease, progressive disease growing by at least 20% annually, and those not amenable to local interventions. We recommend evaluation of the tumor for *RET* mutation status in all patients with medullary thyroid cancer before the start of systemic therapy. Selpercatinib or pralsetinib is recommended in *RET*-mutated medullary thyroid cancer based upon high response rates and better tolerability seen in the seminal trials (LIBRETTO-001, –531 and ARROW). For those with non-*RET* mutated medullary thyroid cancer, we recommend either cabozantinib or vandetanib based upon improvement in progression-free survival seen in randomized phase III double-blind, placebo-controlled trials (Zeta trial for vandetanib, Exam trial for cabozantinib).

Our Patient: In this case, we recommend total thyroidectomy and neck dissection of involved compartments, as well as radiofrequency ablation of solitary liver lesion. She should then be followed postsurgery with serum tumor markers and imaging every three to six months based upon the clinical, biochemical, and imaging findings.

Recommended Readings

Bible, K.C., Kebebew, E., Brierley, J. et al. (2021). 2021 American Thyroid Association guidelines for management of patients with anaplastic thyroid cancer. *Thyroid* 31 (3): 337–386.

Brose, M.S., Robinson, B., Sherman, S.I. et al. (2021). Cabozantinib for radioiodine-refractory differentiated thyroid cancer (COSMIC-311): a randomised, double-blind, placebo-controlled, phase 3 trial. *Lancet Oncol* 22 (8): 1126–1138.

Cabanillas, M.E., McFadden, D.G., and Durante, C. (2016). Thyroid cancer. *Lancet* 388 (10061): 2783–2795.

Elisei, R., Schlumberger, M.J., Müller, S.P. et al. (2013). Cabozantinib in progressive medullary thyroid cancer. *J Clin Oncol* 31 (29): 3639–3646.

Haugen, B.R., Alexander, E.K., Bible, K.C. et al. (2016). 2015 American Thyroid Association management guidelines for adult patients with thyroid nodules and differentiated thyroid cancer: the American Thyroid Association guidelines task force on thyroid nodules and differentiated thyroid cancer. *Thyroid* 26 (1): 1–133.

Huang, J., Harris, E.J., and Lorch, J.H. (2019). Treatment of aggressive thyroid cancer. *Surg Pathol Clin* 12 (4): 943–950.

Schlumberger, M. and Leboulleux, S. (2021). Current practice in patients with differentiated thyroid cancer. *Nat Rev Endocrinol* 17 (3): 176–188.

Schlumberger, M., Tahara, M., Wirth, L.J. et al. (2015). Lenvatinib versus placebo in radioiodine-refractory thyroid cancer. *N Engl J Med* 372 (7): 621–630.

Welch, H.G. and Doherty, G.M. (2018). Saving thyroids – overtreatment of small papillary cancers. *N Engl J Med* 379 (4): 310–312.

Wells, S.A., Jr., Robinson, B.G., Gagel, R.F., Dralle, H. et al. (2012). Vandetanib in patients with locally advanced or metastatic medullary thyroid cancer: a randomized, double-blind phase III trial. *J Clin Oncol* 30 (2): 134–141.

5

Non-Small Cell Lung Cancer: Screening, Staging, and Stage I

Ryan D. Gentzler and Linda W. Martin

University of Virginia Cancer Center, Charlottesville, VA, USA

Introduction

Lung cancer is the second most common malignancy in both men and women, accounting for approximately 235,000 new cases per year. Yet it remains notorious as the leading cause of cancer death in the United States (132,000 estimated deaths annually). There was much celebration in 2021 as overall cancer death rates were reported to be 31% lower between 1999 and 2018. Although the top 4 cancers have shown a gradual decline in mortality rates, the most drastic decrease in mortality has occurred in lung cancer (5% lower death rate between 2014 and 2018). This is attributable to a steady decrease in incidence (2.2%) and large improvements in survival for every stage of lung cancer. The advancements in lung cancer outcomes are the largest contributor to the overall cancer mortality improvements. Unfortunately, the COVID-19 pandemic will negatively affect these statistics, and we will not fully appreciate its impact on diagnosis, treatment, and access to care for several years. This chapter will outline current data for screening and the ever-increasing role of multi-disciplinary treatment for early stage lung cancer. These interventions have the potential to push lung cancer mortality rates in the right direction in the wake of the pandemic.

Case Study 1

A 58-year-old man presents to your clinic accompanied by his wife. He has smoked one pack per day since age 19, and he quit five years ago. He is concerned about lung cancer and is inquiring about screening.

1) Should you recommend a yearly low-dose CT scan of the chest?

Expert Perspective: Yes. Lung cancer is the leading cause of cancer death in the United States. It is responsible for more cancer deaths than breast, prostate, and colon cancer combined. Because early stage lung cancer is usually asymptomatic, most lung cancers are diagnosed at late symptomatic stages. Survival of patients diagnosed with locally advanced or metastatic stages is dismal with five-year survival rates of 16%. Early detection of lung cancer provides the best chance of cure. Only 15% of patients with lung cancer in the United States are diagnosed with curable early stage disease (stages I and II), and those are usually discovered incidentally, by imaging of the chest for other reasons.

Cancer Consult: Expertise in Clinical Practice, Volume 1: Solid Tumors & Supportive Care,
Second Edition. Edited by Syed A. Abutalib, Maurie Markman, Al B. Benson III, and Hope S. Rugo.
© 2024 John Wiley & Sons Ltd. Published 2024 by John Wiley & Sons Ltd.

Over the past four decades, a large amount of research has been performed to evaluate whether conventional radiography or CT scans could be effective screening tests for lung cancer. Previous screening studies with chest radiographs and/or sputum cytology have failed to show any mortality reduction from lung cancer from those tests. The prostate, lung, colorectal, and ovarian cancer-screening trial compared screening with chest radiograph to observation and detected no mortality reduction from lung cancer in the screened population. These earlier randomized controlled trials showed that chest radiographs detected slightly more lung cancers and more stage I tumors but failed to demonstrate decreased mortality from lung cancer or a stage shift, defined as follows: increased detection of early cancer and decreased incidence of late stages.

The advent of low-dose (radiation) computed tomography (LDCT) imaging created renewed interest in screening. In the past 10–15 years, there have been a large number of clinical trials evaluating the role of LDCT screening for asymptomatic lung cancer. Early studies demonstrated that when a chest X-ray was obtained within 30 days of an LDCT scan, the chest X-ray missed 70–80% of the LDCT-detected lung cancers. Many of these early lung cancers detected on these trials were curable by surgical resection. However, these nonrandomized trials have many inherent limitations that hamper our ability to draw definitive conclusions. The limitations include the potential for overdiagnosis bias, lead-time bias, and disease-type bias.

Overdiagnosis bias occurs when a screening test identifies disease that never would have affected the patient's life in the absence of screening. This type of bias might occur if screening identifies indolent lesions that would have never caused clinical disease.

Lead-time bias occurs when screening results in earlier recognition of disease but does not change the patient's eventual lifespan, creating the illusion that the patient's survival time with the disease is longer.

Disease-type bias arises from the observation that any screening test that is applied intermittently is more likely to detect indolent tumors than aggressive, fast-growing tumors that would result in clinical symptoms.

Randomized Controlled Trials in Screening Lung Cancer

Several randomized studies provided evidence on the effect of LDCT screening on lung cancer mortality, of which the National Lung Screening Trial (NLST) and the NELSON trial were the most informative.

2) What were the data from National Lung Screening and NELSON trials?

Expert Perspective: The NLST included 53,454 persons at high risk for lung cancer. Participants were randomly assigned to undergo three annual screenings with either low-dose CT or single-view A/P chest radiography. These three annual rounds of screening (baseline and one and two years later) with LDCT resulted in a 20% relative decrease in deaths from lung cancer versus chest radiographs over a median of 6.5 years of follow-up

($P = 0.004$). In absolute terms, the chance of dying from lung cancer was 33% less over the study period in the LDCT group (87 avoided deaths over 26,722 screened participants).

It is important to know that the rate of positive screening tests was 24.2% with LDCT and 6.9% with radiography over all three rounds. A total of 96.4% of the positive screening results in the LDCT group and 94.5% in the radiography group were false-positive results. This emphasizes the need for careful and structured evaluation protocols for patients with positive screening findings to avoid unnecessary interventions.

The NELSON trial randomly assigned high-risk subjects from the Netherlands and Belgium to CT screening at baseline, 1 year, 3 years, and 5.5 years compared to no screening. Results differed between men and women. For men, suspicious nodules were identified in 2.1% of cases. Lung cancer mortality was reduced by 24% at 10 years. For women, there was a larger impact from screening, and 10-year risk of death was reduced by 33%.

In summary, since the publication of the NSLT results, many organizations, including the American Thoracic Society, the American Society of Clinical Oncology, the National Comprehensive Cancer Network, and the American Cancer Society, have endorsed LDCT screening for high-risk populations, as defined on the NSLT. In March 2021, the United States Preventative Task Force (USPTF) recommended expanding the range of patients eligible for lung cancer screening to include ages 50–80 and 20-pack-per-year smoking history who currently smoke or quit in the last 15 years.

Case Study 2

The wife of the patient in Case Study 1 is also concerned about lung cancer. She is 50 years old and never smoked. Her father developed lung cancer at age 75. She is worried that she was exposed to secondhand smoking through her father and husband.

1) Should you recommend yearly low-dose CT of the chest?

Expert Perspective: The NSLT found that three annual rounds of screening in high-risk individuals with LDCT resulted in a 20% relative decrease in deaths from lung cancer versus chest radiographs over a median of 6.5 years of follow-up ($P = 0.004$). This intervention, however, is not of proven benefit in population at lower risk of developing lung cancer than those included in the NLST. Physicians are occasionally asked to order such a test by individuals who have a family member diagnosed with lung cancer, or those who are generally more concerned about their health. A US survey found that a high proportion of never-smokers would be willing to consider lung CT screening. Besides lack of evidence of benefit in this population, risks of screening should be considered. These risks include the discovery of benign pulmonary nodules (false-positive), resulting in unneeded intervention, and the risk of radiation-induced cancer.

False-positive Results

LDCT identifies both cancerous and benign nodules; the latter are often called "false positives." Based on the study's own size cut-offs, the average nodule detection rate per round of screening was 20%. Most studies reported that more than 90% of nodules were benign.

The NLST found that the rate of positive screening tests was 24.2% with low-dose CT and 6.9% with radiography over all three rounds. A total of 96.4% of the positive screening results in the low-dose CT group and 94.5% in the radiography group were false-positive results. The numbers of false-positive results are likely to be higher in never-smokers, in whom the incidence of cancer is lower. In lower-risk populations, the incidence of false-positive results from screening would be expected to be even higher than that reported in the NLST.

A detected nodule will trigger further imaging. The frequency of further CT imaging among screened individuals ranged from 1 to 44.6%. The frequency of further positron emission tomography (PET) imaging among screened individuals ranged from 2.5 to 5.5% in the NLST. Findings could also result in invasive evaluation. In the NLST, 1.2% of patients who were not found to have lung cancer underwent an invasive procedure such as needle biopsy or bronchoscopy, and 0.7% of patients who were not found to have lung cancer had a thoracoscopy, mediastinoscopy, or thoracotomy. Invasive nonsurgical procedures occurred in 73% of patients with benign lesions in the NLST. Anxiety and unnecessary interventions and complications from these procedures should be weighed against the potential benefit of LDCT screening.

The risk of false positives in lower-risk populations is unknown but is likely to be even higher than the risk seen in the NLST and other trials of individuals with tobacco exposure and higher risk of lung cancer.

Radiation Exposure

The risk of radiation-induced cancer from lung CT screening is small. Most relevant, however, is the relative magnitude of the potential absolute benefit from screening compared with the risk of induced cancer. The effective dose of radiation of LDCT is estimated to be 1.5 mSv per examination, although there is substantial variation in actual clinical practice. Diagnostic chest CT (~6 mSv) or PET–CT (~23 mSv) to further investigate detected lesions accounts for most of the radiation exposure in screening studies. A chest X-ray is about 0.1 mSv, as a point of comparison. It is estimated that NLST participants received approximately 8 mSv per participant over three years, including both screening and diagnostic examinations (averaged over the entire screened population).

Estimates of harms from radiation come from several official bodies and commissioned studies, based on dose extrapolations from atomic bombings and also many studies of medical imaging. Brenner (2004) previously estimated the risk of radiation-induced lung cancer mortality for smokers aged 50 and suggested that lung cancer mortality would need to be reduced by at least 5% to outweigh these risks. This figure is likely to be higher for screening at younger ages because the radiation risks will be higher, due to the longer time available to develop a radiation-induced cancer, whereas the absolute benefit will be lower because lung cancer incidence rates are lower.

Using the NLST data, these models predict that approximately one cancer death may be caused by radiation from imaging per 2,500 persons screened, compared to a benefit of prevention of one cancer death per 320 persons screened reported by the NSLT investigators. The benefit, therefore, in preventing lung cancer deaths in NLST is greater than the radiation risk – which only becomes manifest 10–20 years later.

Younger individuals or those with lower risk of developing lung cancer have less favorable trade-offs. Radiation-induced cancer risk estimates from lung CT screening are not currently available for never-smokers or for screening before age 50. Preliminary modelling studies suggest that potential risks may vastly outweigh benefits in non-smokers or those aged 42 years or younger.

Berrington de Gonzalez et al. (2008) conducted a study to estimate the potential risk of radiation-induced lung cancer from three annual lung CT screens for asymptomatic individuals starting at age 30, 40, and 50 years. They estimated the level of screening efficacy that would be required to outweigh these risks of radiation exposure (Table 5.1). The risk estimates were developed for never-smokers and current smokers. For women, they also estimated the risk of radiation-induced breast cancer. They used the Cancer Prevention Study II to estimate the lung cancer rates for never-smokers. For current smokers, they used the Bach lung cancer risk model, assuming a 40-cigarettes-per-day smoking history, which has been recently validated using data from the Alpha-Tocopherol, Beta-Carotene trial.

Table 5.1 summarizes the mortality reduction required to outweigh the radiation risks for each man and woman depending on their age and smoking status. As illustrated in Table 5.1, for a woman who is 50 years old and a never-smoker, screening has to have a benefit of approximately 75% reduction of mortality to justify the risk of radiation exposure. This is clearly unlikely given the results of the NSLT that demonstrated only a 20% reduction in mortality in the higher-risk screened population.

Table 5.1 Percentage reduction in lung cancer mortality needed to outweigh risk of radiation by smoking status, age, and gender.

Smoking status	Age (years)	% Reduction in lung cancer mortality needed to outweigh risk of radiation (90% CI)	
		Male	Female
Never-smoker	30–32	125 (40–300)	375 (200–800)
	40–42	70 (30–190)	170 (100–300)
	50–52	25 (10–70)	75 (30–130)
Current smoker	30–32	70 (20–120)	170 (100–500)
	40–42	10 (3–20)	30 (10–70)
	50–52	2 (1–4)	4 (2–10)

CI: confidence interval.
Source: Adapted from Berrington de Gonzalez et al. "Low-dose lung computed tomography screening before age 55: estimates of the mortality reduction required to outweigh the radiation-induced cancer risk." *J Med Screen.* 2008;15:153–158.

Case Study 3: Stage I Non-Small Cell Lung Cancer

A 60-year-old man presented to his primary care physician with persistent cough. A chest X-ray revealed a right upper lobe lung 4 cm nodule. Staging work-up revealed no evidence to suggest metastasis. He underwent mediastinoscopy and video-assisted thoracotomy, as well as right upper lobe lobectomy. The surgical pathology report revealed a 4 cm tumor. All margins of resection were negative, and all lymph nodes sampled were negative.

1) Surgical staging was ypT2a, N0, M0 (Stage IB). You now recommend:
    A) Four cycles of adjuvant cisplatin-based chemotherapy
    B) Adjuvant radiation therapy
    C) A and B
    D) None of the above

Expert Perspective: Before 2003, several phase III studies failed to show a significant benefit with adjuvant chemotherapy. Adjuvant chemotherapy after resection of stage II–IIIA non-small-cell lung cancer then became the standard of care based on the results of three phase III studies using cisplatin-based regimens, International Adjuvant Lung Trial (IALT), National Cancer Institute of Canada JBR.10, and Adjuvant Navelbine International Trialist Association (ANITA; see Chapter 6). The role of adjuvant chemotherapy for stage IB (T2 [tumors >3 cm and involvement of the visceral pleura]/N0) disease remains controversial.

The International Adjuvant Lung Trial (IALT), reported in 2004, was the first study to prove a benefit from adjuvant chemotherapy. A statistically significant 4% survival advantage at five years (hazard ratio [HR]: 0.86) with the addition of four cycles of cisplatin-based chemotherapy after complete resection of stage I–III non-small cell lung cancer (NSCLC) was demonstrated. This trial included 1,867 stage I–III patients who were randomized to receive cisplatin-based chemotherapy versus observation. The study was not stratified to evaluate results by stage, but a trend toward increased benefit in patients with stage II–III disease was identified. This study was later updated with seven-year follow-up showing disappearance of the survival benefit with longer-term follow-up.

In 2004, the National Cancer Institute of Canada JBR.10 trial randomized 482 patients with completely resected stage IB–IIB NSCLC to receive four cycles of cisplatin-vinorelbine versus observation. A 15% survival advantage was reported at five years (HR 0.7) with the addition of chemotherapy. This trial was stratified by stage. In subset analysis, no benefit was noted for patients with stage IB disease.

Confirmation of the overall beneficial role of adjuvant therapy was demonstrated in 2005 with the results of the ANITA trial. This study of 840 patients with resected NSCLC, stages IB–IIIA, found a 9% survival advantage at five years (HR 0.79) with four cycles of adjuvant cisplatin-vinorelbine. Once more, however, no benefit was found for the patients with stage IB disease on subset analysis. The Cancer and Leukemia Group B (CALGB) trial 9633 was the only study to focus exclusively on stage IB. In the study, 334 patients with resected stage IB NSCLC were randomized to receive either four cycles of paclitaxel-carboplatin or observation. At an initial report, the CALGB 9633 showed a survival advantage for those receiving adjuvant chemotherapy versus observation. This was the only adjuvant trial to use a carboplatin-based regimen. CALGB 9633 was closed early when the first interim analysis demonstrated a 12% survival advantage at four years (HR 0.62).

With the results of these positive trials, adjuvant chemotherapy was established as the standard of care for completely resected stage II–IIIA NSCLC. The initial positive results of CALGB 9633 were the basis of recommendation of adjuvant chemotherapy for stage IB, despite the negative results from the subset analyses of the other trials.

An update of CALGB 9633, presented at the 2006 annual meeting of the American Society of Clinical Oncology, has further clouded the issue of adjuvant chemotherapy in stage IB disease. The update this year is based on 137 events, now with an HR for overall survival (OS) of 0.8 ($P = 0.1$). The statistically significant survival advantage was lost by the five-year follow-up. Failure-free survival still favors the chemotherapy arm (HR 0.74; $P = 0.03$).

The CALGB 9633 had many shortcomings. First, the study was underpowered to detect survival advantage with an HR of 0.8, which would need more than 1,000 patients. It is worth mentioning that the initial accrual target for the study was 500 patients. In 2000, the sample size was reduced to 384 patients due to slow accrual and was further reduced with early closure of the trial because of the initial positive results at interim analysis. Besides being underpowered, other explanations for the negative results of the CALGB 9633 include a true lack of benefit from adjuvant therapy in patients with stage IB disease, or the use of carboplatin-based (as opposed to cisplatin-based) adjuvant chemotherapy.

An individual patient meta-analysis, the LACE meta-analysis, of the large adjuvant trials conducted since the 1995 meta-analysis (excluding CALGB 9633) was reported by Pignon et al. (2008). A 5.5% survival advantage at five years (HR 0.84; $P < 0.001$) for adjuvant cisplatin therapy was reported. Stage IB subset analysis showed a trend toward benefit (HR 0.92) but failed to reach statistical significance (95% CI 0.73–0.95). Stage IA patients had worse outcomes with adjuvant chemotherapy. This meta-analysis emphasizes that the benefit of platinum agent–based adjuvant chemotherapy, if it exists, in stage IB is small and would require a large trial to be detected.

Table 5.2 summarizes the result of some of the adjuvant clinical trials and meta-analyses.

Tumor Size and Redefining the T Scoring for Staging

Previously, the 6th edition stage IB included T2 (tumor > 3 cm, or involvement of visceral pleura) without an upper limit on size and N0 (no lymphadenopathy). In the TNM, 7th edition classification, the T classification was redefined so that stage IB only included tumors up to 5 cm in size. Further refinement on the TNM 8th edition classifies all tumors > 4 cm as stage IIA.

All the relevant adjuvant clinical trials mentioned here had applied the old TNM classification, 6th edition. Thus, the findings now apply to patients with T2aN0 (IB), T2bN0 (IIA), T3N0 (IIB), and T4N0 (IIIA), according to the new subclassification (see Table 5.3).

The tumor size has been a factor in trying to identify patients who might benefit from adjuvant chemotherapy within the stage IB subgroup. In an unplanned subset analysis, patients on CALGB 9633 with tumors ⩾ 4 cm (approximately 100 patients on each arm) did have an OS advantage, with an HR of 0.66 ($P = 0.04$). The importance of tumor size in stage IB disease was also supported by a long-term follow-up update of the JBR.10. In this report, the OS and disease-specific survival (DSS) data showed persistence of the benefit

Table 5.2 Phase III studies and meta-analyses of adjuvant chemotherapy for early stage NSCLC.

Trial	Stage	Number of patients	Chemotherapy regimen	Hazard ratio	P-value
IALT	I–III	1867	Cisplatin/vinca alkaloid or VP16	0.86	<0.03
IALT (2010)	I–III	1867	Cisplatin/vinca alkaloid or VP16	0.91	0.1
NCIC JBR.10	IB–IIB	482	Cisplatin/vinorelbine	0.7	0.012
CALGB 9633 (2004)	IB	344	Carboplatin/paclitaxel	0.62	0.028
ANITA	IB–IIIA	840	Cisplatin/vinorelbine	0.79	0.013
CALGB 9633 (2008)	IB	344	Carboplatin/paclitaxel	0.8	0.1
LACE[a]	I–III	4584	Platinum doublets	0.89	0.0004

LACE, Lung Adjuvant Cisplatin Evaluation; MVd, mitomycin C/vindestine; NCIC, National Cancer Institute of Canada; VP16, etoposide. [a]Meta-analyses.

Table 5.3 Summary of changes to TNM staging system.

6th edition	7th edition	8th edition
T1 (0–3 cm)	T1a (0–2 cm)	T1a (0–1 cm)
	T1b (>2–3 cm)	T1b (>1–2 cm)
		T1c (>2–3 cm)
T2 (>3 cm)	T2a (3–5 cm)	T2a (>3–4 cm)
		T2b (>4–5 cm)
	T2b (>5–7 cm)	T3 (>5–7 cm)
	T3 (>7 cm)	T4 (>7 cm)
T4 (multiple nodules in the same lobe)	T3	T3
T4 (Malignant pleural effusion)	M1a	M1a
M1 (ipsilateral nodule in a different lobe	T4	T4
M1 (systemic metastases)	M1a (Nodules in contralateral lobes, malignant pleural effusion) M1b (distant metastases)	M1a (Nodules in contralateral lobes, malignant pleural effusion) M1b (single extrathoracic metastasis) M1c (multiple extrathoracic metastases)

of adjuvant chemotherapy that was confined to N1 patients. Within stage IB, however, patients with tumors 4 cm or larger in size derived clinically meaningful benefit from chemotherapy (HR 0.66; 95% CI 0.39–1.14; $P = 0.13$), while those with tumors smaller than 4 cm did not (HR 1.73; 95% CI 0.98–3.04; $P = 0.06$). The five-year survival for patients with tumors 4 cm or larger was 59% on observation versus 79% with chemotherapy.

Both of the subgroup analyses of the CLAGB 9633 and the JBR-10 provide support that a subpopulation of patients with stage IB (i.e. tumors larger than 4 cm) may derive benefit from adjuvant chemotherapy.

A 14-gene expression assay that uses quantitative polymerase chain reaction, runs on formalin-fixed paraffin-embedded tissue samples, and differentiates patients with heterogeneous statistical prognoses was developed in a cohort of 361 patients with nonsquamous NSCLC resected at the University of California, San Francisco UCSF. The assay was then independently validated by the Kaiser Permanente Division of Research in a masked cohort of 433 patients with stage I nonsquamous NSCLC resected at Kaiser Permanente Northern California hospitals, and on a cohort of 1006 patients with stage I–III nonsquamous NSCLC resected in several leading Chinese cancer centers that are part of the China Clinical Trials Consortium (CCTC). The Kaplan–Meier analysis of the Kaiser validation cohort showed five-year overall survival of 71.4% (95% CI 60.5–80.0) in low-risk, 58.3% (48.9–66.6) in intermediate-risk, and 49.2% (42.2–55.8) in high-risk patients (P (trend) = 0.0003). Similar analysis of the CCTC cohort indicated five-year overall survivals of 74.1% (66.0–80.6) in low-risk, 57.4% (48.3–65.5) in intermediate-risk, and 44.6% (40.2–48.9) in high-risk patients (P (trend) < 0.0001). Multivariate analysis in both cohorts indicated that no standard clinical risk factors could account for, or provide, the prognostic information derived from tumor gene expression. The assay improved prognostic accuracy beyond National Comprehensive Cancer Network criteria for stage I high-risk tumors ($P < 0.0001$) and differentiated low-risk, intermediate-risk, and high-risk patients within all disease stages. This assay is now FDA approved under the name DetermaRx.

Zhu et al. (2010), on further analysis of the JBR.10 trial, hypothesized that gene expression profiling may identify stage-independent subgroups who might benefit from adjuvant chemotherapy. A 15-gene expression signature was found to be an independent prognostic marker in early stage, completely resected NSCLC. Furthermore, it has demonstrated the potential to select patients with stage IB–II NSCLC most likely to benefit from adjuvant chemotherapy. This signature separated observation patients into high-risk and low-risk subgroups with significantly different survival (HR 15.02; 95% CI 5.12–44.04; $P < .001$; stage I HR 13.31; $P < .001$; stage II HR 13.47; $P < .001$). The signature was also predictive of improved survival after adjuvant chemotherapy in JBR.10 high-risk patients (HR 0.33; 95% CI 0.17–0.63; $P < .0005$) but not in low-risk patients (HR 3.67; 95% CI 1.22–11.06; $P = .0133$; interaction $P < .001$). Genomic profiling awaits confirmation in prospectively designed clinical trials.

There is currently no FDA-approved use of immunotherapy for stage I surgically resected NSCLC. At the American Society of Clinical Oncology (ASCO) Annual Meeting 2021, data was presented from the Impower 010 trial of adjuvant atezolizumab. This trial randomized patients with stage IB–IIIA (7th edition staging) NSCLC to receive adjuvant atezolizumab for one year after standard chemotherapy versus best supportive care. This study met its primary endpoint of disease-free survival improvement in patients with stage II–IIIA, but not the intention to treat population of stage IB–IIIA. There are numerous other ongoing trials evaluating the use of immunotherapy as neoadjuvant or adjuvant therapy, including patients with stage I disease.

Another important practice changing study was reported in 2020 for *EGFR* mutant patients. The ADAURA trial randomized patients with stage IB–IIIA (7th edition staging) NSCLC with, *EGFR* mutations (exon 19 deletions, and exon 21 L858R) who had completed lobectomy to osimertinib or placebo for three years. Specifically for stage IB disease, the HR for recurrence or death was an impressive 0.39 (95% CI 0.18–0.76). This highlights the importance of testing for *EGFR* mutations even in early stage patients now that there is a meaningful therapeutic intervention.

The research was presented at the 2023 ASCO confirmed these findings. Treatment with osimertinib after surgery significantly lowered the risk of death in adults with completely resected *EGFR*-mutated stage IB, II, or IIIA non–small cell lung cancer (NSCLC).

Osimertinib is a third-generation, central nervous system–active *EGFR* tyrosine kinase inhibitor and is the first targeted agent to be approved by the U.S. Food and Drug Administration as an adjuvant treatment for patients with resected stage IB to IIIA *EGFR*-mutated NSCLC.

Future analyses from ADAURA are underway, Osimertinib is also currently being evaluated in patients with other stages of NSCLC, including as well as neoadjuvantly (See Qs 4–5 next chapter).

In our practice, we generally recommend adjuvant cisplatin-based chemotherapy to fit patients with tumors 4 cm or larger. We have not adopted any of the genomic profiling models or use of adjuvant immunotherapy for patients with stage I NSCLC outside of a trial setting; however, we do routinely check biomarkers regardless of stage.

Correct Answer: A

Conclusion

Screening a population of individuals at a substantially elevated risk of lung cancer most likely could be performed in a manner such that the benefits outweigh the harms. The fear and anxiety that patients can experience once there is even a slight suspicion of lung cancer highlight the need for careful education of LDCT participants and for carefully worded scan interpretations, as well as a structured work-up, evaluation, and follow-up program.

In the setting of increasing health-care costs, the relative cost-effectiveness of LDCT screening compared with other interventions will be a topic of concern. For patients at minimal risk of cancer, the harm of screening could outweigh the potential benefit, and these tests should not be offered outside a clinical trial context.

For patients with stage II–III surgically resected NSCLC, there is convincing evidence for adjuvant cisplatin-based chemotherapy to reduce the risk of death from recurrent lung cancer and immunotherapy to reduce the risk of disease recurrence. Whether immunotherapy will lead to improvements in overall survival for patients with surgically resected lung cancer is not known at this time. Given updates in the staging system, there is no longer a role for adjuvant therapy for most stage IB tumors, except those measuring 4 cm or greater.

Recommended Readings

Arriagada, R., Dunant, A., Pignon, J.P. et al. (2010). Long-term results of the international adjuvant lung cancer trial evaluating adjuvant cisplatin-based chemotherapy in resected lung cancer. *J Clin Oncol* 28 (1): 35–42.

Bach, P.B., Mirkin, J.N., Oliver, T.K. et al. (2012). Benefits and harms of CT screening for lung cancer: a systematic review. *JAMA* 307 (22): 2418–2429.

Brenner DJ. (2004). Radiation risks potentially associated with low-dose CT screening of adult smokers for lung cancer. *Radiology* 231 (2): 440–445.

Butts, C.A., Ding, K., Seymour, L. et al. (2010). Randomized phase III trial of vinorelbine plus cisplatin compared with observation in completely resected stage IB and II non-small-cell lung cancer: updated survival analysis of JBR-10. *J Clin Oncol* 28 (1): 29–34.

Douillard, J.Y., Rosell, R., De Lena, M. et al. (2006). Adjuvant vinorelbine plus cisplatin versus observation in patients with completely resected stage IB–IIIA non-small-cell lung cancer (Adjuvant Navelbine International Trialist Association [ANITA]): a randomised controlled trial. *Lancet Oncol* 7 (9): 719–727.

John, T., Grohé, C., Goldman, J.W. et al. (2023 May 24). Three-year safety, tolerability, and health-related quality of life outcomes of adjuvant osimertinib in patients with resected stage IB-IIIA EGFR-mutated non-small cell lung cancer: updated analysis from the phase 3 ADAURA trial. *J Thorac Oncol.* S1556-0864(23)00574-9. doi: 10.1016/j.jtho.2023.05.015. Epub ahead of print. PMID: 37236398.

Koning, H.J., van der Alst, C.M., de Jong, P.A. et al. (2020). Reduced lung-cancer mortality with volume CT screening in a randomized trial. *NEJM* 382: 503–513.

Tsuboi, M., Herbst, R.S., John, T. et al. (2023 June 4). Overall survival with osimertinib in resected EGFR-mutated NSCLC. *N Engl J Med.* doi: 10.1056/NEJMoa2304594. Epub ahead of print. PMID: 37272535.

Zhu, C.Q., Ding, K., Strumpf, D. et al. (2010). Prognostic and predictive gene signature for adjuvant chemotherapy in resected non-small-cell lung cancer. *J Clin Oncol* 28 (29): 4417–4424.

6

Non-Small Cell Lung Cancer: Stages II and III

Gregory Peter Kalemkerian, Kamya Sankar, and Angel Qin

Division of Hematology/Oncology, Department of Internal Medicine, University of Michigan, MI, USA

Introduction

Non-small cell lung cancer (NSCLC) is the leading cause of cancer-related death and the second most common cancer among both men and women. The high mortality rate associated with NSCLC is primarily due to the advanced stage of the disease at diagnosis in most patients (Chapter 7). Surgical resection, if possible, is still considered the primary curative option for people with early stage disease (Chapter 5). For patients with stage II–III NSCLC, additional modalities such as chemotherapy, radiotherapy, and/or immunotherapy may be beneficial, and studies to optimize these treatments are ongoing. Treatment for stage II–III NSCLC is given with curative intent, but with a historical five-year overall survival rate of only 25–50%, it is clearly evident that better strategies are needed to improve curative therapy.

The current definitions of stage II–III NSCLC are presented in Table 6.1. Surgical resection with lobectomy and mediastinal lymph node sampling/dissection is the recommended treatment for most patients with clinical stage II NSCLC, with adjuvant chemotherapy then given for those with pathologic stage II or III disease. For appropriately selected, biomarker-positive patients, adjuvant immunotherapy or targeted therapy are now approved options. Stage III NSCLC is more heterogeneous in terms of both tumor-node-metastasis (TNM) staging and treatment. Most patients are treated with some form of combined modality therapy, primarily definitive chemoradiotherapy followed by immunotherapy, though select patients with potentially resectable disease may receive neoadjuvant systemic therapy with or without radiotherapy followed by surgical resection.

Cancer Consult: Expertise in Clinical Practice, Volume 1: Solid Tumors & Supportive Care,
Second Edition. Edited by Syed A. Abutalib, Maurie Markman, Al B. Benson III, and Hope S. Rugo.
© 2024 John Wiley & Sons Ltd. Published 2024 by John Wiley & Sons Ltd.

Table 6.1 Lung cancer staging per AJCC 8th edition.

Stage	TNM Subset	TNM Classifier Definition
IA1-3	T1a-c N0 M0	T1: ≤3 cm w/o local invasion [T1a(mi): minimally invasive adenoca; T1a: ≤1 cm; T1b: >1 but no more than 2 cm; T1c: >2 but no more than 3 cm]
IB	T2a N0 M0	T2a: visceral pleural invasion or main bronchus involvement or atelectasis to hilum; and/or >3 but no more than 4 cm
IIA	T2b N0 M0	T2b: visceral pleural invasion or main bronchus involvement or atelectasis to hilum; and/or >4 but no more than 5 cm
IIB	T1-2 N1 M0	N1: hilar or peribronchial or intrapulmonary LN
	T3 N0 M0	T3: >5 but no more than 7 cm or invasion of chest wall, phrenic nerve, parietal pericardium or multiple nodules in same lobe as primary tumor
IIIA	T1-2 N2 M0	N2: ipsilateral mediastinal or subcarinal LN
	T3-4 N1 M0	
	T4 N0 M0	T4: >7 cm; or invasion of diaphragm, mediastinum, heart, great vessels, trachea, recurrent laryngeal nerve, esophagus, vertebral body, carina; or multiple nodules in different ipsilateral lobe than primary tumor
IIIB	T1-2 N3 M0	N3: contralateral mediastinal or contralateral hilar or any supraclavicular LN
	T3-4 N2 M0	
IIIC	T3-4 N3 M0	
IVA	T1-4 N1-3 M1a-b	M1a: contralateral lung nodules or malignant pleural/pericardial nodules/effusion
		M1b: single distant metastasis
IVB	T1-4 N1-3 M1c	M1c: multiple distant metastases

1) What is the role of adjuvant chemotherapy for completely resected stage II–III NSCLC?

Expert Perspective: The standard recommendation for patients with stage II–III NSCLC who have undergone curative resection and have good performance status is adjuvant cisplatin-based chemotherapy. This recommendation is based on randomized phase III studies and meta-analyses that have shown an overall survival benefit with the addition of adjuvant chemotherapy following resection (Table 6.2). Overall, these trials have demonstrated a five-year overall survival benefit of between 4 and 15% (Arriagada et al. 2004, Winton et al. 2005, Douillard et al. 2006). Importantly, all trials supporting adjuvant chemotherapy were done utilizing an older staging system (AJCC 6th edition) in which all patients with N0 disease were considered stage IB regardless of tumor size. Subgroup analyses of the CALGB 9633 and JBR.10 trials found that the use of adjuvant chemotherapy may improve overall survival in patients with lymph node–negative (N0) disease and tumors ≥4 cm, but not in those with smaller tumors. The Lung Adjuvant Cisplatin Evaluation (LACE) meta-analysis pooled data from the five modern, cisplatin-based, adjuvant chemotherapy trials

Table 6.2 Phase III clinical trial of adjuvant chemotherapy for resected stage* I–III NSCLC.

Study	N	Stage*	Arms	Overall Survival			
				Median (months)	5-year	HR (95% CI)	P-value
ALPI	1209	I–IIIA	Mitomycin/vindesine/cisplatin	55.2	+1% over Observation	0.96 (0.81–1.13)	0.589
			Observation	48.0			
IALT	1867	I–III	Cisplatin/etoposide	54	NR	0.86 (0.76–0.97)	0.03
			Cisplatin/vinorelbine		44%		
			Cisplatin/vinblastine				
			Observation	45	40%		
BLT	381	I–III	Mitomycin/vinblastine/cisplatin	33.9	58% (2-yr)	1.02 (0.77–1.35)	0.90
			Mitomycin/ifosfamide/cisplatin				
			Cisplatin/vinorelbine				
			Cisplatin/vindesine				
			Observation	32.6	60% (2-yr)		
JBR.10	482	IB–II	Cisplatin/vinorelbine	94	69%	0.69 (0.49–0.98)	0.002
			Observation	73	54%		
CALGB 9633	344	IB	Carboplatin/paclitaxel	95	60%	0.83 (0.64–1.08)	0.125
			Observation	78	58%		
ANITA	798	IB–IIIA	Cisplatin/vinorelbine	65.7	51%	0.8 (0.66–0.96)	0.013
			Observation	43.7	43%		

* AJCC 6th edition.

involving 4,584 patients (Pignon et al. 2008). With a median follow-up of 5.2 years, the five-year absolute survival benefit from chemotherapy was 5.4%, but this included patients with stage IA disease in whom adjuvant treatment appeared detrimental (HR 1.40 [95% CI 0.95–2.06]); the benefit in those with stage II–III disease was clearly greater (stage II, HR 0.83 [95% CI 0.73–0.95], $p < 0.05$; stage III, HR 0.83 [95% CI 0.72–0.94], $p < 0.05$). Additionally, the benefit did not significantly vary by chemotherapy regimen (Chapter 5).

Based on these data, adjuvant chemotherapy is recommended for patients with stage II–III NSCLC (per the current AJCC 8th edition staging system) who have good performance status following complete resection. For practical purposes, we use an overall survival benefit of 10% when discussing adjuvant chemotherapy with patients with stage II–III disease. In patients with stage IA disease, adjuvant chemotherapy is not recommended, whereas for stage IB disease (T2aN0M0), chemotherapy may be considered for those with tumors 4 cm in diameter.

2) Which chemotherapy regimen would you recommend for completely resected stage II–III NSCLC?

Expert Perspective: The choice of chemotherapy regimen may vary by institutional and clinician preference and is frequently based on the individual patient's tumor histology, comorbid conditions, and anticipated tolerance. The chemotherapy regimens used in the reported phase III adjuvant trials are listed in Table 6.2. The phase II, randomized TREAT trial compared cisplatin/pemetrexed to cisplatin/vinorelbine as postoperative chemotherapy for completely resected, stage IB–III, non-squamous NSCLC. Cisplatin/pemetrexed was less toxic than cisplatin/vinorelbine, and overall survival was similar in both arms (3-year, 75% vs. 77%, $P = 0.858$). The ECOG 1505 phase III trial compared adjuvant chemotherapy plus bevacizumab to chemotherapy alone in people with completely resected stage IB (≥ 4 cm) to IIIA NSCLC (per AJCC 6th edition) and allowed the use of any one of four regimens, cisplatin plus either vinorelbine, docetaxel, gemcitabine, or pemetrexed (non-squamous only). The study found no improvement in survival with the addition of bevacizumab, and although not statistically powered to compare the different chemotherapy regimens, the outcomes in both arms appeared similar regardless of which regimen was utilized, suggesting relative equivalence of two-drug, cisplatin-based regimens.

Based on these findings, we favor four cycles of adjuvant cisplatin/pemetrexed for patients with nonsquamous NSCLC and cisplatin/gemcitabine for those with squamous histology, because these regimens appear to be as beneficial as, and less toxic than, alternative regimens.

3) Can carboplatin be substituted for cisplatin in adjuvant setting?

Expert Perspective: Yes, carboplatin can usually be safely substituted for cisplatin in patients in whom cisplatin is contraindicated or poorly tolerated. Although there is little data on the use of carboplatin in the adjuvant setting, carboplatin-based regimens are equivalent to cisplatin-based regimens in patients with more advanced disease.

4) Is there a role for adjuvant targeted therapy in resected stage II or III NSCLC?

Expert Perspective: Randomized clinical trials have recently reported that both adjuvant targeted therapy and immunotherapy can significantly improve short-term, disease-free survival in patients who have undergone complete resection of stage II or III NSCLC. However, their impact on overall survival and cure rate remains unknown, leading to controversy regarding clinically meaningful, long-term endpoints and challenges in applying early clinical trial data to real-world patients.

Molecular characterization of tumor tissue or circulating tumor DNA (ctDNA) and the use of targeted therapy in patients with tumors harboring targetable driver mutations are now part of the standard care for patients with advanced NSCLC. However, until recently, there was no evidence to support molecular diagnostic testing or the use of targeted therapy in those with early stage disease. The early results of the randomized phase III ADAURA trial, which evaluated adjuvant osimertinib versus placebo in patients with resected, stage IB–IIIA, *EGFR*-mutant NSCLC, has led to substantial controversy regarding the use of osimertinib in the post-operative setting.

Approximately 10% of patients with lung adenocarcinoma have tumors harboring a sensitizing *EGFR* mutation. Prior to the ADAURA trial, three randomized, phase III studies had evaluated *EGFR* tyrosine kinase inhibitor (TKI) therapy versus placebo in the adjuvant setting: RADIANT, BR.19, and ADJUVANT-CTONG. The RADIANT trial evaluated erlotinib versus placebo in patients with resected, stage IB–IIIA, molecularly unselected NSCLC and, unsurprisingly, reported no disease-free survival or overall survival benefit in the overall study population. In the subset of patients with *EGFR*-mutant tumors, there was a numerical improvement in disease-free survival (median, 46.4 vs. 28.5 months, HR 0.61, $P = 0.039$; not significant due to hierarchical testing), but no difference in overall survival. The BR.19 study, which similarly evaluated gefitinib versus placebo in molecularly unselected patients with resected, stage IB–IIIA NSCLC, was stopped early and also failed to demonstrate an improvement in overall survival in the overall study population or in the small subset of patients with *EGFR*-mutant tumors. Of note, neither the RADIANT nor the BR.19 trial was adequately powered to definitively evaluate the *EGFR*-mutant subgroup. The ADJUVANT-CTONG 1104 trial was the first phase III study to exclusively evaluate patients with *EGFR*-mutant, resected, stage II–IIIA (N1–N2) NSCLC. Patients were randomly assigned to adjuvant gefitinib ×2 years versus cisplatin-based chemotherapy ×4 cycles after complete resection. Disease-free survival was significantly higher in the gefitinib arm (30.8 vs. 19.8 months, HR 0.56, $P = 0.001$), but there was no significant difference in overall survival (75.5 vs. 79.2 months, HR 0.96, $P = 0.82$).

ADAURA is a global phase III trial that randomized 682 patients with resected stage IB (≥4 cm) – IIIA lung adenocarcinoma harboring an *EGFR* sensitizing mutation to osimertinib ×3 years or placebo after optional adjuvant chemotherapy (Wu et al. 2020). With median follow-up of 22 months, the 24-month disease-free survival rate in patients with stage II–IIIA disease (the primary endpoint) was significantly higher in the osimertinib group (90% vs. 44%, HR 0.17, $P = 0.001$), a benefit which was seen regardless of whether chemotherapy had been administered prior to osimertinib. A recent update reported continued disease-free survival benefit (median, 66 vs. 22 months; four-year, 70% vs. 29%). Overall survival data remains immature. This data led to the accelerated approval of osimertinib by the U.S. Food and Drug Administration (FDA) for the adjuvant treatment of patients with resected, early stage NSCLC that harbors an *EGFR exon 19* deletion or *exon 21 L858R* mutation, making osimertinib the first targeted therapy available for the adjuvant treatment of NSCLC.

As mentioned previously, the accelerated approval of adjuvant osimertinib based on an improvement in disease-free survival has led to substantial controversy among thoracic oncologists regarding not only the clinical utility of osimertinib as adjuvant therapy, but also the broader question of appropriate endpoints for clinical trials in the curative treatment setting. The ADAURA study has been criticized for not mandating a PET scan and brain MRI at patient screening and for the fact that 40% of enrolled patients did not receive adjuvant chemotherapy, which remains the standard of care for patients with pathologic stage II–III, resected NSCLC Finally, we do not know if the disease-free survival benefit will translate into an overall survival benefit, leading to the important question of whether adjuvant osimertinib is preventing or just delaying disease recurrence. The recent update of the ADAURA trial does suggest a waning of the survival benefit after treatment discontinuation. If, in fact, recurrence is only being delayed, then the initiation of osimertinib at the time of recurrence would potentially result in similar overall survival in both treatment groups despite a significant improvement in disease-free survival (as suggested by the RADIANT trial). In this case, patients who do not have disease recurrence would be spared the potential toxicity of three years of osimertinib treatment. In addition, tumors in patients who recur after receiving adjuvant osimertinib (when they have no disease-associated symptoms) may have developed drug resistance that would limit further benefit from *EGFR* TKI therapy at recurrence when systemic response would be most beneficial for the relief of increasing symptoms of disease.

In the face of these controversial data, oncologists are now faced with the challenge of evaluating the potential risks and benefits of molecular testing and adjuvant osimertinib. Given the profound disease-free survival benefit in the ADAURA trial and recent FDA approval, it is now reasonable to evaluate *EGFR* mutational status in resected, stage II–IIIA lung adenocarcinomas and to discuss the pros and cons of adjuvant osimertinib after adjuvant chemotherapy with patients with tumors harboring a sensitizing *EGFR* mutation. However, analysis of long-term, overall survival will be crucial to determining whether adjuvant osimertinib is truly improving the cure rate in early stage resected NSCLC.

5) Is there a role for adjuvant immunotherapy in resected stage II or III NSCLC?

Expert Perspective: Given the significant improvement in progression-free and overall survival with immune checkpoint inhibitors alone or in combination with chemotherapy in advanced NSCLC, there is a strong rationale for studying the potential use of immunotherapy for the treatment of early stage disease (Chapter 7). Many clinical trials evaluating immunotherapy in the adjuvant setting are ongoing, but mature results have not yet been reported. Early results have been reported from the randomized, phase III IMpower010 trial, which was designed to determine whether the use of atezolizumab, a PD-L1 immune checkpoint inhibitor, after adjuvant chemotherapy would improve outcomes for patients with completely resected, stage IB–IIIA NSCLC (Wakelee et al. 2021). In this study, 1,280 patients who had undergone complete resection and cisplatin-based, adjuvant chemotherapy were randomly assigned to receive atezolizumab every three weeks for up to 16 cycles versus best supportive care. The primary endpoint was disease-free survival with a secondary endpoint of overall survival. At the initial report with median follow-up of 32 months, disease-free survival was improved with atezolizumab in: (a) patients with stage II–IIIA disease and PD-L1 tumor proportional score (TPS) ≥ 1% (HR 0.66; $P = 0.0039$), (b) all patients with stage II–IIIA disease regardless of PD-L1 status (HR 0.79; $P = 0.02$), and (c) the intention-to-treat population with stage IB–IIIA disease (HR 0.81; $P = 0.039$). For patients with stage II–III disease, the disease-free survival benefit was seen primarily in those with PD-L1 TPS ≥ 50% (HR 0.43; 95% CI 0.27–0.68). A recent update of the data with median follow-up of 46 months reported a non-significant trend in overall survival favoring adjuvant atezolizumab in patients with stage II–III disease with PD-L1 TPS ≥ 1% (HR 0.71; 95% CI 0.49–1.03). Overall survival was similar in both arms for all patients with stage II–IIIA disease and in the intention-to-treat population. In addition, 18% of patients in the atezolizumab arm discontinued treatment due to adverse events. Based on these data, the FDA and the European Commission have approved atezolizumab for adjuvant treatment following resection and platinum-based chemotherapy in patients with stage II–IIIA NSCLC whose tumors have PD-L1 TPS ≥ 1% or PD-L1 TPS ≥ 50%, respectively.

The KEYNOTE-091 trial recently reported initial results with median follow-up of 36 months. This study enrolled 1177 patients with completely resected stage IB (≥ 4 cm)–IIIA NSCLC who had undergone guideline-appropriate adjuvant chemotherapy and were randomized to pembrolizumab versus placebo for one year. Disease-free survival was significantly improved with pembrolizumab in all patients (HR 0.76; $P = 0.0014$), but there was no significant difference in overall survival (HR 0.87; $P = 0.17$). Other ongoing trials are evaluating immune checkpoint inhibitor therapy in the adjuvant setting. The ANVIL trial has enrolled 903 patients with stage IB–IIIA resected NSCLC with or without adjuvant chemotherapy and randomized them to receive either adjuvant nivolumab for one year or best supportive care. The BR.31 trial is assessing durvalumab versus placebo in patients with stage IB–IIIA resected NSCLC with or without adjuvant chemotherapy. All of these trials will require several more years to yield mature data. As noted earlier for the ADAURA trial, the focus on early disease-free survival, rather than long-term overall survival, raises significant concerns regarding the actual clinical utility of such treatment in the curative setting. Given the available data and regulatory approvals, it is now reasonable to obtain PD-L1 expression analysis on patients with resected stage II-III NSCLC and to discuss the pros and cons of adjuvant atezolizumab for those with positive expression, particularly those with TPS ≥ 50%. Recently, FDA approved pembrolizumab with platinum-containing chemotherapy as neoadjuvant treatment, and with continuation of single-agent pembrolizumab as post-surgical adjuvant treatment for resectable (tumors ≥4 cm or node positive) NSCLC (KEYNOTE-671).

6) Is there a role for adjuvant radiotherapy in resected stage II or III NSCLC?

Expert Perspective: Historically, postoperative radiotherapy has not been recommended for patients with pathologic stage I–II NSCLC due to data that have suggested a detrimental effect in those with pathologic stage I–II disease. In contrast, despite the lack of prospective data demonstrating an improvement in survival, postoperative radiotherapy has been recommended by some oncologists after complete resection of stage III, N2-positive NSCLC based on retrospective analyses of large patient databases. However, recent prospective, randomized trials have now demonstrated a lack of benefit for post-operative radiotherapy in patients with resected stage IIIA-N2 NSCLC.

In 1998, the PORT Meta-analysis Trialists Group published a meta-analysis of all randomized studies from 1965 to 1995 evaluating the role of postoperative radiotherapy in patients with resected NSCLC (Burdett et al. 1998). This meta-analysis reported an adverse effect of postoperative radiotherapy on overall survival (HR 1.21) in the entire population. However, subgroup analyses had mixed results, finding a detrimental effect of postoperative radiotherapy in patients with stage I–II (N0-1) disease and a nonsignificant trend toward potential benefit in those with stage IIIA (N2-positive) disease.

Retrospective analyses have supported the notion that postoperative radiotherapy is associated with a deleterious effect on survival in early stage NSCLC, though there may be a survival benefit in patients with N2-positive disease. An analysis of the Surveillance, Epidemiology, and End Results (SEER) database of 7,465 patients with pathologic stage II–III NSCLC who underwent complete resection showed that postoperative radiotherapy was associated with a statistically significant detrimental effect on survival in patients with N0 (HR 1.18, $P = 0.04$) and N1 (HR 1.097, $P = 0.02$) disease. However, in patients with N2-positive disease, postoperative radiotherapy was associated with improved overall survival (HR 0.86, $P = 0.008$).

An analysis of the National Cancer Database (NCDB) included patients with pathologic N2-positive NSCLC who had undergone resection and adjuvant chemotherapy plus radiotherapy (≥ 45 Gy) or no postoperative radiotherapy. Postoperative radiotherapy was associated with improved overall survival in patients with N2-positive disease (median, 45.2 vs. 40.7 months; five-year, 39.3% vs. 34.8%, $P = 0.014$). Furthermore, a secondary analysis of the ANITA trial of adjuvant chemotherapy (Table 6.2), in which postoperative radiotherapy could be given at the physician's discretion, found that although postoperative radiotherapy was associated with a deleterious effect on the survival of the overall population, it appeared to improve survival in patients with pathologic N2 disease, both in the chemotherapy (median, 47.4 vs. 23.8 months) and observation (median, 22.7 vs. 12.7 months) arms of the main study.

Until recently, prospective, randomized data on the use of postoperative radiotherapy incorporating modern radiotherapy techniques has been lacking. The phase III PORT-C trial randomized 364 eligible patients with completely resected, stage IIIA, N2-positive NSCLC to either postoperative radiotherapy (50 Gy in 25 fractions) or observation after adjuvant chemotherapy (Hui et al. 2021). There was no significant improvement in disease-free survival (median, 22.1 vs. 18.6 months; HR 0.84, $P = 0.20$) or overall survival (three-year, 78.3% vs. 82.8%; HR 1.02, $P = 0.93$) with the addition of postoperative radiotherapy. Similarly, the phase III LungART trial randomized 501 patients with completely resected stage III, N2-positive NSCLC who may have previously received adjuvant or neoadjuvant chemotherapy to mediastinal postoperative radiotherapy (54 Gy in 27–30 fractions) versus no postoperative radiotherapy (Le Pechoux et al. 2022). After a median follow-up of 4.8 years, the primary endpoint analysis showed that the median disease-free survival was 30.5 months for postoperative radiotherapy versus 22.8 months for observation (HR 0.85; $P = 0.16$), suggesting no significant benefit. In addition, three-year overall survival rates were 67% for post-operative radiotherapy and 69% for observation (HR 0.97; 95% CI 0.73–1.28). The mature analyses of disease-free survival and overall survival data from the LungART trial will provide a more evidence-based assessment of modern postoperative radiotherapy, but based on current data, it appears that there is no role for post-operative radiotherapy in the treatment of patients with pathologic N2-positive NSCLC.

7) Is there a role for neoadjuvant therapy in stage II or IIIA NSCLC?

Expert Perspective: The use of neoadjuvant versus adjuvant therapy for patients with stage II–IIIA, surgically resectable NSCLC continues to be controversial because there are no studies which demonstrate clear superiority of one strategy over the other. An analysis of patients with stage II or III NSCLC from the NCDB showed that chemotherapy improved overall survival compared to surgery alone, but there was no difference in survival between neoadjuvant or adjuvant chemotherapy. In addition, there is little agreement on what constitutes "resectable" stage III disease, with most defining it as T3N1M0 and T1-3N2 (non-bulky) M0, whereas others might add T4N0-1M0. Even the term "non-bulky N2 disease" has multiple definitions with the most common being involvement of one or two ipsilateral mediastinal lymph nodes <3 cm in size.

In the early 1990s, several small, randomized trials demonstrated that neoadjuvant chemotherapy prior to surgery improved overall survival compared to surgery alone in patients with resectable stage III NSCLC. However, the dismal survival of patients in the surgery alone arms of these trials and the emergence of chemoradiotherapy as the standard treatment for stage III NSCLC suggested that surgery alone is the wrong control for these types of studies and raised the question of whether surgery had any role in the care of patients with stage III, N2-positive NSCLC.

Given the high risk of locoregional recurrence associated with N2 disease, the addition of concurrent radiotherapy to neoadjuvant chemotherapy became an attractive strategy. However, in a randomized phase III study of neoadjuvant chemoradiotherapy versus chemotherapy alone evaluating 232 patients with stage IIIA N2-positive NSCLC who were deemed to have surgically resectable disease, the addition of radiotherapy did not result in a significant survival benefit (median, 37 vs. 26 months; $P = 0.67$) (Pless et al. 2015).

The phase III Intergroup 0139 trial randomized 396 patients with T1-3N2M0 NSCLC to concurrent cisplatin/etoposide ×4 cycles plus definitive radiotherapy up to 61 Gy versus neoadjuvant concurrent cisplatin/etoposide ×2 cycles plus radiotherapy to 45 Gy followed by surgical resection and two more cycles of cisplatin/etoposide (Albain et al. 2009). Despite a significant improvement in progression-free survival in the surgical arm (median, 13 vs. 11 months; 5-year, 22% vs. 11%; HR 0.77; $P = 0.017$), surgery did not result in a significant improvement in overall survival (median, 23.6 vs. 22.2 months; five-year, 27% vs 20%; HR 0.87, $P = 0.24$). However, a secondary analysis of patients who only required lobectomy (rather than pneumonectomy) did demonstrate a significant survival benefit in the surgical arm (median, 33.6 vs. 21.7 months; five-year, 36% vs. 18%; $P = 0.002$), leaving open the possibility that neoadjuvant chemoradiotherapy followed by surgery might be a beneficial option for fit patients with non-bulky N2 disease who only required lobectomy to achieve complete resection of the primary tumor.

The recent success of immunotherapy in stage III or IV NSCLC has led to a surge of interest in bringing immune checkpoint inhibitor therapy into the neoadjuvant and adjuvant settings. In the randomized phase II NEOSTAR trial, 44 patients with stage IA–IIIA NSCLC underwent neoadjuvant treatment with either nivolumab alone or nivolumab plus ipilimumab prior to surgical resection. The major and complete pathological response rates were 38% and 29%, respectively, for combination therapy and 22% and 9%, respectively, for nivolumab alone (Cascone et al. 2021).

Other trials have added chemotherapy to neoadjuvant immunotherapy to improve overall tumor response. The NADIM study was a single-arm, phase II trial that added nivolumab to neoadjuvant chemotherapy for stage IIIA NSCLC, resulting in pathological complete response in 63% of patients, and at 24 months, 77% of patients were without recurrence of disease. On the most recent update (Provencio et al. 2022), overall survival at 36 months was 81.9% (95% CI; 66.8–90.6) in the intention-to-treat population and neither tumor mutation burden nor PD-L1 expression was predictive of survival. The subsequent NADIM II trial is a randomized phase II study comparing neoadjuvant chemotherapy plus nivolumab for three cycles followed by adjuvant nivolumab versus chemotherapy alone prior to surgical resection of clinical stage IIIA NSCLC. The pathological complete response rate was 36.2% with chemo-immunotherapy and 6.8% with chemotherapy alone. With median follow-up of 22 months, the two-year progression-free rates were 67.3% and 52.6% (HR 0.56; $P = 0.117$), and overall survival rates were 85.3% and 64.8%, respectively, (HR 0.37; $P = 0.003$), both favoring chemo-immunotherapy.

CheckMate 816 is a randomized, phase III study that compared neoadjuvant chemotherapy to neoadjuvant chemotherapy plus nivolumab in 358 patients with resectable, stage IB–IIIA NSCLC (Forde et al. 2022). The early results show that neoadjuvant chemo-immunotherapy did not delay surgery compared to chemotherapy alone, but only 83% of patients receiving chemo-immunotherapy and 75% receiving chemotherapy went to surgery, a finding that should raise concerns about neoadjuvant therapy potentially jeopardizing the opportunity for curative surgery in patients with early stage NSCLC. Chemo-immunotherapy did significantly increase the pathological complete response rate (24% vs. 2.2%; $P < 0.0001$), major pathologic response rate (37% vs. 9%), and median event-free survival (31.6 vs. 20.8 months; HR 0.63; $P = 0.005$). However, on first interim analysis, overall survival did not meet criteria for significance, so we do not yet know whether these promising surrogate findings will translate into a long-term overall survival benefit. Subset analysis suggests that the most significant benefit is for patients who have stage IIIA disease and PD-L1 TPS $\geq 50\%$, so neoadjuvant chemo-immunotherapy may only be beneficial for specific patients. Nevertheless, the FDA has approved neoadjuvant nivolumab plus platinum-doublet chemotherapy for patients with resectable NSCLC.

Moreover, according to data presented during the ASCO 2023, Neotorch study showed a improvement in event-free survival for patients with resectable stage III (American Joint Committee on Cancer, 8th edition) NSCLC who were treated with toripalimab, a monoclonal antibody targeting the immune checkpoint PD-1, in combination with perioperative chemotherapy vs chemotherapy alone. Despite the promising results, however, caution is advised in interpreting the treatment-emergent adverse events and toxicity profiles, as numerically higher rates of grade 3 to 5 events were noted with the perioperative approach in the Neotorch trial compared with the CheckMate 816 trial. Lastly, new data supporting neoadjuvant pembrolizumab plus chemotherapy followed by surgery and adjuvant pembrolizumab (KEYNOTE-671) as a new treatment option for patients with resectable stage II, IIIA, or IIIB (N2) non–small cell lung cancer (NSCLC) was reported. Among patients with resectable, early-stage NSCLC, neoadjuvant pembrolizumab plus chemotherapy followed by resection and adjuvant pembrolizumab significantly improved event-free survival, major pathological response, and pathological complete response as compared with neoadjuvant chemotherapy alone followed by surgery. Overall survival did not differ significantly between the groups in this analysis.

Overall, the role of neoadjuvant therapy for NSCLC remains to be defined. For patients with clinical stage IB-II disease and negative preoperative mediastinal staging by bronchoscopy with endobronchial ultrasound biopsy and/or mediastinoscopy, we favor initial surgical resection followed by adjuvant systemic therapy for those with pathologic stage II–III disease. This approach avoids the potential for disease progression or treatment toxicity during neoadjuvant therapy that might jeopardize a curative surgical resection. It also allows for accurate pathologic staging and utilization of potentially toxic systemic therapy only in those most likely to benefit from it. For patients with resectable stage III disease who are deemed to be good surgical candidates, we favor neoadjuvant chemo-immunotherapy followed by surgical resection. Neoadjuvant chemo-radiotherapy remains another option for these patients. However, given the favorable data with definitive chemoradiotherapy followed by consolidation immunotherapy, the overall role of surgical resection in stage III disease remains controversial. Decisions regarding surgical resectability must be made prior to the initiation of treatment, because all disease needs to be amenable to safe resection prior to neoadjuvant therapy. Initiating neoadjuvant therapy with the hope of shrinking disease to make it resectable should be discouraged, because it is a strategy that very rarely succeeds.

8) What is the optimal treatment for patients with unresectable, stage III NSCLC?

Expert Perspective: The standard first-line treatment for most patients with unresectable, stage III NSCLC and good performance status is combined modality therapy involving definitive concurrent chemoradiotherapy followed by consolidation immunotherapy based on the outcomes reported from the PACIFIC trial.

Though sequential chemotherapy followed by radiotherapy can minimize overlapping toxicities, randomized, phase III trials have shown that concurrent chemoradiotherapy is superior to sequential therapy. For example, RTOG 9410 showed an improvement in five-year overall survival with use of concurrent chemoradiotherapy (10% vs. 16%, $P = 0.046$), with a higher rate of grade 3–5 acute, non-hematologic toxicity in the concurrent chemoradiotherapy arm, but with similar rates of late toxicity in both arms. The most common (and safest) chemotherapy regimens used in combination with concurrent thoracic radiotherapy are cisplatin (or carboplatin) plus etoposide, weekly carboplatin plus paclitaxel, and cisplatin (or carboplatin) plus pemetrexed (nonsquamous only). The only randomized phase III trial comparing these regimens evaluated cisplatin/etoposide versus cisplatin/pemetrexed concurrently with radiotherapy in patients with nonsquamous, stage III NSCLC and found no difference in survival but greater toxicity with cisplatin/etoposide (Senan et al. 2016). A retrospective review also demonstrated no significant difference in survival between patients with locally advanced NSCLC who were treated with either cisplatin/etoposide or weekly carboplatin/paclitaxel along with concurrent radiotherapy.

Induction chemotherapy prior to chemoradiotherapy has been evaluated in the phase III CALGB 39801 trial in which patients were randomly assigned to chemoradiotherapy alone or induction carboplatin/paclitaxel for two cycles followed by identical chemoradiotherapy. Induction chemotherapy added toxicity but no survival benefit over chemoradiotherapy alone. Therefore, induction chemotherapy prior to chemoradiotherapy is not routinely recommended. However, induction chemotherapy may be considered for patients with bulky tumors that cannot be safely encompassed in a tolerable radiation field.

Consolidation chemotherapy after chemoradiotherapy has also been evaluated. In a randomized phase III study, consolidation chemotherapy with docetaxel did not demonstrate a survival advantage after concurrent chemoradiotherapy with cisplatin/etoposide but did cause increased toxicity and treatment-related deaths. Therefore, consolidation chemotherapy is not favored after treatment with platinum/etoposide-based chemoradiotherapy. In contrast, patients who receive weekly carboplatin/paclitaxel with radiotherapy have typically been considered for consolidation chemotherapy with two to three cycles of full-dose carboplatin/paclitaxel, despite the lack of any clear evidence of benefit in clinical trials. Now, consolidation chemotherapy has largely fallen out of favor since the randomized phase III PACIFIC trial demonstrated an improvement in progression-free survival and overall survival with the addition of one year of consolidation durvalumab following concurrent chemoradiotherapy without consolidation chemotherapy in patients with unresectable, stage III NSCLC (Antonia et al. 2018). The most common concurrent chemotherapy regimens used in PACIFIC were weekly carboplatin/paclitaxel and cisplatin/etoposide, and the regimens were well balanced between the treatment arms. The most recently updated analysis demonstrated a 9.5% absolute five-year overall survival benefit with the addition of durvalumab after concurrent chemoradiotherapy (42.9% vs. 33.4%, HR 0.72 [95% CI 0.59–0.89]; median, 47.5 vs 29.1 months). The improvement in survival was noted with a tolerable toxicity profile and without compromising patient-related outcomes.

Based on these data, the currently accepted optimal treatment for eligible patients with unresectable stage III NSCLC is definitive concurrent chemoradiotherapy followed by one year of consolidation durvalumab. For patient convenience, we favor the durvalumab regimen of 1500 mg every four weeks. For concurrent chemotherapy, we favor weekly carboplatin/paclitaxel for squamous cell carcinoma and either weekly carboplatin/paclitaxel or cisplatin (or carboplatin) plus pemetrexed for adenocarcinoma, without the use of consolidation chemotherapy.

9) **What are the treatment options for patients with stage III NSCLC who are elderly or patients with ECOG performance status of ≥ 2?**

Expert Perspective: Clinical trials usually enroll younger patients with favorable ECOG performance status of 0–1. For example, the median age of patients on most lung cancer trials is 60–65 years, whereas the median age of all patients with lung cancer is 70–75 years. As such, study populations often do not reflect the patients we see in our clinics, and few clinical trials have been conducted with a more realistic patient population. In trials of concurrent chemoradiation therapy for locally advanced NSCLC, this problem is further compounded by the frequent inclusion of strict eligibility criteria regarding weight loss and pulmonary function.

In the elderly population, JCOG 0301 enrolled patients ≥ 70 years of age with unresectable stage III NSCLC and randomized them to either thoracic radiotherapy alone or in combination with concurrent low-dose daily carboplatin; patients with ECOG performance status of 0–2 were included, though only 2% of patients had performance status of 2. The addition of concurrent low-dose chemotherapy resulted in a significant improvement in overall survival compared to radiotherapy alone (median, 22.4 vs 16.9 months, $P = 0.018$). There was a higher incidence of cytopenia (22.9% grade 4 neutropenia) in the chemoradiation therapy group with a concomitant higher incidence of grade 3 infection. Treatment-related death rates were the same in the two study arms. Meta-analyses have also found that there is a benefit for concurrent chemoradiation therapy over radiotherapy alone in fit elderly patients ≥ 70 years of age. It is important to recognize that age alone should not preclude patients from being treated appropriately with concurrent chemoradiation therapy, because age and performance status are independent variables, and fitness is usually a more important indicator of therapeutic tolerance than age.

That said, it is clear to anyone caring for people with lung cancer that age does matter, and that balancing the benefits versus risks of therapy becomes even more challenging in the elderly population. The incidence of most toxicities may not be greater in elderly patients, but their resilience and ability to recover from even moderate degrees of toxicity is not the same as it is in younger patients. Cisplatin should be avoided in patients over 70 years of age due to excessive non-hematologic toxicity. Though consolidation durvalumab appears to be no more toxic in elderly patients, consolidation chemotherapy after concurrent chemoradiation is frequently fraught with excessive complications in those over 80 years of age.

For patients with locally advanced NSCLC and suboptimal performance status, consideration should be given for treatment with sequential chemotherapy followed by radiotherapy or even radiotherapy alone, either definitive or palliative. Although the previously mentioned RTOG 9410 trial comparing sequential to concurrent chemoradiation therapy enrolled only patients with good performance status, it did demonstrate that concurrent chemoradiation therapy causes more grade 3–5 non-hematologic toxicity, a problem that would only be amplified in those with worse performance status. As a rule, treatment should be tailored to the individual patient's overall situation rather than following any stage-based algorithm. For example, patients with clinically significant postobstructive pneumonia from a central lung tumor may start treatment with antibiotics and radiotherapy alone and be reevaluated on a weekly basis to determine if concurrent weekly carboplatin/paclitaxel and/or consolidation durvalumab can be added in once their clinical status improves. In severely debilitated patients, palliative care with or without radiotherapy is usually the most beneficial approach given the potential of more aggressive treatment to cause excessive complications, further impair quality of life, and shorten lifespan.

Conclusion

Numerous controversies persist in the management of patients with stage II–III NSCLC. Although adjuvant chemotherapy after surgical resection of pathologic stage II–III NSCLC is the standard-of-care, recent studies demonstrating improved short-term, disease-free survival with *EGFR* TKIs and immune checkpoint inhibitors have led to the integration of osimertinib and atezolizumab into the adjuvant treatment paradigm and raised questions regarding the optimal endpoints for adjuvant treatment trials. In contrast, recent randomized trials may have finally nailed the coffin shut on postoperative radiotherapy. The heterogeneity of stage III NSCLC has always led to confusion regarding the most appropriate level of aggressiveness in the management of individual patients. Concurrent chemoradiotherapy followed by consolidation durvalumab is now clearly the standard of care for the majority of patients with stage III NSCLC. Yet for those with presumably resectable stage III disease, the roles of surgery and neoadjuvant therapy remain cloudy, with recent promising results from trials of neoadjuvant immune checkpoint inhibitor therapy with or with chemotherapy muddying the waters even further. For the many patients with locally advanced NSCLC who are elderly or unfit, management decisions must be individualized without the benefit of high-quality clinical trial data. In this chapter, we have tried to offer guidance on how best to tailor the many useful and promising available treatment options to optimize outcomes for our individual patients.

Recommended Readings

Albain, K.S., Swann, R.S., Rusch, V.W. et al. (2009). Radiotherapy plus chemotherapy with or without surgical resection for stage III non-small-cell lung cancer: a phase III randomised controlled trial. *Lancet* 374: 379–386.

Antonia, S.J., Villegas, A., Daniel, D. et al. (2018). Overall survival with durvalumab after chemoradiotherapy in stage III NSCLC. *N Engl J Med* 379: 2342–2350.

Arriagada, R., Bergman, B., Dunant, A. et al. (2004). Cisplatin-based adjuvant chemotherapy in patients with completely resected non-small-cell lung cancer. *N Engl J Med* 350: 351–360.

Burdett, S., Parmar, M.K.B., Stewart, L.A. et al. (1998). Postoperative radiotherapy in non-small-cell lung cancer: systematic review and meta-analysis of individual patient data from nine randomised controlled trials. *Lancet* 352: 257–263.

Cascone, T., William, W., Weissferdt, A., et al. (2021). Neoadjuvant nivolumab or nivolumab plus ililimumab in operable non-small cell lung cancer: the phase 2 randomized NEOSTAR trial. *Nature Med* 27:504–514.

Douillard, J.Y., Rosell, R., De Lena, M. et al. (2006). Adjuvant vinorelbine plus cisplatin versus observation in patients with completely resected stage IB–IIIA non-small-cell lung cancer (Adjuvant Navelbine International Trialist Association [ANITA]): a randomised controlled trial. *Lancet Oncol* 7: 719–727.

Forde, P.M., Spicer, J., Lu, S., et al. (2022). Neoadjuvant nivolumab plus chemotherapy in resectable lung cancer. *N Engl J Med* 386:1973–1985.

Hui, Z., Men, Y., Hu, C. et al. (2021). Effect of postoperative radiotherapy for patients with pIIIA-N2 non-small cell lung cancer after complete resection and adjuvant chemotherapy: the phase 3 PORT-C clinical trial. *JAMA Oncol* 7: 1178–1185.

Le Pechoux, C., Pourel, N., Barlesi, F. et al. (2022). Postoperative radiotherapy versus no postoperative radiotherapy in patients with completely resected non-small cell lung cancer and proven mediastinal N2 involvement LungART: an open-label, randomized, phase 3 trial. *Lancet Oncol* 23:104-114. .

Pignon, J.P., Tribodet, H., Scagliotti, G.V. et al. (2008). Lung adjuvant cisplatin evaluation: a pooled analysis by the LACE collaborative group. *J Clin Oncol* 26: 3552–3559.

Provencio, M., Serna-Blasco, R. et al. (2022 May 16). Overall survival and biomarker analysis of neoadjuvant nivolumab plus chemotherapy in operable stage IIIA non-small-cell lung cancer (NADIM phase II trial). *J Clin Oncol* 40:2924-2933.

Senan, S., Brade, A., Wang, L.H. et al. (2016). PROCLAIM: randomized phase III trial of pemetrexed-cisplatin or etoposide-cisplatin plus thoracic radiation therapy followed by consolidation chemotherapy in locally advanced non-squamous non-small-cell lung cancer. *J Clin Oncol* 34: 953–962.

Tsuboi, M., Herbst, R.S., John, T. et al. (2023 June 4). Overall survival with osimertinib in resected EGFR-mutated NSCLC. *N Engl J Med*. doi: 10.1056/NEJMoa2304594. Epub ahead of print. PMID: 37272535.

Wakelee, H.A., Altorki, N.K., Zhou, C. et al. (2021). IMpower010: primary results of a phase III global study of atezolizumab versus best supportive care after adjuvant chemotherapy in resected stage IB–IIIA non-small cell lung cancer. *J Clin Oncol* 39 (15 Suppl.): abstract8500.

Wakelee, H., Liberman, M., Kato, T. et al. (2023 June 3). Perioperative pembrolizumab for early-stage non-small-cell lung cancer. *N Engl J Med*. doi: 10.1056/NEJMoa2302983. Epub ahead of print. PMID: 37272513.

Winton, T., Livingston, R., Johnson, D. et al. (2005). Vinorelbine plus cisplatin vs. observation in resected non-small-cell lung cancer. *N Engl J Med* 352: 2589–2597.

7

Recurrent and Metastatic Non-Small Cell Lung Cancer

Julia Judd, J. Nicholas Bodor, and Hossein Borghaei

Department of Hematology/Oncology, Fox Chase Cancer Center Philadelphia, PA, USA

Introduction

Lung cancer remains the leading cause of cancer related deaths worldwide. In the United States, there were an estimated 235,760 new lung cancer cases and 131,880 lung cancer–related deaths in 2021. Unfortunately, most lung cancer patients are deemed incurable with advanced disease at diagnosis. The number of new lung cancer cases and lung cancer–related deaths continues to decrease each year due to improved smoking cessation rates and implementation of lung cancer screening programs as well as substantial therapeutic advances.

Immunotherapy has revolutionized treatment for patients with recurrent and metastatic NSCLC without actionable mutations. There are several considerations when determining the best front-line therapy. First, broad panel-based molecular testing (NGS) must be performed on tumor tissue. Tumor analysis can be complimented with more timely peripheral blood analysis, while awaiting the tissue-based analysis, or performed on peripheral blood alone if tumor tissue is inadequate. Ideally, molecular testing should be performed prior to initiation of first-line therapy as the identification of a driver alteration would substantially change first-line therapy recommendations. This might be more relevant to the non-squamous histology but should be considered in all cases. Also, there are safety concerns when administering tyrosine kinase inhibitors (TKIs) after immunotherapy. In addition, PD-L1 expression biomarker testing is standard of care and guides therapeutic decisions. Furthermore, assessment of the patient's disease-related symptoms, comorbid conditions, and performance status all need to be performed. Here, we have highlighted the standard treatment options as well as the nuances we consider in our therapeutic decision-making.

Case Study 1

A 64-year-old man, with a 40-pack-year smoking history, who quit five years ago, presents with chest pain and dyspnea. During his work-up, a chest X-ray reveals a right lung mass. CT and PET scans reveal a right lower lobe mass, mediastinal and hilar adenopathy, and hepatic lesions concerning for metastases. CT-guided biopsy of one of the hepatic lesions reveals non-small cell lung cancer (NSCLC), adenocarcinoma histology. MRI of the brain is negative for metastases. The PD-L1 tumor proportion score (TPS) is 50%.

Cancer Consult: Expertise in Clinical Practice, Volume 1: Solid Tumors & Supportive Care,
Second Edition. Edited by Syed A. Abutalib, Maurie Markman, Al B. Benson III, and Hope S. Rugo.
© 2024 John Wiley & Sons Ltd. Published 2024 by John Wiley & Sons Ltd.

1) **Which patients with stage IV NSCLC should receive molecular testing on their tumors?**

Expert Perspective: All patients with stage IV NSCLC, regardless of histology, should have broad, next-generation sequencing panel molecular testing, which includes testing for *EGFR* mutations, *ALK, ROS-1, RET* rearrangements, *MET* exon 14 skipping mutations, *BRAF* V600E mutations, *KRAS* G12C mutations, *NTRK1/2/3* gene fusions, and *HER2* mutations or amplification. This is especially important for never or light smokers and all adenocarcinoma patients. However, it is also important to consider in all squamous cell carcinoma. Although driver mutations are less frequent in squamous cell lung cancers (~4%), it is important to never miss the opportunity to treat with a targeted therapy, which is often well tolerated and very efficacious.

Our patient's NGS profile: The tumor is negative for *EGFR* mutations, *ALK, ROS-1* or *RET* rearrangements, *MET* exon 14 skipping mutation, *BRAF* V600E mutation, or *NTRK1/2/3* gene fusion.

2) **What is the preferred first-line therapy for patients with NSCLC, adenocarcinoma histology, without driver mutations and with PD-L1 of 50% or greater (PD-L1 high)?**

Expert Perspective: The NCCN guidelines includes several standard of care regimens, including checkpoint inhibitor monotherapy, chemo-immunotherapy, and combination immunotherapy with category 1 evidence, which could be considered in this scenario. There are no currently published, randomized clinical trials that directly compare these options. Therefore, the decision of the best personalized therapy is based on both patient and tumor factors as well as the toxicity profile of the regimen. Considerations for the individual patient include the degree of disease-related symptoms, comorbid conditions, and quality of life preferences. Tumor characteristics to consider are the histology, magnitude of PD-L1 expression, and, to a lesser extent currently, the genomic profile (Figure 7.1).

The combination of chemotherapy and immunotherapy should be considered for patients with significant disease related symptoms, visceral crisis, or clinical deterioration. Response rates with chemo-immunotherapy are approximately 60%, compared with approximately 40–45% with checkpoint inhibitor monotherapy, in patients with a PD-L1 TPS ≥50% (Table 7.1). The objective response rate with pembrolizumab and chemotherapy was 62.1% in patients with nonsquamous histology included in the phase III trial KEYNOTE-189 and 60.3% in patients with squamous histology included in the phase III trial KEYNOTE-407. Similar results are seen with atezolizumab combined with chemotherapy in the phase III trial IMpower-131, which included patients with squamous cell histology, but the objective response rate for the phase III trial IMpower-130 (patients with nonsquamous NSCLC) was not reported. Most recently, improved response rates were demonstrated with chemotherapy in combination with cemiplimab (43.3%) compared to chemotherapy with placebo (22.7%) in the phase III trial EMPOWER-Lung 3, which included patients with advanced NSCLC. The response rate in the PD-L1 ≥50% subgroup treated with cemiplimab plus chemotherapy was 53.4%. These rates are higher than those seen with pembrolizumab monotherapy in phase III trials KEYNOTE-024 (44.8%) and KEYNOTE-042 (39%) as well as atezolizumab monotherapy in IMPower-110 (38.3%) and cemiplimab monotherapy in EMPOWER-Lung-1 (39%). The difference in response rates is clinically significant because many patients with advanced NSCLC do not receive second-line therapy due to clinical deterioration.

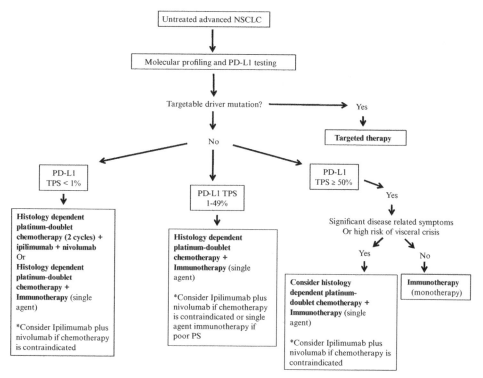

Figure 7.1 NSCLC first-line treatment algorithm.

The median overall survival (mOS) was significantly improved with either chemo-immunotherapy (22 months for nonsquamous patients in KEYNOTE-189 and 15.9 months for squamous patients in KEYNOTE-407) or immunotherapy alone (30 months in KEYNOTE-024 and 20 months in KEYNOTE-042) in this PD-L1 high patient population compared to approximately 12 months with platinum doublet chemotherapy. Of note, different PD-L1 assays were employed with TPS used in the KEYNOTE and EMPOWER-Lung-1 trials, and TC3 plus IC3 was used in the IMpower trials. The combination of chemotherapy with immunotherapy increases the likelihood of treatment response and early clinical benefit for those patients who need the most effective treatment upfront, because they may not survive to receive platinum-doublet chemotherapy in the second line. In addition, it is thought that chemotherapy enhances antitumor immunity. Therefore, the hope is that this combination incites not only a more rapid treatment response but also a durable immunologic response, which translates into long-term survival.

A meta-analysis used indirect comparison of numerous KEYNOTE trials to evaluate the efficacy of pembrolizumab with or without chemotherapy in patients with PD-L1 high advanced NSCLC. While there was only a nonsignificant trend toward improved mOS (HR 0.76, 95% CI 0.51, 1.14; P = 0.184), the ORR (relative risk of 1.62, 95% CI 1.18–2.2.23; P = 0.003) as well as the median progression-free survival (mPFS; HR 0.55, 95% CI 0.51–1.14; P = 0.037) were significantly improved with chemo-immunotherapy compared to pembrolizumab monotherapy. This supports the strategy to offer the regimen with the highest response rate upfront in patients with significant disease related symptoms.

Table 7.1 Summary of trial data in patients with advanced NSCLC and high PD-L1 expression (≥ 50%) vs ITT population.

Study	N PD-L1 high/N ITT	RR%	mPFS months (HR)	mOS months (HR)	P value	ITTmPFS months (HR)	ITTmOS months (HR)	ITTP value
KEYNOTE 024 (P)	305/305	44.8	10.3 (0.5)	30 (0.63)	0.002	NA	NA	NA
KEYNOTE 042 (P) PD-L1 TPS ≧ 50% subgroup	299/1274	39	7.1 (0.81)*	20 (0.69)	0.0003	6.5 vs 5.4 (1.07)	16.7 vs 12.1 (0.81)	0.0018
IMpower 110 (A) TC3 ≧ 50% or IC3 ≧ 10% subgroup	205/572	38.3	8.1 (0.63)	20.2 (0.59)	0.0106	5.7 vs 5.5 (0.77)	17.5 vs 14.1 (0.83)	0.1481
KEYNOTE 189 (P + chemo) PD-L1 TPS ≧ 50% subgroup	202/616	62.1	11.1 (0.36)	Not Reached (0.59)	NR	8.8 vs 4.9 (0.52)	22 vs 10.7 (0.56)	<0.00001
KEYNOTE 407 (P + chemo) PD-L1 TPS ≧ 50% subgroup	146/559	60.3	8.0 (0.37)	Not Reached (0.64)	NR	6.4 vs 4.8 (0.56)	15.9 vs 11.3 (0.64)	<0.001
Impower 130 (A + chemo) TC3 ≧ 50% or IC3 ≧ 10% subgroup	134/723	NR	6.4 (0.51)	17.3 (0.84)	NR	7 vs 5.5 (0.64)	18.6 vs 13.9 (0.79)	0.033
Impower 131 (A + chemo) TC3 ≧ 50% or IC3 ≧ 10% subgroup	154/1021	60.0	10.1 (0.44)	23.4 (0.48)	NR	6.3 vs 5.6 (0.71)	14.2 vs 13.5 (0.88)	0.1581

P, pembrolizumab; P + chemo, pembrolizumab + platinum-doublet chemotherapy; A, atezolizumab; A + chemo, atezolizumab + platinum-doublet chemotherapy; ITT, intention to treat population; NA, not applicable; NR, not reported; RR, response rate; mPFS, median progression-free survival; mOS, median overall survival; TC, tumor cells; IC, immune cells; HR, hazard ration; TPS, tumor proportion score.
* Not statistically significant.
Source: Adapted from Judd, J., Borghaei, H. First-line treatment of patients with advanced NSCLC and high PD-L1 expression: immunotherapy with or without chemotherapy? ASCO Daily News. https://dailynews.ascopubs.org/do/10.1200/ADN.20.200054/full. Published 20 February 2020.

However, the toxicity profiles need to be considered in the context of the individual patient's comorbid conditions, performance status and quality of life preferences. The use of chemotherapy inherently makes a regimen more toxic. If chemotherapy is deployed, treatment-related grade 3–5 adverse events are more frequent than with checkpoint inhibitor monotherapy as seen in the KEYNOTE-024 (31.2% vs 53.3%) and KEYNOTE-042 (18% vs 41%) trials. In addition, these rates are similar whether chemo-immunotherapy or chemotherapy alone is deployed, as observed in KEYNOTE-189 (67.2% vs 65.8%) and KEYNOTE-407 (69.0% vs 68.2%). Furthermore, the rate of grade 3–5 adverse events resulting in treatment discontinuation was doubled with chemo-immunotherapy (approximately 12%) compared with immunotherapy alone (approximately 6–7%). However, the rates of grade 3–5 immune-related adverse events did not increase with the addition of chemotherapy, based on cross-trial comparison in pembrolizumab monotherapy groups (13.2% in KEYNOTE-024 and 8.0% in the KEYNOTE-042) compared to the pembrolizumab plus chemotherapy groups (8.9% in KEYNOTE-189 and 10.8% in the KEYNOTE-407).

Furthermore, the magnitude of PD-L1 expression has been shown to correlate with response rate and survival outcomes based on a retrospective analysis. Patients with PD-L1 TPS of 90–100%, compared with 50–89%, had higher objective response rate (60.0% vs 32.7%), longer mPFS (14.5 vs 4.1 months), and longer mOS (not reached because survival was greater than 50% at last time point vs 15.9 months). However, there is intratumoral heterogeneity of PD-L1 expression that makes this biomarker an imperfect tool. Likewise, there is evidence that tumor genomics may contribute to the discrepancy in outcomes with immunotherapy. Studies have suggested a lack of benefit with pembrolizumab added to platinum doublet in patients with lung adenocarcinoma harboring *STK11* and/or *KEAP1* alterations.

In summary, our group feels the use of single-agent immunotherapy in the group of patients with tumors expressing PD-L1 ≥50% is appropriate. The decision to add chemotherapy in this setting should be made on an individual patient basis. There are three single agents approved in this setting: pembrolizumab, atezolizumab and cemiplimab. Given the consistency in the data, we believe use of any of these agents is suitable.

3) Is there additional benefit of employing dual immunotherapy compared with single-agent immunotherapy in patients with tumors harboring high PD-L1 expression?

Expert Perspective: We do not have complete data directly comparing the potential superiority of dual immunotherapy to checkpoint inhibitor monotherapy in PD-L1 high population in first-line space.

- A phase III trial KEYNOTE-598 sought to evaluate this question by randomizing patients to pembrolizumab plus either ipilimumab or placebo. However, this study was stopped for futility at the time of the first protocol-specified interim analysis with a median study follow up of 20.6 months (range of 12.4–31.7 months). At that time point, the addition of ipilimumab to pembrolizumab did not improve efficacy and increased toxicity compared with the placebo group. There was no significant difference in mOS (21.4 vs 21.9 months), mPFS (8.2 vs 8.4 months), objective response rate (ORR; 45.4% vs 45.4%), or duration of response (16.1 vs 17.3 months). The incidence of grade 3 or higher adverse events was 62.4% with immunotherapy combination compared with 50.2% with pembrolizumab plus placebo. Importantly, this trial may have been discontinued too early to see the magnitude of benefit with combination immunotherapy over monotherapy.

- Long-term follow-up of patients receiving ipilimumab plus nivolumab compared with chemotherapy on the phase III trial CheckMate-227 has demonstrated that the degree of survival advantage with this combination increased at later time points (one-year OS rates in intent to treat population 62% vs 54%; four-year OS rates in the PD-L1 ⩾1% population 29% vs 18% and in the PD-L1 <1% population 24% vs 10%) with a median duration of response of 23.2 months (compared to 6.2 months with chemotherapy). Furthermore, in an exploratory analysis of the PD-L1 high subgroup, the four-year survival rates were 37% (ipilimumab plus nivolumab), 26% (nivolumab alone arm which was not powered for comparison), and 20% (chemotherapy), demonstrating substantial and durable benefit in this population. Ultimately, the authors here would not prefer combination immunotherapy in patients with PD-L1 ⩾ 50% because we have substantial data demonstrating better tolerability with durable survival benefit with single-agent PD-1/PD-L1 inhibition.

In summary, we would favor single-agent immunotherapy in patients with high PD-L1 expression. However, if the patient had significant disease-related symptoms but was otherwise fit, we would employ chemo-immunotherapy.

4) What would be the preferred systemic treatment if his tumor had PD-L1 expression of 1–49%?

Expert Perspective: In our view, pembrolizumab plus histology-dependent platinum-based doublet chemotherapy would be preferred. In this case, we would use carboplatin and pemetrexed for adenocarcinoma histology based on the KEYNOTE-189 trial. Pembrolizumab monotherapy is approved in this subset of patients based on results from KEYNOTE-042, which included advanced NSCLC patients with PD-L1 ⩾1%. However, for the subgroup of patients with PD-L1 expression of 1–49%, there was no significant difference in OS compared with chemotherapy (median OS 13.4 vs 12.1 months; HR 0.92, 95% CI 0.77–1.11). The survival benefit observed in the intent to treat population (mOS 16.7 vs 12.1 months, HR 0.81) was likely driven by those with TPS ⩾ 50% (mOS 20 months, HR 0.69), which comprised nearly half of this cohort. Similarly, there was a PFS improvement for patients with TPS ⩾ 50% (7.1 vs 6.4 months, HR 0.81) but there was no PFS benefit in patients with TPS ⩾ 20% or TPS ⩾ 1% (Table 7.2).

Conversely, trials utilizing either pembrolizumab (KEYNOTE-189 and KEYNOTE-407), atezolizumab (IMpower 130) or cemiplimab (EMPOWER-Lung 3) combined with platinum doublet chemotherapy demonstrated a significant survival benefit over chemotherapy, regardless of PD-L1 expression (Table 7.3). The two-year survival data in patients with nonsquamous histology treated on KEYNOTE-189 showed a significant and similar OS benefit in patients with a PD-L1 TPS <1% (HR 0.52), TPS 1–49% (HR 0.62), and TPS ⩾50% (HR 0.59; Figure 7.2). By cross-trial comparison, response rates in the intent to treat population with chemoimmunotherapy were higher (57.9% in KEYNOTE-407, 47.6% in KEYNOTE-189, 49.2% in IMpower 130) regardless of PD-L1 expression compared with checkpoint inhibitor monotherapy trials with PD-L1 expression ⩾1% (in KEYNOTE-042, the ORR was 27%, the same with pembrolizumab or chemotherapy; in IMpower 110, the objective response rate was 38.3% with atezolizumab). However, for patients with a poor performance status (ECOG performance status 2) who may not tolerate chemotherapy, pembrolizumab monotherapy remains a reasonable option. One must note that these patients were not included in the KEYNOTE-042 trial.

Currently, we do not have data from randomized trials directly comparing immunotherapy with or without chemotherapy. The most effective sequence of these therapies is being studied in ongoing trials (NCT03793179 and NCT04166487) in patients with tumors expressing PD-L1.

In addition, ipilimumab plus nivolumab can be considered as another option in this patient population, particularly if a patient's comorbid conditions preclude chemotherapy use. In the phase III trial CheckMate-227, Ipilimumab plus nivolumab improved OS over chemotherapy regardless of PD-L1 expression (17.1 vs 13.9 months, HR 0.73), including patients with TPS <1% (17.2 vs 12.2 months, HR 0.62). Although the response rate was modestly higher than chemotherapy (35.9% vs 30.0%), the median duration of response was quite robust (23.2 months vs 6.2 months). Currently, we do not have effective biomarkers to guide the use of this combination. Based on current data, patients who appear to benefit most are those with low PD-L1 expression but high tumor mutational burden.

5) **Are there additional considerations if this patient had radiation treated or asymptomatic brain metastases?**

Expert Perspective: There was an unplanned exploratory analysis of CheckMate-227 demonstrating at least equivalent activity of ipilimumab plus nivolumab compared to chemotherapy in the front-line setting in patients with or without baseline brain metastases (treated or stable). The median OS in patients with baseline brain metastasis (median OS 17.4 months, HR 0.60, CI 0.40–0.89) and without brain metastases (median OS 17.1 months, HR 0.77, CI 0.67–0.89) was superior in patients treated with ipilimumab plus nivolumab compared with chemotherapy (median OS approximately 14 months in both groups). Furthermore, the survival benefit with ipilimumab plus nivolumab is durable with a three-year survival rate of 30%, regardless of baseline brain metastasis. This reinforces what is understood in patients with melanoma, for which more prospective data is available than in NSCLC, showing clinically meaningful efficacy with ipilimumab plus nivolumab for intracranial metastasis.

6) **What would be the preferred systemic treatment if his cancer were PD-L1 negative?**

Expert Perspective: There are two good options here, in our opinion, for patients with PD-L1 expression <1%. One is two cycles of histology-based, platinum-doublet chemotherapy combined with ipilimumab plus nivolumab, which can be considered based on results of the CheckMate-9LA trial and what we have learned from prior trials. CheckMate-9LA was designed with the aim of combining the rapid initial disease control, which may be achieved by deploying a short course of chemotherapy, with the durable response and long-term survival observed with ipilimumab plus nivolumab in melanoma patients (at the time the trial was designed) and now in some NSCLC patients (CheckMate-227). The comparator arm was platinum-doublet chemotherapy.

Most recently, a similar regimen of tremelimumab plus durvalumab and chemotherapy for up to four cycles followed by durvalumab maintenance with one additional dose of tremelimumab at week 16/cycle 6 was approved based on the POSEIDON study. This combination, compared to the CheckMate-9LA regimen, contains a longer course of chemotherapy (4 cycles compared to 2 cycles) but a shorter course of CTLA-4 inhibition (5 doses). This regimen also demonstrated benefit in patients with PD-L1 <1%.

Table 7.2 The benefit of I-O monotherapy is established in NSCLC with high PD-L1 expression, but needs remain for PD-L1 low expressors.

Trial	Treatment	PD-L1	ORR	Median PFS (months)	Median OS (months)
Outcomes in NSCLC with high PD-L1 expression					
KEYNOTE-024[1,2]	Pembrolizumab (n = 154)	≥50%	44.8%	10.3	30
IMpower110[3]	Atezolizumab (n = 107)	TC3; IC3	38.3%	8.1	20.2
EMPOWER-Lung 1[4,5]	Cemiplimab (n = 283)	≥50%	39.2%	8.2	NR
Outcomes in NSCLC with lower or unselected PD-L1 expression					
CheckMate 026[6]	Nivolumab (n = 211)	≥5%	26%	4.2	14.4
CheckMate 017[7]	Nivolumab (n = 135)	Any	20%	3.5	9.2
CheckMate 057[8]	Nivolumab (n = 292)	Any	19%	2.3	12.2
KEYNOTE-042[9]	Pembrolizumab (n = 637)	≥1%	27%	6.5	16.7
IMpower110[3]	Atezolizumab (n = 277)	TC1/2/3 IC1/2/3	29%	5.7	17.5
OAK[10]	Atezolizumab (n = 425)	Any	15%	2.8	13.8
POPLAR[11]	Atezolizumab (n = 144)	Any	15%	2.7	12.6

C = tumor-infiltrating immune cell; I-O = immuno-oncology; NR = not reported; NSCLC = non-small cell lung cancer; ORR = objective response rate; OS = overall survival; PD-L1 = programmed cell death-ligand 1; PFS = progression-free survival; TC = tumor cell.
[1] Reck, M. et al. (2016). *N Engl J Med* 375:1823–1833; [2] Reck, M. et al. (2019). *J Clin Oncol.* 37:537–546; [3] Spigel, D. et al. (2019). ESMO. Abstract 6256. 5; [4] Sezer, A. et al. (2020). ESMO. Abstract LBA52; [5] Sezer, A. et al. (2021). *Lancet* 397:592–604; [6] Carbone, D.P. et al. (2017). *N Engl J Med.* 376:2415–2426; [7] Brahmer, J. et al. (2015). *N Engl J Med* 373:123–135; [8] Borghaei, H. et al. (2015). *N Engl J Med* 373:1627–1639; [9] Mok, T.S.K. et al. (2019). *Lancet* 393:1819–1830; [10] Fehrenbacher, L. et al. (2018). *J Thorac Oncol* 13:1156–1170; [11] Fehrenbacher, L. et al. (2016). *Lancet* 387:1837–1846.

Table 7.3 Major trial data combining chemotherapy with immunotherapy in NSCLC.

Name	Description	ORR	mPFS (months)	mOS (months)	HR for OS
Nonsquamous cell					
KeyNote 189	Pembrolizumab + chemotherapy vs chemotherapy	48% vs 19%	8.8 vs 4.9	22.0 vs 10.7 $P < 0.00001$	0.56
IMpower 150	Atezolizumab + chemotherapy/bevacizumab vs chemotherapy/bevacizumab	64% vs 48%	8.3 vs 6.8	19.2 vs 14.7 $P = 0.02$	0.78
IMpower 130	Atezolizumab + chemotherapy vs chemotherapy	49% vs 32%	7.0 vs 5.5	18.6 vs 13.9 $P = 0.033$	0.79
Squamous cell					
KeyNote 407	Pembrolizumab + chemotherapy vs chemotherapy	58% vs 38%	6.4 vs 4.8	15.9 vs 11.3 $P < 0.001$	0.64
IMpower 131	Atezolizumab + chemotherapy vs chemotherapy	59% vs 51%	6.3 vs 5.6	14.0 vs 13.9 $P = 0.6931$	0.96

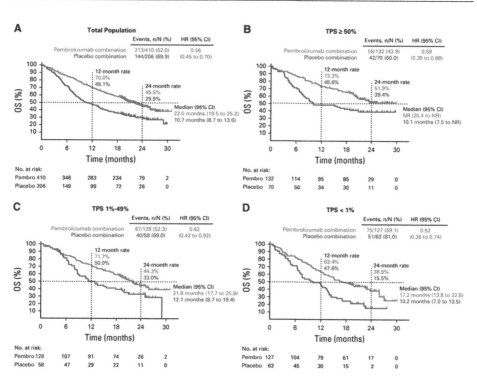

Figure 7.2 Kaplan-Meier analysis of overall survival (OS) in the (A) overall intention-to-treat population and in subsets of patients by tumor proportion score (TPS): (B) ≥ 50%, (C) 1–49%, and (D) <1%. HR, hazard ratio; NR, not reached; pembro, pembrolizumab. *Source:* Published in Gadgeel, S., Rodríguez-Abreu, D., Giovanna Speranza, E.E. et al. (2020). Updated analysis from KEYNOTE-189: Pembrolizumab or placebo plus pemetrexed and platinum for previously untreated metastatic nonsquamous non-small-cell lung cancer. *Clin Oncol* 38:1505–1517. doi:10.1200/JCO.19.03136. Copyright © 2020 American Society of Clinical Oncology.

The magnitude of survival benefit at two years with this regimen was consistent across all PD-L1 subgroups, including the PD-L1 negative population. The HR for death in PD-L1 <1%, ≥1%, 1–49%, and ≥50% were 0.62, 0.64, 0.61, and 0.66, respectively. Prior to approval of the CheckMate-9LA regimen, platinum-doublet chemotherapy plus a PD-1/PD-L1 inhibitor was approved regardless of PD-L1 expression in advanced NSCLC based on the results from KEYNOTE-189, KEYNOTE-407, and IMpower-130. Interestingly, based on subgroup analysis, the clinical activity may be lower when employing these regimens for patients with PD-L1 <1%, compared with subgroups with higher PD-L1 expression or the entire intent to treat population. This was the case with initial follow-up in KEYNOTE-189; however, with longer follow-up, the difference in survival between PD-L1 subgroups dissipated in this trial. The survival discrepancy did persist in patients with squamous cell histology on KEYNOTE-407, where the PD-L1 negative subgroup appears to have inferior survival (PD-L1 negative HR 0.79, CI 0.56–1.11, compared with PD-L1 positive HR 0.67, CI 0.51–0.87). Furthermore, by cross-trial comparison, the addition of a short course of chemotherapy to ipilimumab plus nivolumab overcame the initial inversion of the Kaplan-Meier survival curves followed by crossing of the curves after 6 months of treatment observed with dual immunotherapy (CheckMate-227; Figure 7.3) or pembrolizumab monotherapy (KEYNOTE-042). This implies that there is a patient subgroup that clearly benefits from a short course of platinum-doublet chemotherapy, and PD-L1 negative patients are included in this group. In addition, the toxicities commonly associated with chemotherapy were less frequent with fewer cycles of chemotherapy delivered in CheckMate-9LA. Unfortunately, due to the rapidly changing landscape of lung cancer treatment, the comparator arm in this study was chemotherapy alone rather than the current standard, chemotherapy plus pembrolizumab or atezolizumab. Therefore, we are unable to directly compare which regimen is superior in this patient population. However, this approval does provide another effective treatment option for these patients.

If it was felt that a patient could not tolerate chemotherapy due to organ dysfunction, one should consider ipilimumab plus nivolumab based on an exploratory analysis of patients with PD-L1 <1% expression in CheckMate-227. In this subgroup, more than twice as many patients were alive at four years compared with those who received chemotherapy (24% vs 10%, HR 0.64) and had a numerically superior survival to the nivolumab plus chemotherapy group (13%).

7) **Are there additional treatment considerations if this patient was a never or light smoker with negative comprehensive molecular testing?**

Expert Perspective: It is generally hypothesized that smoking increases tumor neoantigen load, enhancing tumor specific immunity, leading to superior benefit with immune checkpoint inhibitor therapy. An association has been demonstrated between tobacco smoking and improved outcomes in patients with NSCLC treated with immune checkpoint inhibitors, regardless of PD-L1 expression and in different lines of therapy. There have been several challenges with evaluating this theory clinically, including small numbers of never-smokers in phase III trials, variability of definitions for degree of smoking, variability in TMB analysis, and TMB high cutoff, as well as inherent recall and reporting bias.

In the phase I KEYNOTE-001 trial, for which we have long-term follow-up, current/former smokers had improved objective response rate and survival with pembrolizumab monotherapy. Subsequently, a subgroup analysis of the KEYNOTE-024 trial, in which patients with high PD-L1 expression were treated with pembrolizumab monotherapy compared with standard chemotherapy, demonstrated greater OS benefit in former smokers (HR for death 0.59) compared with never smokers (HR 0.90). However, the number of never smokers was quite small (n = 24) compared to former smokers (n = 216) in the overall population (n = 305), creating a large confidence interval crossing 1. A similar trend is seen with dual immunotherapy. A subgroup analysis of CheckMate-227 suggests that ipilimumab plus nivolumab may be inferior to chemotherapy in never-smokers with a HR for death of 1.23 favoring chemotherapy but with a large confidence interval crossing 1 (0.76–1.98). This is compared to current or former smokers with a HR for death of 0.77 (CI 0.64–0.92). Conversely, this pattern was not seen with the addition of chemotherapy to pembrolizumab in KEYNOTE-189; OS subgroup analysis shows significant survival benefit in both never-smokers (HR 0.23, CI 0.10–0.54) and current or former smokers (HR 0.54, CI 0.41–0.71). Similar to patients with PD-L1 expression of <1%, chemotherapy likely generates a more rapid cytotoxic response in never smokers and also augments antitumor immunity. Interestingly, this same pattern was not seen in the CheckMate-9LA never-smoker subgroup. In this study, the hazard ratio favored chemotherapy alone with a large confidence interval crossing 1, but due to the small number of patients in this subgroup, these results are difficult to interpret. Nevertheless, smoking status should be considered in the decision-making process for first line treatment, particularly in patients with a PD-L1TPS ≥50%, when otherwise, single-agent immunotherapy may be favored, based on the clinical scenario.

8) **Would this patient's treatment recommendation change if he had a *KRAS G12C* mutation?**

Expert Perspective: Front-line treatment recommendations would not change based on currently available data. Sotorasib has received accelerated approval in previously treated NSCLC patients with a *KRAS G12C* mutation, based on the efficacy and tolerability demonstrated in the CodeBreaK-100 trial. Of note, this was a heavily pretreated patient population; the median number of prior systemic anticancer therapies for metastatic disease was 2. As of the 15 March 2021 data cutoff, the objective response rate was 37.1% with a median duration of response of 11.1 months, a mPFS of 6.8

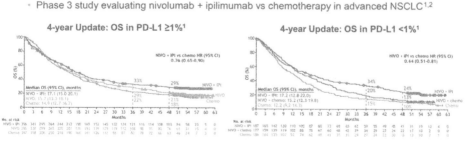

Figure 7.3 CheckMate 227: NIVO + IPI achieved clinically meaningful OS improvement regardless of PD-L1 status. Chemo = chemotherapy; CI = confidence interval; HR = hazard ratio; IPI = ipilimumab; NIVO = nivolumab; NSCLC = non-small cell lung cancer; OS = overall survival; PD-L1 = programmed death-ligand 1; TMB = tumor mutational burden. *Source:* 1. Paz-Ares, L.G. et al. ASCO 2021. Poster 9016; 2. Peters, S. et al. *Ann Oncol.* 2019;30(Suppl. 5):v913–v914.

months, and a median OS of 12.5 months. Adagrasib also received accelerated FDA approval in this setting based on the results of the single arm, KRYSTAL-1 trial. Similar outcomes were seen in this trial compared to CodeBreak-100 with a slighter higher response rate of 42.9%. Previously treated and stable brain metastasis demonstrated an intracranial response rate of 13%. Based on this data, sotorasib or adagrasib would be recommended in the second line over docetaxel ± ramucirumab.

Case Study 2

A 58-year-old woman with a 10-pack-per-year history of smoking presents to her primary care physician with a two-week history of hemoptysis. A chest X-ray reveals a left hilar mass. She undergoes a bronchoscopy with biopsy of the mass, which reveals a squamous NSCLC. CT and PET scans reveal metastases to bone and liver. MRI of the brain is negative for metastases. PD-L1 is <1%.

9) Should molecular testing be performed in this patient?

Expert Perspective: Molecular testing should be considered in all patients with stage IV squamous cell lung cancer and should absolutely be performed in those patients who are light (<10 packs per year) or never-smokers.

10) What is the preferred first-line therapy for patients with squamous cell NSCLC and PD-L1 <1%?

Expert Perspective: In the absence of randomized trials, this is difficult to answer without a bias toward one or the other regimen. Our group would prefer a combination of chemotherapy and immunotherapy in this case. The CheckMate-9LA regimen with platinum-doublet chemotherapy plus dual immunotherapy should be highly considered, based on the patient's performance status and comorbidities. This regimen showed similar efficacy regardless of PD-L1 expression, and unlike the chemoimmunotherapy regimen with single agent immunotherapy (Carboplatin/Paclitaxel + pembrolizumab in KEYNOTE-407), there was no suggestion of inferior efficacy for the PD-L1 negative subgroup. In addition, subgroup analysis from CheckMate-9LA demonstrates similar efficacy regardless of histology, which is not the case (by cross-trial comparison) of patients with squamous cell NSLCLC in KEYNOTE-407 compared with patients with nonsquamous NSCLC in KEYNOTE-189 (Figure 7.4). The HR for death for the squamous cell subgroup in CheckMate-9LA was 0.62 (CI 0.45–0.86) compared with the nonsquamous subgroup 0.69 (CI 0.55–0.87). This echoes the subgroup analysis of CheckMate-227, suggesting greater survival benefit for patients with squamous cell (HR 0.69; CI 0.53–0.92) compared with non-squamous histology (HR 0.85; CI 0.69–1.04) with dual immunotherapy. Therefore, a combination of chemotherapy and dual immunotherapy may be ideal for patients with squamous cell NSCLC with PD-L1 expression of <1%. However, this is based on cross-trial comparison. Of note, the tremelimumab plus durvalumab and chemotherapy regimen (POSEIDON trial) showed a more prominent PFS and OS benefit over chemotherapy alone in patients with nonsquamous, rather than squamous, histology. This may be due to the high rate of gemcitabine-platinum doublet employed in this study compared to patients with squamous cell histology in

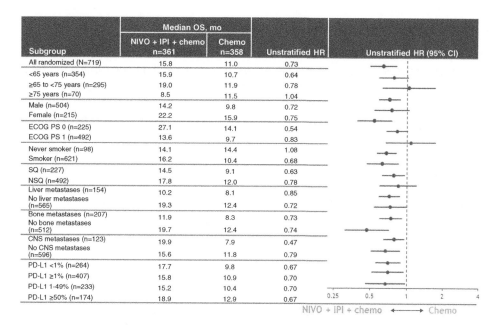

Figure 7.4 CheckMate 9LA: NIVO + IPI + chemo improved OS regardless of PD-L1 level, histology, and CNS metastases. Chemo = chemotherapy; CI = confidence interval; CNS = central nervous system; ECOG PS = Eastern Cooperative Oncology Group performance status; HR = hazard ratio; IPI = ipilimumab; NIVO = nivolumab; NSQ = nonsquamous; OS = overall survival; PD-L1 = programmed death-ligand 1; SQ = squamous. *Source:* Reck M et al. ASCO 2021. Oral presentation 9000.

the CheckMate-9LA trial who received paclitaxel-platinum. Currently, there are no prospective trials comparing pembrolizumab plus histology-dependent platinum-based chemotherapy to dual immunotherapy plus platinum-doublet chemotherapy. Therefore, the options are chemo plus dual immunotherapy or chemo plus single immunotherapy. As a side note, use of palliative radiation for patients who present with hemoptysis should be considered. This case would benefit from a multidisciplinary tumor board discussion.

Case Study 3

A 52-year-old woman with no prior smoking history presents with a dry cough and back pain for the last three months. She takes daily three-mile walks for exercise, although she admits to now having to walk slower to not get short of breath. A CT scan reveals a moderate sized left pleural effusion along with bilateral mediastinal lymphadenopathy and multiple lesions in her thoracic and lumbar vertebrae. A thoracentesis is performed, and 1,000 mL of serosanguineous pleural fluid is drained, with cytology results consistent with adenocarcinoma of the lung. PD-L1 expression assessed via immunohistochemistry reveals a tumor proportion score of 80%, however additional molecular testing was not performed. A brain MRI is performed, which is negative for metastatic disease.

11) What is the next best step in the care of this patient?

Expert Perspective: Obtaining comprehensive molecular testing is the next best step in the care of this patient. A thorough evaluation for the presence of an oncogene alteration in tumors from patients with NSCLC is of the utmost importance. This is especially true for patients who are never-smokers because approximately two-thirds of such patients have tumors that harbor such targetable mutations. An alteration in *EGFR* is the most frequent and is present in approximately 50% of NSCLC tumors from never-smokers. The next most common alteration found is in ALK, which are identified in up to 20% of NSCLC cases from never-smokers. Tissue-based testing is the gold-standard and ideally would include a comprehensive panel evaluating for *EGFR, ALK, ROS1, BRAF V600E, MET, RET, NTRK, HER2, and KRAS* gene alterations. Each of these listed tumor oncogenes now have one or more FDA-approved targeted therapies available listed below (refer to FDA label for precise indication[s]).

- **EGFR** tyrosine kinase inhibitors include osimertinib, erlotinib, gefitinib, and afatinib
- **ALK** inhibitors include crizotinib, ceritinib, alectinib, brigatinib, and lorlatinib
- **ROS1** inhibitors include entrectinib, crizotinib, and ceritinib
- **BRAF V600E mutation**: Combination of dabrafenib plus trametinib or encorafenib and binimetinib
- **MET exon 14 skipping** inhibitors include capmatinib and tepotinib
- **RET** inhibitors include selpercatinib and pralsetinib
- **NTRK** inhibitor include larotrectinib or entrectinib
- **HER2** inhibitors include trastuzumab deruxtecan
- **KRAS G12C** inhibitors include adagrasib and sotorasib

In addition, blood-based circulating DNA (ctDNA) testing, also known as a liquid biopsy, has emerged as an important complement to tissue-based testing to identifying genomic targets. The merits of such blood-based tests are that they are less invasive and usually have a quick turn-around time of one to two weeks. They are especially helpful when there is a delay in completing tissue-based molecular testing or if there are issues with getting sufficient tumor tissue specimens for testing. Research indicates that there is overall greater sensitivity in identifying a targetable mutation when blood-based testing is added to tumor-based testing. However, ctDNA testing may not be sufficiently sensitive when used alone, especially in cases where there is a limited disease burden and insufficient "tumor shed" into the blood stream. Given the greater risk for a false-negative with ctDNA testing, the absence of a target on a liquid biopsy should be confirmed with tissue-based testing. It should also be noted that assessment of tumor PD-L1 expression cannot be performed using blood-based biopsies.

The patient agrees to getting blood drawn for a liquid biopsy but mentions that her uncle also has lung cancer and has been doing well on immunotherapy for the last year. She is eager to begin treatment and asks whether she too should be starting on immunotherapy.

12) What do you recommend to her?

Expert Perspective: Given that she is having relatively minimal symptoms, it is appropriate to wait until the molecular testing returns prior to deciding on a specific form of systemic therapy. Because she is a never-smoker, there is a high likelihood that her tumor will harbor a driver mutation, like an alteration in *EGFR* or *ALK*. Such targets have excellent oral therapies available that should be used in the first line. Moreover, substantial evidence from second-line registration clinical trials and retrospective cohort studies indicates that tumors with such oncogene alterations generally respond poorly to immunotherapy.

If her tumor was noted to have a high PD-L1 expression of 80%, then it may be tempting to start her on a single-agent checkpoint inhibitor. However, if an alteration in *EGFR* or *ALK* is found, PD-L1 expression is not likely to correlate with response to immunotherapy in such oncogene addicted tumors. For instance, prior studies have demonstrated that even among patients with *EGFR* tumors with PD-L1 positivity or high PD-L1 expression, little benefit from single-agent checkpoint inhibitors are typically seen. Furthermore, there is a greater risk for toxicities in situations where a patient receives an immunotherapy agent prior to receiving a tyrosine kinase inhibitor (TKI) targeting a particular oncogene. The greatest evidence for this is in *EGFR*-mutated tumors, where prior data indicate the potential for severe immune-related adverse events when PD-(L)1 blockade is followed by osimertinib. For all these reasons, it is best to wait for the molecular testing results to return prior to deciding on a specific systemic therapy in this patient's case.

In situations where a patient presents more symptomatic or with a large burden of disease, it may be prudent to start systemic therapy immediately while molecular testing results are still pending. In such cases, a cycle of upfront chemotherapy alone (e.g. platinum doublet chemotherapy) without the addition of a checkpoint inhibitor is recommended. It is wise to omit the checkpoint inhibitor with this first cycle to avoid the potential toxicity risk later, in the event that a targetable driver mutation is found and systemic treatment is changed to a TKI.

13) The liquid biopsy report reveals an *EGFR* exon 19 deletion. What should be the first-line therapy for this patient?

Expert Perspective: Several earlier generation TKIs (e.g. erlotinib, afatinib, gefitinib) are approved in the front-line setting for patients with tumors possessing a sensitizing mutations in *EGFR*. However, the third-generation TKI osimertinib is the preferred first-line agent and is recommended for this patient. Osimertinib is approved for the front-line treatment of patients with tumors harboring an *EGFR* exon 19 deletion or exon 21 *L858R* mutation supported by results from the phase III trial FLAURA, which demonstrated superior PFS (18.9 vs 10.2 months; HR 0.46, 95% CI 0.37–0.57) and OS (38.6 vs 31.8 months; HR 0.80, 95% CI 0.64–0.99) as compared with the earlier generation TKIs gefitinib or erlotinib. Prior to the front-line approval, osimertinib was already approved for use in patients with *EGFR* tumors developing *T790M* mutations as a form of acquired resistance to earlier generation TKIs. In addition to the superior outcomes with use of osimertinib in the front line, this drug is generally better tolerated and has better central nervous system penetration as compared with earlier generation TKIs.

Erlotinib in combination with ramucirumab is also an approved front-line regimen for patients with sensitizing *EGFR* tumors. However, the greater central nervous system (CNS) activity of osimertinib, the greater potential toxicities with the vascular endothelial growth factor (VEGF) inhibitor combination, and ultimately the similar PFS times of erlotinib plus ramucirumab when compared with osimertinib alone in cross-trial comparison make osimertinib alone the preferrable front-line choice. Trials examining osimertinib combined with VEGF inhibition or chemotherapy are currently underway, and enrolling in such a trial would also be a reasonable option. Of note, amivantamab, a bispecific antibody directed against epidermal growth factor (EGF) and MET receptors, is approved for adult patients with locally advanced or metastatic NSCLC with EGFR exon 20 insertion mutations. Most recently, the results of PAPILLON study were published. A total of 308 therapy naive advanced NSCLC with EGFR exon 20 insertions patients underwent randomization (153 to receive amivantamab–chemotherapy and 155 to receive chemotherapy alone). Progression-free survival was significantly longer in the amivantamab–chemotherapy group than in the chemotherapy group (median, 11.4 months and 6.7 months, respectively; hazard ratio for disease progression or death, 0.40; 95% confidence interval [CI], 0.30 to 0.53; P<0.001). At 18 months, progression-free survival was reported in 31% of the patients in the amivantamab–chemotherapy group and in 3% in the chemotherapy group; a complete or partial response at data cutoff was reported in 73% and 47%, respectively (rate ratio, 1.50; 95% CI, 1.32 to 1.68; P<0.001).

Case Study continued: The patient starts on osimertinib with good clinical and radiographic response. Unfortunately, two years later, she notes worsening dyspnea and weight loss. CT imaging reveals multiple new pulmonary nodules and several metastatic liver lesions.

14) What is the next best step in her care? And what treatment options should be considered?

Expert Perspective: A repeat tissue biopsy should be considered in nearly all cases of *EGFR*-mutated NSCLC after progression on osimertinib with repeat molecular testing recommended. Such testing may identify certain resistance mechanisms that may allow for the opportunity for specific clinical trials. Off-label use of drugs targeting an identified resistance mechanism while continuing osimertinib can be considered as well. Small cell transformation at the time of progression on an *EGFR* TKI, though a rare entity, needs to also be considered and could be identified with a repeat tissue biopsy.

There are no approved targeted therapies after progression on osimertinib. In the absence of a potential targetable alteration on rebiopsy or a suitable clinical trial, platinum-doublet chemotherapy remains the next best standard of care treatment option. Single-agent immunotherapy can be considered as a later line of treatment and certainly only after platinum-doublet chemotherapy, given the greater resistance to checkpoint inhibitors seen in *EGFR*-mutated disease. Of note, more recent data generated from the phase III trial IMpower150 suggest that therapies that include checkpoint inhibition combined with chemotherapy and VEGF inhibition may overcome the immunotherapy resistance typically seen in such tumors. Subgroup data from this trial demonstrated superior PFS (9.7 vs 6.1 months; HR 0.59, 95% CI 0.37–0.94) and a trend toward better OS (not estimable vs 17.5, HR 0.54, 95% CI 0.29–1.03) with the PD-L1 inhibitor atezolizumab combined with carboplatin + paclitaxel + bevacizumab versus carboplatin + paclitaxel + bevacizumab alone in *EGFR/ALK* tumors. However, no immunotherapy-based combination therapies are currently FDA approved for patients with *EGFR* and *ALK*-mutated tumors, and ongoing clinical trials examining immune-based treatments should always be considered for such patients.

Recommended Readings

Gandhi, L., Rodriguez-Abreu, D., Gadgeel, S. et al. (2018). Pembrolizumab plus chemotherapy in metastatic non-small-cell lung cancer. *N Engl J Med* 378: 2078–2092.

Gogishvili M., Melkadze T., Makharadze T. et al. (2022). Cemiplimab plus chemotherapy versus chemotherapy alone in non-small cell lung cancer: a randomized, controlled, double-blind phase 3 trial. *Nat Med* 28:2374–2380.

Hellmann, M.D., Paz-Ares, L., Bernabe Caro, R. et al. (2019). Nivolumab plus ipilimumab in advanced non-small-cell lung cancer. *N Engl J Med* 381: 2020–2031.

Hong D.S., Fakih M.G., Strickler J.H. et al. (2020). KRAS$_{G12C}$ Inhibition with Sotorasib in Advanced Solid Tumors. *N Engl J Med* 383:1207–1217.

Jänne P.A., Riely G.J., Gadgeel S.M. et al. (2022). Adagrasib in Non-Small-Cell Lung Cancer Harboring a *KRASG12C* Mutation. *N Engl J Med* 387:120–131.

Johnson M.L., Cho B.C., Luft A. et al. (2023). Durvalumab With or Without Tremelimumab in Combination With Chemotherapy as First-Line Therapy for Metastatic Non-Small-Cell Lung Cancer: The Phase III POSEIDON Study. *J Clin Oncol* 41:1213–1227.

Li, B.T., Smit, E.F., Goto, Y., et al. (2022). Trastuzumab deruxtecan in HER2-mutant son-small-cell lung cancer. *N Engl J Med* 386:241–251.

Mok, T.S.K., Wu, Y.L., Kudaba, I. et al. (2019). Pembrolizumab versus chemotherapy for previously untreated, PD-L1-expressing, locally advanced or metastatic non-small-cell lung cancer (KEYNOTE-042): a randomised, open-label, controlled, phase 3 trial. *Lancet* 393: 1819–1830.

Paz-Ares, L., Ciuleanu, T.E., Cobo, M. et al. (2021). First-line nivolumab plus ipilimumab combined with two cycles of chemotherapy in patients with non-small-cell lung cancer (CheckMate 9LA): an international, randomised, open-label, phase 3 trial. *Lancet Oncol* 22: 198–211.

Paz-Ares, L., Luft, A., Vicente, D. et al. (2018). Pembrolizumab plus chemotherapy for squamous non-small-cell lung cancer. *N Engl J Med* 379: 2040–2051.

Reck, M., Rodriguez-Abreu, D., Robinson, A.G. et al. (2019). Updated analysis of KEYNOTE-024: pembrolizumab versus platinum-based chemotherapy for advanced non-small-cell lung cancer with PD-L1 tumor proportion score of 50% or greater. *J Clin Oncol* 37: 537–546.

Sezer, A., Kilickap, S., Gumus, M. et al. (2021). Cemiplimab monotherapy for first-line treatment of advanced non-small-cell lung cancer with PD-L1 of at least 50%: a multicentre, open-label, global, phase 3, randomised, controlled trial. *Lancet* 397: 592–604.

Socinski, M.A., Jotte, R.M., Cappuzzo, F., Orlandi, F., Stroyakovskiy, D. et al. (2018a). Atezolizumab for first-line treatment of metastatic nonsquamous NSCLC. *N Engl J Med* 378: 2288–2301.

Soria, J.C., Ohe, Y., Vansteenkiste et al. (2018). Osimertinib in untreated EGFR-mutated advanced non–small-cell lung cancer. *N Engl J Med* 378: 113–125.

Sun, L., Bleiberg, B., Hwang, W.T. et al. (2023 June 4). Association between duration of immunotherapy and overall survival in advanced non-small cell lung cancer. *JAMA Oncol* e231891. doi: 10.1001/jamaoncol.2023.1891. Epub ahead of print. PMID: 37270700; PMCID: PMC10240399.

8

Small Cell Lung Cancer

Jyoti D. Patel[1] and Husam Hafzah[2]

[1] *Northwestern University – Feinberg School of Medicine, Chicago, IL*
[2] *Chicago Medical School at Rosalind Franklin University of Medicine and Science, Captain James A. Lovell Federal Healthcare Center, North Chicago, IL*

Introduction

Lung cancer is the third most diagnosed cancer in the United States after breast and prostate cancers. Accounting for more than a fifth of all cancer deaths in the United States, lung cancer remains the leading cause of cancer-related death in both men and women. Lung cancer is subclassified based upon histology as small cell lung cancer (SCLC) which accounts for 13% of all cases, and non-small cell lung cancer (NSCLC), which accounts for 84% of lung cancer (Chapters 6 and 7). Because of decreased tobacco consumption, modest uptake of low-dose CT screening, and improvements in treatment, there has been an increase in five-year survival rates and a decline in new cases and death rates in lung cancer in the last 40 years. SCLC occurs almost exclusively in smokers and appears most commonly in heavy smokers. The diagnosis of SCLC is based primarily on light microscopy. Small cell carcinoma is characterized by small "blue" malignant cells that are about twice the size of a lymphocyte. There is sparse cytoplasm, mitotic rates are high, and nuclear molding is characteristic. There are two main subtypes of SCLC that can be differentiated histologically: small cell carcinoma, and combined with NSCLC with other types of histologies such as squamous cells, adenocarcinoma, spindle cell, and large cell neuroendocrine (see Chapter 28). There is no minimal percentage of NSCLC histologic elements required. It is important to note that up to 30% of SCLC specimens show areas of NSCLC differentiation; these patients are preferably treated with an SCLC approach. Several paraneoplastic syndromes are associated with SCLC including endocrine, neurologic, and hematologic syndromes. Endocrine syndromes include syndrome of inappropriate antidiuretic hormone secretion (SIADH), ectopic Cushing syndrome with production of adrenocorticotropic hormone (ACTH) manifesting with hyponatremia, hypertension, and amenorrhea. Neurologic syndromes include Lambert-Eaton myasthenic syndrome, encephalomyelitis, cerebellar degeneration, and sensory neuropathies. Hematologic syndromes include anemia of chronic disease, leukemoid reaction, and Trousseau syndrome. It is important to note that the presence of a paraneoplastic syndrome does not necessarily indicate advanced disease or incurability. SCLC is characterized by early development of widespread metastatic disease, and without treatment, it has the most aggressive course of any type of lung cancer with median survival from diagnosis of only two to four months.

Cancer Consult: Expertise in Clinical Practice, Volume 1: Solid Tumors & Supportive Care,
Second Edition. Edited by Syed A. Abutalib, Maurie Markman, Al B. Benson III, and Hope S. Rugo.
© 2024 John Wiley & Sons Ltd. Published 2024 by John Wiley & Sons Ltd.

SCLC prognosis remains unsatisfactory despite the advances in diagnosis and treatments, so clinical trials inclusion of all SCLC patients should be considered at the time of diagnosis. For patients with limited-stage SCLC treated with chemoradiotherapy and PCI, overall response rates of 80–90%, including 50–60% complete response rates, are typically reported. Median survival is approximately 17 months, and the five-year survival rate is approximately 20%. The overall survival rate of extensive stage SCLC patients at five years is only 5–10%. SCLC is highly sensitive to chemotherapy and radiation therapy. Current treatment modalities include surgery, chemotherapy, radiation therapy, and immunotherapy. The selection of a treatment modality is highly dependent on cancer staging, which utilizes the AJCC TNM staging system, whereas other societies utilize the older Veteran Administration (VA) scheme for SCLC.

Case Study 1

A 50-year-old woman is being evaluated for chronic nonresolving cough and new-onset dyspnea. Her medical history is significant for hypertension and cigarette smoking for more than 30 years. She also reports an unintentional weight loss over the past six months. She was found to have a large right upper lung mass on a chest X-ray. A CT chest demonstrates a 7.5 cm right upper lobe mass and ipsilateral mediastinal adenopathy. EBUS is performed, and right lung mass and right paratracheal node with SCLC. Her PET scan reveals right supraclavicular adenopathy, right paratracheal and hilar adenopathy, and right upper lobe mass. No distant disease is detected. An MRI of the brain is negative for metastases.

She is believed to have limited-stage SCLC. You recommend definitive treatment with chemoradiation. She starts cisplatin and etoposide.

1) What radiation schedule to the primary site do you recommend in limited-stage SCLC?

Expert Perspective: Twice daily schedule. Although the ideal schedule for radiation therapy is unclear, hyperfractionation of radiation has been shown to improve survival in patients with limited-stage SCLC receiving concurrent chemotherapy.

- In the study from A. T. Turrisi et al. (1999), patients on the twice-daily radiation schedule with concurrent cisplatin and etoposide had a five-year survival rate of 26%, compared with 16% for those treated once daily radiation. There was increased toxicity, specifically a higher rate of acute esophagitis with twice-daily dosing (27% vs. 11%). It should be noted that the more appropriate once-daily dose is now considered to be 60–70 Gy.
- Another randomized clinical trial (CONVERT) showed no difference in the survival outcomes or toxicity between twice-daily and once-daily radiation therapy in the limited-stage SCLC with concurrent chemotherapy. However, because the study was designed to show superiority and not equivalence, twice-daily regimen is still considered a standard of care.
- A recent meta-analysis did not show a statistically significant difference in survival, but a trend toward better outcomes was noted. For patients able to comply with a twice-daily schedule, a hyperfractionation approach is reasonable.

- The phase III CALGB 30610 (Alliance)/RTOG 0538 study (started March 2008, estimated completion date June 2023) is exploring a boost approach that delivers 70 Gy in seven weeks compared with 61.2 Gy concomitant boost over five weeks or standard dose of 45 Gy twice a day over three weeks. Patients with limited stage SCLC were assigned to receive four cycles of cisplatin and etoposide chemotherapy with one of three thoracic radiation schedules starting with either the first or second cycle of chemotherapy. Early results show that higher doses of radiation to the primary tumor did not significantly improve overall survival (median, 29 vs. 31 months; HR 0.94, P = 0.59) compared with the standard total dose of 45 Gy divided twice daily over 21 days. Rates of grade 3 or higher adverse events were also similar between the arms.
- In a randomized phase II trial in which 182 patients were assigned to concurrent chemoradiotherapy at either 45 Gy twice daily in 30 fractions or 65 Gy once daily in 26 fractions, the once-daily group experienced improved progression-free survival (median, 13.4 vs. 17.2 months; HR 0.67, 95% CI 0.46–0.96). Median OS was not statistically different between the two arms.

In summary, the dose and schedule of concurrent chemoradiation in limited-stage SCLC is unclear. The data support both 45 Gy twice daily or 60–70 Gy daily radiation therapy, with the possibility of escalating the dose to 60 Gy twice daily, in select patients.

2) What are the risk factors for developing SCLC?

Expert Perspective: Smoking cigarettes is the leading cause of SCLC, and it is not uncommon to diagnose this type of lung cancer in current smokers. The risk of developing lung cancer is proportional to the cumulative duration of smoking and the number of cigarettes smoked daily. High-risk patients are those with a history of more than 20–30 pack years. As the prevalence of smoking is declining, so is the incidence of SCLC in the United States. Other risk factors include radon exposure, occupational exposure to asbestos, exposure to ionizing radiation, and industrial exposure to arsenic, nickel, chromium, and environmental air pollution. Research has not found known genetic syndromes that are associated with lung cancer.

3) How do patients with SCLC present?

Expert Perspective: SCLC is often incidentally found during regular workup for other conditions, and most patients will presents with hematogenous metastases. Only about one-third of cases will have the disease confined to the chest cavity. Symptoms depend on the location and the bulk of the primary tumor and have a rapid onset. Signs and symptoms may be related to the primary tumor growth, which can cause coughing, wheezing, hemoptysis, fever, and dyspnea. They may indicate tumor invasion or regional lymphatic metastases such as hoarseness, dysphagia, chest pain, SVC syndrome, and pericardial effusion, or they may be related to extrathoracic hematogenous metastases including headache, weakness, confusion, slurred speech, diplopia, gait instability, back pain, right upper quadrant pain, bone pain, anorexia, weight loss, and fatigue. Lastly, signs and symptoms may indicate a paraneoplastic syndrome, but this does not necessarily indicate advanced disease or incurability.

4) Are there any current screening tests for SCLC?

Expert Perspective: Currently there is no effective screening test for the detection of early stage SCLC, but the National Lung Screening Trials (NLST) reports that screening with annual low-dose spiral CT scan decreases lung cancer mortality in asymptomatic high-risk individuals. Although this screening test can detect early stage NSCLC, it was not found to be useful in detecting early stage SCLC. These findings are likely related to the aggressiveness, rapid doubling time, high growth fraction, and the fact that symptomatic disease can develop in between annual scans (Chapter 5).

5) What staging system is used for SCLC, and what significance does it have on treatment options?

Expert Perspective: Treatment of SCLS is highly dependent on the stage of the disease. However, systemic therapy is essential for all patients with SCLC.

The current NCCN SCLC Panel adopts a combined approach for staging SCLC using both AJCC TNM staging system and the older VA scheme for SCLC. This older system defines two stages: limited-stage disease is when the disease is confined to the ipsilateral hemithorax, and extensive-stage disease is when the disease is beyond the ipsilateral hemithorax, including malignant effusions (pleural and pericardial) or hematogenous metastases. The main criteria in this VA system determines whether a reasonable radiation plan can encompass the disease extent.

With the use of these two staging systems, limited-stage SCLC is defined as stage I–III (T any, N any, M0), which can be treated with definitive radiation therapy, excluding T3 and T4. Extensive-stage disease is defined as stage IV (T any, N any, M1a/b/c) or T3 and T4 due to multiple lung nodules. The TNM staging system more useful for patients who are candidates for surgery. Proper staging includes a history and physical examination, CT scan with contrast of the chest and abdomen, and brain imaging. MRI with intravenous contrast and PET-CT scan may be useful in limited-stage disease. Of note, once extensive-stage disease is found, no further staging is required except for brain imaging.

6) What is the role of surgery, adjuvant chemotherapy, and radiation therapy in early (T1–2 and N0) limited-stage SCLC?

Expert Perspective: Although generally considered a systemic disease at diagnosis, there is a small subset of patients with limited disease SCLC who appear to benefit from surgery. Several retrospective analyses report five-year survival rates approaching 50% for patients with pathologic stage I SCLC treated with resection. Despite a lack of data, most experts suggest adjuvant chemotherapy for patients who have undergone a complete resection for SCLC. The role of adjuvant radiation therapy in patients found to have early (N1) nodal disease postoperatively is unclear. Of note, these data also demonstrate a significant discordance between clinical and pathologic staging. Although surgical resection should be considered for patients with stage I SCLC, proper staging workup, including PET–CT and mediastinoscopy, must be completed prior to resection.

7) What is the appropriate platinum, cisplatin or carboplatin?

Expert Perspective: As mentioned, systemic therapy is essential for all patients with SCLC as either as primary or adjuvant therapy. Single-agent and combination chemotherapy regimens have shown effectiveness in treating SCLC. In clinical practice, carboplatin is preferred and is frequently substituted for cisplatin due to reduced risk of nonhematologic toxicity (nausea, vomiting, ototoxicity, neuropathy, and nephropathy). However, carboplatin use puts patients at a higher risk of hematologic toxicity (myelosuppression). A meta-analysis from four randomized studies compared cisplatin-based and carboplatin-based regimens in SCLC treatment found no significant difference in response rate, progression-free survival, or overall survival. Other studies suggest less subsequent health-care use and equivalent efficacy between the two platins in treating SCLC.

8) What is the role of immunotherapy in front-line setting for limited- and extensive-stage SCLC?

Expert Perspective: Currently there is no data supporting the use of immunotherapy in limited-stage SCLC, although several trials incorporating immunotherapy with chemoradiation are ongoing. The use of platinum and etoposide plus immunotherapy in extensive-stage SCLC is considered the standard of care. A randomized phase III trial (IMpower133) demonstrated and improvement in survival when atezolizumab (PD-L1 targeted immune checkpoint inhibitor) was added to carboplatin plus etoposide. A phase III trial (CASPIAN) assessed durvalumab with and without tremelimumab in combination with etoposide plus platinum as a first-line therapy for extensive-stage SCLC also showed similar improvements in overall survival with the addition of durvalumab, and it is also considered a standard of care. A Chinese phase III trial (CAPSTONE-1) found that the addition of adebrelimab, a novel anti–PD-L1 antibody, to carboplatin and etoposide significantly improved overall survival as a first-line treatment for patients with extensive-stage SCLC. Median overall survival was 15.3 versus 12.8 months with and without immunotherapy, respectively. Both atezolizumab and durvalumab have FDA approvals when combined with a platinum agent and etoposide during induction and continued as maintenance therapy in extensive-stage SCLC.

A recent report of phase II S1929 trial, conducted by the SWOG Cancer Research Network showed that among patients with extensive-stage SCLC positive for expression of the Schlafen-11 gene (SLFN11), those who received maintenance treatment with the immune checkpoint inhibitor atezolizumab plus the PARP inhibitor talazoparib had significantly longer progression-free survival (4.2 months) than those who received atezolizumab alone (2.8 months). Patients receiving atezolizumab plus talazoparib experienced significantly more hematologic adverse events than those receiving only atezolizumab—50% vs 4%—although this increased rate of hematologic toxicity was expected. Nonhematologic adverse event rates were similar between the two arms: 15% vs 13%, respectively.

9) What is the role of prophylactic cranial irradiation (PCI) in limited- and extensive-stage SCLC?

Expert Perspective: Because the natural history of SCLC is of dissemination, PCI for patients without detectable central nervous system (CNS) disease can decrease intracranial relapse and improve survival for patients with limited-stage SCLC. The administration of PCI after chemotherapy has demonstrated a decrease in the incidence of brain metastases and an increase in overall survival in limited-stage SCLC. The role of PCI is unclear in patients with surgically resected or unresected early stage (T1–2/N0) SCLC because they have a lower incidence of brain metastases. Current guidelines recommend PCI for limited-stage SCLC with complete remission or partial response even in stage I SCLC. There have been multiple conflicting data regarding PCI efficacy in extensive-stage SCLC and most recent guidelines recommend considering either PCI or surveillance MRI imaging depending on individual patient factor. Late neurological sequelae have been reported after PCI limiting its use in patients with poor performance status or impaired neurocognition. The use of PCI for this group should be discussed with the patient and decided on an individual basis. Another important issues with regard to PCI is whether sparing the hippocampus mitigates the deterioration of cognitive function in patients with SCLC. In the Spanish phase III PREMER trial, Rodríguez de Dios et al. found that hippocampal avoidance during PCI SCLC was associated with better preservation of cognitive function versus PCI alone and did not increase the risk of brain metastasis.

10) Should patients with CNS metastases receive stereotactic radiotherapy?

Expert Perspective: SCLC patients with CNS metastases are typically treated with whole brain radiation therapy (WBRT). Adding WBRT to the chemotherapy regimen in SCLC treatment has showed increased response rate but did not improve survival. WBRT can be considered in patients who develop CNS metastases after PCI. The data on stereotactic radiotherapy (or stereotactic radiosurgery) remain limited, but it is the preferred method for limited CNS metastases from most types of cancer, where WBRT is still the standard of care for CNS metastases in patients with SCLC.

The FIRE-SCLC study compared the outcomes of first-line stereotactic radiotherapy with WBRT. The study showed that WBRT offered no overall survival advantage (median of 5.2 months for WBRT and 6.5 months for stereotactic radiosurgery). The results were also stratified by the number CNS lesions and indicated an increase in the median overall survival for fewer lesions. The advantage of stereotactic radiosurgery comes from the decreased neurocognitive adverse effects and similar overall survival when compared with WBRT. The study shows that stereotactic radiotherapy/radiosurgery may be appropriate in treating selected patients with a small number (one to four) of CNS metastases.

11) What are appropriate second-line therapies for patients with SCLC?

Expert Perspective: SCLC is very sensitive to chemotherapy and radiation therapy, but most patients will relapse with resistant disease. Therapeutic second-line options include reinduction or a single-agent chemotherapy but depend on duration of response to the first-line agents. The preferred regimen when relapse occurs more than six months after initial therapy is reinduction with the original regimen. When the relapse occurs in less than six months, preferred agents are topotecan or lurbinectedin, an alkylating agent and a selective inhibitor of oncogenic transcription that binds preferentially to guanine residues in the minor groove of DNA. Other agents are being studied as second-line agents, including paclitaxel, docetaxel, irinotecan, temozolomide, CAV (cyclophosphamide/doxorubicin/vincristine), and other immunotherapies such as nivolumab and pembrolizumab.

Conclusion

It is important to be reminded of the sobering fact that less than 40% of limited-stage and less than 5% of extensive-stage patients survive two years. Patient should be offered clinical trial options whenever available.

Recommended Readings

Aupérin, A., Arriagada, R., Pignon, J.P. et al. (1999). Prophylactic cranial irradiation for patients with small-cell lung cancer in complete remission. Prophylactic Cranial Irradiation Overview Collaborative Group. *N Engl J Med* 341 (7): 476–484. https://doi.org/10.1056/NEJM199908123410703.

Bogart, J., Wang, X., Masters, G. et al. (2023 May 1). High-dose once-daily thoracic radiotherapy in limited-stage small-cell lung cancer: CALGB 30610 (Alliance)/RTOG 0538. *J Clin Oncol* 41 (13): 2394-2402. doi: 10.1200/JCO.22.01359. Epub 2023 Jan 9. PMID: 36623230; PMCID: PMC10150922.

Cheng, Y., Han, L., Wu, L. et al. (2022). Effect of first-line Serplulimab vs Placebo added to chemotherapy on survival in patients with extensive-stage small cell lung cancer: the ASTRUM-005 randomized clinical trial. *JAMA* 328 (12): 1223–1232. doi:10.1001/jama.2022.16464.

Faivre-Finn, C., Snee, M., Ashcroft, L. et al. (2017). Concurrent once-daily versus twice-daily chemoradiotherapy in patients with limited-stage small-cell lung cancer (CONVERT): An open-label, phase 3, randomised, superiority trial. *Lancet Oncol* 18 (8): 1116–1125. https://doi.org/10.1016/S1470-2045(17)30318-2.

Horn, L., Mansfield, A.S., Szczęsna, A. et al. (2018). IMpower133 study group. First-line atezolizumab plus chemotherapy in extensive-stage small-cell lung cancer. *N Engl J Med* 379 (23): 2220–2229. doi: 10.1056/NEJMoa1809064. Epub 2018 Sep 25. PMID: 30280641.

Johnson, B.E., Grayson, J., Makuch, R.W. et al. (1990). Ten-year survival of patients with small-cell lung cancer treated with combination chemotherapy with or without irradiation. *J Clin Oncol* 8 (3): 396–401. doi: 10.1200/JCO.1990.8.3.396. PMID: 2155310.

National Lung Screening Trial Research Team, Aberle, D.R., Adams, A.M. et al. (2011). Reduced lung-cancer mortality with low-dose computed tomographic screening. *N Engl J Med* 365 (5): 395–409. https://doi.org/10.1056/NEJMoa1102873.

Paz-Ares, L., Dvorkin, M., Chen, Y. et al. (2019). CASPIAN investigators. Durvalumab plus platinum-etoposide versus platinum-etoposide in first-line treatment of extensive-stage small-cell lung cancer (CASPIAN): a randomised, controlled, open-label, phase 3 trial. *Lancet* 394 (10212): 1929–1939. doi: 10.1016/S0140-6736(19)32222-6. Epub 2019 Oct 4. PMID: 31590988.

Slotman, B.J., Mauer, M.E., Bottomley, A. et al. (2009). Prophylactic cranial irradiation in extensive disease small-cell lung cancer: short-term health-related quality of life and patient reported symptoms: results of an international phase III randomized controlled trial by the

EORTC Radiation Oncology and Lung Cancer Groups. *J Clin Oncol* 27 (1): 78–84. doi: 10.1200/JCO.2008.17.0746. Epub 2008 Dec 1. Erratum in: J Clin Oncol. 2009 Feb 20;27(6):1002.PMID: 19047288; PMCID: PMC2645093.

Trigo, J., Subbiah, V., Besse, B. et al. (2020). Lurbinectedin as second-line treatment for patients with small-cell lung cancer: a single-arm, open-label, phase 2 basket trial. *Lancet Oncol* 21 (5): 645–654. doi: 10.1016/S1470-2045(20)30068-1. Epub 2020 Mar 27. Erratum in: Lancet Oncol. 2020 Dec;21(12):e553.PMID: 32224306.

Turrisi, A.T., 3rd, Kim, K., Blum, R. et al. (1999). Twice-daily compared with once-daily thoracic radiotherapy in limited small-cell lung cancer treated concurrently with cisplatin and etoposide. *N Engl J Med* 340 (4): 265–271. doi: 10.1056/NEJM199901283400403. PMID: 9920950.

Wang, J., Zhou, C., Yao, W. et al. (2022 June). Adebrelimab or placebo plus carboplatin and etoposide as first-line treatment for extensive-stage small-cell lung cancer (CAPSTONE-1): a multicentre, randomised, double-blind, placebo-controlled, phase 3 trial. *Lancet Oncol* 23 (6): 739–747. doi: 10.1016/S1470-2045(22)00224-8. Epub 2022 May 13. PMID: 35576956.

9

Mesothelioma

Harvey I. Pass, David Chen, and Jack Donaghue

NYU Langone Medical Center, New York University, New York, NY

Introduction

Malignant mesothelioma is an insidious neoplasm arising from the mesothelial surfaces. A total of 80% of all cases are pleural in origin, termed malignant pleural mesothelioma. In the past few years, there have been several major advances in the management of patients with malignant pleural mesothelioma, including more accurate staging and patient selection, improvements in surgical techniques and postoperative care, novel chemotherapy regimens with definite activity such as pemetrexed plus platinum combinations, and new radiotherapy techniques such as intensity-modulated radiation therapy. Treatment for early stage disease with surgery and radiation is potentially curative, but many patients either are too sick to undergo aggressive surgery or present with advanced disease. Results of second-line therapy have been disappointing, yet novel treatment such as immunotherapy and gene therapy present a window of hope. Palliative care remains an important component of the management.

Case Study

You are asked to see a 67-year-old female after an abnormal chest X-ray shows a unilateral pleural effusion and pleural-based mass. She is an otherwise healthy woman who is a nonsmoker, and she works from home selling pottery and taking care of her family. Her husband retired 5 years ago after working 40 years as an insulator. She reports right-sided chest pain and weight loss but no cough, hemoptysis, or other symptoms. How would you approach making a diagnosis of malignant pleural mesothelioma in this patient?

1) What is the relative importance of environmental exposures, and what have we learned about the pathogenesis of malignant pleural mesothelioma?

Expert Perspective: The link between asbestos exposure and malignant pleural mesothelioma has been well documented in both human studies and animal models, and it is estimated that up to 5% of asbestos miners will develop malignant pleural mesothelioma. The mechanism of asbestos-induced mesothelioma is thought to involve inhalation of insoluble fibers, which lead to chronic inflammation, genetic changes, and subsequent cellular oncogenic dysregulation. The incidence of malignant pleural mesothelioma is about 3,500 cases per year in the United States and reflects a 25-to-40-year latency between exposure and tumor development. Outside of the United States, death rates from mesothelioma mirror national asbestos exposure, with high rates seen in Australian, New Zealand, Western Europe, and the United Kingdom. Although a dose-response relationship exists with all types of asbestos fibers in animal models of carcinogenicity, epidemiologic studies in humans suggest that amosite and crocidolite carry a higher risk that chrysotile fibers. Human studies have demonstrated that exposure to asbestos fibers create reactive oxygen species that cause oxidative stress to mesothelial cells, which can overwhelm the cell's antioxidant defense mechanisms and lead to malignant pleural mesothelioma carcinogenesis. Other nonasbestos mineral fibers, such as erionite (found in high levels in areas of Turkey as well as in regions of the western United States), also show a strong relationship to malignant pleural mesothelioma prevalence.

The threshold exposure level below which malignant pleural mesothelioma will not develop remains unclear. Professions other than miners with lower-level exposure, such as plumbers, insulators, and carpenters, may also develop mesothelioma from asbestos exposure that is higher than that of the general population, but the exposure is still much lower than that experienced by miners. As in our hypothetical patient, reports have shown that even spouses of insulators have developed mesothelioma, presumably through exposure to the contaminated clothing. Other professions with cases of documented asbestos exposure include aircraft mechanics, aerospace workers, electricians, shipyard workers, auto mechanics, pipe fitters, construction workers, boilermakers, railway workers, mining, asbestos removal, and sheet metal workers. While the relationship between asbestos exposure and the development of malignant pleural mesothelioma is incontrovertible, the level and type of exposure that leads to mesothelioma formation are unclear and remain a topic of research.

Although over 80% of malignant pleural mesothelioma is attributable to asbestos exposure by patient histories, other factors may also predispose people to mesothelioma formation, including radiation and chronic inflammation of the pleura, such as tuberculosis, collagen vascular disease, and empyema thoracis. Most recently, chronic use of talc powder contaminated with fibers has been implicated. Tobacco exposure's role in mesothelioma formation remains controversial, but it is generally not considered a strong risk factor for malignant pleural mesothelioma formation, unless there is a history of consumption of Kent cigarettes, whose micronite filter was constructed with asbestiform fibers. Simian virus 40 (SV40) is a DNA tumor virus that has also been associated with the formation of mesothelioma. Although animal studies show that pleurally injected SV40 alone can lead to malignant pleural mesothelioma formation, human studies that suggest that SV40 may act as a co-carcinogen in asbestos-exposed individuals remain extremely controversial.

Genetics also clearly plays a key role in cancer formation. Recent data continue to suggest that malignant pleural mesothelioma has a lower mutation burden compared to other solid tumors and is primarily driven by inactivation of tumor suppressor genes *BAP1*, *TP53*, *NF2*, and *CDKN2A*. Familial mesothelioma can be seen in the *BAP1* syndrome in which *germline BAP1* mutations have been associated with families with high incidence of mesothelioma, uveal melanomas. *BAP1* germ line malignant pleural mesothelioma patients seem to have a longer survival and are younger in age. Individuals with malignant pleural mesothelioma have also been found to have significantly higher probability of heterozygous germline Bloom Syndrome mutations *BLM* mutations compared with the general population, suggesting that *BLM* mutation carriers are at a higher risk of developing malignant pleural mesothelioma and may have their risk increased upon asbestos fiber exposure.

2) How is malignant pleural mesothelioma diagnosed?

Expert Perspective: Diagnosis of malignant pleural mesothelioma is suggested by history and associated risk factors, clinical presentation, physical exam, and radiographic imaging, but it ultimately depends on tissue diagnosis. The most common presenting symptoms are non-pleuritic chest pain (60%) and dyspnea (50–70%). Patients typically report several months of symptoms before seeking attention, with as many as 25% reporting more than six months of symptoms. On physical exam, evidence of effusion is common, and digital clubbing may reflect poor respiratory function secondary to entrapped lung. Weight loss (cachexia) is common in late-stage disease.

Mesothelioma can have a diverse radiographic appearance and may be confused with benign entities, such as pleural plaques or parenchymal pulmonary fibrosis. Chest radiograph classically shows pleural effusion, diffuse pleural thickening, and nodularity and more commonly affects the right side (60%). Often the lower chest demonstrates a loculated effusion, which may encase and trap the lung. Chest CT can more clearly demonstrate the nature of the pleural thickening and effusion. CT accurately visualizes the involvement of the pericardium, diaphragm, and extrathoracic organs, such as the liver and stomach, but is poor in other regards. Although certain radiographic "patterns" suggest malignant disease, CT radiographic criteria are insensitive and prevent the use of CT as the sole method of diagnosis. PET and the radionuclide imaging agent [^{18}F] fluorodeoxyglucose (FDG) can be used to identify pleural malignancies and predict prognosis in patients with mesothelioma as well as to help in staging to make sure that there are no suspicious extrathoracic sites. However, studies of FDG-PET have shown poor sensitivity in identifying lymph node metastases, and therefore FDG-avid lesions should be pathologically confirmed before proceeding with a stage-defined treatment algorithm.

Soluble markers for mesothelioma are being explored as a promising new strategy for screening patients at risk for mesothelioma and improving diagnostic accuracy in patients with unclear diagnoses. The Mesomark assay (Fujirebio, Malvern, PA) is a commercially available assay that measures soluble mesothelin-related proteins (SMPRs); it has a high specificity (95%) but low sensitivity (32%), limiting its use as a screening test. Osteopontin is another protein biomarker that may be used for diagnosis, but due to low sensitivity, it may be better utilized as a prognostic biomarker because patients with elevated osteopontin have been associated with unfavorable outcomes. Other recent markers under investigation include Fibulin-3 and Calretinin; however, further validation in large prospective cohorts is necessary before any use other than for research.

Pathologic confirmation ultimately establishes the diagnosis of malignant pleural mesothelioma, but it also carries a risk of equivocation. Patients with unexplained pleural effusions should undergo thoracentesis, and then if reactive mesothelial cells are seen, or if immunohistochemistry suggests mesothelioma, tissue diagnosis must be obtained. Modern cell-block techniques have improved the diagnostic accuracy of pleural fluid analysis, but they remain imperfect with a reported sensitivity of only 70–80%. Patients who have negative pleural fluid and biopsy (or whose effusions recur after initial drainage) should undergo thoracoscopic evaluation. Video-assisted thoracoscopic surgery (VATS) is invaluable in providing diagnostic information and is the method of choice in acquiring tissue for analysis. VATS is also useful prognostically in that patients with more widespread disease on thoracoscopic evaluation have shown consistently worse outcomes. In patients whose disease precludes the use of VATS due to obliteration of the pleural space, open (but limited) pleural biopsy is necessary, preferably in line with a potential cytoreductive incision for later removal.

Given the phenotypic heterogeneity of malignant pleural mesothelioma, pathologic evaluation of pleural specimens is complex and outside the scope of this review. In general, evidence of stromal invasion remains the gold standard in diagnosis. However, the number of proliferating cells, their distribution, inflammation, and the presence of necrosis are important factors to consider. Although significant controversy exists over the use of antibody panels, immunohistochemistry, and fluorescence *in situ* hybridization (FISH), the use of these adjunctive stains can facilitate diagnosis in certain cases, and usually reveals tumor cells that stain for *BAP1*, cytokeratins, calretinin, and Wilms tumor 1.

3) **How is malignant pleural mesothelioma staged, and what are the prognostic implications of staging?**

Expert Perspective: Multiple staging systems have existed for malignant pleural mesothelioma, which reflects the controversial nature of the diagnosis and treatment of this disease. The oldest system proposed by Butchart, which has now fallen out of use, was based on the location of the primary tumor but did not account for extent of disease. The Brigham system is defined by extent and resectability of disease. The American Joint Committee on Cancer (AJCC) staging system for mesothelioma (see Table 9.1) is the most common staging system used in the United States. It was proposed by the International Mesothelioma Interest Group (IMIG) in 1995 based on data regarding prognosis associated with tumor size and presence of disease in lymph nodes. The most recent revision of the AJCC staging was established with the 8th edition of the TNM (tumor, node, metastasis) classification system after the International Association for the Study of Lung Cancer (IASLC) and the IMIG established consensus changes in 2016 based on a large, multinational database established in 2009. Important changes were made to the T and N components because the 2016 study found that the 7th edition failed to differentiate the prognosis for stage T1a versus T1b, T2 versus T1, N1 versus N2, and stage I versus II. In the 8th edition, T1a and T1b were collapsed into one T1 category. In addition, N3 has been removed while N1 and N2 have been combined into a single N1 category. The study also reemphasized several factors associated with good prognosis: epithelioid histology (vs sarcomatoid), whether the patient underwent a procedure "with curative intent" (vs palliation; median survival 18 vs 12 months; $P < 0.0001$), and, among patients who received surgery, whether they received multimodal treatment (vs surgery alone; median survival 20 vs 11 months; $P < 0.0001$). Further analysis of other features including immunohistochemistry, genomic, and immune-based biomarkers are ongoing.

Table 9.1 AJCC staging, 8th edition of the TNM.

Primary Tumor Site (T)	
Tx	Primary tumor not assessable
T0	No evidence of a primary tumor
T1	Tumor involving the ipsilateral parietal pleura (including mediastinal and diaphragmatic pleura) with or without involvement of visceral pleura
T2	Tumor involving each of the ipsilateral pleural surfaces (parietal, mediastinal, diaphragmatic, and visceral pleura) with at least one of the following features: • Confluent visceral pleural tumor (including fissures) • Involvement of diaphragmatic muscle • Invasion of the lung parenchyma
T3	Tumor involving all of the ipsilateral pleural surfaces (parietal, mediastinal, diaphragmatic and visceral pleura) with at least one of the following features: • Invasion of the endothoracic fascia • Extension into the mediastinal fat • Solitary, completely respectable focus invading soft tissues of the chest wall • Nontransmittal involvement of the pericardium
T4	Tumor involving all of the ipsilatural pleural surfaces with at least one of the following features: • Diffuse or multi focal invasion of soft tissues of the chest wall • Any rib involvement • Invasion of the peritoneum through the diaphragm • Invasion of any mediastinal organ • Direct extension to the contra lateral pleura • Invasions of the spine or brachial plexus • Transmural invasion of the pericardium (with or without pericardial effusion) or myocardium invasion
Nodule Metastases (N)	
Nx	Regional lymph nodes not assessable
N0	No regional lymph node metastases
N1	Metastasis in the ipsilateral bronchopulmonary, hilar, or mediastinal lymph nodes (including the internal mammary, peridiaphragmatic, pericardial fat pad, or intercostal lymph nodes)
N2	Metastasis in the contralateral bronchopulmorary, hilar, or mediastinal lymph nodes or ipsilateral or contralateral supraclavicular lymph nodes
Distant Metastases (M)	
Mx	Presence of distant metastases not assessable
M0	No evidence of distant metastases
M1	Evidence of distant metastases

(Continued)

Table 9.1 (Continued)

Staging			
Stage	T	N	M
IA	T1	N0	M0
IB	T2/T3	N0	M0
II	T1/T2	N1	M0
IIIA	T1/T2	N1	M0
IIIB	T1/T2/T3	N2	M0
IV	T4	N0/N1/N2	M0
	Any T	Any N	M1

Staging as determined by cross sectional or functional imaging continues to have its limitations. While studies have shown that PET–CT can identify malignant pleural mesothelioma with high sensitivity and specificity, PET–CT has a low sensitivity for N2 and T4 disease; in summary, imaging has utility in identifying macroscopic disease but as with most malignancies, detection of microscopic disease remains elusive. The gold standard for diagnosis of metastatic disease continues to rely on tissue analysis.

Our Patient: The patient in the case study returns to your office with core needle biopsy, which confirmed malignant pleural mesothelioma and radiographic evidence of diaphragmatic involvement. She is otherwise in excellent physical health and has a good performance status. How should you approach her treatment?

4) What are the available treatments for locoregional malignant pleural mesothelioma?

Expert Perspective: Surgical therapy for treatment of mesothelioma remains controversial as there are insufficient randomized trials to guide decision-making with regard to surgical intervention. The MARS randomized trial was an attempt to compare multimodality therapy for malignant pleural mesothelioma with and without extrapleural pneumonectomy but failed to accrue the prespecified number of patients required for adequate power. It was critiqued for lack of prerandomization criteria, patient crossover, and a higher than expected surgical mortality. Therefore, although it is clear that patients with widespread disease do not benefit from surgical intervention, the threshold at which patients may benefit from surgical resection is not well defined, including the optimal surgical approach. Currently enrolling is the MARS-2 trial, designed to answer the question of whether surgery plus chemotherapy is superior to chemotherapy alone. Patients receive two cycles of pemetrexed-platinum chemotherapy. Those who do not demonstrate progression on CT scan will then be randomized to either (a) up to four more cycles of pemetrexed-platinum chemotherapy or (b) extended pleurectomy/decortication followed by up to four cycles of adjuvant pemetrexed-platinum chemotherapy. The estimated study will reach completion soon.

Unfortunately, the growth patterns of malignant pleural mesothelioma can make complete surgical excision difficult. Unlike other solid tumors, nodular invasion and the irregular anatomy of the thoracic cavity often prevent surgical resection from removal of all microscopic disease (R0 resection). Instead, surgery is an integral part of a "multimodal" treatment approach, which, when correctly applied, can reduce the bulk of the tumor to microscopic levels that are then treated with adjuvant therapy. A consensus statement (IASLC plus IMIG 2011) has been published to standardize the nomenclature for mesothelioma operations. Two operations are routinely used in this cytoreductive tactic to provide complete "macroscopic" complete resection: extrapleural pneumonectomy (en bloc resection of parietal and visceral pleura with ipsilateral lung, pericardium, and diaphragm) and pleurectomy decortication (parietal and visceral pleurectomy without resection of diaphragm or pericardium). In addition, two additional terminologies were defined—extended pleurectomy decortication (pleurectomy decortication plus resection of pericardium or diaphragm) and partial pleurectomy (partial removal of parietal and/or visceral pleura for diagnostics or palliation, leaving gross tumor unresected).

Extrapleural pneumonectomy is associated with considerable morbidity, but it has improved from unacceptably high mortality (>30%) in the 1970s to 3–8% mortality and 20–40% morbidity in modern series, which is comparable to other major oncologic surgeries (esophagectomy, hepatectomy, and pancreatic duodenectomy). The surgical results of extrapleural pneumonectomy have been generally disappointing and overall offer limited benefit in survival relative to nonsurgical therapies. Median survival after surgery alone ranges from 9 to 17 months in most series. The longest survival is generally seen among patients with early stage (stage I or II) disease and among patients with epithelioid histology, where median survival of greater than 17 months is possible. There are also functional consequences to extrapleural pneumonectomy, as pneumonectomy limits a patient's ability to receive treatment upon tumor progression, leading to a median time to death of three months once there is recurrence after extrapleural pneumonectomy. The difficulty in widespread application of extrapleural pneumonectomy to mesothelioma, therefore, has been reconciling the high morbidity of surgery with its marginal benefit and long-term sequelae.

Pleurectomy decortication is a "lung-conserving" approach to surgery for malignant pleural mesothelioma, and it has been repopularized as a potential therapeutic cytoreductive modality. The goal of pleurectomy decortication is to achieve an equivalent surgical resection while avoiding the high morbidities associated with extrapleural pneumonectomy that are discussed in this chapter. Although controversial, it gained increasing acceptance after the initial report of a retrospective study of 663 patients from three institutions demonstrated that patients undergoing pleurectomy decortication had a survival that was at least equivalent to those who received extrapleural pneumonectomy. Given the lack of appropriate prospective surgical trials, there are no consensus recommendations for the timing and extent of surgical therapy except that any patient who is considered a surgical candidate must be able to undergo a maximal cytoreduction of the disease. Nonetheless, physicians who encounter patients who may have a surgical option for malignant pleural mesothelioma should consider referring the patient to an experienced mesothelioma surgeon at a known mesothelioma center, where the surgical procedure will reflect surgeon experience, patient characteristics, and emerging evidence of surgical benefit.

Surgery is one component of a multimodal approach. Radiation has been used as an adjuvant therapy after surgery as mesothelioma is relatively radiosensitive; doses higher than 45 Gy have been successful at reducing the risk of local recurrence after extrapleural pneumonectomy among selected patients. High-dose radiation therapy after pleurectomy decortication has, in the past, been limited by radiation injury to the ipsilateral lung, which prevents its widespread application to these patients. Neoadjuvant radiotherapy is being investigated as a novel approach, termed Surgery for Mesothelioma After Radiation Therapy (SMART); data from 69 patients at the University of Toronto show a median survival of 34 months versus 22 months (SMART vs neoadjuvant chemotherapy plus extrapleural pneumonectomy) in patients with epithelioid malignant pleural mesothelioma and an association with CD8 + tumor infiltrating lymphocyte activity. Standard practice at this time is to deliver radiation in the adjuvant setting with intensity modulated radiation therapy (IMRT). In 2019, an IASLC expert consensus established that radiation should be indicated primarily in three settings: (1) post-extrapleural pneumonectomy, (2) post-pleurectomy decortication, and (3) palliative treatment. Hemithoracic radiation with intact lung or using proton therapy should be restricted to experienced centers or in context of a clinical trial.

Although malignant pleural mesothelioma was previously considered to be chemo-resistant, newer platinum-based therapy has shown benefit as an adjuvant therapy for malignant pleural mesothelioma. The efficacy of platinum and pemetrexed (antifolate agent) was established in 2003 in a multicenter randomized trial of patients with unresectable disease, which demonstrated improved median survival time (12.1 vs 9.3 months; $P = 0.012$) and longer median time to disease progression (5.7 vs 3.9 months; $P = 0.001$) in the combination therapy group compared with cisplatin alone. Although trials of chemotherapy have shown improved survival, objective partial response or stabilization of disease, chemotherapy alone is not considered a curative option.

Trials focusing on the use of trimodality therapy are associated with improvement in survival. In a multicenter trial of induction pemetrexed and cisplatin, followed by extrapleural pneumonectomy and radiation (54 Gy), patients who completed all modes of therapy were associated with a median survival of 29.1 months. Complete or partial response to chemotherapy was associated with improved median survival (26 vs 13.9 months; $P = 0.05$). The problem however with the trimodality trials is that only 50% of the intent to treat patients receive all components of the therapy. Overall, no clear superior treatment algorithm has been established, and all patients with malignant pleural mesothelioma should be considered for referral to clinical trials.

5) What are the treatments available for widespread disease?

Expert Perspective: Patients with unresectable disease generally have poorer prognoses. As mentioned in this chapter, cisplatin- and pemetrexed-based chemotherapy can improve median survival in unresectable patients. Prospective studies have also examined the use of pemetrexed and carboplatin with similar results. Small studies have shown good response rates with the use of gemcitabine in combination with platinum agents, but small sample sizes have limited the applicability of these results. Radiation can also be used in the palliative setting to reduce chest wall pain, with side effects of fatigue, nausea, and skin irritation. Palliative surgery has been utilized to control pleural effusions either through talc pleurodesis or by indwelling pleural drainage catheters with good effect. Palliation of ascites can be accomplished with a valved intraperitoneal catheter to help the patient be more functional for second-line therapy.

The landscape for treatment, however, has now changed significantly. In October 2020, there was a landmark FDA approval for systemic treatment of malignant pleural mesothelioma with unresectable disease. The combination of the immune checkpoint modulators nivolumab and ipilimumab demonstrated an improvement in median overall survival (18 vs 14 months, combination nivolumab plus ipilimumab vs chemotherapy) in a randomized controlled trial CheckMate 743. This is the first drug regimen approved for mesothelioma in 16 years and the second FDA-approved systemic therapy treatment for mesothelioma. The reuslts of IND227 trial of chemotherapy with or without pembrolizumab was reported. This trial showed that, in patients with treatment-naive unresectable pleural mesothelioma, cisplatin and pemetrexed with pembrolizumab improved median overall survival with acceptable tolerability. This disease, like all the many other solid epithelial malignancies, is undergoing a change in treatment paradigm because immunotherapy has demonstrated significant improvement in long-term durability of responses.

Three years after undergoing extended pleurectomy decortication (with no radiographic evidence of disease), the patient returns to your office with new-onset ascites and a new contralateral pleural effusion.

6) What novel therapies and targeted molecular agents are being studied?

Expert Perspective: Several targeted molecular agents have been studied in the treatment of malignant pleural mesothelioma with disappointing results. Malignant pleural mesothelioma expresses high levels of *epidermal growth factor receptor (EGFR)*, but targeted therapies with erlotinib and gefinitib used in a phase II clinical trial have not shown promise. A phase II, multicenter, placebo-controlled, randomized trial of an anti-VEGF (vascular endothelial growth factor) monoclonal antibody, bevacizumab, or placebo in combination with gemcitabine-cisplatin did not improve progression-free or overall survival relative to placebo. However, an international Phase III Study indeed revealed an overall survival advantage when bevacizumab was added to cisplatinum-pemetrexed. Most recently, a large international study demonstrated no efficacy for the use of deacetylating agents (i.e. Vorinostat). Phase I and II trials of various agents are underway, including antimesothelin monoclonal antibodies, peptide vaccination against Wilms tumor, recombinant antimesothelin immunotoxins. Promising but early results with autologous gene modified cellular therapy using chimeric antigen receptor T cells (CAR T cells) directed against mesothelin has been reported.

7) What is the best "second-line" therapy for recurrent malignant pleural mesothelioma?

Expert Perspective: Sites of recurrence after surgery are often found in the abdomen, and after extrapleural pneumonectomy, diaphragmatic and pericardial margins are often involved. There is no standard therapy for recurrent malignant pleural mesothelioma, and patients who recur should be considered for enrollment in a clinical trial. Combination or single-agent therapies of gemcitabine, vinorelbine, paclitaxel, and docetaxel have been used with limited success. Single agent vinorelbine and pemetrexed have both been studied specifically among patients who have received prior therapies and had disappointing results. In the pemetrexed study, relative to best supportive care, chemotherapy improved disease control rate (59.3% vs 19.2%) but was not associated with improved survival (8.4 months for pemetrexed plus best supportive care vs 9.7 months for best supportive care alone; $P = 0.74$). For patients who have epithelial histologies, the standard of care has moved to chemotherapy and immunotherapy, while patients with biphasic and sarcomatoid histologies benefit more from dual immunotherapy as described above. Recently, a phase II study found *EZH2* inhibitor, tazemetostat is active in patients with relapsed or refractory *BRCA*-associated protein 1 (*BAP1*)-inactivated malignant pleural mesothelioma. Tazemetostat produced a disease control rate of 54% at 12 weeks and tumor shrinkage was observed in 35% of evaluable patients.

Palliative surgical options include chest wall debulking (controversial) and insertion of valved pleural and abdominal drainage catheters, which have been used with success.

Recommended Readings

Gomez, D.R., Rimner, A., Simone, C.B. et al. (2019). The use of radiation therapy for the treatment of malignant pleural mesothelioma: expert opinion from the National Cancer Institute Thoracic Malignancy Steering Committee, International Association for the Study of Lung Cancer, and Mesothelioma Applied Research Foundation. *J Thorac Oncol* 14 (7): 1172–1183. doi: 10.1016/j.jtho.2019.03.030. Epub 2019 May 22. PMID: 31125736.

Janne, P.A. and Baldini, E.H. (2004). Patterns of failure following surgical resection for malignant pleural mesothelioma. *Thoracic Surg Clin* 14: 567–573.

Lim, E., Darlison, L., Edwards, J. On behalf of MARS 2 Trialists et al. (2020). Mesothelioma and Radical Surgery 2 (MARS 2): Protocol for a multicentre randomised trial comparing (extended) pleurectomy decortication versus no (extended) pleurectomy decortication for patients with malignant pleural mesothelioma. *BMJ Open* 10: e038892. doi: 10.1136/bmjopen-2020-038892*.

Pass, H., Giroux, D., Kennedy, C. et al. (2016). IASLC staging and prognostic factors committee, advisory boards and participating institutions. The IASLC mesothelioma staging project: improving staging of a rare disease through international participation. *J Thorac Oncol* 11 (12): 2082–2088. doi: 10.1016/j.jtho.2016.09.123. Epub 2016 Sep 23. PMID: 27670823.

Pass, H.I., Levin, S.M., Harbut, M.R. et al. (2012). Fibulin-3 as a blood and effusion biomarker for pleural mesothelioma. *New Engl J Med* 367: 1417–1427.

Rice, D., Rusch, V., Pass, H. et al. (2011). Recommendations for uniform definitions of surgical techniques for malignant pleural mesothelioma: a consensus report of the International Association for the Study of Lung Cancer International Staging Committee and the International Mesothelioma Interest Group. *J Thorac Oncol* 6: 1304–1312.

Steele, J.P., Walley, T., and Edwards, J. (2012). A randomized trial of extended pleurectomy and decortication with pemetrexed and platinum chemotherapy versus pemetrexed and platinum chemotherapy in patients with malignant pleural mesothelioma. Paper presented at: International Mesothelioma Interest Group Meeting; October 2012; Boston, MA.

Sugarbaker, D.J. and Wolf, A.S. (2010). Surgery for malignant pleural mesothelioma. *Exp Rev Resp Med* 4: 363–372.

Zahid, I., Sharif, S., Routledge, T. et al. (2011). What is the best way to diagnose and stage malignant pleural mesothelioma? *Inter Cardio Thorac Surg* 12: 254–259.

Zalcman G, Mazieres J, Margery J, et al. A; French Cooperative Thoracic Intergroup (IFCT). Bevacizumab for newly diagnosed pleural mesothelioma in the Mesothelioma Avastin Cisplatin Pemetrexed Study (MAPS): a randomized, controlled, open-label, phase 3 trial. Lancet. 2016 Apr 2;387(10026):1405–1414. doi: 10.1016/S0140-6736(15)01238-6. Epub 2015 Dec 21. Erratum in: Lancet. 2016 Apr 2;387(10026):e24. PMID: 26719230.

Part 3

Breast Cancer

10

DCIS and LCIS

Amanda Nash[1], Rita Mukhtar[2], and Shelley Hwang[3]

[1] Department of Surgery, Duke University Medical Center, Durham, NC
[2] Department of Surgery, University of California, San Francisco, San Francisco, CA
[3] Department of Surgery, Duke University School of Medicine, Durham, NC

Introduction

The widespread adoption of screening mammography has led to a dramatic increase in the incidence of ductal carcinoma *in situ* (DCIS) in the last several decades. DCIS currently represents 20–30% of all screen-detected breast cancers and has historically been considered a precursor lesion to invasive cancer. As such, it is treated aggressively with surgical excision with or without adjuvant radiation and endocrine therapy, resulting in a 10-year survival rate of over 98%. However, despite the rise in DCIS treatment, the incidence of invasive cancer has not fallen, calling into question the prevailing understanding of the pathogenesis of breast cancer. In addition, the excellent outcomes associated with treatment make DCIS, and breast cancer generally, an ideal proving ground for de-escalation in cancer care with the goal of "right-sizing" therapies to reduce toxicities and treatment-related sequelae without sacrificing outcomes. At the present time, the mainstay of treatment for DCIS remains surgery.

Another *in situ* lesion, lobular carcinoma *in situ* (LCIS), can also lead to questions about the best management approach. Although it is not considered a precursor lesion, LCIS can be found associated with a malignancy and can indicate the presence of elevated baseline breast cancer risk.

Key management considerations for DCIS and LCIS are highlighted in the following sections and summarized in Figure 10.1.

10 DCIS and LCIS

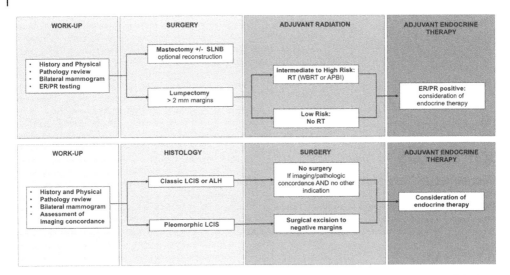

Figure 10.1 Treatment guidelines for (A) DCIS and (B) LCIS. Ongoing clinical trials (COMET, LORIS, LORD, LORETTA) may add observation as an option for primary treatment of DCIS. In addition, ongoing biomarker research may add molecular testing as part of the workup for some or all DCIS patients to determine benefit from adjuvant radiation.

Case Study 1

A 55-year-old woman presents to your clinic with newly diagnosed grade 2 estrogen receptor positive (ER+) DCIS. The estimated extent of her DCIS on mammogram is 3 cm. She is large breasted and therefore potentially a candidate for breast-conserving therapy. She mentions that she has a friend with breast cancer who required axillary surgery. The patient asks you if she is going to need to have her nodes removed as well.

1) How should ipsilateral axilla be managed in DCIS patients undergoing breast-conserving surgery and mastectomy?

Expert Perspective: The National Comprehensive Cancer Network (NCCN) recommends against routine axillary staging in patients undergoing breast-conserving therapy for DCIS without evidence of invasive disease, or in whom future ability to perform sentinel lymph node biopsy is not compromised. Because sentinel lymph node biopsy is not generally feasible after mastectomy due to division of the breast tissue from the lymphatic channels, patients undergoing mastectomy for DCIS warrant upfront axillary staging to avoid the morbidity of an axillary lymph node dissection should the mastectomy specimen contain invasive disease (upstaging). For unselected populations of patients with DCIS, the upstaging rate is about 20%.

Hung et al. (2019) retrospectively analyzed 1,992 patients aged 67–94 from the SEER database with final pathology showing pure DCIS who underwent sentinel lymph node biopsy. Using matching, they found no difference in treated recurrence, invasive recurrence, or breast cancer mortality between those who underwent sentinel lymph node biopsy and those who did not. Francis et al. (2015) similarly reported no difference in survival among patients with pure DCIS with and without positive sentinel lymph nodes, suggesting that sentinel lymph node biopsy, even if positive, has no prognostic value even in such patients with a presumed occult invasive component. Therefore, sentinel lymph node biopsy should not be routinely performed with breast-conserving therapy because in these patients, sentinel lymph node biopsy may still be performed if an initial lumpectomy results in upstaging.

Case Study 2

A 70-year-old otherwise healthy patient presents with ER+ DCIS. You discuss treatment options, and she elects to proceed with breast-conserving therapy. Her final pathology returns with DCIS within 1 mm of the final inferior margin. She returns to clinic to discuss next steps.

2) What is the appropriate margin width in DCIS?

Expert Perspective: A great deal of research has focused on quantifying the appropriate margin width in DCIS because it is one of the few modifiable risk factors for recurrence. Consensus guidelines published in 2016 by the Society of Surgical Oncology, the American Society for Radiation Oncology, and the American Society of Clinical Oncology recommend 2 mm margins. This recommendation was based on a meta-analysis that included 7,883 patients, most of whom underwent lumpectomy with radiation, which found a significant reduction in ipsilateral breast tumor recurrence with 2 mm margins compared to >0 or 1 mm margins (HR 0.51; CI 0.31–0.85). However, the authors found that a margin of >0 or 1 mm significantly reduced the risk of recurrence when compared to positive margins (HR 0.45; CI 0.32–0.61). When a 2 mm margin was compared to smaller negative margins (>0 or 1 mm) there was a nonsignificant reduction in the risk of ipsilateral breast tumor recurrence. Thus, the panel felt that there was sufficient evidence to support a margin of 2 mm providing optimal local control.

The guidelines stipulated that in cases of narrower but negative margins, clinical judgment should be used in determining the appropriateness of re-excision, taking into consideration residual calcifications, location of the positive margin, impact on cosmesis, and overall health of the patient. In this case, where the patient is otherwise healthy and the positive margin is at a location where additional breast tissue can be easily excised, the most appropriate course of action would likely be re-excision.

A recent analysis of 1,491 DCIS patients treated at MD Anderson Cancer Center supported the conclusion that women with margin width <2 mm have an increased risk of recurrence (Tadros et al. 2019). However, when analyzed by receipt of radiation, the authors found that this association disappeared in those patients who were treated with radiation therapy. Within the limits of the retrospective methodology, these results suggest that in patients who are poor candidates for or who decline re-excision, radiation therapy may limit recurrence risk. Of note, endocrine therapy did not mitigate this effect.

Case Study 3

A 50-year-old woman presents to you with ER+ DCIS. The total extent of disease is 2 cm; however, she is small breasted and will require a mastectomy. There is no clinical or radiographic evidence of nipple involvement. She asks you about a nipple-sparing mastectomy and reconstruction.

3) What is the opinion about nipple-sparing mastectomy and reconstruction in DCIS?

Expert Perspective: The greatest concern in nipple-sparing mastectomy as compared with skin-sparing mastectomy is the risk of occult nipple-areolar complex involvement. Factors that increase the risk of nipple-areolar complex involvement, according to a study by Mallon et al. (2013), include tumor-to-nipple distance of less than 2 cm, high grade, ER/progesterone receptor (PR) negativity, tumor size greater than 5 cm, retro-areolar/central location, and multicentricity. The authors found similar rates of nipple involvement across tumor types including DCIS, LCIS, and invasive carcinomas. The NCCN guidelines mandate nipple margin assessment, but there are no other strict exclusion criteria. As long as this patient meets other criteria for nipple-sparing mastectomy, a DCIS diagnosis is not a reason to withhold it as an appropriate surgical option. As in all patients considering nipple-sparing mastectomy, the patient should be counseled of the risk of nipple loss secondary to necrosis or its involvement with disease on final pathology.

Case Study 4

A 63-year-old woman presents with new suspicious calcifications on a recent screening mammogram. Core needle biopsy reveals ER+ and low-grade DCIS with minimal necrosis. She opts for breast conserving therapy. The final surgical pathology report shows atypical ductal hyperplasia and biopsy site changes from the core biopsy, which appears to have removed the entire DCIS lesion. A follow up mammogram reveals no residual calcifications. The patient asks you about forgoing radiation because she is concerned about the side effects and time commitment.

4) What is the benefit of adjuvant radiation therapy in DCIS? Does it improve the overall survival?

Expert Perspective: The benefit of adjuvant radiation following lumpectomy for DCIS is well documented in high quality randomized studies including the NSABP B-17 and B-24 protocols. As seen in Table 10.1, radiation reproducibly reduces the risk of ipsilateral recurrence by half in patients with DCIS regardless of margin status, age, tumor size, focality, hormone receptor status, use of tamoxifen, presence of comedonecrosis, histologic type, and grade. To date, there has never been a population of patients with DCIS shown to not benefit from radiation in a randomized study. However, radiation therapy has also never been shown to improve overall survival in DCIS patients. Consequently, the decision to undergo radiation therapy is one that balances the risk of recurrence with the potential side effects and its impact on quality of life. Therefore, there has been an active pursuit to identify low-risk patients who may be able to forego radiation therapy. The 15-year risk of contralateral breast cancer in DCIS patients without endocrine therapy is approximately 10–11% (Wapnir et al. 2011), so this seems a reasonable threshold at which radiation therapy may be omitted.

In this case, the lesion was screen detected, small, and low grade, and it was excised with widely negative margins. It therefore falls into a lower risk category. Table 10.2 compares the outcomes of DCIS patients who underwent lumpectomy without radiation therapy in prospective trials. Among low-risk patients, the recurrence rate is 6.7–15.5% at 7–12 years follow-up. Mushen et al. (2017) examined patients with minimal volume DCIS,

Table 10.1 Comparison of outcomes among clinical trials for patients with DCIS who underwent excision alone.

Study	Study design	Accrual	Patients, n[a]	Time to recurrence[b] (median years)	Local recurrence rate	Pathologic inclusion criteria	Endocrine Therapy[c]
NSABP B-17	Double arm RCT	1985–1990	403	17.25	35%	Grade 1–3, tumor-free margins	0%
EORTC 10853	Double arm RCT	1986–1996	503	10	26%	≤5 cm, Grade 1–3, tumor-free margins[d]	Not Recommended[e]
SweDCIS	Double arm RCT	1987–1999	520	5	22%	Grade 1–3, tumor-free margins[f]	3%
UK/ANZ	2×2 factorial RCT	1990–1998	508	10	19.4%	Grade 1–3, tumor-free margins	52%
DFCI	Single arm nonrandomized trial	1995–2002	158	10	15.5%	≤2.5 cm, Grade 1–2, 1 cm margins	0%
E5194	Double arm nonrandomized trial	1997–2002	Cohort 1: 561	12	14.4%	≤2.5 cm, Grade 1–2, 3 mm margins	31%
			Cohort 2: 104	12	24.6%	≤1 cm, Grade 3, 3 mm margins	24%
RTOG 9804	Double arm RCT	1998–2006	298	7	6.7%	≤2.5 cm, Grade 1–2, 3 mm margins	62%[g]

[a] Number of patients in excision alone arm.
[b] Time to recurrence curves in years, calculated by the Kaplan-Meier method unless otherwise noted.
[c] Percentage of patients receiving endocrine therapy in excision only arm of study, unless otherwise specified.
[d] 22% positive margins.
[e] Percentage of patients receiving endocrine therapy not quantified.
[f] 10.7% positive margins.
[g] Percentage of patients receiving endocrine therapy in both arms.

Table 10.2 Outcomes in randomized clinical trials evaluating the use of radiation in patients with DCIS.

Study	Study design	Accrual	Patients, n[a]	Follow-up (median years)	Local recurrence rate, no RT	Local recurrence rate, RT	Pathologic inclusion criteria	Endocrine therapy[b]
NSABP B-17	Double arm RCT	1985–1990	813	17.25	35%	19.8%	Grade 1–3, tumor-free margins	0%
EORTC 10853	Double arm RCT	1986–1996	1,010	10	26%	15%	≤5 cm, Grade 1–3, tumor-free margins[c]	Not recommended[d]
SweDCIS	Double arm RCT	1987–1999	1,046	5	22%	7%	Grade 1–3, tumor-free margins[e]	3%
UK/ANZ	2×2 factorial RCT	1990–1998	1,030	10	19.4%	7.1%	Grade 1–3, tumor free margins	54%
RTOG 9804	Double arm RCT	1998–2006	585	7	6.7%	0.9%	≤2.5 cm, Grade 1–2, 3 mm margins	62%

[a] Number of patients enrolled in both arms.
[b] Percentage of patients in both arms receiving endocrine therapy unless otherwise stated.
[c] 22% positive margins.
[d] Percentage of patients receiving endocrine therapy not reported.
[e] 10.7% positive margins.

defined as DCIS completely excised on core needle biopsy, as in the case presented here. They found a 10-year ipsilateral breast tumor recurrence rate of 13.9% among patients with low grade lesions who did not receive radiation therapy. The NCCN permits the exclusion of radiation in patients who are at low risk (not defined further) of recurrence. This patient's risk of ipsilateral breast tumor recurrence is likely slightly higher than her risk of contralateral breast cancer. Although this patient might benefit from radiation, her absolute risk reduction would be small. It is therefore reasonable to discuss omission of radiation in the context of shared decision-making with this patient. Alternatively, one could consider molecular testing or other risk stratification methods to better assess this patient's need for radiation.

Role of accelerated partial breast irradiation in DCIS: If the patient wishes to proceed with radiation, she is also eligible to receive accelerated partial breast irradiation because she meets RTOG 9804 criteria. The benefits of accelerated partial breast irradiation include a lower total dose of radiation and fewer treatment days. Potential drawbacks include the possibility of leaving occult disease in the breast untreated. This is of particular concern in DCIS where skip lesions increase the risk of residual disease. The largest and most mature clinical trial investigating the use of accelerated partial breast irradiation For DCIS is the NSABP B-39/RTOG 0413 study, which randomized 4,216 patients to WBRT or accelerated partial breast irradiation. About 24% of included patients had DCIS. At 10 years of follow-up, there was no increased risk of ipsilateral breast tumor recurrence in the DCIS patients who received accelerated partial breast irradiation (HR 1.01; CI 0.61–1.68). The RAPID trial randomized DCIS patients with tumors ≤3 cm to either accelerated partial breast irradiation or WBRT. At a median follow-up of 8.6 years, there was no difference in ipsilateral recurrence between the study groups, which included 18% DCIS patients (HR 1.27; 90% CI 0.84–1.91).

In summary, this patient is young and otherwise healthy and has a slightly elevated risk of ipsilateral breast tumor recurrence as compared with contralateral breast cancer if she does not receive radiation. Therefore, any benefit from adjuvant radiation would be small. Reasonable treatment options include APBI or traditional WBRT, additional risk stratification (DCIS Score, DCISionRT), or omission of radiation with close monitoring.

Case Study 5

You are seeing a 52-year-old postmenopausal woman who had a lumpectomy and radiation for DCIS two years ago. She had been taking her prescribed tamoxifen therapy but tells you she stopped it recently due to side effects. She asks you if she can remain off it or try a different medication.

5) What is the added value of antihormonal therapy in DCIS?

Expert Perspective: Two large, randomized studies have evaluated the use of tamoxifen in patients with DCIS, shown in Table 10.3. In the UK/ANZ study, tamoxifen reduced the risk of any new breast event by approximately 30%, primarily driven by decreased recurrent ipsilateral DCIS and contralateral invasive disease. Subgroup analysis showed that this benefit was restricted to those patients not receiving radiotherapy, likely due to relatively small numbers of patients who received radiation. The NSABP B-24 study

Table 10.3 Outcomes in randomized trials evaluating the use of tamoxifen in DCIS.

Study	Study design	Accrual	Patients, n[a]	Follow-up (median years)	All new breast events, no tamoxifen[b]	All new breast events, tamoxifen[b]	Pathologic inclusion criteria	Radiation therapy[c]
NSABP B-24[d]	Double arm RCT	1991–1994	732	14.5	31%	20%	Grade 1–3, 25.8% positive or unknown margins	100%
UK/ANZ[e]	2×2 factorial RCT	1990–1998	1,576	10	24.6%	18.1%	Grade 1–3, tumor-free margins	33%

[a] Total number of patients enrolled in both arms.
[b] Recurrence rate for all patients in each arm, regardless of radiation treatment.
[c] Percentage of patients receiving radiation therapy in both arms.
[d] Data from subgroup analysis of patients with ER positive DCIS.
[e] Trial did not include estrogen receptor testing.

randomized patients to breast conserving therapy with radiation therapy with or without tamoxifen. In an analysis of ER+ patients, tamoxifen reduced the risk of any breast event by 42% (HR 0.58; CI 0.42–0.81). Tamoxifen is therefore routinely offered to ER+ patients undergoing breast-conserving therapy for DCIS.

Table 10.4 compares the results from two clinical trials evaluating the differential effects of tamoxifen and anastrozole in postmenopausal women with DCIS. Anastrozole and tamoxifen have similar efficacy, with a potential small advantage to anastrozole in women under 60, per NSABP B-35. In addition, the Tam01 trial demonstrated that patients with intraepithelial neoplasia can be treated with a reduced dose and duration of tamoxifen (5 mg/d for three years) while still achieving similar risk reduction as traditional tamoxifen therapy (20 mg/d for five years) with fewer side effects (HR 0.48; CI 0.26–0.92 vs placebo).

It is therefore reasonable to recommend dose reduction of tamoxifen or switching from tamoxifen to an aromatase inhibitor for the remainder of this patient's course. If she is unable to tolerate either of these, cessation of endocrine therapy could be considered.

6) **What is the status of risk-prediction models and sequencing to better identify the low-risk DCIS?**

Expert Perspective: The goal of prediction models in DCIS is to identify a population of patients who are at low risk of recurrence to help guide management decisions and prevent overtreatment. The first of these, the Van Nuys Prognostic Index (VNPI), was created using a large single institution database. The index takes into consideration four factors: age, extent of DCIS, histology and necrosis, and margin width.

Unfortunately, the VNPI had poor validity and discriminatory power in external populations, limiting its clinical utility. An alternative is the Memorial Sloan Kettering Cancer Center nomogram. Using 10 clinical, pathologic, and treatment variables, this nomogram predicts

Table 10.4 Outcomes in randomized clinical trials evaluating the efficacy of tamoxifen vs anastrozole in DCIS.

Study	Study design	Accrual	Patients, n[a]	Follow-up (median years)	All new breast events, tamoxifen[b]	All new breast events, anastrozole[b]	P-value	Pathologic inclusion criteria	Menopausal status	Radiationtherapy[c]
IBIS-II DCIS	Double arm RCT	2003–2012	2,938	7.2	5%	5%	NS	Grade 1–3, tumor-free margins, ER/PR+	Postmenopausal	71%
NSABP B-35	Double arm RCT	2003–2006	3,077	9	7.9%	5.8%	.02[d]	Grade 1–3, tumor-free margin, ER/PR+	Postmenopausal	100%

[a] Total number of patients enrolled in both arms.
[b] Recurrence rate for all patients in each arm, regardless of radiation treatment.
[c] Percentage of patients receiving radiation therapy in both arms.
[d] On subgroup analysis, result only significant for patients younger than 60 years old.

the probability of local recurrence at 5 and 10 years after breast-conserving therapy. Multiple attempts at external validation have found this nomogram to have imperfect discrimination and calibration, as model performance likely differs based on patient population.

In general, the ability of clinical, pathologic, and treatment variables alone to discriminate between high- and low-risk DCIS is limited. This has spurred a more recent focus on molecular markers as predictors of local recurrence. The DCIS Score is a 12-gene assay for DCIS that estimates the 10-year risk of recurrence following breast conserving therapy without radiation. The DCIS Score was initially tested in a cohort of patients enrolled in the ECOG-ACRIN 5194 study. In this low-risk population, the 10-year risks of an ipsilateral breast event were 10.6%, 26.7%, and 25.9% for the low-, intermediate-, and high-risk groups, respectively. The rates of invasive cancer were 3.7%, 12.3%, and 19.2%, respectively. These findings were confirmed in a larger cohort by Rakovitch et al. (2015). In the study, 718 patients were included in the final analysis, which demonstrated that the DCIS Score correlated with local recurrence (low, 12.7%; intermediate, 33%; high, 27.8%), albeit with less discrimination than in the E5194 dataset.

Another scoring system, the DCISionRT, has recently been shown to have prognostic as well as potential predictive value in DCIS. The test uses seven protein markers and four clinicopathologic factors to create a numeric score from 0 to 10 according to the 10-year recurrence/progression risk to help inform treatment decisions. A cutoff of 3 separates the low- and high-risk groups. The authors have also shown that the low-risk decision score group derives minimal benefit from radiation, with a 10-year risk of any ipsilateral breast event of 8% without radiation compared to 7% with radiation. External validation has confirmed the test's prognostic value for 10-year recurrence and its ability to identify a population with minimal benefit from radiotherapy.

7) **What is the existing evidence for active surveillance alone as a management option for low-risk DCIS?**

Expert Perspective: Because DCIS is almost always surgically excised at the time of diagnosis, there are sparse data in patients managed without surgery. However, retrospective registry data suggest that the risk of invasive progression may be less than 10% at 10 years in some favorable risk populations (Ryser et al. 2019). Four major clinical trials are underway to investigate the safety of active monitoring for low-risk DCIS lesions as opposed to standard surgical and adjuvant therapies: LORIS, COMET, LORD, and LORETTA. These studies will enroll both low- and intermediate-grade ER+ DCIS. The primary endpoint of all four studies is progression to ipsilateral invasive breast cancer. These trials will help determine whether the range of treatment options for DCIS may be expanded in the future to include close monitoring, with or without endocrine therapy.

Lobular carcinoma *in situ* (LCIS)

Case Study 6

A 47-year-old perimenopausal woman has a first screening mammogram that identifies calcifications. Subsequent diagnostic mammogram demonstrates a 1 cm span of pleomorphic calcifications, and stereotactic core needle biopsy shows classic lobular carcinoma *in situ* (LCIS).

8) Should this patient be recommended to undergo excisional biopsy?

Expert Perspective: Multiple studies demonstrate that the presence of LCIS constitutes a risk factor for future breast cancer development in either breast; as such, LCIS is not thought to be a precursor lesion, and surgical removal of the area of LCIS does not reduce baseline breast cancer risk. However, LCIS can be found concurrently with DCIS or invasive malignancy, so excisional biopsy should be considered. The upgrade rate of LCIS depends on radiology-pathology concordance as well as the morphologic features of the LCIS. For classic LCIS, which is identified as a small area of calcifications or is identified incidentally when another lesion is being biopsied, upgrade rates to malignancy are reported to be less than 5%. However, when LCIS is found upon biopsy of a mass, upgrade rates are higher. In addition, when core biopsy shows LCIS in addition to other high-risk lesions such as atypical ductal hyperplasia, upgrade rates to malignancy upon excision can reach nearly 30%. For this patient, where imaging and pathology results are felt to be concordant, the span of calcifications is small, and LCIS has classic morphology, the risk of upgrade is low and excisional biopsy could be omitted after discussion of risks and benefits. Many patients with LCIS pursue high-risk screening, and as such the lesion will undergo close monitoring for change.

9) If the core biopsy showed pleomorphic (nonclassic) LCIS, should the patient be recommended to undergo excisional biopsy?

Expert Perspective: When LCIS has central comedonecrosis or marked pleomorphism of the nuclei, pathologists may describe these lesions as florid LCIS or pleomorphic LCIS. These nonclassic forms of LCIS appear to be biologically distinct, with a higher risk of associated malignancy and risk of recurrence. An institutional analysis of 76 nonclassic LCIS lesions found that the upgrade rate to malignancy on excisional biopsy was 36%, with no radiographic features being associated with malignancy. As such, nonclassic LCIS such as pleomorphic LCIS should be treated with surgical excision. Although the optimal margin width when excising nonclassic LCIS is unknown, small series suggest that positive margins may be associated with higher risk of local recurrence. As such, excision to negative margins is warranted.

10) Should women with LCIS undergo risk reduction or high-risk screening?

Expert Perspective: Yes; a diagnosis of LCIS confers high lifetime risk of future breast cancer development in both ipsilateral and contralateral breast, with an analysis of the SEER database showing a cumulative incidence of breast malignancy of 11.3% at 10 years and 19.8% at 20 years in women with prior LCIS. NCCN guidelines from January 2021 recommend risk reduction for those with LCIS and at least 10-year life expectancy, with endocrine therapy preferred over surgical risk reduction.

Recommended Readings

Early Breast Cancer Trialists' Collaborative Group (2010). Overview of the randomized trials of radiotherapy in ductal carcinoma in situ of the breast. *J Natl Cancer Inst Monogr* 41: 162–177.

Francis, A.M., Haugen, C.E., Grimes, L.M. et al. (2015). Is sentinel lymph node dissection warranted in patients with a diagnosis of ductal carcinoma in situ? *Ann Surg Oncol* 22 (13): 4270–4279.

Hoffman, D.I., Zhang, P.J., and Tchou, J. (2019). Breast-conserving surgery for pure non-classic lobular carcinoma in situ: a single institution's experience. *Surg Oncol* 28: 190–194.

Hung, P., Wang, S.Y., Killelea, B.K. et al. (2019). Long-term outcomes of sentinel lymph node biopsy for ductal carcinoma in situ. *JNCI Cancer Spectr* 3 (4): pkz052.

Rakovitch, E., Nofech-Mozes, S., Hanna, W. et al. (2015). A population-based validation study of the DCIS Score predicting recurrence risk in individuals treated by breast-conserving surgery alone. *Breast Cancer Research and Treatment* 152 (2): 389–398. https://doi.org/10.1007/s10549-015-3464-6

Mallon, P., Feron, J.G., Couturaud, B. et al. (2013). The role of nipple-sparing mastectomy in breast cancer: a comprehensive review of the literature. *Plast Reconstr Surg* 131 (5): 969–984.

Morrow, M., Van Zee, K.J., Solin, L.J. et al. (2016). Surgical Society of Oncology – American Society for Radiation Oncology – American Society of Clinical Oncology consensus guideline on margins for breast-conserving surgery with whole breast irradiation in ductal in situ. *Pract Radiat Oncol* 6 (5): 287–295.

Muhsen, S., Barrio, A.V., Miller, M. et al. (2017). Outcomes of women with minimal volume ductal carcinoma in situ completely excised on core biopsy. *Ann Surg Oncol* 24 (13): 3888–3895.

Nakhlis, F., Harrison, B.T., Giess, C.S. et al. (2019). Evaluating the rate of upgrade to invasive breast cancer and/or ductal carcinoma in situ following core biopsy diagnosis of non-classic lobular carcinoma in situ. *Ann Surg Oncol* 26 (1): 55–61.

Rendi, M.H., Dintzis, S.M., Lehman, C.D. et al. (2012). Lobular in-situ neoplasia on breast core needle biopsy: imaging indication and pathologic extent can identify which patients require excisional biopsy. *Ann Surg Oncol* 19 (3): 914–921.

Ryser, M.D., Weaver, D.L., Zhao, F. et al. (2019). Cancer outcomes in DCIS patients without locoregional treatment. *JNCI* 111 (9): djy220.

Tadros, A.B., Smith, B.D., Shen, Y. et al. (2019). Ductal carcinoma in situ and margins <2 mm: contemporary outcomes with breast conservation. *Ann Surg* 269 (1): 150–157.

Wapnir, I.L., Dignam, J.J., Fisher, B. et al. (2011). Long-term outcomes of invasive ipsilateral breast tumor recurrences after lumpectomy in NSABP B-17 and B-24 randomized clinical trials for DCIS. *JNCI* 106 (6): 478–488.

Wong, S.M., King, T., Boileau, J.M. et al. (2017). Population-based analysis of breast cancer incidence and survival outcomes in women diagnosed with lobular carcinoma in situ. *Ann Surg Oncol* 24 (9): 2509–2517.

11

Early-Stage ER/PR–Positive, HER2-Negative Breast Cancer

William J. Gradishar

Northwestern University – Feinberg School of Medicine, Chicago, IL

Introduction

Adjuvant endocrine therapy of early stage, hormone sensitive breast cancer continues to evolve with unanswered questions regarding the optimal duration of both tamoxifen and aromatase inhibitors as well as integration of newer targeted therapies for those with high-risk disease. These questions remain germane because estrogen receptor (ER)–positive breast cancer has an ongoing risk of recurrence 20 years after the original diagnosis, with a greater absolute risk for late recurrence especially for those with higher risk features at diagnosis (Chapter 12). In an era where de-escalation of therapy is an important focus, knowing which patients require more therapy remains important and is the subject of multiple recent trials in both pre- and post- menopausal women with hormone sensitive breast cancer. The cases in this chapter highlight some of the important issues.

Case Study 1

A 62-year-old postmenopausal female presents following a routine mammogram identified a 2 cm spiculated right-sided mass. Due to the COVID-19 pandemic, she missed her last two annual screening mammograms. She had an ultrasound of the axilla that revealed one suspicious appearing node. Biopsy of the breast and node were positive for ER+/progesterone receptor (PR)+/HER2− invasive ductal carcinoma with a proliferation index (Ki67) of 15%. She underwent a lumpectomy and sentinel lymph node biopsy (SLNB), which revealed a 2.2 cm invasive ductal carcinoma and two of three involved axillary nodes. The patient's past medical history was unremarkable, and there was no family history of breast cancer or ovarian cancer.

1) **How would you proceed with recommendations for adjuvant systemic therapy in addition to the planned breast irradiation?**
   A) Chemotherapy with an anthracycline-based regimen followed by adjuvant endocrine therapy
   B) Oncotype Dx™ to determine whether chemotherapy is required

---

Cancer Consult: Expertise in Clinical Practice, Volume 1: Solid Tumors & Supportive Care,
Second Edition. Edited by Syed A. Abutalib, Maurie Markman, Al B. Benson III, and Hope S. Rugo.
© 2024 John Wiley & Sons Ltd. Published 2024 by John Wiley & Sons Ltd.

C) Adjuvant endocrine therapy with the addition of abemacilib
D) Consider the addition of olaparib if the patient has a germline *BRCA* mutation

Expert Perspective: The critical choice in this case is whether or not the patient will require adjuvant chemotherapy. Until relatively recently, a patient in this age group with positive axillary nodes would have automatically received a recommendation for systemic chemotherapy in addition to adjuvant endocrine therapy. We learned from the use of molecular assays such as Mammaprint™ and Oncotype Dx™ that we could identify patients with ER+/HER2-, early stage breast cancer with 1–3 positive nodes who may avoid adjuvant chemotherapy without compromising the patient's overall outcome. For instance, in node-negative breast cancer, based on the TAILORx study, the 21-gene assay, Oncotype Dx™, has been shown to be predictive of chemotherapy benefit in node-negative, ER+ disease. With Mammaprint™, it can be argued that it is possible to identify a patient with a prognosis so good that little if any additional benefit could be derived from adjuvant chemotherapy, but only the Oncotype Dx™ had a confirmed predictive value for chemotherapy. If biology trumps clinical characteristics, it was postulated that the recurrence score could potentially identify similar patients with axillary node-positive disease who may safely avoid chemotherapy and be treated with endocrine therapy alone. The SWOG 8814 trial, though small and statistically underpowered, suggested that the recurrence score may indeed identify such patients. Recently the results of the RxPONDER trial were reported at ESMO 2021 showing that subgroup of patients can be identified that derive no benefit from adjuvant chemotherapy. The RxPONDER trial, which examined the ability of the 21-gene recurrence score to identify patients with ER+, HER2− disease with up to three positive axillary lymph nodes and a recurrence score of ≤ 25 who could safely avoid adjuvant chemotherapy and be treated with endocrine therapy alone. The patient described does not have sufficient risk to meet the eligibility for the monachE trial with abemaciclib and similarly does not meet the criteria for olaparib in the OLYMPIA trial.

Correct Answer: B

2) **Which of the following statements about RxPONDER study is correct?**
   A) RxPONDER enrolled patients with one to four positive axillary nodes
   B) Only patients with an intermediate recurrence score were randomized to endocrine therapy with and without chemotherapy
   C) Ovarian suppression was used in a majority of premenopausal patients
   D) Approximately one-third of patients were premenopausal, and two-thirds were postmenopausal

Expert Perspective: RxPONDER enrolled patients with one to three positive axillary nodes who would have been able to receive standard adjuvant chemotherapy. The 5,083 patients with a recurrence score of 0–25 were randomized to endocrine therapy alone or with chemotherapy (50% received TC [docetaxel/cyclophosphamide]). At the third prespecified interim analysis, 410 invasive, disease-free survival events had occurred, triggering the report of the data.

Ovarian suppression was used in a minority of premenopausal patients (16% in the endocrine therapy alone arm, 3% in the endocrine therapy plus chemotherapy arm).

Approximately one-third of patients were premenopausal, and two-thirds were postmenopausal; 43% had a recurrence score of 0–13, and 57% had a recurrence score of 14–25; and 66% had one positive node, 25% had two nodes, and only 9% had three positive nodes. The investigators reported that there was no interaction between the benefit of chemotherapy and recurrence score; in other words, the relative benefit was not smaller with a lower recurrence score and not greater with a higher recurrence score. At a median follow-up of 5.1 years, the invasive disease-free survival (iDFS) (primary endpoint) for the entire population, was improved by 1.4% in those receiving chemotherapy.

Correct Answer: D

3) What was the outcome differences between premenopausal and postmenopausal patients in the RxPONDER study?

Expert Perspective: Approximately, 70% of patients < 50 years and 30% of those ≥ 50 years were premenopausal. There was no benefit from chemotherapy in postmenopausal patients, whereas there was a 5.2% absolute difference in iDFS favoring chemotherapy in premenopausal patients with the reduction of DFS events being in distant metastatic sites. In postmenopausal patients, the effect of adjuvant chemotherapy did not differ among those with a recurrence score of 0–13 or 14–25 (no benefit in either group), though in premenopausal patients, there was a numerical increase in the benefit derived from chemotherapy in those with a recurrence score of 14–25 compared with a recurrence score of 0–13 (6.2% vs. 3.9 %, respectively). In premenopausal patients, the absolute improvement in iDFS was similar whether they had one or two to three positive nodes. There was no difference in overall survival for those who were postmenopausal, and the addition of chemotherapy conferred roughly a 1.3% improvement in outcome.

These data suggest that in postmenopausal patients with one to three nodes, there would be little benefit to the addition of chemotherapy. An important caveat is that only 9% of patients had three positive nodes, so one must have a discussion with the patient regarding the role of chemotherapy in this particular group. Only a minority of premenopausal patients received ovarian suppression, which raises the question of whether optimizing endocrine therapy in premenopausal patients could have resulted in similar outcomes to what chemotherapy conferred. Finally, these data suggest that premenopausal patients with one to three positive lymph nodes will derive benefit from chemotherapy. At the 2021 SABCS, updated data on the RxPONDER data in premenopausal women were presented. In the original study, roughly 5,000 pre- and post- menopausal women with breast cancer were randomized to endocrine therapy with or without chemotherapy. At a median five-year follow-up, premenopausal women had a 5.2% absolute benefit in iDFS with the addition of chemotherapy (94.2% for the endocrine therapy plus chemotherapy group vs. 89.0% for the endocrine therapy group). The postmenopausal women had no benefit.

In updated data presented at 2021 SABCS and with a median six-year follow-up, the absolute benefit for iDFS among premenopausal women who underwent chemotherapy increased to 5.9%. Chemotherapy was also associated with a 3.3% absolute benefit in distant DFS. With chemotherapy, premenopausal women with a recurrence score of 0–13 had a 2.3% absolute improvement in the distant recurrence-free interval, and those with a score of 14–25 had a 2.8% improvement.

Rates of iDFS were not statistically different among those who did and did not undergo ovarian function suppression. The RxPONDER trial design was amended to exclude patients with axillary micro-metastases, but prior to the change, 206 premenopausal women were included with an exploratory analysis suggesting an improvement in five-year iDFS of 7.3%. Furthermore, almost 60% of patients in the endocrine therapy alone arm and 80% in the chemo-endocrine arm stopped having regular menstrual periods in the first 24 months, with an associated improvement in iDFS in both arms. It remains unclear from these data whether optimal endocrine therapy with ovarian suppression function suppression can substitute for chemotherapy.

4) **What should be the duration of endocrine therapy in early stage HR+/HER2-negative breast cancer?**

Expert Perspective: There are many options for adjuvant endocrine therapy which are outlined in the National Comprehensive Cancer Network (NCCN) guidelines. For most postmenopausal women an aromatase inhibitor would be chosen and continued for a minimum of five years though several trials have explored longer durations. There is an ongoing risk of recurrence in ER+ disease that continues to increase over 20 years regardless of initial stage (Figure 11.1; Pan et al. 2018).

Most clinical trials evaluating longer durations of an aromatase inhibitor beyond five years show no, or minimal, effect on the development of distant disease recurrence. The effect that is observed with longer durations of aromatase inhibitor therapy is largely a prevention effect on the development of a second breast cancers. Longer durations of adjuvant endocrine therapy, with either tamoxifen or an aromatase inhibitor, must be individualized, taking into account the ongoing risk of recurrence and tolerance to prior therapy.

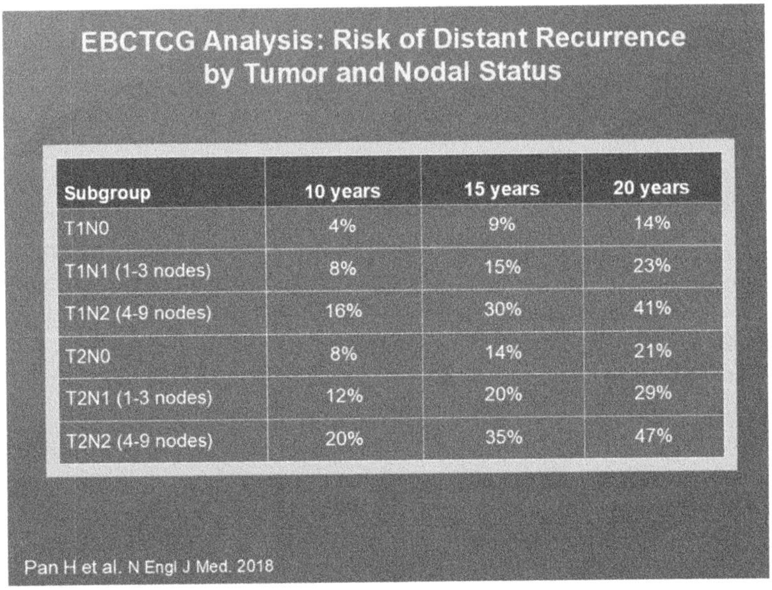

EBCTCG Analysis: Risk of Distant Recurrence by Tumor and Nodal Status

Subgroup	10 years	15 years	20 years
T1N0	4%	9%	14%
T1N1 (1-3 nodes)	8%	15%	23%
T1N2 (4-9 nodes)	16%	30%	41%
T2N0	8%	14%	21%
T2N1 (1-3 nodes)	12%	20%	29%
T2N2 (4-9 nodes)	20%	35%	47%

Pan H et al. N Engl J Med. 2018

Figure 11.1 EBCTCG analysis – Risk of distant recurrence by tumor and nodal status.

Introduction | 133

In a higher-risk patient such as the one in Case Study 1, extending the duration of aromatase inhibitor therapy to 7.5–8 years can be justified, particularly if the patient is tolerating treatment. There are individuals who cannot tolerate aromatase inhibitor therapy. In such cases, tamoxifen should be continued for a total of 10 years based on the ATLAS and aTTom trials showing an improvement in survival with durations of therapy beyond five years (Figures 11.2 and 11.3).

5) **What would be the role of cyclin-dependent kinase 4/6 (CDK 4/6) inhibitor in patient presented in case study 1?**

Expert Perspective: The patient presented case study 1 has an increased risk of recurrence, the only other consideration that might be put forth is whether she would be a candidate for a cyclin-dependent kinase 4/6 (CDK 4/6) inhibitor. The monarchE trial demonstrated that patients with four or more lymph nodes had an improved outcome when abemaciclib was added to adjuvant endocrine therapy.

As noted, eligibility for the monarchE trial included patients viewed as high risk and eligible for the trial if they had four or more positive axillary nodes. In addition, patients with one to three positive axillary nodes and either a tumor greater than 5 cm or a histologic grade 3 or centrally tested Ki-67 greater than 20% were eligible (Figure 11.4).

As noted, the entire group who received abemaciclib had an improved outcome compared with those who received endocrine therapy alone. In addition, those with high proliferation, or Ki-67, also had improved outcome with abemaciclib (Figure 11.5). The NCCN guidelines have now endorsed the use of abemaciclib selectively for patients who fit the criteria for eligibility into the monarchE trial. There is an increase in gastrointestinal symptoms for those receiving abemaciclib, including diarrhea. Most of these side effects can be well controlled, but the toxicity profile of the combination is different compared to endocrine therapy alone and the treatment duration with abemaciclib is two years.

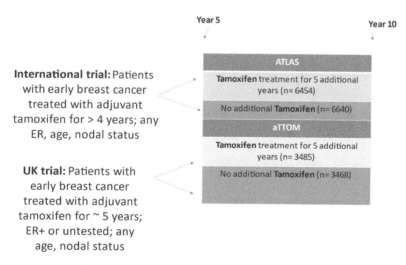

Figure 11.2 Tamoxifen duration in ATLAS and aTTom trials in early breast cancer.

Pooled Analysis ATLAS & aTTom
Breast Cancer Mortality

10 vs 5 years BC mortality RR by period in ER+ ve (or unknown) patients	ATLAS[1] ER+ve n = 10543* HR (95% CI)	aTTom[2] ER+ ve n+ 6934 In UK HR (95% CI)	Combined ER+ve n = 17477 HR (95% CI)
Years 5-9	0.92 (0.77- 1.09)	1.08 (0.85- 1.38)	0.97 (0.84-1.15)
Years 10+	0.75 (0.63-0.90) p= .002	0.75 (0.63-0.90) p= .007	0.75 (0.65-0.86 p= .00004
All years	0.83 (0.73-0.94) p= .004	0.88 (0.74-1.03) p= .1	0.85 (0.77-0.94) p= .001

Also, significant improvements in **overall survival**

5-9 yrs   HR 0.99   (0.89-1.10)
10-14 years HR 0.84 (0.77-0.93)   (p= 0.0007)
All yrs   HR 0.91   (0.84-0.97)   (p= 0.008)

*IPCW (Inverse probability of censoring weighted) estimate of effect in ER+
Gray RG et al. ASCO 2013 (Abstract 5); 1 ATLAS- Smith ASCO 2014; 2aTTom: Gray ASCO 2013

Figure 11.3 Outcome analysis of ATLAS and aTTom trials in early breast cancer.

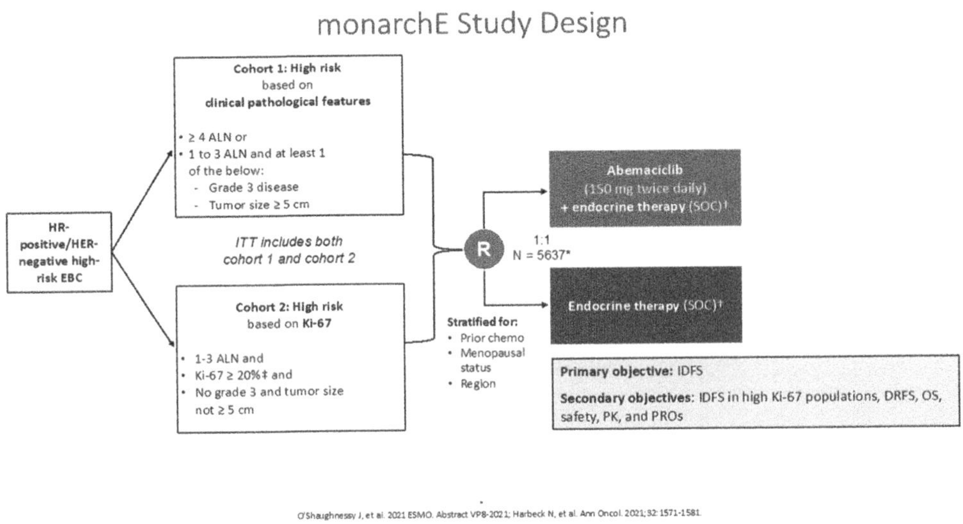

monarchE Study Design

O'Shaughnessy J, et al. 2021 ESMO. Abstract VP8-2021; Harbeck N, et al. Ann Oncol. 2021;32: 1571-1581.

Figure 11.4 monarchE study design.

6) What is the role of Poly (ADP-ribose) polymerase inhibitors in early stage HR+/HER2-negative breast cancer?

Expert Perspective: At present, only a fraction of newly diagnosed breast cancer patients who are eligible for genetic testing, based on guidelines, get tested. The gap is more glaring for those without insurance and among underserved and minority populations. Another important, underappreciated statistic is there are more patients with germline (g)BRCA mutations in ER-positive/HER-negative breast cancer (~10,000 annually) compared with those with triple-negative breast cancer (TNBC, ~4,800 annually) even though gBRCA mutations occur at a

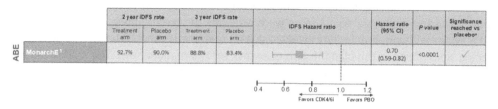

Figure 11.5 Summary of monarchE trial.

higher rate in TNBC (14.8% vs. 5%, respectively). The Poly (ADP-ribose) polymerase (PARP) inhibitors, olaparib and talozaparib have been approved as treatment for metastatic, *BRCA*-mutated breast cancer, but now data from the OLYMPIA trial with olaparib confirms significant benefit for those with high-risk, *HER2*-negative/*gBRCA*-mutated, early stage breast cancer (Figure 11.6).

Early stage, *HER2*-negative breast cancer patients with a *gBRCA* mutation and deemed at high risk for recurrence were eligible to participate. High risk was defined for those receiving neoadjuvant chemotherapy as follows: (1) TNBC with non-pCR, (2) ER-positive with a non-pCR and a clinical-pathologic-stage and estrogen receptor and histologic grade (CPS-EG) score of > 3. CPS-EG considers both the pre- and post-surgery stage as well as ER status and nuclear grade. For those receiving adjuvant chemotherapy, high risk was defined as follows: (1) TNBC with pT2 or ≥ pN1, (2) ER-positive with at least four nodes. Patients were randomized to receive olaparib or placebo for one year. Most patients received an anthracycline/taxane regimen, in ~24% a platinum was included, and ~18% had ER-positive tumors. With a median follow-up of 2.5 years, the three-year invasive, disease-free survival was 85.9% versus 77.1% for those receiving olaparib compared to placebo, respectively. The three-year overall survival, though not statistically significant, showed a numerical

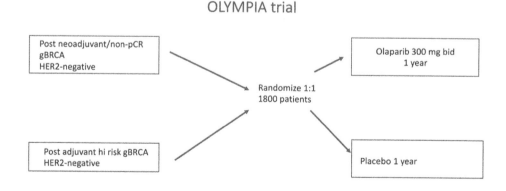

- Geyer CE Jr, et al. Ann Oncol. 2022:S0923-7534(22)04165-5; Tutt A, et al. J Clin Oncol. 2021;39(suppl 15): Abstract LBA1.

Figure 11.6 Design of OLYMPIA trial.

advantage for those receiving olaparib (92% vs. 88.3%). A Forest plot of all subsets showed an advantage to treatment with olaparib, though the confidence intervals for ER-positive tumors and those exposed to platinum were wide due to small numbers. The reduction in iDFS events with olaparib largely involved distant metastatic events. There were no unexpected side effects in the olaparib arm or excess second malignancies. The magnitude of benefit in patients receiving olaparib is clinically relevant and practice changing. Both American Society of Clinical Oncology (ASCO) and NCCN practice guidelines were immediately updated to reflect this data. One of the downstream effects of this trial will be an increase in genetic testing to identify patients eligible to receive olaparib. In the patient described in this case, she would not be a candidate for olaparib even if she was *BRCA* positive because she did not fit the eligibility criteria for the OLYMPIA trial.

7) **Which statement about the TAILORx trial is correct?**
   A) The trial evaluated hormone receptor+ (HR+), *HER2*-negative, axillary node-positive breast cancer
   B) Among women with a high recurrence score of ≥ 26, all of whom received chemotherapy, the invasive disease-free survival was 90%
   C) Women older than 50 years with axillary node-negative disease derived no benefit from chemotherapy and could be treated with endocrine therapy alone if recurrence scores are ≤ 25
   D) All of the above

Expert Perspective: The TAILORx study evaluated outcomes in 9719 women with HR+, *HER2*-negative, axillary node-negative breast cancer. The trial confirmed that women older than 50 years with axillary node-negative disease with low recurrence score (≤ 10), all of whom received endocrine therapy without chemotherapy, the rate of iDFS at nine years was 84%. Among 6700 women with recurrence scores between 11 to 25, those randomly assigned to endocrine therapy alone had the same iDFS outcomes as those randomized to chemotherapy and endocrine therapy (83 vs. 84% at nine years; HR 1.08; 95% CI 0.94–1.24). Among almost 1400 women with a high recurrence score of ≥ 26, all of whom received chemotherapy (typically taxane- and/or anthracycline-containing regimens), the iDFS was 76% at nine years, and the rate of freedom from distant recurrence was 87%.

Correct Answer: C

Case Study 2

A 33-year-old premenopausal female presents after self-detection of a left-sided breast lump. She has no other relevant medical history or family history. Mammogram and ultrasound confirm the mass measuring ~1.7 cm, but no axillary nodes were identified by exam or imaging. A biopsy confirms an ER+/PR+/ HER2-negative tumor. Genetic testing is negative. The patient undergoes a lumpectomy and SLNB, and a 1.6 cm primary is removed with clear margins. One of three axillary lymph nodes was positive with no extranodal extension.

8) **You would recommend the following for adjuvant therapy in addition to radiation therapy:**
   A) Oncotype Dx™ to determine the need for chemotherapy
   B) Aromatase inhibitor therapy for at least 7.5 years

C) Ovarian function suppression plus tamoxifen or an aromatase inhibitor
D) Adjuvant chemotherapy followed by adjuvant endocrine therapy with ovarian function suppression if the patient remains premenopausal.

Expert Perspective: As noted in the discussion with the first case, there is evidence that adjuvant chemotherapy confers benefit to premenopausal woman with node-positive disease, and there is no recurrence score that one could confidently identify in which chemotherapy could be safely avoided. Chemotherapy may have an ovarian suppression effect to achieve a reduction in the risk of recurrence. Although optimal endocrine therapy with ovarian suppression may confer a similar benefit to chemotherapy, the RxPONDER trial did not formally address this in the design of the trial, and as a result adjuvant chemotherapy would still be viewed as optimal evidence-based option for a patient in this age group with node-positive disease.

An aromatase inhibitor alone would not be effective in a premenopausal woman, and as noted earlier, chemotherapy would be viewed as a standard adjuvant therapy recommendation. Ovarian function suppression plus endocrine therapy has not been directly compared to chemotherapy in patients like the one described. If the patient was unable to receive chemotherapy, or refused, then one could justify an optimal endocrine therapy approach with ovarian function suppression (OFS) using a GnRH agonist (i.e. goserelin or triptorelin) plus either tamoxifen or an aromatase inhibitor (once postmenopausal status was confirmed). Ovarian function suppression can also be achieved with oophorectomy.

For premenopausal women with hormone receptor–positive, early breast cancer such as the patient in this case, adjuvant therapy with exemestane plus ovarian function suppression is superior to tamoxifen plus ovarian function suppression at 12 years, according to an updated analysis of roughly 4,700 participants in the TEXT and SOFT trials.

- In the TEXT trial, patients were randomized within 12 weeks of surgery to five years of either exemestane or tamoxifen, plus OFS; chemotherapy was optional and at the discretion of the clinician.
- In the SOFT trial, patients were similarly randomized within 12 weeks of surgery, or within 8 months of completing chemotherapy. After a median of nine years' follow-up, DFS and distant, recurrence-free interval were both improved with exemestane plus ovarian function suppression versus tamoxifen plus ovarian function suppression

In the latest analysis presented at 2021 SABCS, 12-year DFS continued to favor exemestane over tamoxifen (80.5% vs. 75.9%). Secondary outcomes, including 12-year invasive breast cancer–free interval and distant recurrence-free interval, also favored exemestane. Overall survival was high in both groups and did not differ significantly between the two (90.1% vs. 89.1%). In patients with high-risk features, particularly those for whom adjuvant chemotherapy is recommended, endocrine therapy with an aromatase inhibitor and OFS confers a clinically relevant improvement in outcome. In addition, clinicians will need to have a discussion with patients regarding potential toxicities associated with OFS, including menopausal symptoms and risk of fractures.

Correct Answer: D

Recommended Readings

Burstein, H.J., Lacchetti, C., Anderson, H. et al. (2019). Adjuvant endocrine therapy for women with hormone receptor-positive breast cancer: ASCO clinical practice guideline focused update. *J Clin Oncol* 37: 423–438.

Francis, P.A., Pagani, O., Fleming, G.F. et al. (2018). SOFT and TEXT investigators and the international breast cancer study group. Tailoring adjuvant endocrine therapy for premenopausal breast cancer. *N Engl J Med* 379: 122–137.

Johnston, S.R.D., Harbeck, N., Hegg, R. et al. (2020). monarchE committee members and investigators. Abemaciclib combined with endocrine therapy for the adjuvant treatment of HR+, HER2−, node-positive, high-risk, early breast cancer (monarchE). *J Clin Oncol* 38: 3987–3998.

Kalinsky, K., Barlow, W.E., Gralow, J.R. et al. (2021). 21-Gene assay to inform chemotherapy benefit in node-positive breast cancer. *N Engl J Med* 385: 2336–2347.

Kunkler, I.H., Williams, L.J., Jack, W.J.L. (2023 February 16). Breast-conserving surgery with or without irradiation in early breast cancer. *N Engl J Med* 388 (7): 585–594. doi: 10.1056/NEJMoa2207586. PMID: 36791159.

National Comprehensive Cancer Network. Breast Cancer (Version 2.2022). http://www.nccn.org/professionals/physician_gls/pdf/breast.pdf (accessed 3 January 2022).

Pagani, O., Francis, P.A., Fleming, G.F. et al. (2020). SOFT and TEXT investigators and international breast cancer study group. Absolute improvements in freedom from distant recurrence to tailor adjuvant endocrine therapies for premenopausal women: results from TEXT and SOFT. *J Clin Oncol* 38: 1293–1303.

Pan, H., Gray, R., and Hayes, D.F. (2018). Early Breast Cancer Trialists' Collaborative Group. Breast-cancer recurrence after stopping endocrine therapy. *N Engl J Med* 378: 870–871.

Ribnikar, D., Sousa, B., Cufer, T., and Cardoso, F. (2017). Extended adjuvant endocrine therapy – A standard to all or some? *Breast* 32: 112–118.

Sparano, J.A., Gray, R.J., Makower, D.F. et al. (2018). Adjuvant chemotherapy guided by a 21-gene expression assay in breast cancer. *N Engl J Med* 379: 111–121.

Sparano, J.A., Gray, R.J., Makower, D.F. et al. (2020). Clinical outcomes in early breast cancer with a high 21-gene recurrence score of 26 to 100 assigned to adjuvant chemotherapy plus endocrine therapy: A secondary analysis of the TAILORx randomized clinical trial. *JAMA Oncol* 6: 367–374.

Tutt, A.N.J., Garber, J.E., Kaufman, B. et al. (2021). OlympiA Clinical Trial Steering Committee and investigators. Adjuvant olaparib for patients with *BRCA1*- or *BRCA2*-mutated breast cancer. *N Engl J Med* 384: 2394–2405.

Geyer CE, et al. Overall survival in the OlympiA phase III trial of adjuvant olaparib in patients with germline pathogenic variants in *BRCA1/2* and high risk, early breast cancer Ann Oncol https://doi.org/10.1016/j.annonc.2022.09.159

O'Shaughnessy, Joyce A. et al. "Abstract GS1-01: Primary Outcome Analysis of Invasive Disease-Free Survival for monarchE: Abemaciclib Combined with Adjuvant Endocrine Therapy for High Risk Early Breast Cancer." Cancer research (Chicago, Ill.) 81.4_Supplement (2021): GS1-01–GS1-01. Web.

Early Breast Cancer Trialists' Collaborative Group (EBCTCG). Electronic address: bc.overview@ctsu.ox.ac.uk; Early Breast Cancer Trialists' Collaborative Group (EBCTCG). (2023 April 15). Anthracyclinecontaining and taxane-containing chemotherapy for early-stage operable breast cancer: a patient-level meta-analysis of 100 000 women from 86 randomised trials. *Lancet* 401 (10384): 1277–1292. doi: 10.1016/S0140-6736(23)00285-4. PMID: 37061269.

12

ER/PR-Positive, HER2-Negative Metastatic Breast Cancer

Sara Nunnery, Laura Kennedy, and Sonya Reid

Vanderbilt Ingram Cancer Center, Nashville, TN

Introduction

Hormone receptor positive (HR+) breast cancer comprises tumors that express estrogen receptors (ER+) and/or progesterone receptors (PR+) as indicated by positive staining on immunohistochemistry. HR+ breast cancer is the most common type of breast cancer, making up 65–75% of all cases, and has a better prognosis than HR negative (HR−) tumors. Several large cohort studies have shown that the five-year overall survival for patients with HR+ cancers is approximately 10% better than those with HR− cancers. The majority of cases of HR+ metastatic breast cancer (MBC) develop as a recurrence of earlier stage disease, whereas 5–20% represent *de novo* metastatic disease at diagnosis.

The main goals of treating HR+ MBC are to prolong survival by slowing disease progression and to control symptoms while maintaining quality of life and minimizing complications from both the disease and treatment. Endocrine therapy has remained the backbone of treatment for patients with HR+ MBC for over the past four decades. Improvements in systemic treatment with the development of newer targeted therapies have improved survival of patients with HR+ MBC over the past 10 years. The choice of systemic treatment should take into consideration various patient and disease characteristics. Patient factors that can impact treatment selection include age, menopausal status, comorbidities, performance status, and social factors that might affect the ability to receive and adhere to certain treatments. Sites of metastatic disease, disease burden, disease-free interval, prior systemic treatment, and symptoms are important clinical features to consider when deciding on endocrine therapy, targeted therapies, or cytotoxic chemotherapy. Identifying germline and/or somatic mutations in the tumor, such as *PIK3CA*, *BRCA1/2*, and *ESR1* mutations, also has important implications for treatment, and it is now mandatory per the National Comprehensive Cancer Network (NCCN) guidelines to perform tumor profiling either through next-generation sequencing (NGS) on tumor tissue or through circulating tumor DNA (ctDNA) from plasma for all patients with metastatic breast cancer.

There are many treatments, including hormonal treatments, targeted treatments, and cytotoxic chemotherapy, currently approved for first-line and subsequent-line therapies in HR+ MBC. The following cases illustrate current treatment practices based on evidence from randomized trials and aim to provide insightful information to the practicing medical oncologist for the clinical management of HR+ MBC.

Case Study 1

A postmenopausal 60-year-old woman presents to her primary care physician for evaluation of three weeks of right hip pain. She has a history of stage I HR+ breast cancer diagnosed at age 46 that was treated with lumpectomy, adjuvant radiation, and five years of adjuvant tamoxifen. Her hip pain continues to worsen despite two weeks of conservative management. Her primary care physician orders an MRI of the hip given her history of breast cancer, which reveals three lytic lesions in the right pelvis. Biopsy of one of the lesions confirms metastatic adenocarcinoma of breast origin, strongly ER/PR positive, HER2 negative. Staging CT scan of the chest, abdomen, and pelvis and bone scan reveal three additional sites of metastatic disease in the lumbar spine but no other evidence of visceral metastatic disease.

1) **How do you select first-line treatment for newly diagnosed HR+ metastatic disease?**

Expert Perspective: The preferred initial treatment for HR+ MBC consists of combination endocrine therapy with a targeted CDK4/6 inhibitor (CDK4/6i) due to the overall survival advantage seen in first- and second-line phase III trials. Three CDK4/6 inhibitors, palbociclib, ribociclib, and abemaciclib, are currently approved for the first-line treatment of metastatic HR+, HER2 negative breast cancer in combination with endocrine therapy. The PALOMA-2 phase III trial compared palbociclib plus letrozole to letrozole plus placebo and found a median progression-free survival of 24.8 months in the palbociclib plus letrozole arm compared with 14.5 months for letrozole plus placebo. Palbociclib was the first CDK4/6i approved based on these results. Both the MONALEESA-2 and MONARCH-3 placebo-controlled phase III trials had similar designs and results leading to the approvals of ribociclib and abemaciclib, respectively.

The main differences between the three approved CDK4/6 inhibitors are the side effect profile (Table 12.1). Both palbociclib and ribociclib are associated with myelosuppression. This mainly tends to manifest as neutropenia, but both anemia and thrombocytopenia can also be seen. Abemaciclib is more strongly associated with gastrointestinal toxicity, including diarrhea, nausea, vomiting, and loss of appetite. All of these toxicities respond well to dose adjustments, and the diarrhea associated with abemaciclib typically improves after about six months. Palbociclib and ribociclib are both given once daily for three weeks, followed by one week off over 28-day cycles. Abemaciclib, in contrast, is the only CDK4/6 inhibitor that is administered twice daily on a continuous schedule. It is also the only CDK4/6 inhibitor that is FDA approved as monotherapy in women with HR+ MBC whose disease progressed following chemotherapy and endocrine therapy.

CDK4/6 inhibitors have efficacy with multiple different endocrine therapies, so the endocrine therapy partner likely has much less impact on the progression-free survival and overall survival (OS) advantage seen. For patients who have not had any prior endocrine therapy or had a long disease-free interval prior to developing metastatic

Table 12.1 The CDK 4/6 inhibitors and their key differences.

	Palbociclib(Ibrance, Pfizer)		Abemaciclib(Kisqali, Novartis)		Ribociclib(Verzenio, Eli Lilly)	
Dosing	125 mg daily (3 weeks on, 1 week off)		200 mg twice daily (continuously)		600 mg daily (3 weeks on, 1 week off)	
Phase III trial leading to FDA approval for metastatic disease	PALOMA-2		MONALEESA-2		MONARCH-3	
Activity as monotherapy	No		Yes		No	
CNS penetration	No		Yes		No	
Common toxicities in the advanced setting (%)*	All grades	Grade 3/4	All grades	Grade 3/4	All grades	Grade 3/4
Neutropenia	80	66	41	22	75	60
Anemia	24	5	28	6	18	1
Thrombocytopenia	16	1	10	2	29	1
Fatigue	37	2	46	3	37	2
Diarrhea	26	1	81	9	35	1
Creatinine increased	NR	NR	98	2	20	1
QTc prolongation	NR	NR	NR	NR	8	0
Drug Discontinuation	7.4%		20%		7.5%	

* Toxicities adapted from Braal et al. (2021). Inhibiting CDK4/6 in breast cancer with palbociclib, ribociclib, and abemaciclib: Similarities and differences. *Drugs* 81(3): 317–331.

disease, CDK4/6i can be combined with an aromatase inhibitor for first-line treatment. If the patient had a short disease-free interval with prior treatment with aromatase inhibitor, CDK4/6i should be combined with fulvestrant in the first line.

It is also reasonable to start treatment for metastatic disease with single-agent endocrine therapy and defer CDK4/6i to second-line treatment for patients who presented with *de novo* metastatic disease, oligometastatic disease, or a long disease-free interval after initial treatment with endocrine therapy. The FALCON phase III trial of fulvestrant compared with aromatase inhibitor alone in the first line setting found a median progression-free survival of 16.6 months with fulvestrant versus 13.8 months with aromatase inhibitor and an even greater median progression-free survival of 22.3 months with fulvestrant versus 13.8 months with aromatase inhibitor in patients without any visceral disease. Median OS was not yet reached. The SWOG0226 phase III trial of fulvestrant combined with aromatase inhibitor compared with aromatase inhibitor alone as first-line treatment had similar results with a median progression-free survival of 15 months with fulvestrant plus aromatase inhibitor versus 13 months with aromatase inhibitor alone. The median OS for the fulvestrant plus aromatase inhibitor arm was

49.8 months compared with 42 months for aromatase inhibitor alone. The patient in this case could start treatment with an aromatase inhibitor alone given her minimal disease burden, no prior exposure to aromatase inhibitor, and a long disease-free interval from her previous treatment with tamoxifen. If the patient had previously been treated with aromatase inhibitor, we could also start endocrine therapy with fulvestrant alone or fulvestrant combined with aromatase inhibitor.

2) **What is the preferred second-line treatment for HR+ MBC after progression on first-line endocrine therapy?**

Expert Perspective: After disease progression on endocrine therapy alone, CDK4/6i can be combined with fulvestrant for second-line treatment. Multiple phase III placebo-controlled trials (PALOMA-3, MONARCH-2, MONALEESA-3) showed improved progression-free survival with CDK4/6 inhibitor combined with fulvestrant compared to fulvestrant alone in patients who had progression after previous response to endocrine therapy. If the patient was on fulvestrant alone as first line therapy, a CDK4/6i can be added to fulvestrant for second line treatment.

Case Study 2

A 44-year-old premenopausal woman with history of an 8 mm intermediate grade ER+/PR−/HER2-invasive ductal carcinoma of the right breast, treated with lumpectomy three years prior, presents to urgent care with a two-week history of nonproductive cough, dyspnea, and right flank pain. Plain films of the chest show bilateral infiltrates. She is started on a course of antibiotics and prednisone. At follow-up with her family physician one week later, her symptoms have failed to improve, and she now complains of pain in her right breast. Given her history of ductal carcinoma *in situ*, CT of the chest, abdomen, and pelvis is ordered and reveals scattered nodules throughout both lungs, poorly defined lytic lesions in the thoracic spine, right axillary lymphadenopathy, and hepatomegaly with innumerable nodules seen throughout the liver. Labs are notable for mildly elevated ALT, AST, alkaline phosphatase 1,800, and a total bilirubin of 5.2. Biopsy of a liver lesion shows metastatic carcinoma consistent with breast origin, ER/PR+, HER2−.

3) **How do you approach treatment for a patient with newly diagnosed HR+ MBC in visceral crisis?**

Expert Perspective: Patients who present with extensive visceral metastases and evidence of severe organ dysfunction, such as dyspnea, pancytopenia, or elevated liver function tests, are considered to have visceral crisis. Visceral crisis is associated with a worse survival compared with patients presenting without visceral crisis. Liver dysfunction, poor performance status, and prior treatment with multiple lines of systemic therapy correlate with a worse prognosis in patients presenting with visceral crisis.

For patients in visceral crisis, initiation of endocrine therapy alone is unlikely to provide a prompt clinical response, so starting treatment with combination chemotherapy for three to six months or until clinical response is seen is warranted. Chemotherapy would also be appropriate for a patient who is started on endocrine therapy but continues to have rapid disease progression. Chemotherapy is given without any combination of endocrine therapy because prior evidence shows that the combination is not more effective than chemotherapy alone. Once an adequate clinical response is seen with improvement in organ function and disease symptoms, patients can transition to endocrine therapy combined with CDK4/6i or single-agent chemotherapy for patients with disease that was refractory to prior lines of endocrine therapy.

The chemotherapy choice is dictated by the patient's prior treatment history and medical comorbidities, as well as the presence of any hepatic or renal dysfunction. Anthracycline-based regimens are associated with higher response rates in patients with previously untreated MBC. Doxorubicin plus cyclophosphamide (AC) or doxorubicin plus a taxane (docetaxel or paclitaxel) have response rates ranging from 40 to 54%. Doxorubicin is contraindicated with severe hepatic impairment (bilirubin > 5 mg/dL or Child-Pugh class C). For patients who are not a candidate for anthracycline, alternative regimens include gemcitabine plus paclitaxel or capecitabine plus docetaxel. However, taxanes are also hepatically cleared and require dose adjustments with hepatic impairment. Use of docetaxel is not recommended with any elevation of bilirubin above the upper limit of normal.

Platinum-containing regimens, such as gemcitabine plus carboplatin or carboplatin plus paclitaxel, are also an option for younger patients and patients with a good performance status and higher disease burden. However, no prospective trials have shown an OS advantage for platinum-containing regimens compared to non-platinum-containing regimens. Gemcitabine plus carboplatin can be safely administered to patients with hepatic dysfunction. Platinum-containing regimens may also have some benefits in patients with somatic or germline *BRCA1* or *BRCA2* mutations, making these regimens a reasonable choice when a rapid response is needed.

There has been recent interest in using the combination of endocrine-based therapies and CDK4/6 inhibitors in patients with visceral crisis due to the rapid responses and survival advantage that can be seen with this combination. There is limited data for CDK4/6 inhibition in this setting, however, because patients with visceral crisis were explicitly excluded from the phase III clinical trials that validated the survival benefit of endocrine therapy in combination with CDK4/6 inhibitors. Because of this, the current standard of care for HR+ breast cancer in visceral crisis remains chemotherapy.

Case Study 3

A 58-year-old postmenopausal woman with metastatic ER+/PR+ breast cancer has been on an aromatase inhibitor and CDK4/6i for over one year with stable disease. She develops a right-sided headache with nausea and vomiting. MRI of the brain reveals a new 2 cm metastatic lesion in the right temporal lobe. CT scan of the chest, abdomen, and pelvis does not reveal any new sites of metastatic disease or other disease progression.

4) How should you treat new CNS metastasis in a patient who has no other evidence of systemic disease progression?

Expert Perspective: Aggressive local treatment of new brain metastases is indicated for patients with a good performance status, younger age (generally age < 65), and otherwise adequately controlled systemic disease. Many factors such as number of brain metastases, size, location, and extent of edema and mass effect influence the treatment choice between surgical resection, stereotactic radiosurgery, or whole-brain radiation therapy. Patients who have a single, potentially resectable brain metastasis should be referred for surgical resection because patients who undergo resection have a longer overall survival.

More than half of patients who develop brain metastases develop intracranial disease while their extracranial disease is stable or even responding to systemic therapy. For such patients with new intracranial disease but stable extracranial disease, the current systemic therapy can be continued while intracranial disease is treated with local therapy. The same aromatase inhibitor and CDK4/6i combination therapy can be continued in this patient because she does not have any evidence of extracranial disease progression. A change in systemic therapy is warranted once there is evidence of systemic disease progression on future scans.

Case Study 4

A 62-year-old woman presents with a 6 cm mass in her right breast along with palpable, axillary lymphadenopathy and right rib pain. She has a history of intermediate grade, ER/PR+ invasive mammary carcinoma of the right breast treated seven years prior with lumpectomy followed by radiation and five years of adjuvant aromatase inhibitor. Biopsy of the right breast mass and lymph nodes confirms high grade invasive mammary carcinoma, strongly ER/PR+, HER2−. CT scan of the chest, abdomen, and pelvis shows multiple enlarged axillary nodes and lesions in her right ribs and thoracic spine. Bone scan again shows lesions in the right ribs and thoracic spine consistent with metastatic disease. She is started on treatment with an aromatase inhibitor and CDK4/6 inhibitor.

5) **Is there a role for locoregional treatment of the primary breast tumor in patients with metastatic disease?**

Expert Perspective: The question of whether removal of the primary tumor in addition to systemic treatment in patients with MBC prolongs survival has been a topic of increasing research interest in recent years. Multiple retrospective studies from the early 2000s suggested that surgical resection of the primary tumor improved overall survival, with one retrospective analysis from the Surveillance, Epidemiology, and End Results (SEER) data base reporting an improvement in OS by as much as 15 months. Many of these retrospective studies were small, single-institution reviews that were subject to the limitations of selection bias and other confounding factors, and many reported conflicting results.

The ECOG 2108 trial was a prospective, randomized phase III trial evaluating whether surgery and radiation combined with systemic treatment compared to systemic treatment alone improved OS for patients with MBC. The long-awaited results from this prospective trial were reported in May 2020 and found that local treatment in addition to systemic treatment did not provide any additional benefit to OS, nor was there any quality of life (QoL) advantage based on patient-reported QoL measures between the two groups. Another randomized, controlled trial with a similar study design conducted in Mumbai, India, also found no difference in OS between patients receiving locoregional treatment in addition to systemic treatment and those receiving systemic treatment alone. Given these results from prospective trials, local treatment of the primary breast tumor in patients with metastatic disease is reserved for patients in need of palliation of local symptoms such as pain, ulceration, or infection.

Introduction | 145

Case Study 5

A 61-year-old man was diagnosed with stage III, low-grade, invasive mammary carcinoma of the right breast, ER/PR+, HER2−, six years ago after he noticed a palpable mass in the right axilla. He is a lifelong smoker with chronic obstructive pulmonary disease that is managed with inhalers. He underwent a right mastectomy with axillary dissection and was found to have multiple lymph nodes involved by metastatic carcinoma. Genetic testing did not reveal any pathologic germline mutations. He completed adjuvant chemotherapy with doxorubicin, cyclophosphamide, and weekly paclitaxel followed by adjuvant radiation. He completed one year of adjuvant tamoxifen and then stopped because of joint pain and muscle aches. He now presents with new lymphadenopathy in the left axilla and skin lesions on the right anterior chest. Skin biopsy of one of the lesions shows metastatic adenocarcinoma consistent with breast primary, strongly ER/PR+. CT scan shows left axillary lymphadenopathy, and bone scan shows multiple small rib metastases.

6) What is the preferred first-line treatment for a male patient with newly diagnosed HR+ MBC?

Expert Perspective: Management of metastatic disease in male patients is similar to that in women. Male patients with breast cancer have not been included in most large clinical trials, and evidence for treatment is primarily based on real-world data and extrapolation from trials in women. For HR+ MBC in men, CDK4/6 inhibitors can be started in combination with tamoxifen or in combination with an aromatase inhibitor and gonadotropin-releasing hormone (GnRH) agonist. Unlike in postmenopausal women, aromatase inhibitor does not block testicular production of estrogen in men, so use of a GnRH agonist with aromatase inhibitor is required for estrogen blockade. Palbociclib is the only CDK4/6i that has formal approval by the US Food and Drug Administration (FDA) for use in men with HR+ MBC, but ribociclib and abemaciclib are also appropriate for off-label use in men.

It is also reasonable to start treatment with endocrine therapy alone in male patients who have a low burden of disease, comorbidities, or other personal preferences that impact treatment. Because this patient has a low burden of metastatic disease without any visceral organ involvement and was treated with adjuvant tamoxifen for one year, he could start treatment with an aromatase inhibitor and GnRH agonist. After progression on endocrine therapy alone, fulvestrant with GnRH agonist can be used as a subsequent-line endocrine therapy combined with CDK 4/6i. Fulvestrant and newer agents, such as mTOR inhibitors and *PIK3CA* inhibitors, have not been evaluated in male patients with breast cancer in clinical trials. However, published case reports and other real-world evidence have shown similar efficacy and safety in men with breast cancer compared to women (see Chapter 18).

Case Study 6

A 65-year-old postmenopausal woman presents with lower back pain that has been progressively worsening over the past two months. MRI reveals multiple bony lesions in her L-spine, sacrum, and pelvis. CT scan shows a few small pulmonary nodules but no other evidence of metastatic disease. She has a history of stage I HR+ breast cancer of the right breast that was treated with lumpectomy, adjuvant radiation, and five years of adjuvant letrozole completed just one year ago. Biopsy of one the L-spine lesions confirms metastatic adenocarcinoma of breast origin, strongly ER/PR positive and HER2 negative. She is started on treatment with letrozole and palbociclib and maintains stable disease control for 18 months until a repeat CT scans show a new liver lesion. NGS of her previous bone biopsy shows a *PIK3CA* mutation.

7) What is the significance of a *PIK3CA* mutation in HR+ breast cancer?

Expert Perspective: Activation of the PI3K/AKT/mTOR pathway allows cancer cells to develop estrogen-independent survival and creates acquired resistance to endocrine therapy. Mutation of the *PIK3CA* gene is one of the most common activating mutations for this pathway found in breast cancer, and approximately 30–40% of advanced HR+ breast cancer has an activating *PIK3CA* mutation. Alpelisib was the first PI3K inhibitor approved for the treatment of HR+, *PIK3CA* mutated MBC based on the results of the phase III SOLAR-1 trial, which showed prolonged progression-free survival in this patient population after progression on endocrine therapy. Since the approval of alpelisib for *PIK3CA* mutant HR+ MBC and the approval of PARP inhibitors for germline *BRCA* mutant MBC, the NCCN guidelines recommend that tumor profiling be performed on all patients with MBC, especially HR+ MBC, either by NGS on tumor tissue or by ctDNA from plasma.

8) When do you start treatment with a PI3K inhibitor in *PIK3CA* mutant ER+ MBC?

Expert Perspective: PI3K inhibitors can be given as second-line or later therapy to patients with HR+ MBC who have progressed on either endocrine therapy alone or endocrine therapy combined with CDK4/6 inhibitors. Two phase III trials (SOLAR-1 and BYlieve) showed a modest but real improvement in progression-free survival when PI3K inhibitors were given in the second-line or later line of therapy. Patients with *PIK3CA* mutations should be treated with alpelisib in combination with fulvestrant based on results from these trials. For patients without *PIK3CA* mutations, the mTOR inhibitor, everolimus, can be given with endocrine therapy. The partner endocrine therapy likely does not matter for everolimus because it has been shown to have efficacy with multiple different agents. Although these therapies have not demonstrated an overall survival advantage, these therapies offer disease control and the opportunity to delay chemotherapy which are important goals for many patients.

Case Study 7

A 35-year-old premenopausal woman presents with a metastatic recurrence of ER+, HER2− breast cancer with bone and lung involvement. She was first diagnosed with stage II strongly ER+, HER2−, intermediate grade, invasive mammary carcinoma of the right breast two years prior. She declined genetic testing at the time but underwent bilateral mastectomies with sentinel lymph node biopsies, which found one positive lymph node on the right side. She declined adjuvant chemotherapy and ovarian suppression and was started on tamoxifen for endocrine therapy. She presented to clinic three weeks ago with worsening left hip pain that was limiting her mobility. MRI revealed multiple pelvic and sacral lesions. A CT scan of the chest also showed multiple lung nodules. Bone biopsy results confirm metastatic carcinoma consistent with breast primary, again strongly ER+, HER2−. She agrees to genetic testing, which reveals a germline *BRCA2* mutation.

9) What is the appropriate first-line therapy for patients with ER+ MBC and germline BRCA mutations?

Expert Perspective: Women who have a *BRCA1/2* mutations have a lifetime risk of breast cancer of 50–85% compared with only 12% in the general population. Almost 70% of *BRCA1* mutated breast cancers are triple negative cancers, whereas 77% of *BRCA2* mutated breast cancers are ER+. The OlympiaD trial was a large, randomized, phase III trial of the PARP inhibitor olaparib as monotherapy compared with single agent chemotherapy in patients with a germline *BRCA* mutation and metastatic, HER2− breast cancer. Results showed an improved response rate and improved progression free survival in the olaparib group compared with standard therapy and led to the approval by the US FDA of olaparib for patients with HER2− MBC and germline *BRCA* mutations.

The optimal sequence of PARP inhibitors in the treatment of ER+ MBC has not been established in prospective trials. OlympiaD included HR+ MBC patients who had previously been treated with endocrine therapy, and these patients did have benefit from olaparib after prior treatment with endocrine therapy. For patients with *BRCA* mutations and prior platinum agent exposure in the metastatic setting, PARP inhibitors may have limited efficacy, particularly if the platinum agent was discontinued due to disease progression. This can be related to the development of *BRCA* reversion mutations.

Best recommendation based on the current evidence is to start patients with germline *BRCA* mutations and MBC on endocrine therapy combined with CDK4/6 inhibitor as first-line therapy and treat with PARP inhibitor after progression. Because this patient has already been treated with adjuvant tamoxifen, she should start treatment with an aromatase inhibitor and GnRH agonist for ovarian suppression combined with a CDK4/6 inhibitor.

10) Can you treat with a PARP inhibitor in patients with HR+ MBC and somatic BRCA mutations but no germline mutation?

Expert Perspective: The TBCRC048 phase II trial evaluated olaparib in a small cohort of patients with metastatic *HER2* negative breast cancer with somatic *BRCA1/2* mutations or germline non-*BRCA* mutations. This trial had encouraging results with 50% of patients achieving a partial response and 67% of patients having clinical benefit. Although somatic *BRCA* mutations are not a current FDA-approved indication for treatment with PARP inhibitors, these trial results suggest that olaparib could provide clinical benefit and be a reasonable treatment option as a later line of therapy for patients with ER+ MBC and a tumor with a *BRCA* mutations identified on tumor profiling (Chapters 45 and 46).

Conclusion

Multiple options for single-agent or combination therapies are approved for first-line and subsequent-line therapies in patients with metastatic HR+, HER2− breast cancer. No optimal sequence for these various therapies has been clearly established, and randomized clinical trials further investigating the sequence of these therapies are needed. The initial targeted therapy that is preferred for metastatic disease is combination endocrine therapy

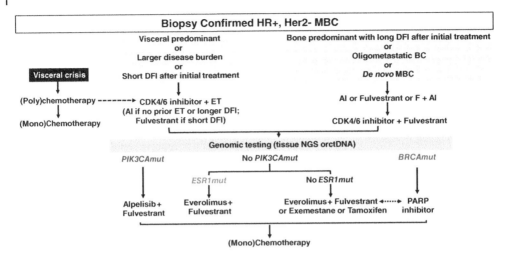

Figure 12.1 Treatment approach to HR+ MBC.

with a CDK 4/6i due to the overall survival advantage of this regimen demonstrated in multiple phase III trials (Figure 12.1). There is currently no data to support continuation of therapy with an alternative CDK4/6i after disease progression on endocrine therapy with CDK 4/6i, although several clinical trials are ongoing.

Patients should have genomic profiling of their tumor through NGS on tumor tissue, through ctDNA at the point of disease progression, or even before progression to identify actionable mutations that could guide subsequent line treatments. Following endocrine therapy and CDK4/6i, subsequent-line therapy with endocrine therapy should be combined with either everolimus (if *PIK3CA* wild-type) or with alpelisib (if *PIK3CA* mutation in identified in the tumor). Recently, in a phase 3, randomized, double-blind trial, investigators enrolled eligible pre-, peri-, and postmenopausal women and men with HR+/HER2− advanced breast cancer who had relapse or disease progression during or after treatment with an aromatase inhibitor, with or without previous CDK4/6 inhibitor therapy. Capivasertib–fulvestrant therapy resulted in significantly longer progression-free survival than treatment with fulvestrant alone. In addition, the identification of *ESR1* mutations in tumors have treatment implications because the presence of this mutation is associated with the development of resistance to endocrine therapy, especially aromatase inhibitors. Some data suggests that tumors with *ESR1* mutations have improved response to treatment with fulvestrant-containing regimens rather than aromatase inhibitor regimens. Efficacy was evaluated in EMERALD, a randomized, open-label, active-controlled, multicenter trial that enrolled 478 postmenopausal women and men with HR+/HER2− advanced or metastatic breast cancer. In the 228 (48%) patients with ESR1 mutations, median progression-free survival was 3.8 months (95% CI confidence interval [CI] = 2.2–7.3) in the elacestrant arm and 1.9 months (95% CI = 1.9–2.1) in the fulvestrant or aromatase inhibitor arm (hazard ratio [HR] = 0.55, 95% CI = 0.39–0.77, two-sided P-value = .0005). On January 27, the FDA approved elacestrant for postmenopausal women or adult men with HR+/HER2−, ESR1-mutated advanced or metastatic breast cancer with disease progression following at least one line of endocrine therapy. Finally, the transition to treatment with cytotoxic chemotherapy should be considered after disease progression on more than three prior lines of endocrine therapy including combination with a targeted agent as well as the presence of rapidly progressive visceral disease.

Recommended Readings

André, F., Ciruelos, E., Rubovszky, G. et al. (2019). Alpelisib for PIK3CA-mutated, hormone receptor-positive advanced breast cancer. *N Engl J Med* 380 (20): 1929–1940. (In eng). doi: 10.1056/NEJMoa1813904.

Awada, A., Gligorov, J., Jerusalem, G. et al. (2019). CDK4/6 inhibition in low burden and extensive metastatic breast cancer: summary of an ESMO open-cancer horizons pro and con discussion. *ESMO Open* 4 (6): e000565. (In eng). doi: 10.1136/esmoopen-2019-000565.

Braal, C.L., Jongbloed, E.M., Wilting, S.M. et al. (2021). Inhibiting CDK4/6 in breast cancer with palbociclib, ribociclib, and abemaciclib: similarities and differences. *Drugs* 81 (3): 317–331. (In eng). doi: 10.1007/s40265-020-01461-2.

Burstein, H.J., Somerfield, M.R., Barton, D.L. et al. (2021). Endocrine treatment and targeted therapy for hormone receptor-positive, human epidermal growth factor receptor 2-negative metastatic breast cancer: ASCO guideline update. *J Clin Oncol* 39 (35): 3959–3977. (In eng). doi: 10.1200/jco.21.01392.

Kalinsky, K., Accordino, M.K., Chiuzan, C. et al. (2023 May 19). Randomized phase II trial of endocrine therapy with or without ribociclib after progression on cyclin-dependent kinase 4/6 inhibition in hormone receptor-positive, human epidermal growth factor receptor 2-negative metastatic breast cancer: MAINTAIN trial. *J Clin Oncol* JCO2202392. doi: 10.1200/JCO.22.02392. Epub ahead of print. PMID: 37207300.

Kennedy, L.C. and Mayer, I.A. (2021). New targets in endocrine-resistant hormone receptor-positive breast cancer. *Clin Adv Hematol Oncol* 19 (8): 511–521. (In eng).

McAndrew, N.P. and Finn, R.S. (2021). Clinical review on the management of hormone receptor-positive metastatic breast cancer. *JCO Oncol Pract* Op2100384. (In eng). doi: 10.1200/op.21.00384.

Reddy, P.M., Martin, J.M., and Montero, A.J. (2021). CDK 4/6 inhibitors: evolution and revolution in the management of ER+ metastatic breast cancer. *JCO Oncol Pract* Op2100611. (In eng). doi: 10.1200/op.21.00611.

Robson, M., Im, S.A., Senkus, E. et al. (2017). Olaparib for metastatic breast cancer in patients with a germline BRCA mutation. *N Engl J Med* 377 (6): 523–533. (In eng). doi: 10.1056/NEJMoa1706450.

Rugo, H.S., Bianchi, G.V., Chia, S.K.L., and Turner, N.C. (2018). BYLieve: A phase II study of alpelisib (ALP) with fulvestrant (FUL) or letrozole (LET) for treatment of *PIK3CA* mutant, hormone receptor-positive (HR+), human epidermal growth factor receptor 2-negative (HER2–) advanced breast cancer (aBC) progressing on/after cyclin-dependent kinase 4/6 inhibitor (CDK4/6i) therapy. *J Clin Oncol* 36 (15).

Turner, N.C., Oliveira, M., Howell, S.J. et al. (2023 June 1). Capivasertib in hormone receptor-positive advanced breast cancer. *N Engl J Med* 388 (22): 2058–2070. doi: 10.1056/NEJMoa2214131. PMID: 37256976.

13

Early-Stage HER2-Positive Breast Cancer

Erin Roesch and Jame Abraham

Taussig Cancer Institute, Cleveland, OH

Introduction

HER2 overexpression occurs in 15–20% of breast cancers and historically has been associated with a more aggressive subtype. The advent of HER2-targeted therapies has favorably impacted outcomes for patients with early stage HER2-positive breast cancer. Although the advances have led to improvements in survival endpoints, approximately 15–25% still experience a relapse. Furthermore, the central nervous system serves as a sanctuary site in these patients, and therefore they are at higher risk for development of brain metastases compared to other breast cancer subtypes. HER2-positive breast cancer exhibits heterogeneity, leading to variable treatment responses and outcomes. Research is focused on identification of biomarkers of response and resistance, which may assist in therapy de-escalation in the appropriate clinical scenario, as well as determination of patients who are in need of novel therapies. pCR has emerged as a valuable endpoint in clinical trials and can facilitate tailoring adjuvant therapy for early HER2-positive breast cancer.

Adjuvant Therapy

1) **What is the impact of trastuzumab in early stage HER2-positive breast cancer?**

Expert Perspective: Trastuzumab is a monoclonal antibody against the HER2 receptor which inhibits ligand-independent HER2 signaling, prevents HER2 activation by extracellular domain shedding, and activates antibody-dependent cellular cytotoxicity. Trastuzumab significantly reduces risk of recurrence and death for early HER2-positive breast cancer. A meta-analysis conducted by The Early Breast Cancer Trialists' Collaborative group (EBCTCG) including seven randomized trials (n = 13,864 patients) demonstrated significant reductions in risk of recurrence (relative risk 0.66; $P < 0.0001$) and mortality related to breast cancer (relative risk 0.67; $P < 0.0001$) with the addition of trastuzumab to chemotherapy. Absolute 10-year reductions in recurrence risk and breast cancer mortality were 9.0% and 6.4%, respectively (EBCTCG 2021).

Cancer Consult: Expertise in Clinical Practice, Volume 1: Solid Tumors & Supportive Care,
Second Edition. Edited by Syed A. Abutalib, Maurie Markman, Al B. Benson III, and Hope S. Rugo.
© 2024 John Wiley & Sons Ltd. Published 2024 by John Wiley & Sons Ltd.

Combined results of two trials (National Surgical Adjuvant Breast and Bowel Project B-31 and North Central Cancer Treatment Group trial N831) further demonstrated the longevity of trastuzumab benefit. At 8.4 years median follow-up, the addition of trastuzumab to paclitaxel after anthracycline-based therapy led to a 37% relative improvement in overall survival (OS; HR 0.63; absolute benefit in 10-year OS of 8.8%) and improvement in disease-free survival (DFS) of 40% (HR 0.60; absolute benefit in 10-year DFS of 11.5%) (Perez et al. 2014).

The Breast Cancer International Research Group 006 (BCIRG-006) study investigated the role of trastuzumab with non-anthracycline-based therapy. Patients were randomized to doxorubicin and cyclophosphamide followed by docetaxel with or without trastuzumab (AC/TH or AC/T), or docetaxel, carboplatin, and trastuzumab (TCH). No significant differences in efficacy were found between the two trastuzumab-containing regimens, although both were better than AC/T without trastuzumab. Estimated five-year DFS rates for AC/T, AC/TH, and TCH were 75%, 84%, and 81%, respectively; estimated OS rates were 87%, 92%, and 91%, respectively (Slamon et al. 2011).

2) What were the risks of leukemia and congestive heart failure in using anthracycline with trastuzumab in the adjuvant setting?

Expert Perspective: Rates of congestive heart failure and acute leukemia were higher in the anthracycline arms. At 10.5 years of follow-up, 0.2% developed leukemia in the AC/TH arm, 2% had heart failure (vs 0.4% in TCH arm), and nearly 20% had a 10% relative reduction in ejection fraction. Although not designed nor powered to compare the two trastuzumab-containing arms, DFS rates were similar (74.6% and 73% for AC/TH and TCH, respectively).

3) What are the data on duration of trastuzumab therapy?

Expert Perspective: A total of one year of trastuzumab therapy has historically been, and remains, the standard of care in the adjuvant setting. However, various trials have addressed both shorter and longer durations. The FinHER trial, which included 232 patients with early HER2-positive breast cancer (total study population, n = 1,010), randomized patients to docetaxel or vinorelbine with or without nine weeks trastuzumab followed by three cycles of fluorouracil, epirubicin, and cyclophosphamide (FEC). Treatment with trastuzumab led to improved distant DFS compared to chemotherapy alone (HR 0.65, 95% CI 0.38–1.12; $P = 0.12$). This trial prompted interest in consideration for shorter duration of adjuvant trastuzumab therapy, because it demonstrated similar DFS results as initial pivotal studies. Joint analysis of NSABP-B31 and NCCTG-N9831 showed a DFS benefit of 11.8% at three years, whereas in FinHER, DFS benefit was 11.7% at three years.

Two trials (SOLD AND SHORTHer) explored nine weeks versus one year of trastuzumab with chemotherapy and failed to demonstrate non-inferiority with shorter duration. Interestingly, in the SHORTHer trial, at median follow-up of 8.7 years, there was similar DFS benefit with nine weeks versus one year of trastuzumab treatment in patients who were considered low or intermediate risk of recurrence, comprising 83.9% of the study population. In the low- and intermediate-risk groups, HR for DFS was 0.91 (90% CI 0.60–1.38) and 0.88 (90% CI 0.63–1.21), respectively, with short versus long treatment duration of trastuzumab. Furthermore, nine-year OS was 90% with short treatment versus 91% with one year of trastuzumab (HR 1.18, 90% CI 0.86–1.62).

Trials of 6 compared with 12 months of trastuzumab treatment have shown mixed results. The phase III PHARE trial included 3,380 patients with HER2-positive early breast cancer, and at a median follow-up of 7.5 years, it failed to show non-inferiority of 6 months versus 12 months of trastuzumab (DFS events occurring in 20.4% in the 12-month group and 21.2% in the 6-month group); adjusted HR for DFS was 1.08 (95% CI 0.93–1.25; $P = 0.39$). The non-inferiority margin was included in the 95% CI. The smaller (n = 481) Hellenic Oncology Research Group (HORG) study also failed to show non-inferiority of 6 versus 12 months of adjuvant trastuzumab therapy (3-year DFS was 95.7% vs 93.3% in favor of 12-month group: HR 1.57, 95% CI 0.86–2.10; $P = 0.137$; non-inferiority margin set at 1.53).

The phase III PERSEPHONE trial randomized over 4,000 patients to 6 or 12 months of adjuvant trastuzumab therapy and has reported results with a median follow-up of 5.4 years. Four-year DFS was 89.4% in the 6-month group and 89.8% in the 12-month group (HR 1.07, 90% CI 0.93–1.24; non-inferiority $P = 0.011$). Trastuzumab for six months led to fewer adverse events or early discontinuation due to cardiotoxicity (3% vs 8%, $P < 0.0001$). This trial demonstrated that 6 months trastuzumab therapy is non-inferior to 12 months.

Potential reasoning for the differences seen between these studies (PHARE and HORG compared to PERSEPHONE) is the different prespecified non-inferiority criteria. The HRs for PHARE at 7.5 years' follow-up (1.08) and PERSEPHONE at 5.4 years' follow-up (1.07) are notably similar; however, each trial reported results adherent to their respective prespecified statistical analysis plan and therefore had different conclusions. In addition, longer follow-up is warranted and planned. For example, risk of recurrence is higher for ER+/HER2+ subtype after five years compared with those with ER-/HER2+ breast cancer, and PERSEPHONE included a high percentage of patients with ER+ disease. Importantly, treatment of HER2-positive early breast cancer is very dynamic, and it is unclear how these changes may impact trials that were designed in earlier times. The evolution of novel HER2-targeted therapies and other de-escalation strategies may make it challenging to accurately apply trial results such as PERSEPHONE to current clinical practice. For example, only 10% of patients in PERSEPHONE received non-anthracycline-containing regimens (which is standard practice in recent times), and with few events reported, conclusions cannot be drawn regarding shorter duration in these patients. In the subset of the PERSEPHONE trial that is most reflective of current practice with trastuzumab given concurrently vs sequentially, there was a benefit for 12 over 6 months of trastuzumab (HR 1.53, 95% CI 1.16–2.01).

Regarding trastuzumab beyond one year, results from the phase III HERA trial after a median follow-up of 11 years demonstrated similar outcomes between 1 and 2 years of trastuzumab, and both were better compared to observation. Ten-year DFS was 69% in both arms (HR 1.02), versus 63% in the observation arm; OS was 79% and 80% in the one- and two-year trastuzumab groups, respectively, versus 73% in the observation arm (Cameron et al. 2017).

Trastuzumab, along with other anti-HER2 therapies, is associated with potential cardiac toxicity and requires echocardiogram monitoring while patients are receiving therapy. In HERA, the incidence of cardiac endpoints was 7.3% and 4.4% in the two- and one-year trastuzumab groups, respectively, compared with 0.9% in observation arm. Most cases of cardiac dysfunction are asymptomatic and reversible, and the majority of patients are able to resume trastuzumab-based therapy.

In summary, although one year duration of trastuzumab remains standard of care, results from trials including PERSEPHONE and updated DFS and OS outcomes of SHORTHer provide support for consideration of shorter course of trastuzumab in select cases. These may include patients deemed at low risk of relapse where access may be limited, or tolerance related to cardiac toxicity arises.

4) Is de-escalation therapy possible for small (≤3 cm) HER2-positive, node-negative tumors?

Expert Perspective: The single-arm phase II APT trial investigated a de-escalation strategy for small HER2-positive tumors (≤3 cm) that were node-negative, for patients who may do well with a less intensive chemotherapy with trastuzumab regimen. Among 410 patients who received adjuvant weekly paclitaxel plus trastuzumab for 12 weeks, followed by trastuzumab to complete one year, the three-year DFS rate was 98.7%. Longer-term follow-up of this study maintained these excellent outcomes, with ten-year invasive DFS, OS and breast cancer-specific survival (BCSS) of 91.3%, 94.3% and 98.8%, respectively (Tolaney et al. 2023). Seven-year DFS and OS of 93% and 95%, respectively (Tolaney et al. 2019). These favorable outcomes have led to the adoption of paclitaxel plus trastuzumab in the clinic and National Comprehensive Cancer Network guidelines as a standard regimen for small (≤3 cm), node-negative, HER2-positve tumors in the adjuvant setting.

5) What is the role of ado-trastuzumab emtansine in the adjuvant setting?

Expert Perspective: Ado-trastuzumab emtansine (T-DM1) is an antibody-drug conjugate composed of trastuzumab linked to a cytotoxic anti-microtubule agent, emtansine (DM1), which is released into target cells upon degradation of the HER2-DM1 complex in lysosomes. T-DM1 has shown DFS and OS benefit in the metastatic setting after disease progression on trastuzumab therapy. A large aim of evaluation of T-DM1 in the curative space is to improve efficacy and lower toxicity, using T-DM1 versus chemotherapy.

The phase II ATEMPT trial was designed to determine whether T-DM1 caused less toxicity with similar efficacy compared with paclitaxel plus trastuzumab (TH) per the APT regimen. In the trial, 497 patients with stage I HER2-positive breast cancer were randomized to receive T-DM1 for 17 cycles or paclitaxel plus trastuzumab for 12 weeks followed by trastuzumab to complete one year duration. Clinically relevant toxicities were similar between the two groups (46% in the T-DM1 arm vs 47% in the TH arm, $P = 0.83$). However, more patients discontinued T-DM1 for adverse events compared to TH (17% versus 6%). The study was not powered to discern efficacy differences, although at a median follow-up of 3.9 years, 3-year invasive DFS for T-DM1 was 97.8% (95% CI 96.3–99.3) versus 93.4% (95% CI 88.7–98.2) for paclitaxel plus trastuzumab. Considering the short-term follow-up and fairly high discontinuation rate with T-DM1, this agent is not viewed as standard in this setting. T-DM1 may be considered as an alternative in very select situations for patients who are concerned about specific risks associated with paclitaxel plus trastuzumab (such as neuropathy, alopecia, or use of steroid premedication).

KAITLIN was a randomized, phase III trial including 1,846 patients with high-risk early HER2-positive breast cancer (either node-positive or node-negative/HR-negative/> T2 [> 5 cm or any size growing into the chest wall or skin]) who received adjuvant anthracycline-based chemotherapy followed by TDM-1 plus pertuzumab for 18 cycles (AC-KP) or 3–4 cycles of taxane plus trastuzumab plus pertuzumab (AC-THP). In both the lymph-node-positive and intention-to-treat populations, there was no significant difference in invasive

DFS between the two arms. In patients with lymph node involvement, three-year invasive DFS was 94.1% with AC-THP and 92.7% with AC-KP. (HR 0.97, 95% CI 0.71–1.32). Similarly, in the ITT population, three-year invasive DFS was 94.2% versus 93.1% (HR 0.98, 95% CI 0.72–1.32). There was a similar incidence of adverse events in each arm, although more patients discontinued T-DM1 or trastuzumab because of adverse events in the AC-KP arm versus AC-THP (26.8% vs 4.0%). Results of this study did not show improved efficacy or toxicity via replacement of taxane plus trastuzumab with T-DM1, and as such, taxane chemotherapy remains the standard backbone for HER2-targeted therapy.

6) What is the role of pertuzumab in the adjuvant setting?

Expert Perspective: Pertuzumab is a monoclonal antibody that binds to an alternative epitope on HER2 than trastuzumab, and it blocks the formation of HER2 dimer pairs, activates antibody-dependent cellular cytotoxicity, and suppresses multiple HER2 signaling pathways, leading to a more comprehensive HER2 blockade.

The role of pertuzumab in the adjuvant setting was studied in the phase III APHINITY trial including over 4,800 patients with early HER2-positive breast cancer, who were randomized to chemotherapy plus trastuzumab with or without pertuzumab. The pertuzumab group experienced a modest improvement in invasive DFS versus placebo (three-year estimates of invasive DFS were 94.1% in the pertuzumab group and 93.2% in the placebo group; HR 0.81, 95% CI 0.66–1.00; $P = 0.045$). The greatest benefit was seen in the node-positive subgroup: three-year rate of invasive DFS was 92.0% in the pertuzumab group, as compared with 90.2% in the placebo group (HR 0.77, 95% CI 0.62–0.96; $P = 0.02$). Longer follow-up of APHINITY at approximately six years demonstrated invasive DFS rates of 91% versus 88% for pertuzumab and placebo groups, respectively (HR 0.76), and 88% versus 83% (HR 0.72) among those with node-positive disease (Piccart-Gebhart et al. 2021).

In our opinion, considering the relatively modest benefit, toxicities including diarrhea, and financial cost, adjuvant pertuzumab should be selected for those patients deemed high risk. In addition, there are no clear guidelines on the adjuvant treatment of patients who received prior pertuzumab in the neoadjvuant setting, particularly those who achieved a pathologic complete response.

Neoadjuvant Therapy

Potential advantages of a neoadjuvant chemotherapy approach include the goal of downstaging to achieve more surgical options, as well as assessment of the biology of the cancer itself via response to systemic therapy that can have prognostic and therapeutic implications. There is no difference in survival outcomes between pre- and postoperative chemotherapy, and thus this a favorable option in many scenarios. This includes early HER2-positive breast cancer with primary tumor ≥ 2 cm ($\geq$T2) or with lymph node involvement. Achievement of a pCR has been supported by various studies as a surrogate marker for long-term outcome. In addition, the neoadjuvant space is desirable for investigation of novel agents because it provides a more rapid means of evaluation compared with the adjuvant setting.

7) What is the role of trastuzumab in neoadjuvant setting?

Expert Perspective: Trastuzumab added to chemotherapy has been shown to improve pCR. The phase II NOAH trial included 235 patients with locally advanced HER2-positive breast cancer who received neoadjuvant chemotherapy with an anthracycline and taxane and demonstrated a higher pCR rate with the addition of trastuzumab compared to chemotherapy alone (38% vs 19%). At a median follow-up of 5.4 years, the trastuzumab arm experienced improved event-free survival versus chemotherapy alone (58% vs 43%, HR 0.64, 95% CI 0.44–0.93; $P = 0.016$), and of those achieving a pCR, receipt of trastuzumab was strongly associated with event-free survival (HR between those with and without trastuzumab was 0.29; 95% CI 0.11–0.78).

A pooled analysis including 12 trials and nearly 12,000 patients (n = 1,989 with HER2-positive tumors) demonstrated improvement in pCR with the addition of trastuzumab for both hormone-receptor positive and hormone-receptor negative disease (for HER2+/HR+, pCR was 30.9% and 18.3% with and without trastuzumab, respectively; for HER2+/HR−, pCR was 50.3% and 30.2% with and without trastuzumab, respectively). Furthermore, pathologic complete response was associated with long-term outcomes in HER2-positive cases, irrespective of hormone receptor status (event-free survival: HR 0.39, 95% CI 0.31–0.50; OS: HR 0.34, 95% CI 0.24–0.47).

8) What is the role of pertuzumab in the neoadjuvant setting?

Expert Perspective: In neoadjuvant treatment, pertuzumab is given in combination with trastuzumab and chemotherapy for patients diagnosed with locally advanced or early stage breast cancer that is ≥ 2 cm or involves lymph nodes. The addition of pertuzumab in the pre-operative setting has been shown to improve pCR without significant cumulative cardiotoxicity.

The phase II NeoSphere trial randomized 417 patients with HER2-positive early breast cancer to one of four treatments arms: (A) trastuzumab plus docetaxel, (B) pertuzumab plus trastuzumab plus docetaxel, (C) pertuzumab plus trastuzumab, or (D) pertuzumab plus docetaxel. Those receiving arm B had a significant improvement in pCR rate compared with those given arm A (45.8% vs 29.0%, $P = 0.0141$). The pCR rate was 24.0% in arm D and 16.8% in arm C (Gianni et al. 2012). Because pertuzumab blocks heterodimerization and resultant signaling via *EGFR* and HER2, diarrhea and skin rash can be observed. In arm C of this study, diarrhea and rash occurred in 28% and 11%, respectively, and were mostly low grade. Notably, there did not appear to be an increase in cardiac safety events with the addition of pertuzumab.

The phase II TRYPHAENA trial, including 225 patients with early HER2-positive breast cancer, was designed to investigate cardiac safety of trastuzumab and pertuzumab added to neoadjuvant chemotherapy, with pCR as a secondary endpoint. Group A received FEC plus trastuzumab plus pertuzumab followed by docetaxel plus trastuzumab plus pertuzumab, group B received FEC followed by docetaxel plus trastuzumab plus pertuzumab, and group C received docetaxel plus carboplatin plus trastuzumab plus pertuzumab. Rates of cardiac toxicity were similar in the two anthracycline-containing arms and lower in arm C. The pCR rates were high across all three treatment arms (61.6%, 57.3%, and 66.2% in groups A, B, and C, respectively). The findings from this study led to the FDA accelerated approval for pertuzumab in the neoadjuvant setting. Long-term analysis of TRYPHAENA demonstrated similar progression-free survival (three-year estimates were 89%, 89%, and 87%) and DFS (three-year estimates were 87%, 88%, and 90%). Furthermore, rates of left ventricular dysfunction remained relatively low (2.8%, 4.0%, and 5.4%).

The optimal chemotherapy backbone to combine with dual HER2-targeted therapy has been studied in various trials. Anthracyclines have potential risk of cardiac toxicity, and therefore, efforts have been made to investigate whether a non-anthracycline chemotherapy backbone may attain similar favorable outcomes and spare toxicity. The phase III TRAIN-2 study randomized 438 patients to FEC followed by carboplatin plus paclitaxel or carboplatin plus paclitaxel, with both groups receiving concurrent trastuzumab plus pertuzumab. The pCR rate was 67% in the anthracycline arm and 68% in the non-anthracycline arm ($P = 0.95$). At a median follow-up of four years, three-year event-free survival estimates were 92.7% and 93.6%, and three-year OS estimates were 97.7% and 98.2% for the anthracycline and non-anthracycline arms, respectively. The anthracycline group had higher incidence of LVEF decline (8.6% vs 3.2%) and grade 3 or worse febrile neutropenia (10% vs 1%), and two patients developed acute leukemia in this arm. Long-term follow-up of TRAIN-2 further supports a neoadjuvant regimen including carboplatin plus taxane with dual HER2-targeted therapy, because this regimen is associated with similar efficacy and less toxicity compared with an anthracycline-containing regimen.

The West-German Study Group phase II ADAPT trial randomized 134 patients with early HER2+/HR− breast cancer to 12 weeks of neoadjuvant trastuzumab plus pertuzumab with or without paclitaxel chemotherapy. The aim of this study was to determine whether patients with a strong early response to dual HER2 blockade (defined as low cellularity and/or Ki67 decrease > 30% after three weeks) achieve similar pCR rates as those receiving chemotherapy plus dual HER2-targeted therapy. Of note, 60% of patients had tumors that were cT2–T4, and 42% were clinically node-positive. The pCR rate in the trastuzumab plus pertuzumab plus paclitaxel arm was 90.5%, compared with 36.3% in the dual blockade arm. After a median follow-up of approximately five years, invasive DFS was 98% with trastuzumab plus pertuzumab plus paclitaxel and 87% with dual HER2 blockade alone (HR 0.32; $P = 0.144$). The rate of distant DFS was 98% versus 92%, respectively (HR 0.34; $P = 0.313$), and the OS rate was 98% versus 94% (HR 0.41; $P = 0.422$). Furthermore, achievement of a pCR was strongly associated with invasive DFS benefit at five years, irrespective of arm (98% vs 82%, HR 0.18, $P = 0.011$). The excellent outcomes seen in both the chemotherapy and dual HER2-targeted therapy arms raises the question of whether antibody treatment alone can be considered for select patients in the neoadjuvant setting. At the present time, it remains standard practice to give combination chemotherapy and HER2-targeted therapy for neoadjuvant treatment; however, biomarker studies will be integral to address this clinical question. This trial also supports the concept that regardless of how a pCR is achieved, it has meaningful value in terms of outcomes, including in settings where de-escalation strategies are being studied.

9) What is the role of ado-trastuzumab emtansine in the neoadjuvant setting?

Expert Perspective: The phase III KRISTINE trial randomized 444 patients with stage II–III early HER2-positive breast cancer to six cycles of preoperative T-DM1 plus pertuzumab or docetaxel plus carboplatin plus trastuzumab plus pertuzumab (TCHP). Efficacy favored the TCHP regimen, with a pCR rate of 55.7% compared with 44.4% in the T-DM1 plus pertuzumab arm. The T-DM1 arm was better tolerated then TCHP with fewer grade 3–4 adverse events (13% vs 64%); notably, TCHP had higher frequencies of grade 3–4 neutropenia (25% vs <1%), diarrhea (15% vs <1%), and febrile neutropenia (15% vs 0%). Final analysis of this study reported three-year event-free survival (EFS) rates of 94.2% with TCHP compared with 85.3% with T-DM1 plus pertuzumab (HR 2.61, 95% CI 1.36–4.98), driven mostly by locoregional recurrences in the T-DM1 group, which were found to have HER2 mRNA expression below the median. The three-year invasive DFS rates were 92.0% and 93.0% with TCHP and T-DM1, respectively (HR 1.11, 95% CI 0.52–2.40). Neoadjuvant chemotherapy in combination with HER2-targeted therapy remains standard, although there is reason to hypothesize that some patients may not require traditional systemic chemotherapy.

Post-Neoadjuvant Therapy

10) What is the role of ado-trastuzumab emtansine following neoadjuvant setting?

Expert Perspective: Patients with residual disease after neoadjuvant chemotherapy have inferior prognosis compared with those who have minimal residual disease present or achieve a pCR. The phase III KATHERINE trial randomized 1,486 patients who had residual disease after receipt of neoadjuvant systemic therapy, including a taxane (with or without an anthracycline) and trastuzumab, to either T-DM1 or trastuzumab for 14 cycles. The absolute invasive DFS benefit at three years was 11.3% in favor of T-DM1 (three-year invasive DFS rate was 88.3% in the T-DM1 arm vs 77.0% in the trastuzumab arm; HR for invasive disease or death 0.50; 95% CI 0.39–0.64; $P < 0.001$) (von Minckwitz et al. 2019). Distant recurrence as first event occurred in 10.5% and 15.9% in the T-DM1 and trastuzumab arms, respectively. There were higher rates of serious adverse events (12.7% vs 8.1%) and discontinuation of the drug due to adverse events (18% vs 2.1%) in the T-DM1 arm. Decreased platelet count, elevated liver function tests, peripheral neuropathy, and decreased ejection fraction were the most common adverse events leading to T-DM1 discontinuation. Results from KATHERINE support T-DM1 as the standard of care for patients with HER2-positive early breast cancer with residual disease after preoperative chemotherapy including a taxane and trastuzumab.

Extended Adjuvant Therapy

11) What is the role of neratinib as an extended adjuvant therapy?

Expert Perspective: Neratinib is an oral, potent, irreversible pan-HER (HER1, HER2, and HER4) tyrosine kinase inhibitor. The role of neratinib for early HER2-positive breast cancer is in the extended adjuvant setting. The phase III ExteNET trial included 2,840 patients diagnosed with stage II–III early HER2-positive breast cancer, with randomization to one year of neratinib versus placebo after completion of trastuzumab-based adjuvant therapy. Neratinib treatment was associated with a significant improvement in five-year invasive DFS versus placebo (five-year invasive DFS was 90.2% in the neratinib group vs 87.7% in the placebo group; HR 0.73; 95% CI 0.57–0.92; $P = 0.0083$). There appears to be greater benefit with neratinib in the HR+ population and those who initiated neratinib treatment 1 year after completion of trastuzumab. In the HR+ group, the absolute invasive DFS benefit at five years was 5.1% (HR 0.58, 95% CI 0.41–0.82) and was 1.3% (HR 0.74, 95% CI 0.29–1.84) for those initiating neratinib ≤1 year versus >1 year post-trastuzumab, respectively. In the HR+ group who initiated ≤1 year after trastuzumab, neratinib was associated with a numerical improvement in OS at 8 years (absolute benefit 2.1%; HR 0.79; 95% CI 0.55–1.13). Furthermore, in the HR+ ≤1 year group, those with residual disease after neoadjuvant therapy derived more benefit (absolute benefits of 7.4% at five-year invasive DFS [HR 0.60, 95% CI 0.33–1.07] and 9.1% at eight-year OS [HR 0.47; 95% CI 0.23–0.92]) (Chan et al. 2021). Importantly, there were fewer CNS events with neratinib. The cumulative incidence of first CNS recurrences at five years was 0.7% with neratinib and 2.1% with placebo. At five years, 98.4% (95% CI 96.8–99.1) of patients in the neratinib group and 95.7% (95% CI 93.6–97.2) of patients in the placebo group were alive and did not report a CNS recurrence (HR for CNS disease-free survival 0.41; 95% CI 0.18–0.85).

Diarrhea is the most common toxicity associated with neratinib, and without prophylaxis, grade 3 diarrhea occurred in 40% (prophylaxis in ExteNET was not mandatory, and 17% discontinued due to diarrhea). The phase II CONTROL trial evaluated various antidiarrheal prophylaxis strategies, including loperamide, loperamide plus budesonide, colestipol plus loperamide, colestipol plus as needed loperamide, and dose-escalation. The rates of grade 3 diarrhea, discontinuation due to diarrhea, and duration were lower with prophylaxis. Notably, the rate of grade 3 diarrhea in the dose-escalation arm was 15% with a 3% diarrhea-related discontinuation rate. These mechanisms have favorably impacted tolerability of neratinib and may facilitate patients' ability and motivation to complete the planned one-year treatment course.

Based on the ExteNET study, the FDA approved neratinib in the extended adjuvant setting for patients with early HER2-positive breast cancer after completion of trastuzumab-based therapy. Based on available data, the activity and benefit of neratinib appears to be greatest among those with high-risk HR+ disease, if initiated within one-year post-trastuzumab, and in the presence of residual disease. The role of neratinib after receipt of pertuzumab or T-DM1 is not yet elucidated.

The HER2-targeted therapies including trastuzumab, pertuzumab, ado-trastuzumab emtansine, and neratinib each have designated time points to be given or considered in the treatment algorithm for early HER2-positive breast cancer (Figure 13.1).

12) **What is the role of lapatinib as an extended adjuvant therapy?**

Expert Perspective: Lapatinib is an oral, small-molecule tyrosine kinase inhibitor that binds selectively and reversibly to *EGFR* and HER2. Lapatinib has an indication in the metastatic setting either in combination with chemotherapy or trastuzumab. There have been various trials conducted in the early stage setting, and although improvement in pCR has been seen with the addition of lapatinib to trastuzumab, this has not translated to significant survival benefit. Toxicity is also greater with lapatinib.

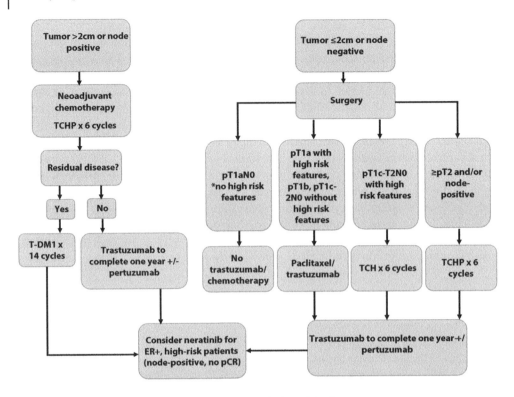

Figure 13.1 Treatment algorithm for early stage HER2-positive breast cancer.
*High risk features: ER-negative, high grade, young age
TCH: Docetaxel/Carboplatin/Trastuzumab
TCHP: Docetaxel/Carboplatin/Trastuzumab/Pertuzumab.

The phase III NeoALTTO study evaluated the role of dual HER2-targeted therapy with lapatinib plus trastuzumab in the neoadjuvant setting. In the study, 455 patients were randomized to 6 weeks of lapatinib, trastuzumab, or the combination; this period was followed by the addition of paclitaxel for 12 weeks to each of the arms prior to surgery, and subsequently FEC chemotherapy in the adjuvant setting. The dual HER2-targeted treatment group experienced a significantly higher pCR compared with the trastuzumab alone group (51.3% vs 29.5%, $P = 0.0001$), and there was no significant difference found between the lapatinib (pCR rate 24.7%) and trastuzumab groups ($P = 0.34$). After a median follow-up of 6.3 years, EFS and OS were not significantly different when comparing lapatinib versus trastuzumab or the combination versus trastuzumab.

NSABP B-41 was a phase III trial that included 519 patients with early HER2-positive breast cancer. The chemotherapy backbone was AC for four cycles followed by weekly paclitaxel; lapatinib plus trastuzumab versus lapatinib or trastuzumab alone was added to paclitaxel. After surgery, patients went on to complete one year of trastuzumab therapy. Rates of pCR in the breast were 52.5% in the trastuzumab group, 53.2% in the lapatinib group ($P = 0.9852$); and 62.0% in the combination group ($P = 0.095$). Similar to other studies, dual HER2-targeted therapy with lapatinib plus trastuzumab compared with single-agent led to a numerically improved pCR rate that did not reach statistical significance. Longer-term follow-up of NSABP B-41 showed numerically better relapse-free interval and OS with lapatinib plus trastuzumab versus either alone, but the differences were not statistically significant.

The phase III Adjuvant Lapatinib and/or Trastuzumab Treatment Optimization (ALTTO) trial evaluated one year of adjuvant trastuzumab, lapatinib, their sequence, or combination among 8,381 patients with early HER2-positive breast cancer. At a median follow-up of 4.5 years, there was no significant difference in DFS with inclusion of lapatinib compared with trastuzumab alone (L+T vs T; HR 0.84; 97.5% CI 0.70–1.02; $P = 0.048$; T→L vs T: HR 0.96; 97.5% CI 0.80–1.15; $P = 0.61$) (Piccart-Gebhart et al. 2016). Lapatinib treatment was associated with more diarrhea, rash, and hepatic toxicity. Longer-term follow-up (median 6.9 years) yielded similar findings.

Future Research

Although significant progress has been made in the treatment for early HER2-positive breast cancer, there is a desire to continue development of strategies that will further improve outcomes and minimize side effects that can impact patients' quality of life. Described in Table 13.1, these include novel therapy combinations, de-escalation studies, and evaluation in the curative space of agents demonstrating efficacy in the metastatic setting.

Table 13.1 Ongoing and future trials for early stage HER2-positive breast cancer.

Clinical trial	Phase	Treatment setting	Regimen being investigated
PALTAN (NCT02907918)	II	Neoadjuvant; ER+	Palbociclib + letrozole (GnRH if premenopausal) + T
TOUCH (NCT03644186)	II	Neoadjuvant; ER+, node-positive	Palbociclib + letrozole + T + P
neoHIP (NCT03747120)	II	Neoadjuvant	Pembrolizumab + paclitaxel + T + P
DECRESCENDO (NCT04675827)	II	Neoadjuvant	Paclitaxel + T + P; adjuvant T + P (yes pCR) vs T-DM1 (no pCR)
DESTINY-Breast05 (NCT04622319)	III	Adjuvant; residual disease post-neoadjuvant therapy	Trastuzumab-deruxtecan vs T-DM1
CompassHER2 RD (NCT04457596)	III	Adjuvant; residual disease post-neoadjuvant therapy	T-DM1 + tucatinib vs T-DM1

T = trastuzumab, P = pertuzumab.

Conclusions

In summary, there have been significant advances in the area of early stage HER2-positive breast cancer, beginning with development and application of trastuzumab, to more recent studies with novel therapies and combinations. The aggressive biology of HER2-positive breast cancer has been offset by the successful outcomes seen in various pivotal clinical trials with anti-HER2 therapies. The value of pCR is certainly relevant in this subtype of breast cancer, and the personalization of treatment is a goal in this setting. This dynamic landscape will likely continue to evolve, and identification of biomarkers and predictors of response and resistance will be key to further improving outcomes for patients with early HER2-positive breast cancer.

Recommended Readings

Cameron, D., Piccart-Gebhart, M.J., Gelber, R.D. et al. (2017). 11 years' follow-up of trastuzumab after adjuvant chemotherapy in HER2-positive early breast cancer: Final analysis of the HERceptin Adjuvant (HERA) trial. *Lancet* 389 (10075): 1195–1205.

Chan, A., Moy, B., Mansi, J., et al. (2021). Final efficacy results of neratinib in HER2-positive hormone receptor-positive early-stage breast cancer from the phase III ExteNET trial. *Clin Breast Cancer* 21 (1): 80–91.e7.

EBCTCG (Early Breast Cancer Trialists' Collaborative Group). (2021). Trastuzumab for early-stage, HER2-positive breast cancer: A meta-analysis of 13,864 women in seven randomised trials. *Lancet Oncol* 22 (8): 1139–1150.

Gianni, L., Pienkowski, T., Im, Y.H., et al. (2012). Efficacy and safety of neoadjuvant pertuzumab and trastuzumab in women with locally advanced, inflammatory, or early HER2-positive breast cancer (NeoSphere): A randomised multicentre, open-label, phase 2 trial. *Lancet Oncol* 13 (1): 25–32.

Perez, E.A., Romond, E.H., Suman, V.J. et al. (2014). Trastuzumab plus adjuvant chemotherapy for human epidermal growth factor receptor 2-positive breast cancer: Planned joint analysis of overall survival from NSABP B-31 and NCCTG N9831. *J Clin Oncol* 32 (33): 3744–3752.

Piccart-Gebhart, M., Holmes, E., Baselga, J. et al. (2016). Adjuvant lapatinib and trastuzumab for early human epidermal growth factor receptor 2–positive breast cancer: Results from the randomized phase III adjuvant lapatinib and/or trastuzumab treatment optimization trial. *J Clin Oncol* 34 (10): 1034–1042.

Piccart-Gebhart, M., Procter, M., Fumagalli, D. et al. (2021). Adjuvant pertuzumab and trastuzumab in early HER2-positive breast cancer in the APHINITY trial: 6 years' follow-up. *J Clin Oncol* 39 (13): 1448–1457.

Slamon, D., Eiermann, W., Robert, N. et al. (2011). Adjuvant trastuzumab in HER2-positive breast cancer. *N Engl J Med* 365 (14): 1273–1283.

Tolaney, S.M., Tarantino, P., Graham, N. et al. (2023). Adjuvant paclitaxel and trastuzumab for node-negative, HER2-positive breast cancer: final 10-year analysis of the open-label, single-arm, phase 2 APT trial. *Lancet Oncol* 24 (3): 273–285.

von Minckwitz, G., Huang, C.S., Mano, M.S. et al. (2019). Trastuzumab emtansine for residual invasive HER2-positive breast cancer. *N Engl J Med* 380 (7): 617–628.

14

HER2 Positive Metastatic Breast Cancer

Reshma L. Mahtani, Naomi G. Dempsey, and Ana Sandoval

Miami Cancer Institute, Baptist Health South Florida, Member, Memorial Sloan Kettering Cancer Alliance, Plantation, FL

Introduction

Since the advent of trastuzumab over 20 years ago, the outlook for patients with HER2-positive metastatic breast cancer has improved considerably. Historically, this subtype of breast cancer was associated with an aggressive phenotype, high recurrence rates, and inferior survival outcomes. By 2006, chemotherapy and trastuzumab became standard treatments in both early and advanced stage disease, based on landmark trials that established improvements in efficacy. Despite these gains, long-term follow-up data from large adjuvant trials indicate that up to 25% of patients with early stage disease will experience disease relapse within 10 years postdiagnosis, and patients with metastatic disease inevitably develop resistance to HER2-directed therapies. As such, further improvements in patient outcomes are needed. Research has focused on strategies to overcome resistance, ultimately intending to develop additional treatment options. Recently the treatment landscape has further evolved, with the approval of several new agents in the metastatic setting. Currently, there are eight FDA-approved HER2-targeted therapies in the (neo)adjuvant and/or metastatic setting: trastuzumab; the humanized HER2-targeted monoclonal antibody, pertuzumab; the HER1 and HER2 tyrosine kinase inhibitor (TKI) lapatinib; the pan-HER TKI, neratinib; the selective HER2-targeted TKI, tucatinib; two antibody-drug conjugates (ADCs), trastuzumab emtansine (T-DM1) and trastuzumab deruxtecan (T-DXd; DS-8201a); and most recently, the Fc-engineered monoclonal antibody, margetuximab. Given the rapidly evolving data, the authors hope to provide guidance on sequencing therapies based on randomized data and pivotal trials.

Case Study 1: *De novo* HER2-positive metastatic breast cancer

A 64-year-old woman noticed a rapidly enlarging right breast mass. A mammogram documented a 4 × 6 cm mass and multiple abnormal appearing right axillary lymph nodes. Biopsy of the breast mass and lymph node both revealed poorly differentiated, hormone receptor negative, HER2-positive (3+ by immunohistochemistry), invasive ductal carcinoma. Staging CT scans identified multiple hypodense liver lesions measuring up to 6 cm and sclerotic-appearing bone lesions with an osteoblastic appearance on nuclear medicine bone scan. Biopsy of a liver lesion confirmed hormone receptor-positive and HER2+ metastatic breast cancer.

Cancer Consult: Expertise in Clinical Practice, Volume 1: Solid Tumors & Supportive Care,
Second Edition. Edited by Syed A. Abutalib, Maurie Markman, Al B. Benson III, and Hope S. Rugo.
© 2024 John Wiley & Sons Ltd. Published 2024 by John Wiley & Sons Ltd.

14 HER2 Positive Metastatic Breast Cancer

1) What is the optimal first-line treatment for *de novo* HER2-positive metastatic breast cancer?

Expert Perspective: This patient has metastatic disease upon initial presentation, which is not uncommon in HER2-positive disease. In fact, around 50% of patients with HER2-positive metastatic breast cancer present with *de novo* metastatic disease (Tripathy et al. 2020). The Systemic Therapies for HER2-Positive Metastatic Breast Cancer Study (SystHERs) was a prospective, observational cohort study designed to provide real-world insights into current treatment patterns, long-term survival, and patients' experiences with initial and subsequent treatments for HER2-positive metastatic breast cancer. In this study, Tripathy et al. reported patients with *de novo* HER2-positive metastatic breast cancer more commonly had hormone receptor-negative disease with bone and liver metastasis, and less commonly presented with central nervous system (CNS) metastases, compared with patients who had received treatment for early stage disease. As compared with patients with recurrent disease, those with *de novo* disease had longer median progression-free survival and overall survival (OS).

Standard first-line therapy for patients with HER2-positive metastatic breast cancer is taxane chemotherapy (docetaxel or paclitaxel), trastuzumab, and pertuzumab. This standard was established by the CLEOPATRA trial (Swain et al. 2020). This was a phase III randomized, placebo-controlled trial that enrolled 808 patients with HER2-positive metastatic breast cancer who were previously untreated in the metastatic setting. Patients were randomized to docetaxel, trastuzumab, and pertuzumab versus docetaxel, trastuzumab, and placebo. The study met its primary endpoint with a progression-free survival of 18.7 months in the pertuzumab group compared with 12.4 months in the placebo group (HR 0.69; 95% CI 0.59–0.81, $P < 0.0001$). Even more impressive was the secondary endpoint of eight-year landmark OS, which was 57.1 months in the pertuzumab group versus 40.8 months in the placebo group (HR 0.69; 95% CI 0.58–0.82; $P < 0.0001$), even though crossover was allowed (Figure 14.1). Of note, only 11% of patients on the trial had previously been treated with trastuzumab in the localized setting, and therefore the patient in Case 1 with *de novo* metastatic disease was well represented in the CLEOPATRA trial.

The option to use a taxane other than docetaxel was evaluated in the PERUSE study. Among 1,436 patients with HER2-positive metastatic breast cancer treated with physician's

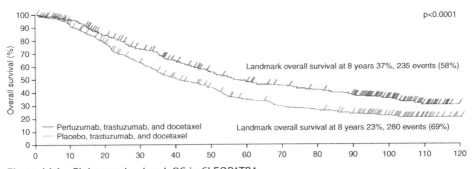

Figure 14.1 Eight-year landmark OS in CLEOPATRA.

choice of taxane, median progression-free survival was comparable between docetaxel, paclitaxel, and nanoparticle albumin-bound paclitaxel. Compared with docetaxel-containing therapy, paclitaxel-containing therapy was associated with more neuropathy but less febrile neutropenia and mucositis. A limitation in the interpretation of these data is that patients were not randomly assigned to different taxanes. The authors concluded that paclitaxel is a viable alternative to docetaxel, which is now reflected in the National Comprehensive Cancer Network (NCCN) guidelines (NCCN 2023). We generally continue taxane plus trastuzumab, and pertuzumab until the best response or intolerable side effects, before dropping the taxane and continuing trastuzumab and pertuzumab until progression. For hormone receptor positive patients, we add endocrine therapy after we stop the taxane, further discussed later in the chapter. A similar approach was taken in the CLEOPATRA trial, where docetaxel was given for a median of eight cycles.

Ongoing trials are seeking to improve upon the current first-line standard of care. The DESTINY-Breast09 trial is currently ongoing, and is seeking to establish trastuzumab deruxtecan as the first-line standard of care. The antibody-drug conjugate trastuzumab deruxtecan has demonstrated impressive activity and is now the current standard of care in the second-line setting for most patients. The ongoing DESTINY-Breast09 trial is evaluating the efficacy and safety of trastuzumab deruxtecan, alone or with pertuzumab, compared with the standard of care treatment with taxane (docetaxel or paclitaxel), trastuzumab, and pertuzumab. This trial is currently accruing and will enroll 1,100 patients with a plan to complete accrual in July 2025.

Case Study 2: Recurrent metastatic HER2-positive breast cancer

A 61-year-old woman presented with an erythematous enlarged left breast that did not improve with antibiotics. A mammogram identified a 6.7 cm irregular mass and multiple abnormal appearing axillary lymph nodes. Biopsy of the breast mass and lymph node revealed poorly differentiated, hormone receptor negative, HER2-positive (3+ by immunohistochemistry) invasive ductal carcinoma. Staging CT scans were negative for metastatic disease. She received neoadjuvant docetaxel, carboplatin, trastuzumab, and pertuzumab for six cycles with excellent clinical response, and at the time of modified radical left mastectomy, she was found to have a pathologic complete response. She received adjuvant postmastectomy radiation and completed one year of adjuvant trastuzumab and pertuzumab. Three years later, she developed right hip pain, and imaging showed bone and liver lesions. Biopsy of a liver lesion confirmed hormone receptor-negative and HER2-positive metastatic breast cancer.

2) **In addition to bone modifying agents, what is the optimal first-line treatment for HER2-positive metastatic breast cancer that recurs more than one year after previously treated early stage disease?**

Expert Perspective: The CLEOPATRA trial is also informative to guide therapy in patients with recurrent HER2-positive metastatic breast cancer, with an important caveat. Patients previously untreated in the metastatic setting were enrolled in this study and stratified according to prior receipt of neo(adjuvant) therapy. However, the study was conducted in an era before the routine use of pertuzumab in the neo(adjuvant) setting, so none of the patients enrolled had prior exposure to pertuzumab. Therefore, the efficacy demonstrated in this pivotal trial may not reflect what is demonstrated in patients with prior exposure to pertuzumab, such as in the case presented. The study did permit patients to enroll who developed metastatic disease after treatment in the early stage setting, as long as the disease-free interval was at least 12 months from the completion of treatment for early breast cancer. In a subgroup analysis of the 46.5% of patients who had previously received any type of treatment in the localized setting, OS was longer in the pertuzumab group compared with placebo (53.8 months vs 46.6 months; HR 0.86; 95% CI 0.51–1.43), although the study was not powered to detect a difference in this subgroup (Swain et al. 2020). Therefore, although the patient in Case 2 was not reflective of the population of patients enrolled on CLEOPATRA, given the three-year disease-free interval, it would be reasonable to rechallenge with a pertuzumab-based regimen.

It would also be reasonable to offer the antibody-drug conjugate trastuzumab deruxtecan (T-DXd) in this clinical scenario. Trastuzumab deruxtecan first received accelerated approval for HER2-positive MBC based on the single arm non-randomized phase 2 DESTINY-Breast01 trial (Modi et al. 2020) in which patients who were intolerant or had progressed on trastuzumab emtansine received T-DXd. In this heavily pre-treated population (median number of prior lines of therapy 6), there was an impressive overall response rate of 61% and an unprecedented median duration of response of 20.8 months (Figure 14.2). This benefit was confirmed in the phase 3 DESTINY-Breast02 trial, which randomized patients who had progressed on T-DM1 to trastuzumab deruxtecan versus treatment of physician's choice (options to include trastuzumab and capecitabine or lapatinib and capecitabine). The trial met the primary endpoint, with a progression-free survival of 17.8 months in the T-DXd arm and 6.9 months in the treatment of physician's choice arm (HR 0.36 95% CI 0.28-0.45; $P<0.0001$) (Andre et al. 2023). Although these trials firmly established the efficacy of T-DXd after T-DM1, most patients will receive T-DXd prior to T-DM1 based on the

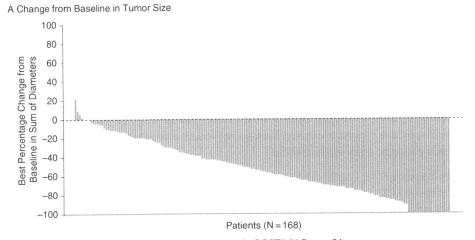

Figure 14.2 Waterfall plot for overall response in DESTINY-Breast01.

phase 3 DESTINY-Breast03 trial. This study randomized patients who had progressed on a taxane and trastuzumab to T-DXd vs T-DM1, and firmly established T-DXd as the preferred ADC in the second line for the majority of patients. Given these data, in this patient who had previously received taxane, trastuzumab, and pertuzumab in the early stage setting we would also consider trastuzumab deruxtecan as first-line therapy in the metastatic setting.

3) **How would you treat the patient in Case 2 if she was to be diagnosed with recurrent HER2-positive metastatic breast cancer less than one year after treatment of early breast cancer?**

Expert Perspective: The DESTINY-Breast03 was a phase III head-to-head trial of trastuzumab deruxtecan versus trastuzumab emtansine in patients with HER2-positive MBC previously treated with trastuzumab and a taxane. Of note, the trial included patients who had progressed within six months after (neo)adjuvant treatment involving a regimen including trastuzumab and taxane. At a median follow-up of about 27 months (28.4 for T-DXd and 26.5 for T-DM1), median progression-free survival by blinded independent central review was 28.8 months with trastuzumab deruxtecan and was 6.8 months with trastuzumab emtansine (HR 0.33; 95% CI 0.26–0.43; $P < 0.0001$).

The benefit was observed across all prespecified subgroups. Although median overall survival has not yet been reached in either arm, there was a significant improvement in 24-month OS with T-DXd (77.4% vs 69.9%). Fewer overall survival events occurred in the T-DXd arm as compared to T-DM1 (28% vs 37%; HR 0.64; $P = 0.0037$) (Figure 14.3) (Hurvitz et al. 2023). We would recommend trastuzumab deruxtecan for a patient with a disease-free interval of 12 months or less from the treatment of early HER2-positive breast cancer and diagnosis of metastatic disease. NCCN guidelines were updated in early 2022 to include trastuzumab deruxtecan as the preferred second-line therapy. The American Society of Clinical Oncology (ASCO) guidelines also support this recommendation (Giordano et al. 2022).

Case Study 3: HER2-positive metastatic breast cancer in a patient who received trastuzumab emtansine in the adjuvant setting

A 61-year-old woman was diagnosed with clinical stage T3 N2 M0 hormone receptor–negative and HER2-positive breast cancer and received six cycles of neoadjuvant docetaxel, carboplatin, trastuzumab, and pertuzumab. At the time of her surgery, there was significant residual disease in the breast and lymph nodes. She received one year of adjuvant trastuzumab emtansine per the KATHERINE trial. Unfortunately, two years later she developed right hip pain, and imaging showed widespread bone and liver lesions. Biopsy of a liver lesion confirmed metastatic hormone receptor–negative and HER2-positive breast cancer.

4) **What is the first-line treatment of metastatic HER2-positive breast cancer when trastuzumab emtansine was given for residual disease after neoadjuvant therapy?**

Expert Perspective: The KATHERINE trial has changed the treatment paradigm for early stage HER2-positive breast cancer patients who do not achieve a pathologic complete response. Patients in this trial received neoadjuvant therapy for HER2-positive early stage breast cancer. Those who had residual disease at the time of surgery were randomized to one year of adjuvant trastuzumab emtansine versus trastuzumab alone. The absolute difference in invasive disease-free survival between the two arms was 11%, favoring the use of trastuzumab emtansine. In the event these patients develop metastatic disease, trastuzumab deruxtecan would be the preferred regimen, because there is documented activity of this agent in patients who progress on trastuzumab emtansine based on the DESTINY-Breast01 and DESTINY-Breast02 trials. In a patient with CNS involvement in addition to systemic disease at recurrence, the combination of tucatinib, capecitabine, and trastuzumab could be considered, although current approval is after one line of therapy in the metastatic setting. However, there is a rationale to consider this approach, given patients included in the pivotal HER2CLIMB trial that led to the approval of the tucatinib regimen (discussed below) had all progressed on prior trastuzumab, pertuzumab, and trastuzumab emtansine. Moving forward, it will be essential for investigators to focus on understanding mechanisms of resistance to current therapies. Patients who receive neoadjuvant treatment and have residual disease requiring adjuvant trastuzumab emtansine and then develop metastatic disease will have unique biology which, to date, has not been represented in any of our completed trials.

Case Study 4: Second-line treatment of metastatic HER2-positive breast cancer

A 64-year-old woman with a history of *de novo* hormone receptor–negative and HER2-positive metastatic breast cancer with metastases to liver and bone received paclitaxel, trastuzumab, and pertuzumab as first-line therapy, as well as zoledronic acid. After six cycles, she had an excellent response with normalization of liver enzymes, and a response was noted on imaging. The taxane was dropped, and she continued to receive trastuzumab, and pertuzumab alone, for another year, at which time new liver lesions were noted on follow-up scans.

5) **What is considered the standard second-line treatment for HER2-positive metastatic breast cancer?**

Expert Perspective: As previously reviewed, the DESTINY-Breast03 trial established trastuzumab deruxtecan as the preferred regimen in the second-line setting and has now replaced the previous standard of trastuzumab emtansine. Another option in the second line would be the combination of tucatinib, capecitabine, and trastuzumab, but this regimen would generally be considered prior to T-DXd only in a patient who develops significant CNS disease early in the course of treatment (see below).

There are ongoing studies evaluating other treatment options in the second line. The HER2CLIMB-02 trial is enrolling patients with advanced HER2-positive breast cancer who have previously received trastuzumab and taxane, (in the metastatic or early stage setting). Patients are randomized to receive trastuzumab emtansine with either tucatinib or placebo. Patients who previously received trastuzumab emtansine are ineligible, but patients with brain metastases (both active and stable) are eligible. Given that trastuzumab emtansine is no longer the preferred second-line treatment, if this study is positive, it will be challenging to clarify how to incorporate the results into our treatment paradigm, given the impressive results of the DB-03 trial.

Introduction | 169

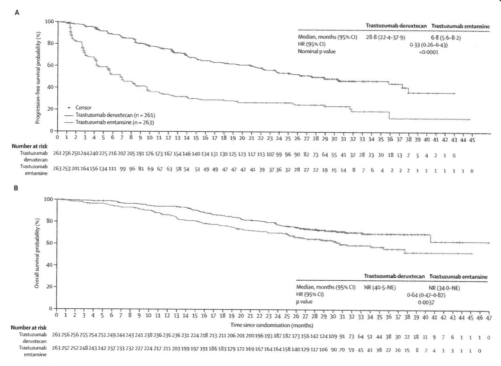

Figure 14.3 Progression-free survival in DESTINY-Breast03. Copyright Elsevier.

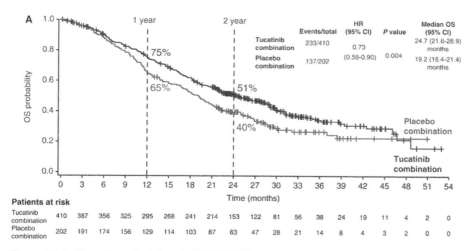

Figure 14.4 Overall survival data for HER2CLIMB.

6) What if the patient in Case 4 had well-controlled disease in the liver and bones after first-line taxane plus trastuzumab and pertuzumab, but two small new brain metastases were incidentally discovered on imaging?

Expert Perspective: For patients who develop CNS metastases while still maintaining systemic control of disease, ASCO guidelines (Ramakrishna et al. 2018) recommend local therapy to be utilized with the continuation of the same systemic therapy. Local therapy options ultimately depend on the number and size of the brain lesions but include surgery, stereotactic radiosurgery (SRS), fractionated stereotactic radiotherapy, and whole brain radiotherapy (WBRT). However, these guidelines were developed in an era before the availability of agents with significant CNS penetration. The combination of tucatinib, capecitabine, and trastuzumab is approved in the second line and beyond, based on the HER2CLIMB trial. This large phase II randomized trial included patients who had progressed on prior treatment with trastuzumab, pertuzumab, and trastuzumab emtansine, and the trial was unique in allowing patients with both stable as well as active brain metastatic disease (< 2 cm and not requiring immediate local therapy). For patients with CNS metastatic disease, CNS progression-free survival (defined as the time from random assignment to disease progression in the brain or death resulting from any cause) was 9.9 months in the tucatinib arm versus 4.2 months in the placebo arm (HR 0.39; 95% CI 0.27–0.56). A similar benefit was noted for those with active brain metastasis at enrollment. In addition, the intracranial overall response rate was higher in the tucatinib arm (47.3%; 95% CI 33.7–61.2) versus the placebo arm (20.0%; 95% CI 5.7–43.7), and the median duration of response was 8.6 months (95% CI 5.5–10.3) versus 3.0 months (95% CI 3.0–10.3). Therefore, even in the absence of progressive systemic disease, one could make a case to utilize this very active regimen in patients with a significant burden of CNS disease in the second-line setting. In the case presented, given the overall low disease burden in the CNS with well-controlled systemic disease, we would continue systemic therapy with trastuzumab and pertuzumab and refer to radiation oncology for consideration of local therapy.

Case Study 5: Trastuzumab deruxtecan toxicity

A 62-year-old woman with HER2-positive metastatic breast cancer with bone and liver involvement progressed on first-line docetaxel, trastuzumab, and pertuzumab and was treated with trastuzumab deruxtecan as second-line therapy. She has never smoked, has no underlying pulmonary condition, and at baseline did not have lung metastases. During the fourth cycle, she began to develop shortness of breath and a dry cough. A chest CT was done and revealed interstitial lung disease/pneumonitis. Trastuzumab deruxtecan was discontinued and steroids were initiated, and her symptoms improved.

7) How is interstitial lung disease related to trastuzumab deruxtecan managed?

Expert Perspective: In the phase II DESTINY-Breast01 trial, 13.6% of patients developed interstitial lung disease of any grade, and most unfortunately, four patients (2.2%) developed interstitial lung disease that was fatal (Modi et al. 2020). Symptom identification and investigation at the first sign of interstitial lung disease/pneumonitis are key to diagnosis and monitoring. Signs and symptoms can include cough, dyspnea, fever, and new or worsening respiratory symptoms. Prompt investigation is recommended and may include an evaluation with high-resolution CT, blood cultures, ABG as indicated, and pulmonary consultation for consideration of bronchoscopy. For asymptomatic (grade 1) events, consider steroids (⩾0.5 mg/kg/day prednisolone or equivalent) and interrupt treatment until resolved to grade 0. If resolution occurs in 28 days or fewer, the same dose can be maintained. If it takes longer than 28 days for resolution, a dose level reduction is recommended. For symptomatic interstitial lung disease (grade 2 or greater), prompt treatment with steroids (⩾1 mg/kg/day prednisolone or equivalent) is recommended for at least 14 days followed by gradual taper over at least four weeks. Permanent discontinuation of the drug is recommended in patients who are diagnosed with any symptomatic interstitial lung disease/pneumonitis. As a result, it is our practice to obtain re-staging imaging after the third cycle of treatment to include an assessment for grade 1 interstitial lung disease. Figure 14.5 shows the treatment algorithm for trastuzumab deruxtecan-related interstitial lung disease.

Case Study 6: Third-line treatment of HER2-positive metastatic breast cancer

A 58-year-old postmenopausal woman was diagnosed with *de novo* hormone receptor–negative and HER2-positive metastatic breast cancer with bone and liver metastasis. She received docetaxel, trastuzumab, and pertuzumab and had a complete response. Then she continued on trastuzumab, and pertuzumab alone. The disease was controlled for 18 months, followed by the development of progression in the liver and bone. She received trastuzumab emtansine (before the availability of results from DESTINY-Breast03) and had a partial response. Eight months later, she developed progression again with worsening liver metastases and new asymptomatic brain metastases.

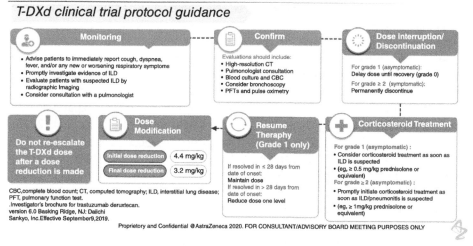

Figure 14.5 Management of interstitial lung disease caused by trastuzumab deruxtecan.

8) **What are the options for the third-line treatment of metastatic HER2-positive breast cancer?**

Expert Perspective: Under the current HER2-positive metastatic breast cancer treatment paradigm, most patients will have received T-DXd in the second line. Some patients with CNS involvement may have received the HER2CLIMB regimen of trastuzumab, tucatinib, and capecitabine in the second line setting per the FDA label. If HER2CLIMB regimen was not used in the second line, it is the preferred therapy in the third line. HER2CLIMB was a large phase II study that randomized patients to capecitabine and trastuzumab with either tucatinib or placebo. This trial met all of its primary and secondary endpoints with an improvement in progression-free survival and overall survival in patients with or without brain metastasis (Figure 14.4) (Murthy et al. 2020). In the final analysis by Curigliano et al 2022, the addition of tucatinib resulted in an improvement in progression-free survival from 4.9 months to 7.6 months (HR 0.57; 95% CI 0.47–0.70; $p < 0.001$) and overall survival from 19.2 months to 24.7 months (HR 0.73; 95% CI 0.59–0.90; $p = 0.004$).

Given the rapid development of new agents for the treatment of HER2-positive metastatic breast cancer, there are now multiple HER2-directed therapies approved for use in the fourth line and beyond, and optimal sequencing of these agents is unknown. Trastuzumab emtansine was studied in the salvage therapy setting in the TH3RESA trial, which was a phase 3 randomized trial comparing trastuzumab emtansine to treatment of physician's choice (TPC) in the third line or beyond setting. All patients had received prior trastuzumab, lapatinib, and taxane. Median overall survival was significantly improved with trastuzumab emtansine vs TPC (22.7 months vs 15.8 months; HR 0.68; $P = 0.0007$), and progression free survival was 6.2 vs 3.3 months (HR 0.528; 95% CI 0.422–0.661; $P = 0.0034$). Trastuzumab emtansine has not been studied after the use of trastuzumab deruxtecan, and it is unknown whether trastuzumab emtansine would remain efficacious in that setting. NCCN guidelines state that the HER2CLIMB regimen is the preferred third line option, and they also list T-DM1 as an option (NCCN 2023). However, whether there will be activity of trastuzumab emtansine in patients who have experienced disease progression on trastuzumab deruxtecan is unknown, and studies evaluating mechanisms of resistance to ADCs will be needed to help inform optimal sequencing.

Margetuximab, a novel chimeric Fc-engineered HER2 antibody, was studied in the phase III SOPHIA trial. Patients were randomized to chemotherapy with one of four chemotherapies (capecitabine, eribulin, gemcitabine, or vinorelbine) plus margetuximab or trastuzumab. There was a statistically significant, although quite modest, improvement in progression-free survival of approximately five weeks. An exploratory analysis showed that the benefits were enhance in patients with a low-affinity CD16A genotype (85% of patients) (Rugo et al. 2021).

Neratinib has an indication in the early stage setting and received an expanded indication in the metastatic setting based on the phase III NALA study by Saura et al. (2020). Patients who had progressed after two or more prior therapies were randomized to the combination of neratinib/capecitabine or lapatinib/capecitabine. There was about a two-month improvement in progression-free survival by restricted means analysis. Patients with stable, asymptomatic CNS disease were eligible for the study. A numeric benefit of neratinib/capecitabine in overall survival was observed but did not achieve statistical significance. Perhaps most meaningful, a delay in time to intervention for CNS metastatic disease was observed in the neratinib arm (Saura et al. 2020).

Introduction | 173

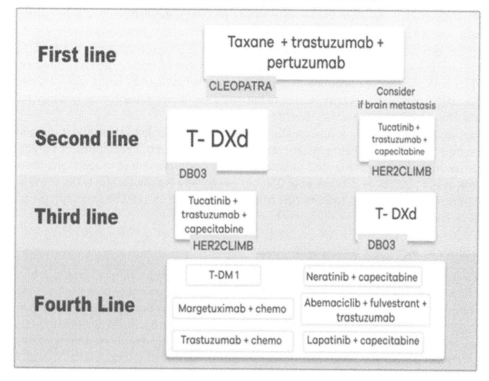

Figure 14.6 Algorithm for the approach to the treatment of metastatic HER2-positive breast cancer. *Source:* Bardia et al. 2022/Oxford University Press/CC BY 4.

NCCN guidelines list neratinib plus capecitabine and margetuximab plus chemotherapy as fourth-line and beyond options, also including the combination of trastuzumab with other chemotherapy backbones in this category. For patients with CNS metastases, tucatinib is preferred (NCCN 2023).

Given the presence of brain metastases in the patient in Case 5, we would recommend capecitabine with trastuzumab and tucatinib as third-line therapy.

Figure 14.6 shows a suggested treatment algorithm for metastatic HER2-positive breast cancer.

Case Study 7: Tucatinib toxicity

The patient from Case 6 started treatment with trastuzumab, capecitabine, and tucatinib. At the time of the third cycle, she reported diarrhea up to four times per day, redness and pain in her palms and soles, nausea, and fatigue. Routine labs revealed grade 1 elevations in AST and ALT. She was advised to use loperamide as needed. Despite the use of loperamide, diarrhea did not improve. The dose of capecitabine was reduced and the patient's symptoms improved considerably.

9) How is the toxicity of the HER2CLIMB regimen managed?

Expert Perspective: Some of the more problematic common adverse reactions occurring in at least 20% of patients in the HER2CLIMB study were diarrhea and palmar-plantar erythrodysesthesia. These are known side effects of capecitabine. Patients also reported nausea, vomiting, fatigue, and stomatitis, but these were not significantly different between the two arms. In contrast to neratinib, which is a pan-HER inhibitor, tucatinib is highly selective for HER2, and this may account for improved tolerability and less frequent need for anti-diarrheal medications. In patients who develop diarrhea while receiving the HER2CLIMB regimen, it is recommended to initially dose reduce capecitabine and to start antidiarrheal medications such as loperamide.

Transaminitis was higher in the tucatinib arm but did not result in treatment discontinuation and no dose adjustments are required for grade 1 and 2 elevations. For grade 3 transaminitis, it is recommended to hold tucatinib until recovery to grade 1 and then resume at the next lower dose level of 250 mg twice daily. Finally, tucatinib can cause a rise in creatinine that is due to inhibition of tubular secretion of creatinine and not due to renal toxicity. Therefore, dose adjustments are not required.

Case Study 8: Metastatic triple-positive breast cancer

An 85-year-old woman with hypertension, hyperlipidemia, type 2 diabetes, and a history of NSTEMI presents with mid-back pain. She reports a palpable breast mass that she has ignored over the past year. Imaging revealed diffuse bone metastases. Biopsy of the breast and a bony site identifies poorly differentiated invasive ductal carcinoma, hormone receptor–positive and HER2-positive. The patient lives alone and has been requiring more help with ADLs. She wishes to maintain her independence and is concerned about the side effects she may experience from chemotherapy.

10) What are the options for first-line treatment of metastatic triple-positive breast cancer?

Expert Perspective: As previously detailed, first-line treatment with taxane (docetaxel or paclitaxel), trastuzumab, and pertuzumab has become the standard of care based on the CLEOPATRA trial. In this study, a benefit from the addition of pertuzumab was identified regardless of hormone receptor status, and patients received a minimum of six cycles of taxane therapy (Swain et al. 2020) with the continuation of dual antibody thereafter. Although endocrine therapy was not started after discontinuation of chemotherapy in the CLEOPATRA trial, this is the usual approach in practice and is coined "maintenance endocrine therapy". However, for some patients who are felt to not be appropriate candidates for chemotherapy, it may be reasonable to consider a different strategy, which includes upfront hormonal therapy plus HER2 targeted therapy. This approach is supported by the ASCO guidelines (Giordano et al. 2022). Although this approach has not been directly compared against chemo plus trastuzumab, and pertuzumab, some trials are informative in this subgroup of patients.

The phase II PERTAIN trial examined first-line aromatase inhibitor (AI) with trastuzumab with or without pertuzumab in triple-positive patients. The random assignment was to pertuzumab plus trastuzumab and a nonsteroidal AI, or trastuzumab and a nonsteroidal AI. Induction chemotherapy with taxane-based chemo for 18–24 weeks at the investigator's discretion was permitted, and the primary endpoint was progression-free survival. Patients were stratified by whether they received induction chemotherapy and their time since adjuvant hormone therapy. Progression-free survival was 20.6 months for the dual antibody arm and 15.8 months for the trastuzumab alone arm (HR 0.7; 95% CI 0.5–0.9, P = 0.006), and median overall survival was 60.2 months versus 57.2 months (HR 1.05; P = 0.78), respectively (Arpino et al. 2023). Of note, these numbers are very similar to those reported in the CLEOPATRA trial, and there was a potentially enhanced treatment effect observed by the addition of P to H + an AI in patients who did not receive induction chemotherapy.

The use of HER2-directed therapy alone is often considered in patients who are elderly or not otherwise felt to be appropriate for chemotherapy. The EORTC 75111 was designed to specifically evaluate this approach. Patients who were 70 years or older, or 60 years or older with confirmed functional restrictions defined by protocol, were randomized to receive metronomic oral cyclophosphamide 50 mg per day plus trastuzumab and pertuzumab, or trastuzumab and pertuzumab alone. Hormone receptor status was a stratification factor. Progression-free survival with trastuzumab and pertuzumab alone was 5.6 months and improved to 12.7 months (HR 0.65, 95% CI 0.37–1.12; P = 0.12) with the addition of metronomic cyclophosphamide. This study highlighted the importance of including chemo with trastuzumab and pertuzumab and provides the option to use a less toxic chemo approach in those patients who are not felt to be candidates for taxane-based chemo.

Finally, the ongoing PATINA trial addresses the addition of a CDK4/6 inhibitor to endocrine therapy plus trastuzumab and pertuzumab following induction chemotherapy plus trastuzumab and pertuzumab. In this study, patients with triple-positive metastatic breast cancer receive induction chemotherapy, and after four to eight cycles of a taxane or vinorelbine plus trastuzumab and pertuzumab, patients are randomized to palbociclib or placebo in combination with endocrine therapy and anti-HER2 therapy. This study is no longer recruiting, and results are awaited.

11) **What are the options after first-line treatment of metastatic triple-positive breast cancer?**

Expert Perspective: There are many options after first-line treatment for metastatic triple-positive breast cancer. Trastuzumab deruxtecan is the preferred second-line option, and as stated earlier, there are multiple third-line and beyond options. It is important to note that the 2022 ASCO guidelines list the combination of fulvestrant, abemaciclib, and trastuzumab as a third-line option. This is based on monarcHER, a phase II study for patients with hormone receptor-positive, HER2-positive advanced breast cancer who had received at least two HER2-targeted therapies for advanced disease. Patients were randomized 1:1:1 to the combination of abemaciclib, trastuzumab, and fulvestrant (group A); abemaciclib with trastuzumab (group B); or standard of care chemotherapy with trastuzumab (group C). A total of 237 patients were randomized. Patients in group A had a better progression-free survival compared with group C (8.3 months vs 5.7 months; HR 0.67; 95% CI 0.45–1.00, P = 0.05). The MonarcHER regimen provides an important chemotherapy-free option which is not FDA approved in this setting but can be considered in select situations.

Case Study 9: Novel therapies

The patient from Case 6 develops progression of disease and has received prior treatment with docetaxel, trastuzumab, and pertuzumab, trastuzumab emtansine, trastuzumab deruxtecan, and the HER2CLIMB regimen. Combinations of trastuzumab plus various chemotherapy agents, including vinorelbine, eribulin, and gemcitabine, have been used with further progression noted. The patient maintains a good performance status and wishes to continue on treatment and expresses an interest in participating in a clinical trial.

12) What novel therapies or investigational agents are under investigation in HER2-positive metastatic breast cancer?

Expert Perspective: Many new therapies are currently being developed for HER2-positive breast cancer, and clinical trials are ongoing. One such promising agent is trastuzumab duocarmazine, or SYD985. This is a novel HER2-targeting antibody-drug conjugate consisting of trastuzumab covalently bound by cleavable linker to drug duocarmazine. The phase III TULIP trial randomized patients with pretreated advanced HER2-positive breast cancer after progression on two or more prior lines of therapy to trastuzumab duocarmazine versus physician's choice to include trastuzumab plus chemo or lapatinib plus capecitabine. Results presented at ESMO 2021 showed an improvement in median PFS with trastuzumab duocarmazine of 7.0 months vs 4.9 months in the chemotherapy arm (HR 0.64; 95% CI 0.49-0.84; $P = 0.002$). The main safety signal has been ocular toxicity, including keratitis, conjunctivitis, and dry eye. Trastuzumab duocarmazine is also being studied in combination with niraparib in HER2-positive advanced setting and as neoadjuvant treatment in the early stage HER2 low population.

Immunotherapy has been studied in HER2-positive metastatic breast cancer in an effort to improve outcomes, however there has been low antitumor activity demonstrated to date. Results in heavily pre-treated patients have not been impressive, with the exception of a possible signal in PD-L1+ tumors. The phase 1b/2 PANACEA trial evaluated the combination of pembrolizumab and trastuzumab in patients who progressed on trastuzumab. In those with PD-L1+ tumors, the objective response rate (ORR) was 15%, while there were no responses noted in the PD-L1 negative tumors. A similar correlation between checkpoint inhibitor antitumor efficacy and expression of PD-L1 was observed in the randomized phase 2 KATE2 trial. In this study, patients with PD-L1+, HER2+ pretreated MBC had improved PFS when treated with T-DM1 and atezolizumab compared with T-DM1 alone (HR = 0.82 [95% CI: 0.55, 1.23]; $P = 0.3332$). One interesting therapeutic strategy being studied is a HER2-specific CAR T cell. Animal models have shown that HER2-specific CAR T cells can successfully combat antibody-resistant tumors. A phase I study of anti-HER2 CAR T for patients with any solid tumor with HER2 overexpression is ongoing. There is a close interplay between HER2-targeting therapies and the immune system, and several new immunotherapeutic strategies, including immune checkpoint inhibitors, CAR-T cells and therapeutic vaccines, are under investigation.

Case Study 10: HER2-low metastatic breast cancer

A 62-year-old woman with *de novo* hormone receptor–positive and HER2-negative (IHC 1+) metastatic breast cancer to bone received treatment with a CDK4/6 inhibitor and endocrine therapy for 25 months. At the time of progression, no PIK3CA or ESR1 mutation was identified, and she received single-agent fulvestrant followed by exemestane plus everolimus upon progression when new bone lesions and two small liver lesions were noted. She was treated with capecitabine, and after six months, several new liver lesions were noted with progression in the bone as well.

13) What is the best option for the next systemic therapy?

Expert Perspective: The results of the DESTINY-Breast04 trial have changed the nomenclature for MBC by defining a new subtype of tumors, HER2-low, that derive significant benefit from the use of trastuzumab deruxtecan. HER2-low is defined as HER2 1+ or 2+ by IHC with a negative *in situ* hybridization results per ASCO and College of American Pathologists guidelines and includes both hormone receptor positive and negative tumors. These tumors would previously be considered HER2-negative. The phase III DESTINY-Breast04 trial enrolled 557 patients with hormone receptor–negative or hormone receptor–positive MBC and centrally confirmed HER2-low expression. All patients had been previously treated with one or two prior lines of chemotherapy for metastatic breast cancer and were required to have endocrine therapy–refractory disease. Patients who experienced disease recurrence within six months of completion of adjuvant chemotherapy were also eligible. Patients were randomly assigned in a 2:1 ratio to receive either trastuzumab deruxtecan or the physician's choice of standard chemotherapy (capecitabine, eribulin, gemcitabine, paclitaxel, or nab-paclitaxel). The primary endpoint was progression-free survival in patients with hormone receptor–positive disease. Key secondary endpoints were progression-free survival in patients with either hormone receptor–positive or hormone receptor–negative disease, as well as OS in all patients and in those with hormone receptor–positive disease. At a median follow-up of 18.4 months, in the hormone receptor–positive cohort, the median progression-free survival was 10.1 months for the trastuzumab deruxtecan–treated patients versus 5.4 months for those treated with standard chemotherapy ($P < .0001$). Among all 557 patients enrolled in the study, the median progression-free survival was 9.9 months vs 5.1 months, respectively ($P < .001$). In the patients with hormone receptor positive disease, the median OS was 23.9 months versus 17.8 months, respectively. Median OS in the total study population was 23.4 months for trastuzumab deruxtecan recipients versus 16.8 months for standard chemotherapy recipients, significant gain in survival of 6.6 months favoring trastuzumab deruxtecan ($P = .001$). In an exploratory analysis of the hormone receptor negative patients, median progression-free survival was 8.5 months with trastuzumab deruxtecan versus 2.9 months with standard therapy. Also, in this group, the median OS was 18.2 months versus 8.3 months, respectively. Given these dramatic improvements, the patient in Case 8 would be an excellent candidate for treatment with trastuzumab deruxtecan as the next systemic therapy.

The incorporation of HER2-targeted treatment has changed the natural history of what was once thought to be one of the most aggressive subtypes of breast cancer. There is a reason for further optimism because even more options are on the horizon.

Recommended Readings

Andre, F., Park, Y.-H., Kim, S.-B., et al. (2023) Trastuzumab deruxtecan versus treatment of physician's choice in patients with HER2-positive metastatic breast cancer (DESTINY-Breast02): a randomized, open-label, multicentre, phase 3 trial. *Lancet* (online first).

Arpino, G., de la Haba-Rodriguez, J., Ferrero, J., et al. (2023) Pertuzumab, Trastuzumab, and an Aromatase Inhibitor for HER2-Positive and Hormone Receptor-Positive Metastatic or Locally Advanced Breast Cancer: PERTAIN Final Analysis. *Clin Cancer Res* 29: 1468–1476.

Bardia, A., Harnden, K., Mauro, L., et al. (2022). Clinical practices and institutional protocols on prophylaxis, monitoring, and management of selected adverse events associated with trastuzumab deruxtecan. *Oncologist* 27(8): 637–645.

Cortes, J., Kim, S.-B., Chung, W.P. et al. (2022). Trastuzumab deruxtecan versus trastuzumab emtansine for breast cancer (DESTINY-Breast03). *N Engl J Med* 386: 1143–1154.

Curigliano, G., Mueller, V., Borges, V., et al. (2022) Tucatinib versus placebo added to trastuzumab and capecitabine for patients with pretreated HER2+ metastatic breast cancer with and without brain metastases (HER2CLIMB): final overall survival analysis. *Ann Oncol* 33(3): 321–329.

Giordano, S., Franzoi, M., Temin, S. et al. (2022). Systemic therapy for advanced human epidermal growth factor receptor 2-positive breast cancer: ASCO guideline update. *Journal of Clinical Oncology*. Epub ahead of print.

Hurvitz, S., Hegg, R., Chung, W.-P., et al. (2023) Trastuzumab deruxtecan versus trastuzumab emtansine in patients with HER2-positive metastatic breast cancer: updated results from DESTINY-Breast03, a randomized, open-label, phase 3 trial. *Lancet* 401: 105–117.

Modi, S., Saura, C., Yamashita, T. et al. (2020). Trastuzumab deruxtecan in previously treated HER2-positive BC (DESTINY-Breast01). *N Engl J Med* 382: 610–621.

Modi, S., Jacot, T., Yamashita, T. et al. (2022). Trastuzumab deruxtecan in previously treated HER2-low advanced breast cancer (DESTINY-Breast04). *N Engl J Med* 387: 9–20.

National Comprehensive Cancer Network (NCCN). (2023). NCCN clinical practice guidelines in oncology. BC version 4.2023. National Comprehensive Cancer Network. [Online]. http://www.nccn.org/professionals/physician_gls/pdf/breast.pdf (accessed 24 May 2023).

Ramakrishna, N., Temin, S., Chandarlapaty, S. et al. (2018). Recommendations on disease management for patients with advanced human epidermal growth factor receptor 2-positive BC and brain metastases: ASCO clinical practice guideline update. *J Clin Oncol* 36 (27): 2804–2807.

Rugo, H., Im, S., Cardoso, F. et al. (2021). Efficacy of margetuximab vs trastuzumab in patients with pretreated ERBB2-positive advanced BC (SOPHIA). *JAMA Oncol* 7 (4): 573–584.

Saura, C., Oliveira, M., Feng, Y. et al. (2020). Neratinib plus capecitabine versus lapatinib plus capecitabine in HER2-positive metastatic BC previously treated with ≥ 2 HER2-directed regimens: Phase III NALA trial. *J Clin Oncol* 38 (27): 3138–3149.

Swain, S., Miles, D., Kim, S. et al. (2020). Pertuzumab, trastuzumab, and docetaxel for HER2-positive metastatic BC (CLEOPATRA): End-of-study results from a double-blind, randomized, placebo-controlled phase 3 trial. *Lancet* 21 (4): 519–530.

Tripathy, D., Brufsky, A., Cobleigh, M. et al. (2020). De novo versus recurrent HER2-positive metastatic BC: patient characteristics, treatment, and survival from the SystHERs Registry. *Oncologist* 25 (2): e214–e222.

Verma, S., Miles, D., Gianni, L. et al. (2012). Trastuzumab emtansine for HER2-positive advanced BC (EMILIA). *N Engl J Med* 367: 1783–1791.

15

Early-Stage Triple-Negative Breast Cancer

Tiffany A. Traina[1], Carlos dos Anjos[2], and Elaine Walsh[1]

[1] *Memorial Sloan Kettering Cancer Center, New York*
[2] *Hospital Sírio-Libanês, São Paulo, Brazil*

Introduction

Triple-negative breast cancer (TNBC) is a subtype of breast cancers that do not express estrogen receptor (ER), progesterone receptor (PR), or human epidermal growth factor receptor 2 (HER2). Current American Society of Clinical Oncology/College of American Pathologists (ASCO/CAP) guidelines define TNBC as tumors with ER < 1%, PR < 1% and HER2 negative (0 to 1+ by immunohistochemistry [IHC], or IHC 2+ and fluorescence *in situ* hybridization not amplified).

TNBC accounts for 15% of all breast cancer diagnosed, accounting for 200,000 cases per year worldwide. It is more commonly diagnosed in young (<40 years) and in African American women when compared with hormone receptor (HR)–positive breast cancer. It is associated with a poor prognosis in both the early and advanced settings, in part due to a more aggressive intrinsic behavior and due to fewer systemic treatment options, compared with HR-positive or HER2-enriched breast cancer (Chapter 16).

In the early stage setting, TNBC is treated according to tumor stage (tumor size and nodal status), and treatment typically consists of both local and systemic therapy given to reduce risk of recurrence and improve survival. More recently, therapeutic advances in the fields of immunotherapy and targeted therapy have changed the treatment landscape for a subset of patients with early stage TNBC, as outlined in this chapter. Further work is needed to improve outcomes for all patients with TNBC, and clinical trial development remains a critical component of these future goals.

1) What are the main prognostic markers in early stage TNBC?

Expert Perspective: Like other breast cancer subtypes, the main prognostic factors in early stage TNBC represent anatomic tumor burden, namely tumor size and nodal involvement. Studies have also shown that an increased immune infiltrate in early stage TNBC, evaluated on standard diagnostic hematoxylin and eosin (H&E) slides, is associated with significantly improved clinical outcomes. In 2019, Loi et al. published a pooled analysis of nine randomized trials including more than 2,000 patients with early stage TNBC. Correlation between baseline stromal tumor infiltrating lymphocytes and disease outcomes were evaluated. Patients with early stage TNBC with high stromal tumor infiltrating lymphocytes were found to have excellent rates of survival after adjuvant chemotherapy. For example, patients with pT1–2 pN0 tumors and baseline stromal tumor infiltrating lymphocytes ≥30% who had been treated with an anthracycline or anthracycline-taxane regimen in the adjuvant setting had three-year invasive, disease-free survival of 93%, three-year distant disease-free survival of 98%, and three-year overall survival (OS) of 99%.

Gene/mRNA/protein expression has also been shown to provide prognostic information in TNBC. Through gene expression cluster analysis of tumor samples from patients with TNBC, molecular subtyping of TNBC has been performed. More than one TNBC subtype classification has been proposed, with differing responses to neoadjuvant chemotherapy, differing rates of recurrence, and differing survival rates seen among the different subtypes. These gene-expression classifications are not currently used in routine clinical practice, but ongoing work may lead to these prognostic markers being incorporated into clinical decision making.

2) **Which patients with early stage TNBC should be considered for germline testing?**

Expert Perspective: The most recent National Comprehensive Cancer Network (NCCN) guidelines recommend that all patients with both early stage and metastatic TNBC, irrespective of age at diagnosis, should have a consultation with a genetic counseling team for discussion and consideration of germline testing (Chapters 45 and 46).

3) **How will the presence of a pathogenic germline variant affect treatment of early stage TNBC?**

Expert Perspective: Approximately 7–10% of patients with a diagnosis of TNBC harbor a pathogenic germline variant in *BRCA1/2*. Another 3–5% will harbor mutations in other homologous recombination repair (HRR) genes such as *PALB2*. The presence of pathogenic germline variants can influence both surgical planning and systemic therapy options for patients with TNBC.

Patients with pathogenic variants in *BRCA1/2* or other HRR genes have a significantly increased risk of developing a second primary breast cancer. In these patients, even if breast conservation is feasible, a therapeutic mastectomy is often considered. In addition, these patients often elect for a prophylactic contralateral mastectomy. This strategy has been shown to significantly decrease the risk of developing a second primary breast cancer, although there are limited data pertaining to improvements in OS.

Patients with germline pathogenic variants in *BRCA1/2* have additional systemic therapy options for the management of their early stage disease. In the metastatic setting, Poly (ADP-ribose) polymerase (PARP) inhibitors (PARPi) have been shown to improve progression-free survival in *BRCA1/2*-associated tumors because PARPi target cancers with defects in homologous recombination repair by synthetic lethality. These advances were recently brought to the early stage setting when Tutt et al. (2021) reported on the pivotal phase III, double-blind, OlympiA trial. In this study, patients harboring germline pathogenic or likely pathogenic variants in *BRCA1/2* who had a diagnosis of an early stage, HER2-negative breast cancer with high-risk clinicopathological features were randomized to one year of the PARPi, olaparib, versus placebo after completion of definitive local and systemic therapy. In this study, 81% of the patients had TNBC. After a median follow-up of 2.5 years, olaparib was shown to significantly improve 3-year invasive disease-free survival (DFS) over placebo (85.9% vs 77.1% for olaparib vs placebo; HR 0.58). Secondary endpoints of distant DFS and OS also favored olaparib. Olaparib has been approved by the US Food and Drug Administration (FDA) in this setting, and both the NCCN and the American Society of Clinical Oncology (ASCO) recommend one year of adjuvant olaparib for patients harboring germline pathogenic *BRCA1/2* mutations and a diagnosis of a high-risk, HER2-negative breast cancer.

4) Do all patients with early stage TNBC require treatment with chemotherapy? Or can certain low-risk patients potentially omit chemotherapy?

Expert Perspective: Systemic therapy is an integral part of the management of early stage TNBC, and the majority of patients will receive neoadjuvant or adjuvant chemotherapy. Typically, patients with tumors ≥ 1 cm should receive chemotherapy to reduce their risk of distant recurrence. However, patients with tumors < 1 cm have largely been excluded from phase III trials. Population-based data suggests that small, lymph-node negative tumors have good outcomes when treated with local therapy alone without the addition of systemic therapy. Two population-based studies retrospectively evaluated the potential benefit of adjuvant chemotherapy for small, lymph-node negative TNBCs. One study conducted, using data from the National Cancer Database, included >16,000 patients with pT1a–bN0 TNBC. The other study was conducted with a Dutch data bank incorporating >4,000 patients with pT1a–cN0 TNBC. Both studies suggested a potential detrimental effect of adjuvant chemotherapy for small, lymph-node negative tumors ≤0.5 cm (pT1aN0) but a potential survival benefit of chemotherapy for patients with tumors > 0.5 cm (pT1bN0).

Current NCCN guidelines do not recommend chemotherapy for pT1aN0 TNBCs but suggest consideration of adjuvant chemotherapy for tumors pT1bN0 and recommend chemotherapy for ≥pT1cN0 tumors (Figure 15.1).

5) If chemotherapy is deemed necessary for the treatment of early stage TNBC, should it be given in a neoadjuvant or adjuvant setting?

Expert Perspective: TNBCs are associated with a considerable risk of distant recurrent/ metastatic disease, and therefore systemic chemotherapy is considered early in the treatment course. As outlined earlier, chemotherapy is recommended for patients with TNBC whose primary tumor measures > 0.5 cm and in those patients with lymph-node positive disease, irrespective of tumor size.

Neoadjuvant chemotherapy has been the preferred approach for patients with locally advanced breast cancer or for those patients where breast conservation surgery is not feasible. Historical data suggests that the timing of chemotherapy, whether neoadjuvant or adjuvant, does not influence overall survival. In addition, recent data from a randomized phase III trial demonstrated the benefit of adjuvant capecitabine for patients with early stage TNBC who had residual disease after neoadjuvant chemotherapy. Therefore, we typically consider neoadjuvant treatment for patients with ≥ cT2cN0 TNBC or any TNBC with

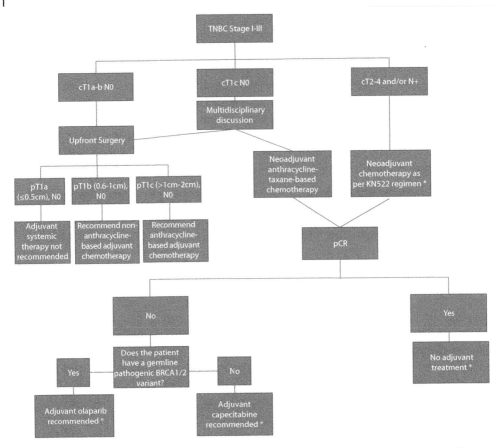

Figure 15.1 Proposed algorithm for patients with early stage TNBC. TNBC, Triple negative breast cancer; KN522, KEYNOTE-522 trial; pCR, pathological complete response. * Patients on KN522 received neoadjuvant anthracycline, taxane, carboplatin, and pembrolizumab. Pembrolizumab was continued adjuvantly for nine cycles independently of pathological response. Patients on KN522 did not receive adjuvant olaparib or capecitabine. Although there are safety data for the combination of pembrolizumab with both olaparib and capecitabine, the optimal adjuvant regimen for these patients remains unknown.

clinical evidence of lymph-node involvement in order to guide additional treatments in the adjuvant setting. In addition, because the presence of residual disease after neoadjuvant chemotherapy is an important prognostic marker for early stage TNBC, this strengthens the argument for considering neoadjuvant chemotherapy. As discussed in more detail later (Question 7), immune checkpoint inhibitors now also play a role in the neoadjuvant therapy of select patients with high-risk TNBC.

6) **What are the standard chemotherapy regimens for early stage TNBC? Does platinum play a role?**

Expert Perspective: Anthracycline-taxane-based chemotherapy remains the standard of care chemotherapy backbone for early stage TNBC. Prior phase III trials (pooled together in the ABC trial) were designed to evaluate the hypothesis that anthracycline-free regimens (taxane-based regimens) would be non-inferior to anthracycline-taxane-based regimens. These studies failed to demonstrate non-inferiority, reemphasizing the importance of anthracyclines in the management of early stage TNBC. However, in a subset of patients with small lymph-node negative tumors (e.g. pT1bN0), it is reasonable to consider an anthracycline-free regimen. This particular subset of patients has a lower risk of disease recurrence and was found to derive minimal benefit with the addition of anthracyclines in a subgroup analysis of the ABC trial (four-year invasive DFS of 89.5% and 87% for anthracycline and non-anthracycline containing regimens, respectively). In addition, for patients in whom anthracyclines might be medically contraindicated, an anthracycline-free regimens, such as docetaxel-cyclophosphamide (TC) or a platinum-containing regimen such as docetaxel-carboplatin may be considered. A recent meta-analysis by Early Breast Cancer Trialists' Collaborative Group (EBCTCG) provides a reliable evidence base to inform that incorporation of an anthracycline into a taxane-based regimen reduced breast cancer recurrence rates. Direct comparisons between anthracycline and taxane regimens showed that a higher cumulative dose and more dose-intense schedules were more efficacious. The proportional reductions in recurrence for taxane plus anthracycline were similar in estrogen receptor-positive and estrogen receptor-negative disease, and did not differ by age, nodal status, or tumor size or grade.

There is controversy about the benefit of adding platinum agents to a neoadjuvant anthracycline-taxane-based regimen. Three randomized trials in the neoadjuvant setting have shown that the addition of carboplatin to a neoadjuvant regimen can increase the rates of pathologic complete response. However, none of these studies was powered to demonstrate overall survival benefit with added platinum, and survival benefit with platinum has not been consistently demonstrated. The largest study, a phase III, randomized, three-arm study (Brightness trial) was presented at ESMO Annual Congress (September 2021) and published at Annals of Oncol early 2022. Data suggests the potential benefit, in event-free survival, with the addition of carboplatin to an anthracycline/taxane/cyclophosphamide backbone. The main benefit in this study was the decrease in locoregional recurrence, including breast and axillary recurrence. Further studies are needed to determine whether improvements in pathologic complete response rates will correspond to improvements in long-term outcomes, especially overall survival.

7) What is the role of immune checkpoint inhibition in the treatment of early stage TNBC?

Expert Perspective: Yes, in patients with stage II and III TNBC. In July 2021, the FDA approved the anti-PD-1 antibody pembrolizumab for the neoadjuvant treatment of high-risk, early stage TNBC in combination with chemotherapy. This approval was based on the results of the phase III, randomized, double-blind, placebo-controlled KEYNOTE-522 trial. In this study, patients with previously untreated stage II or stage III TNBC were randomized to receive 12 weeks of neoadjuvant paclitaxel and carboplatin followed by four cycles of anthracycline and cyclophosphamide with or without pembrolizumab. The two co-primary endpoints of this study were rates of pathologic complete response and event-free survival. After a median follow-up of 39.1 months, KEYNOTE-522 demonstrated the benefit of pembrolizumab in the neoadjuvant treatment of stage II and III TNBC. The addition of pembrolizumab significantly increased the rate of pathologic complete response by 7.5% (63% for pembrolizumab-chemotherapy vs 55.6% for placebo-chemotherapy). The three-year event-free survival was significantly increased by 7.7% (84.5% for pembrolizumab-chemotherapy versus 76.8% for placebo-chemotherapy). The incorporation of immunotherapy also increased distant recurrence-free survival (87% vs 80.7% favoring pembrolizumab), and although OS data is not mature, there appears to be a numerical trend favoring pembrolizumab. Interestingly, and unlike the data observed in the metastatic setting, the clinical benefits with the addition of pembrolizumab to chemotherapy were observed irrespective of PD-L1 status: improvements in pathologic complete response rates and event-free survival were noted in patients with both PD-L1 positive and negative tumors.

In KEYNOTE-522, patients continued pembrolizumab adjuvantly to complete a total of one year of therapy. At this time, it remains unclear whether the event-free survival benefits observed with the addition of pembrolizumab are driven by neoadjuvant or adjuvant therapy, meaning that the optimal or required duration of immune checkpoint inhibition remains uncertain. In addition, for this study, patients were not permitted to receive either adjuvant capecitabine or olaparib for the treatment of residual disease after neoadjuvant treatment, meaning that the benefit of both adjuvant pembrolizumab and capecitabine/olaparib is unknown.

Notably, the addition of pembrolizumab to chemotherapy resulted in increased rates of toxicities: 13% more patients treated with pembrolizumab discontinued at least one drug while on study. Close monitoring of patients is required while on checkpoint inhibition and early management of toxicities is essential (Chapter 50). NCCN guidelines have already incorporated the KEYNOTE-522 regimen into their recommendation for the management of patients with stage II–III TNBC.

8) What are the side effects of systemic treatment? Are these short-term or long-term side effects?

Expert Perspective: Chemotherapy side effects are drug dependent. As noted, most patients with early stage TNBC will receive chemotherapy regimens containing an anthracycline, an alkylator, and a taxane. All three agents can induce alopecia, nausea, vomiting, bone marrow suppression (including anemia, leucopenia/neutropenia, and thrombocytopenia), and fatigue. These side effects are usually acute, improving once chemotherapy is discontinued.

With respect to longer-term toxicity, anthracyclines are associated with a risk of cardiotoxicity, increasing the risk of heart failure and associated with significant morbidity and mortality. Risk factors for anthracycline-induced cardiotoxicity include older age (>65 years), preexisting cardiovascular disease, hypertension, smoking, hyperlipidemia, obesity, diabetes, and high cumulative lifetime dose of anthracycline exposure. Pre-evaluation of heart function with an echocardiogram or a MUGA scan is imperative for patients receiving anthracycline-based regimens.

Both anthracyclines and alkylator agents are associated with a small risk of secondary malignancies, including acute myeloid leukemia (AML), myelodysplastic syndrome (MDS), and myeloproliferative neoplasms. There are limited data about potential risk factors for chemotherapy-induced secondary malignancies, but cumulative chemotherapy dose is an important risk factor. Patients should be counseled about this and all potential side effects before anthracycline and/or alkylator treatment.

Taxanes, including docetaxel, paclitaxel, and nab-paclitaxel, can potentially cause neurotoxicity, namely peripheral sensory and motor neuropathies, that are typically acute and reversible but may be prolonged or permanent. Risk factors for developing neurotoxicity include cumulative taxane dose, older age, prior history of peripheral neuropathy, diabetes mellitus, and possibly obesity. There are limited data about prevention strategies for taxane-induced peripheral neuropathy. Dose adjustment or even treatment discontinuation should be considered for high-grade neurotoxicity. Taxanes also cause nail changes, including discoloration, brittle nails, ridging, and onycholysis. The use of ice packs during taxane infusion may decrease the risk of nail toxicity and is usually recommended if tolerated. Less commonly, taxanes may cause pneumonitis, which could be fatal in a small percentage of patients. Finally, the risk of infusion related reaction associated with both paclitaxel and docetaxel infusions requires routine steroid and antihistamine premedication.

Like taxanes, platinum agents can also cause neurotoxicity, including sensory and motor neuropathy and ototoxicity, specifically with the use of cisplatin. Platinum agents can also cause hypersensitivity reactions, which is related to prolonged use over multiple infusions. Platinum agents can also cause nephrotoxicity, requiring the dose to be calculated based on creatinine and estimated glomerular filtration rate (GFR).

As previously discussed, capecitabine is considered standard of care adjuvant therapy for patients with residual disease after neoadjuvant treatment. Capecitabine is known to cause gastrointestinal side effects, namely nausea, vomiting, diarrhea and mucositis, bone marrow toxicity, and hand-foot syndrome. Hand-foot syndrome is dose dependent and can be seen with cumulative dosing, frequently necessitating dose modification, dose delay, or even drug discontinuation. As a 5-fluorouracil pro-drug, capecitabine is also associated with a risk of coronary artery vasospasm. However, this is rare and typically does not require any specific cardiac evaluation prior to starting the drug.

The most common side effects of olaparib are gastrointestinal symptoms (nausea, vomiting, and diarrhea) and myelosuppression, often requiring dose modification. PARPi are also associated with a risk of developing secondary hematological malignancies such as AML and MDS, which is related to dose and duration of PARPi treatment. In the OlympiA study, although longer follow-up is awaited, the incidence of AML/MDS did not appear increased with the use of adjuvant olaparib for one year.

Pembrolizumab can be associated with immune-related adverse events (irAEs), resulting from off-target effects of an activated host immune system. Approximately 10% of patients receiving anti-PD-1 antibodies will develop grade ≥3 irAE, most often occurring within the first six months of treatment. Virtually any organ or tissue may be affected by irAE, but most frequently these side effects occur in the skin, liver, endocrine glands, and gastrointestinal tract. Fatal irAE are rare (<1%) and usually involve the lungs (pneumonitis), the heart (myocarditis), or the neurologic system. In the recent KEYNOTE-522 study, the most commonly observed toxicities related to the addition of immunotherapy to chemotherapy were hypothyroidism, hyperthyroidism, and skin toxicity. Adrenal and hypophysis insufficiency were rare but appeared to be more frequent in the immuno-chemotherapy arm. Patients and providers must be educated about the potential for irAE toxicities because early management and intervention is critical. This topic is discussed in detail in Chapter 50.

9) What is the impact of systemic breast cancer therapies on fertility?

Expert Perspective: As already discussed, most patients with early stage TNBC will receive polychemotherapy as part of their curative intent therapy. When compared with HR-positive breast cancer, TNBC is more commonly diagnosed in women <40 years. Polychemotherapy may permanently impair future fertility, so it is imperative that patients considering such therapy are counseled about their options for fertility preservation. (See Chapter 19).

The most effective technique for fertility preservation is cryopreservation, including freezing of embryos, oocytes, or ovarian tissue. Ovarian induction and tissue collection can be conducted quickly in a matter of days to weeks. Discussion about fertility preservation and a referral to a reproductive medicine team should be conducted at diagnosis prior to starting chemotherapy for all patients of childbearing age, if that is in line with their wishes.

Gonadotropin-releasing hormone (GnRH) agonists have been shown to be safe when given concurrently with systemic treatment. In a phase III randomized trial of premenopausal patients with early stage, HR-negative breast cancer (85% of whom had early stage TNBC), patients were randomized to receive adjuvant chemotherapy with or without GnRH agonists. The primary end point was rate of ovarian failure at two years with secondary end points of disease-free survival and OS. This study demonstrated a statistically significant improvement in disease-free survival and OS with the use of GnRH agonists (four-year disease-free survival of 89% vs 78%, favoring GnRH agonists). Although we do not use these data to endorse GnRH agonist use as part of the treatment paradigm for early stage TNBC, the safety data are reassuring. Trials of coadministration of a GnRH agonist with perioperative chemotherapy for the purpose of protecting ovarian function have shown mixed results. Most of these trials have focused on return of menstrual function and not on fertility capacity or chances of future pregnancies. Therefore, cryopreservation remains the gold standard technique for fertility preservation.

10) **Postoperatively, what prognostic markers are evaluated with the final surgical pathology? How can postsurgical findings impact disease management?**

Expert Perspective: Patients with early stage TNBC who have residual invasive breast cancer after neoadjuvant chemotherapy have an elevated risk of relapse. Both the presence and the volume of residual disease are important prognostic markers and can influence adjuvant treatment decisions. Invasive residual disease can be measured as a binary outcome (pathologic complete remission versus invasive residual disease) or via a residual cancer burden scale that takes multiple factors in account, including primary tumor bed area, overall cancer cellularity, percentage of cancer that is *in situ* disease, number of lymph nodes, and diameter of the largest lymph node. Residual cancer burden can classify patients into four different residual disease categories that in turn can correlate with the risk of disease recurrence and overall mortality.

Because patients with invasive residual TNBC after neoadjuvant treatment have a substantial risk of disease relapse, studies have been designed to test adjuvant strategies with the intention to mitigate the risk of disease recurrence. Currently, we have data to support the use of capecitabine as adjuvant treatment for patients with early stage TNBC with residual invasive disease after neoadjuvant treatment. In the CREATE-X trial, patients with HER2-negative breast cancer and any amount of residual disease after neoadjuvant chemotherapy were randomized to standard adjuvant therapy plus six to eight cycles of capecitabine versus standard adjuvant therapy alone. This study was shown to significantly improve DFS in the overall population, demonstrating the benefit of adjuvant capecitabine for early stage HER2-negative breast cancer and residual invasive disease. Notably, the subgroup of patients with TNBC and residual disease after neoadjuvant chemotherapy were found to derive the most benefit from adjuvant capecitabine: five-year disease-free survival was 69.8% versus 56.1%, favoring capecitabine. The OS benefit was also observed in patients with TNBC: the five-year OS increased from 70.3% to 78.8% with the addition of capecitabine.

In the adjuvant setting, an ECOG-ACRIN Cancer Research group study compared the role of platinum agents to capecitabine in patients with early stage TNBC and residual disease after neoadjuvant treatment. This study was closed early due to futility with increased toxicities observed in the platinum arm. Based on this data, there is currently no role for platinum agents as adjuvant treatment for patients with residual disease after neoadjuvant treatment.

As previously discussed, olaparib has demonstrated invasive, disease-free survival benefit for patients with a germline pathogenic or likely pathogenic *BRCA1/2* variant and a HER2-negative early stage breast cancer. Notably, about 81% of the patient population in the OlympiA study had TNBC, and about 50% of these TNBC patients were included based on the presence of residual disease after neoadjuvant treatment.

Multiple other strategies to treat patients with residual disease after neoadjuvant therapy are being evaluated, such as the role of immune checkpoint inhibition and antibody drug conjugates.

11) What is the optimal way to monitor for disease recurrence after definitive systemic therapy?

Expert Perspective: Most patients with early stage TNBC will be cured after their multi-modality treatment. Long-term management of breast cancer survivors should focus not only on identifying signs and symptoms concerning for disease recurrence but also on the patient's overall medical health, including adherence to lifestyle recommendations, treatment of medical and psychological consequences of cancer and its therapy, and screening for other primary tumors, including new breast cancers.

There are no data supporting intensive laboratory and/or radiologic surveillance for asymptomatic breast cancer survivors. In one meta-analysis, routine follow-up was compared with intensive surveillance strategies without any overall survival benefit observed in the group followed with a more aggressive approach. NCCN and ASCO guidelines favor clinical history and physical exams as principal means of detecting a breast cancer recurrence, and both guidelines recommend against the use of intensive labs (including tumor markers and circulating tumor cells) and/or body images (CT, bone scans, PET-CT) for monitoring asymptomatic breast cancer survivors. Randomized trials with modern images technologies are testing whether radiologic surveillance can improve overall survival in high-risk early stage triple-negative breast cancer.

Patients who underwent either breast conservation surgery or unilateral mastectomy should have regular clinical breast examinations and an annual mammogram, starting 6–12 months after local treatment. Patients with shortened life expectancy due to comorbidities or age can omit routine breast imaging because this intervention is not expected to have an effect on their overall survival. There are limited data favoring the use of routine breast ultrasound or breast MRI as complementary imaging modalities. These studies may be conducted as per physician's discretion.

Prior treatment for breast cancer is a risk factor for the development of osteopenia and osteoporosis. Patients who meet criteria for a bone density examination, namely those >65 years old or those with premature menopause, should have routine bone-density examinations performed. Furthermore, prior Early Breast Cancer Trialists' Collaborative Group (EBCTCG) meta-analysis has suggested the potential benefit of using bisphosphonates in the management of early stage HER2 negative breast cancer. In this meta-analysis, adjuvant bisphosphonate was associated with a decrease in breast cancer specific mortality, with an absolute reduction in 10-year breast cancer specific mortality of 3.3%. The benefit was present irrespectively of ER status, but only in postmenopausal patients. The use of adjuvant bisphosphonates can be discussed with post-menopausal early stage TNBC.

An area of ongoing developments for breast cancer surveillance pertains to the use of tumor guided circulating tumor DNA (ctDNA). The ability to detect patients with molecular evidence of residual disease that has not been eradicated by systemic therapy could facilitate clinical trials of adjuvant therapies focused on those specific patients at highest risk. To this point, a UK study conducted across five centers evaluated 170 patients with early stage breast cancer, irrespective of HR or HER2 status. Patients underwent DNA sequencing of their primary breast tumor. If a somatic mutation was identified in the tumor, a personalized digital polymerase chain reaction assay was designed to track this somatic mutation in the plasma, which was collected from the patient every three months in the first year of follow-up and every six months between years two to five. Detection of ctDNA during follow-up was associated with a statistically significant increased risk of relapse (HR 25.2) demonstrating the role of ctDNA as a prognostic biomarker. Further prospective studies are needed to determine the full potential of ctDNA as a means of detecting molecular relapse and to guide adjuvant therapy and patient follow-up.

12) What lifestyle recommendations should be considered for a patient after treatment for early stage TNBC?

Expert Perspective: Certain lifestyle modifications can be implemented after a diagnosis of TNBC that may improve a patient's long-term survival. Lifestyle changes in breast cancer survivors not only can improve physical and mental health but also have been shown to have a potential benefit in overall and breast cancer specific mortality. Health-care providers should encourage patients to engage in regular physical activity, maintain a healthy body weight, minimize alcohol intake, and stop smoking.

Several clinical trials have evaluated the feasibility and potential benefit of increasing physical activity after a diagnosis of breast cancer. Most of these trials have not been large enough to evaluate whether such interventions improve breast cancer outcomes among survivors. However, these trials have shown that exercise can improve other clinical outcomes such as mental health (anxiety/depression), cancer-related fatigue, physical function, muscle strength, body image, and body composition.

Systematic reviews and meta-analyses support the data that patients who are overweight/obese at the time of diagnosis of early stage TNBC have a poorer prognosis with shorter disease-free survival and OS compared with those patients who are normal body weight at diagnosis. Despite the data linking overweight/obesity with poorer outcomes in TNBC, there have been few studies evaluating the impact of weight-loss interventions in breast cancer survivors. Nevertheless, such as is observed with physical activity, maintaining a healthy body weight can positively impact a series of health metrics, including physical and mental health.

Data suggest that alcohol intake is associated with an increased risk of breast cancer recurrence. In the Life after Cancer Epidemiology (LACE) study, patients who drank more than six grams of alcohol daily had significantly higher rates of recurrence (HR 1.35) compared with those who drank less than 0.5 grams daily. Limited alcohol intake should be suggested for patients with early stage TNBC in survivorship.

Some data suggest that reducing dietary fat intake after a cancer diagnosis could improve breast cancer outcomes in cancer survivors, but the data have not been consistent, and dietary modification is not a standard part of adjuvant therapy for women with breast cancer at this time. Nevertheless, guidelines for cancer survivors from the American Cancer Society and the American College of Sports Medicine support the indication of eating a healthy diet rich in plant sources.

13) What are future areas of development in the management of early stage TNBC?

Expert Perspective: Several strategies focusing on immune manipulation, novel antibody drug conjugates, and targeted therapies are under development for the treatment of early stage TNBC. An area of highest unmet need are those patients who fail to achieve pathologic complete response, particularly following anthracycline, taxane, and platinum-based regimens that include checkpoint inhibition. This population could benefit from novel approaches, beyond traditional cytotoxic therapy, that may alter the microenvironment or leverage other signaling pathways activated in the setting of chemotherapy resistance. In addition, studying molecular residual disease, using ctDNA testing, is another therapeutic strategy that may allow for early intervention that may change the natural history of this disease. Presently, sacituzumab-govitecan (an antibody drug conjugate approved by the FDA for metastatic TNBC) and pembrolizumab are being evaluated in phase III randomized clinical trials for the adjuvant treatment of patients with residual invasive TNBC after neoadjuvant treatment. The results of these studies could potentially be practice-changing.

Efforts are also needed to evaluate de-escalation therapeutic strategies in low-risk, early stage TNBC utilizing biomarkers in conjunction with targeted, non-chemotherapy agents. Patient and tumor selection is a critical component of de-escalation strategies, and appropriate biomarker-driven regimens would incorporate agents proven to demonstrate benefit without adding excessive toxicity.

Recommended Readings

Burstein, M.D., Tsimelzon, A., Poage, G.M. et al. (2015). Comprehensive genomic analysis identifies novel subtypes and targets of triple-negative breast cancer. *Clin Cancer Res* 21 (7): 1688–1698.

Cortazar, P., Zhang, L., Unch, M. et al. (2014). Pathological complete response and long-term clinical benefit in breast cancer: the CTNeoBC pooled analysis. *Lancet* 384 (9938): 164–172.

Loi, S., Drubay, D., Adams, S. et al. (2019). Tumor-infiltrating lymphocytes and prognosis: A pooled individual patient analysis of early-stage triple-negative breast cancers. *J Clin Oncol* 37 (7): 559–569.

Loibl, S., O'Shaughnessy, J., Untch, M. et al. (2018). Addition of the PARP inhibitor veliparib plus carboplatin or carboplatin alone to standard neoadjuvant chemotherapy in triple-negative breast cancer (BrighTNess): A randomised, phase 3 trial. *Lancet Oncol* 19 (4): 497–509.

Masuda, N., Lee, S.J., Ohtani, S. et al. (2017). Adjuvant capecitabine for breast cancer after preoperative chemotherapy. *N Engl J Med* 376 (22): 2147–2159.

Mayer, I.A., Zhao, F., and Arteaga, C.L. (2021). Randomized phase III postoperative trial of platinum-based chemotherapy versus capecitabine in patients with residual triple-negative breast cancer following neoadjuvant chemotherapy: ECOG-ACRIN EA1131. *J Clin Oncol* 39 (23): 2539–2551.

Moore, H.C.F., Unger, J.M., Phillips, K.A. et al. (2015). Goserelin for ovarian protection during breast-cancer adjuvant chemotherapy. *N Engl J Med* 372 (10): 923–932.

Oladure, O.T., Singh, A., and Ma, S.J. (2020). Association of adjuvant chemotherapy with overall survival among women with small, node-negative, triple-negative breast cancer. *JAMA Netw Open* 3 (9): e2016247.

Schmid, P., Cortes, J., Pusztai, L. et al. (2020). Pembrolizumab for early triple-negative breast cancer. *N Engl J Med* 382 (9): 810–821.

Tutt, A.N.J., Garber, J.E., Kaufman, B. et al. (2021). Adjuvant olaparib for patients with BRCA1- or BRCA2-mutated breast cancer. *N Engl J Med* 384 (25): 2394–2405.

Early Breast Cancer Trialists' Collaborative Group (EBCTCG). Electronic address: bc.overview@ctsu.ox.ac.uk; Early Breast Cancer Trialists' Collaborative Group (EBCTCG). (2023 April 15). Anthracycline-containing and taxane-containing chemotherapy for early-stage operable breast cancer: a patient-level meta-analysis of 100 000 women from 86 randomised trials. *Lancet* 401 (10384): 1277–1292. doi: 10.1016/S0140-6736(23)00285-4. PMID: 37061269.

16

Triple-Negative Metastatic Breast Cancer

Azadeh Nasrazadani[1], Juan Gomez[2], and Adam Brufsky[3]

[1] MD Anderson Cancer Center, Division of Breast Medical Oncology, Houston, TX
[2] Lenox Hill Hospital, New York City, NY
[3] UPMC Hillman Cancer Center, University of Pittsburgh School of Medicine, Pittsburgh, PA

Introduction

Triple-negative breast cancer (TNBC) is a subtype of breast cancer that accounts for approximately 15% of all breast cancer cases as per national population-based studies. Among other clinical features, TNBC is characterized as being highly invasive and prone to metastasis and relapse. Although patients achieving a pathological complete response (pCR) after neoadjuvant chemotherapy have an estimated five-year overall survival of 92%, this significantly decreases to 58% in patients not achieving pCR, reflecting the high likelihood of distant recurrence in earlier years after diagnosis compared with other breast cancer subtypes (Chapter 15). TNBC is more frequently seen in younger patients compared with other types of breast cancer. It mostly presents in young premenopausal women and has a predilection for development in African American women.

From a pathologic standpoint, this subtype is characterized by the lack of expression of estrogen receptor (ER), progesterone receptor (PR), and human epidermal growth factor receptor 2 (HER2). Given the lack of upregulation of these targets, TNBC is not sensitive to endocrine therapy or HER2-targeted therapies, thus limiting treatment options. As a result, chemotherapy continues to be the main treatment approach, although recent successes have been achieved owing to the incorporation of immunotherapy and/or targeting of DNA damage pathways in appropriate cases. Ongoing efforts are focused on identification of potential targets to expand treatment options, with novel agents currently in clinical trials including inhibitors of PI3K/AKT signaling pathways. Most recently, sacituzumab govitecan, which consists of a Trop-2-directed antibody conjugated to a topoisomerase inhibitor, has demonstrated overall survival (OS) benefit in metastatic TNBC and is approved for patients having received at least two prior lines of therapy. In ASCENT III, in which sacituzumab govitecan was compared with single-agent chemotherapy of physician's choice (eribulin, vinorelbine, capecitabine, or gemcitabine), OS was extended to 12.1 from 6.7 months (HR 0.48; 95% CI 0.38–0.59; $P < 0.001$). In general, however, there remains an unmet need for effective therapies for the management of these patients.

Cancer Consult: Expertise in Clinical Practice, Volume 1: Solid Tumors & Supportive Care,
Second Edition. Edited by Syed A. Abutalib, Maurie Markman, Al B. Benson III, and Hope S. Rugo.
© 2024 John Wiley & Sons Ltd. Published 2024 by John Wiley & Sons Ltd.

16 Triple-Negative Metastatic Breast Cancer

Case Study 1

A 43-year-old premenopausal woman presents after recent diagnosis of a 4 cm invasive ductal carcinoma of the left breast with triple-negative pathology (ER–, PR–, HER2–) involving left axillary lymph nodes and staging CT chest, abdomen, and pelvic scans demonstrating multiple hepatic and osseous sclerotic lesions. Biopsy of a hepatic lesion was consistent with metastatic triple negative invasive ductal carcinoma.

1) What is the standard chemotherapy regimen recommended for use in the first line?

Expert Perspective: The general approach to treatment of metastatic TNBC involves sequential utilization of single-agent chemotherapy until progression of disease. In cases in which tumor burden is high and there is concern for visceral crisis, combination chemotherapy can be considered given higher response rates achieved with this approach. However, overall survival has not been found to be improved using combinatorial versus single-agent chemotherapy, and thus combination chemotherapy should be reserved for cases in which achieving response is more critical (i.e. in visceral response). Choice of initial chemotherapy agent is reliant on prior therapies received in the non-metastatic setting, and thus there are no formal recommendations on specific agent to choose. Paclitaxel is commonly favored in *de novo* metastatic cases, and capecitabine may be preferred in patients who have previously received an anthracycline and taxane.

2) When should immunotherapy be considered?

Expert Perspective: At time of diagnosis of metastatic disease, programmed cell death ligand 1 (PD-L1) expression should be determined in addition to tumor mutational burden (TMB) and microsatellite instability (MSI)/mismatch repair deficiency (dMMR) status if resources allow. In cases of PD-L1 positivity or in the presence of high MSI (MSI-H) or dMMR, the addition of immunotherapy should be considered.

Utilizing the VENTANA PD-L1 (SP142) assay, PD-L1 is considered positive if 1% or more tumor infiltrating immune cells stain positive on immunohistochemistry analysis. Results from Impassion130 led to initial accelerated US Food and Drug Administration (FDA) approval of atezolizumab to be used for first-line therapy in metastatic TNBC if the intratumoral PD-L1 > 1% criteria is met. In the study, the addition of atezolizumab versus placebo to nab-paclitaxel in Impassion130 led to numerical improvement in OS to 25 months versus 18 months in patients with PD-L1 positive tumors; however, that was not statistically significant. Atezolizumab was given at 840 mg intravenous every two weeks, 1,200 mg intravenous every three weeks, or 1680 mg intravenous every four weeks, with nab-paclitaxel administered at 100 mg/m^2 on days 1, 8, and 15 until disease progression or unacceptable toxicity was encountered. Impassion131 had the same trial design but used paclitaxel instead of nab-paclitaxel as the chemotherapy backbone. This trial did not demonstrate similar benefit and thus is not recommended for combination with atezolizumab in lieu of nab-paclitaxel. Interestingly, as of 27 August 2021, the sponsor (Roche) voluntarily withdrew the indication of atezolizumab with nab-paclitaxel for management of first-line therapy in metastatic TNBC after discussions with the US FDA.

Pembrolizumab is a second immunotherapy agent with FDA approval for use in metastatic TNBC in which the PD-L1 combined positive score (CPS) in tumor and immune cells is 10% or more utilizing the PD-L1 IHC 22C3 pharmDx test. In KEYNOTE-355, the addition of pembrolizumab (200 mg intravenous every three weeks) versus placebo to chemotherapy (nab-paclitaxel 100 mg/m^2 on days 1, 8, and 15, every 28 days; paclitaxel 90 mg/m^2 on days 1, 8, and 15; or gemcitabine 1000 mg/m^2 plus carboplatin AUC 2 on days 1 and 8, every 21 days) significantly extended the median progression-free survival to 9.7 versus 5.6 months (HR 0.65; 95% CI 0.49–0.86; one-sided $P = 0.0012$) in patients with CPS of 10% or more. Most recently, OS was reported to be significantly improved in the pembrolizumab arm in cases where CPS > 10. This index is obtained from the number of PD-L1 positively stained cells divided by the total number of viable tumor cells multiplied by 100.

Although pembrolizumab was not found to be superior to chemotherapy in previously treated metastatic TNBC with regard to overall response rates, progression-free survival, or OS in KEYNOTE-119, pembrolizumab monotherapy does have FDA approval for treatment of metastatic solid tumors with high tumor mutational burden (TMB) ≥ 10 mutations/megabase.

3) Are there contraindications to immunotherapy?

Expert Perspective: There are no firm contraindications to pembrolizumab use in the management of metastatic TNBC. However, patients with active autoimmune diseases are at high risk of worsening autoimmune symptoms and should be appropriately counseled. In general, patients with multiple sclerosis or history of transplant are not thought to be ideal candidates for immunotherapy (Chapter 50).

4) Which adverse events should be monitored during immunotherapy for breast cancer, and how?

Expert Perspective: Immune-mediated adverse events may develop in any organ system or tissue with variable time in onset after initiation of immunotherapy, although median onset is typically several weeks depending on agent and site of immune-mediated adverse. Laboratory tests of liver enzymes, creatinine, and thyroid function should be obtained at baseline and periodically during the course of treatment, in addition to close monitoring for symptoms and signs that may be clinical manifestations of immune-mediated adverse. Among immune-mediated adverse, hypothyroidism is notable in incidence followed by immune-mediated colitis, hepatitis, and less common although potentially fatal pneumonitis. Rare yet potential other immune-mediated endocrinopathies include adrenal insufficiency and hypophysitis (Chapter 50).

5) Which of the following statements about *BRCA1/2* genes in breast cancer is correct?
   A) Complete loss of *BRCA1/2* function leads to a variety of genomic instability
   B) Cumulative risk of *BRCA2* breast cancer by the age of 70 is 25%
   C) Somatic *BRCA1/2* mutations are seen in around 8% of cases
   D) Among patients with TNBC, germline *BRCA1* mutations are diagnosed at later ages than what is seen with germline *BRCA2* mutations.

Expert Perspective: The *BRCA* genes are tumor suppressors involved in homologous recombination repair of DNA double-stranded breaks, cell cycle checkpoint control, and regulation of key mitotic steps. A complete loss of BRCA1/2 function leads to a variety of genomic instability. In the setting of germline BRCA mutations, when one allele is affected, the other allele leads to protein truncation of BRCA1 and BRCA2 and dysfunctional regulation of cell cycle and DNA repair. In these cases, the cumulative risk of BRCA1 and BRCA2 breast cancer by the age of 70 is 80% and 50%, respectively.

Germline BRCA mutations are seen in roughly 8% of breast cancer cases and to a significantly lower extent, seen as somatic mutations in tumor in around 3% of cases. Among patients with TNBC, there is a higher propensity for underlying BRCA1 vs BRCA2 mutation, whereas BRCA2 is more predominant in ER+/HER2− tumors. Among patients with TNBC, germline BRCA2 mutations are diagnosed at later ages than what is seen with germline BRCA1 mutations. In contrast, patients with TNBC and germline BRCA1 mutations tend to have higher nuclear grade disease than their counterparts with non-TNBC subtypes of breast cancer. A recent report also suggested that BRCA1/2 mutations impacted survival only in the TNBC subgroup but not among non-TNBC subtypes.

Given the role of BRCA genes in DNA damage pathways, patients with underlying BRCA1/2 mutations are uniquely positioned to benefit from poly adenosine diphosphate-ribose polymerase (PARP) inhibitors, which lead to accumulation of double-stranded breaks by initially hindering the repair of single-stranded breaks and eventual apoptosis of cancer cells. It is thus imperative to identify patients eligible for this treatment approach. (Also refer to Chapters 19 and 46.)

Correct Answer: A

6) **Who should be referred for genetic counseling for consideration of germline BRCA mutation testing?**

Expert Perspective: In line with NCCN recommendations, all patients with metastatic HER2 negative breast cancer are recommended to undergo testing for presence of germline BRCA testing given potential for benefit utilizing a PARP inhibitor in this population (Chapters 45 and 46).

7) **When should PARP inhibitors be considered?**

Expert Perspective: PARP inhibitors are approved for use in patients with germline BRCA mutated, HER2 negative metastatic breast cancer. Olaparib monotherapy (300 mg orally twice daily) in this setting was found to improve progression-free survival when compared with single-agent chemotherapy (capecitabine 2,500 mg/m^2 days 1–14 every 21 days, or vinorelbine 30 mg/m^2 day 1 and 8 every 21 days, or eribulin 1.4 mg/m^2 day 1 and 8 every 21 days) from 4.2 to 7 months (HR 0.58; 95% CI 0.43–0.80; $P < 0.001$) in the OlympiAD trial. However, OS data was not significant (HR 0.90; 95% CI 0.66–1.23, $P = 0.513$). The study investigators did find clinically meaningful differences favoring olaparib in patients who had not received prior chemotherapy in the metastatic setting (HR 0.51; 95% CI 0.29–0.90; $P = 0.02$). OlympiAD results did not appear to reflect that PARP inhibitors were as effective as second- or third-line therapy (HR 1.13; 95% CI 0.79–1.64).

Talazoparib (1 mg once daily) is similarly approved in this setting for use in patients with germline BRCA mutation based on data from EMBRACA showing improvement in progression-free survival when compared with single-agent physicians' choice of chemotherapy (capecitabine, eribulin, gemcitabine, or vinorelbine) from 5.6 to 8.6 months (HR 0.54; 95% CI 0.41–0.71; $P < 0.001$). No significant improvement in OS was reported, although quality of life measures were additionally improved with talazoparib.

BROCADE3 is currently ongoing and evaluating the addition – rather than monotherapy – of veliparib (120 mg orally twice daily on days 2–5) to carboplatin and paclitaxel in patients having previously received up to two prior lines of chemotherapy. This study compares veliparib versus placebo in combination with carboplatin and paclitaxel. The design included veliparib or placebo continuation as monotherapy until disease progression if the doublet chemotherapy was discontinued. The primary endpoint from this phase III trial was progression-free survival per Response Evaluation Criteria in Solid Tumors (RECIST) v1.1. Reported interim analysis revealed an increased progression-free survival derived from veliparib use (HR 0.71; 95% CI 0.57–0.88; $P = 0.0016$). Remarkably, most of the benefit appeared to be derived from veliparib maintenance post-chemotherapy, because the survival curves appeared to diverge after chemotherapy was completed. Findings are in line with prior trials with regard to progression-free survival benefit with addition of veliparib, although this agent has not yet received FDA approval.

8) Are PARP inhibitors effective in tumors with somatic *BRCA* mutation?

Expert Perspective: In the phase II TBCRC 048 trial, olaparib was found to be effective in patients with tumors harboring somatic *BRCA* mutation with a reported overall response rate of 50%. This is comparable to overall response rate reported with talazoparib in EMBRACA (62.2%) and olaparib in OlympiAD (52%). Therefore, PARP inhibitors are an appropriate option for patients harboring somatic *BRCA* mutations.

9) How should one approach somatic *BRCA* mutations designated as a variant of uncertain significance?

Expert Perspective: The pathological impact of a mutation designated as a variant of uncertain significance (VUS) on genetic analysis is unclear. With ongoing research, VUS mutations may over time be reclassified as benign or pathogenic based on emerging clinical data. However, preclinical data show that saturation genome editing (SGE) could functionally classify thousands of variants in *BRCA1* (and possibly *BRCA2*). These tools may allow development and attribution of a function score based on the newly observed variants that may guide future management. In the interim, clinical decision making should not be influenced by the presence of VUS mutations.

10) What other mutations related to DNA deficiency may benefit from PARP inhibitors?

Expert Perspective: There is accumulating evidence for homologous recombination deficiency (HRD) tumors demonstrating a response to PARP inhibitors in tumors other than breast, and efficacy and current FDA approvals are limited for use in metastatic prostate and advanced epithelial ovarian, fallopian tube, and primary peritoneal cancers. Multiple studies are investigating the role of additional homologous recombination repair (HRR) pathway proteins including *PALB2*, notable for the phase II TBCRC 048 trial demonstrating high response rate (82%) to olaparib in patients with metastatic HER2 negative breast cancer harboring a germline *PALB2* mutation.

Role of Next Generation Sequencing

Next generation sequencing (NGS) allows for the detection of a variety of aberrations within the tumor genome, which may indicate mechanisms of tumor resistance and ideally reveal intervenable targets if the corresponding agent is commercially available. Commercially available assays such as Foundation One testing (Foundation Medicine), TempusXT (Tempus), PCDx (Paradigm), GPS Cancer (NantOmics), CancerPlex (Kew), or the Oncomine Comprehensive Assay (ThermoFisher) evaluate panels of DNA from tumor tissue. Others have integrated their own NGS toolkit internally; such is the case of the Memorial Kettering-Integrated Mutation Profiling of Actionable Cancer Targets (MSK-IMPACT) assay. Whereas most, such as FoundationOne or Caris CDx, perform only tumor analysis, providing information on CNV, gene fusions, microsatellites, and TMB, others such as TempusXT develop techniques where tumor genomics is compared to normal tissue genomics. Detailed information regarding the distribution and type of mutations is provided in addition to whether a specific targeted agent is recommended. Liquid biopsies have also come into favor over recent years and rely on the detection of cell-free circulating-tumor DNA (ctDNA) obtained from peripheral blood. Guardant360 CDx, FoundationOne Liquid, and TempusXT, among others, are frequently utilized liquid biopsy-mediated assays that provide comprehensive genomic profiling of ctDNA from which mutations are presumed to be promoting tumor progression and invasive qualities. Assays based on NGS data from tumor tissue may have a higher yield of detecting aberrancies. Initial selection of assay may be contingent on whether tumor tissue is available for analysis, although data yielded from liquid biopsy is informative in its own right and should be considered when resources are available.

11) How should one approach PD-L1 negative tumors in patients without germline *BRCA* mutations?

Expert Perspective: Sequential utilization of single-agent chemotherapy is standard in patients who are not candidates for either immunotherapy or PARP inhibitors. Combination chemotherapy may be considered in cases in which visceral crisis is of concern and need for immediate response is more critical. Given overall poor prognosis of these patients, upfront consideration of available clinical trials is appropriate, as is investigation of intervenable targets utilizing commercially available NGS-based assays on either tumor tissue or ctDNA from liquid biopsy.

Metastatic Pattern of Spread in TNBC

Women with TNBC often have poorer prognosis than women with other subtypes of breast cancer. This may be due to the rapid onset of recurrence and aggressive metastatic spread observed in this subtype. Recurrence may occur at an accelerated mean of 2.6 years.

Women with TNBC are four times more likely to experience a visceral metastasis within five years after diagnosis, although they are comparatively less likely to develop bone metastasis than other breast cancer subtypes. In addition, TNBC is highly prone to cause central nervous system (CNS) involvement at comparable rates as seen in HER2 positive breast cancer, as well as possessing a high propensity for lung metastasis.

12) Should staging workup at diagnosis include surveillance for CNS involvement?

Expert Perspective: There should be a high index of clinical suspicion for presence of CNS involvement of metastatic TNBC in patients reporting congruent signs or symptoms such as new or worsening headaches, gait disturbances, visual changes, or other neurologic deficits. In the absence of a supportive history or pertinent physical examination findings, surveillance CT or MRI imaging of the brain is not necessary.

13) What are novel therapies to consider that are approved for use in later lines of therapy and that are currently in development?

Expert Perspective: The antibody drug conjugate (ADC) sacituzumab govitecan is FDA approved for use in metastatic TNBC for patients who have received two prior lines of therapy for metastatic disease. When compared to physician's choice of single-agent chemotherapy (eribulin, vinorelbine, capecitabine, or gemcitabine), sacituzumab govitecan significantly improved OS from 6.7 to 12.1 months (HR 0.48; 95% CI 0.38–0.59; $P< 0.001$) in the ASCENT III trial. The addition of the AKT inhibitor capivasertib versus placebo to paclitaxel has also been shown to improve OS in the first-line setting in untreated women with metastatic TNBC, as reported in the phase II PAKT trial. OS was extended from 12.6 to 19.1 months (HR, 0.61; 95% CI 0.37–0.99; 2-sided $P= 0.04$). In the phase III IPATUNITY trial of paclitaxel and ipatasertib versus paclitaxel alone, there was no significant improvement in progression-free survival. However, capivasertib is currently undergoing evaluation in a phase III trial. Most recently, fam-trastuzumab deruxtecan-nxki (Enhertu) was granted FDA approval in patients with unresectable or metastatic HER2 low breast cancer which includes patients with TNBC based on the results of DESTINY-Breast04 which included a small cohort of TNBC patients (N = 63). Enhertu was given at 5.4mg/kg every 3 weeks versus physician's choice of chemotherapy. The median progression free survival in the overall population was 9.9 months in the Enhertu arm versus 5.1 months in the comparator arm, concordant with improvement in median overall survival which was 23.9 months in the Enhertu arm and 17.5 in the chemotherapy arm, respectively. It is important to note; however, that the benefit of Enhertu is unclear in patients who have already received Sacituzumab govitecan and should be utilized in the absence of other more favorable options to include clinical trials in this context. Other agents of interest being explored for use in metastatic TNBC include inhibitors of PI3K and mTOR pathways, which have already gained approval in hormone-positive breast cancer with promising preclinical data in TNBC models (Chapters 11 and 12).

14) Is there a role for CDKIs in metastatic TNBC?

Expert Perspective: The introduction of cyclin-dependent kinase inhibitors (CDKIs) has dramatically changed the landscape of therapy for patients with metastatic hormone receptor positive disease in recent years (Chapter 12). However, the role of these agents in HER2-positive and TNBC remains unclear. Studies are ongoing specifically examining luminal subtypes of TNBC that are positive for the androgen receptor and may be sensitive to not only androgen receptor antagonists but also CDKIs. Currently, however, there is no role for CDKI in TNBC outside of clinical trials.

15) Is there a role for metastatectomy in metastatic TNBC?

Expert Perspective: In general, the topic of metastatectomy in metastatic breast cancer remains highly controversial, with conflicting reports regarding benefit with regard to outcomes. Surgical resection of oligometastatic disease is not commonly performed, particularly in metastatic TNBC; however, it may be considered on a case-by-case basis upon multidisciplinary tumor board discussion.

Conclusion

TNBC is an aggressive subtype of breast cancer that confers a particularly poor prognosis in the metastatic setting. Given lack of upregulation in ER, PR, or HER2 receptors, options for targeted therapy are severely limited in this setting. Cytotoxic chemotherapies are heavily relied upon in the management of metastatic TNBC; however, outcomes have been significantly improved in recent years with the addition of immunotherapy and PARP inhibitors for subgroups within this population. Most recently, the ADC sacituzumab govitecan and fam-trastuzumab deruxtecan-nxki has proven highly effective in patients having progressed on two prior therapies with significant extension of OS. Despite these advances, outcomes of patients with metastatic TNBC remain poor and significantly inferior compared to patients with other breast cancer subtypes (also refer to Chapters 11–14). Clinical trial participation is encouraged for patients with otherwise good performance status given the urgent need for more effective therapies in this space.

Recommended Readings

Anders, C.K., Abramson, V., Tan, T., and Dent, R. (2016). The evolution of triple-negative breast cancer: From biology to novel therapeutics. *Am Soc Clin Oncol Educ Book* 35: 34–42.

Bardia, A., Hurvitz, S.A., Tolaney, S.M. et al. (2021). ASCENT clinical trial investigators. Sacituzumab govitecan in metastatic triple-negative breast cancer. *N Engl J Med* 384 (16): 1529–1541. doi: 10.1056/NEJMoa2028485. PMID: 33882206.

Cortes, J., Cescon, D.W., Rugo, H.S. et al. (2020). KEYNOTE-355 Investigators. Pembrolizumab plus chemotherapy versus placebo plus chemotherapy for previously untreated locally recurrent inoperable or metastatic triple-negative breast cancer (KEYNOTE-355): A randomised, placebo-controlled, double-blind, phase 3 clinical trial. *Lancet* 396 (10265): 1817–1828. doi: 10.1016/S0140-6736(20)32531-9. PMID: 33278935.

Foulkes, W.D., Smith, I.E., and Reis-Filho, J.S. (2010). Triple-negative breast cancer. *N Engl J Med* 363 (20): 1938–1948. doi: 10.1056/NEJMra1001389. PMID: 21067385.

Lin, N.U., Vanderplas, A., Hughes, M.E. et al. (2012). Clinicopathologic features, patterns of recurrence, and survival among women with triple-negative breast cancer in the National Comprehensive Cancer Network. *Cancer* 118 (22): 5463–5472. doi: 10.1002/cncr.27581. Epub 2012 Apr 27. PMID: 22544643; PMCID: PMC3611659.

Martins, F., Sofiya, L., Sykiotis, G.P. et al. (2019). Adverse effects of immune-checkpoint inhibitors: Epidemiology, management and surveillance. *Nat Rev Clin Oncol* 16 (9): 563–580. doi: 10.1038/s41571-019-0218-0. PMID: 31092901.

Mavaddat, N., Barrowdale, D., Andrulis, I.L. et al. (2012 January). Pathology of breast and ovarian cancers among BRCA1 and BRCA2 mutation carriers: Results from the Consortium of Investigators of Modifiers of BRCA1/2 (CIMBA). *Cancer Epidemiol Biomarkers Prev* 21 (1): 134–147. doi: 10.1158/1055-9965.EPI-11-0775. Epub 2011 Dec 5. PMID: 22144499; PMCID: PMC3272407.

Robson, M.E., Tung, N., Conte, P. et al. (2019). Final overall survival and tolerability results: Olaparib versus chemotherapy treatment of physician's choice in patients with a germline

BRCA mutation and HER2-negative metastatic breast cancer. *Ann Oncol* 30 (4): 558–566. doi: 10.1093/annonc/mdz012. PMID: 30689707; PMCID: PMC6503629.

Merck. (2021, July 27). Merck announces phase 3 KEYNOTE-355 trial met primary endpoint of overall survival (OS) in patients with metastatic triple-negative breast cancer whose tumors expressed PD-L1 (CPS ≥10) [Press release]. https://www.merck.com/news/merck-announces-phase-3-keynote-355-trial-met-primary-endpoint-of-overall-survival-os-in-patients-with-metastatic-triple-negative-breast-cancer-whose-tumors-expressed-pd-l1-cps-%E2%89%A510.

Schmid, P., Adams, S., Rugo, H.S. et al. (2018). IMpassion130 trial investigators. Atezolizumab and Nab-Paclitaxel in advanced triple-negative breast cancer. *N Engl J Med* 379 (22): 2108–2121. doi: 10.1056/NEJMoa1809615. Epub 2018 Oct 20. PMID: 30345906).

17

Inflammatory Breast Cancer – A Distinct Entity

Massimo Cristofanilli[1] and Elena Vagia[2]

[1] *Weill Cornell Medicine, New York, NY*
[2] *Northwestern University Feinberg School of Medicine, Chicago, IL*

Introduction

Breast cancer remains the most common malignancy diagnosed among women in the world. Inflammatory breast cancer (IBC) is an uncommon virulent subset of disease that accounts for up to 2% of all breast cancers in the United States. Patients with IBC are often younger at the age at diagnosis, are more often black, and by definition, present with inoperable disease. Compared with patients diagnosed with noninflammatory locally advanced breast cancer, patients with IBC have as high as a twofold increased risk of dying of disease, with OS rates being consistently less than 50%. Approximately, 40% of patients with IBC have evident metastatic disease at the time of presentation.

1) What is the definition of Inflammatory Breast Cancer?

Expert Perspective: Inflammatory breast cancer (IBC) is the most aggressive form of breast cancer characterized by unique clinical, radiographic, and pathological features. The term "Inflammatory" was first introduced nearly one century ago, to describe a different clinical pattern observed in some breast cancer patients. Later on, IBC was established as a distinct entity of breast malignancies, and the definition remained as an accurate description of the clinical manifestation.

IBC is a rare disease, counting for approximately 5% of all breast cancers with significantly higher morbidity and mortality rates compared to non-IBC. The classification of a breast tumor as IBC is primarily based on the clinical presentation. Typical appearance consists of rapidly progressing breast engorgement associated with warmth, tenderness, and dark red or purple skin discoloration and thickening commonly reported as "peau d'orange," (meaning "orange peel") affecting more than one-third of the breast. The affected breast is visibly larger and firm. It is suggested that the underlying mechanism responsible for the breast and skin changes is the drainage obstruction of dermal lymphatics caused by tumor emboli.

The symptoms usually develop within days or weeks, but at most they develop within six months. A primary breast mass may not always be present; nonetheless, in either case a histological confirmation of the malignancy is required.

2) Are there any predisposing factors responsible for IBC?

Expert Perspective: Small retrospective epidemiologic studies have reported various reproductive and lifestyle risk factors associated with IBC. For example, age at first birth, number of children, duration of breastfeeding, smoking, and body mass index (BMI) are the most frequently reported factors.

Women younger than 26 years old at first pregnancy were at higher risk for all types of IBC. Increased number of children was associated with higher risk of triple negative and HER2+ IBC. A history of breastfeeding was associated with lower risk of triple negative and HR+ IBC.

BMI was associated with an increased risk of all subtypes of IBC in both premenopausal and postmenopausal women. History of smoking was associated with increased risk of HER2+ and luminal subtype IBC. Higher level of education was associated with lower risk of IBC.

3) What is the prognosis of IBC?

Expert Perspective: Despite the progress that has been made for the diagnosis and treatment of IBC, the prognosis remains poorer compared to non-IBC. The dismal prognosis is partially related with the aggressive nature of IBC and the advanced stage at disease presentation, including approximately 30% with *de novo* stage IV. Moreover, the peculiar initial locally advanced presentation of breast involvement is defined separately in the staging system (T4d) to reflect the unique clinical aspects of the disease. The majority of IBC patients have lymph node involvement early in the disease course including axillary, internal mammary, infraclavicular, and supraclavicular regions, and there is an increased risk for distant metastatic spread. However, lack of uniformity in diagnostic criteria and treatment guidelines is also responsible for the higher recurrence and death rates.

According to retrospective studies, the five-year overall survival (OS) rate for IBC patients was approximately 41% for all tumor stages and 56% and 19% for stage III and stage IV, respectively. When stratified by hormone receptor (HR) and human epidermal receptor (HER2) status, of note, HR+ status is not a favorable prognostic marker, as is the case for non-IBC, and TN tumors have the worst prognosis.

For stage III tumors, the recurrence rate is significantly higher for IBC patients compared to locally advanced non-IBC. The most common sites of recurrence are lymph nodes, chest wall, bone, and brain. Of note, IBC patients have higher incidence of developing brain metastases compared to those with non-IBC. These results are drastically improving in the era of modern drug development such as anti-HER2-targeted therapies, CDK4/6, and immune checkpoint inhibitors.

4) What are the diagnostic criteria for IBC?

Expert Perspective: The diagnosis of IBC is primarily based on the clinical presentation. Rapid onset of breast swelling and diffuse skin edema and erythema that involve more than one-third of the affected breast are concerning for IBC. The symptoms usually develop within a few weeks but at most in six months. In certain cases, the absence of an underlying breast mass can be misleading, and the breast findings can be misdiagnosed as mastitis, which will delay adequate treatment for IBC.

In addition to the clinical findings, diagnostic imaging including mammogram and/or breast MRI may reveal breast enlargement, diffuse skin thickening, and the underlying breast lesion if present (Figure 17.1).

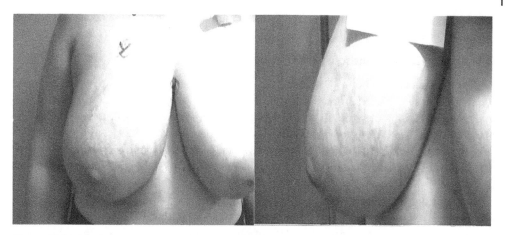

Figure 17.1 Illustration of skin changes in inflammatory breast cancer.

Lastly, a biopsy of the breast mass if present or other suspicious areas is required to confirm histologic diagnosis of IBC. A skin punch biopsy when performed can reveal tumor emboli in the dermal lymphatics supporting IBC diagnosis. Whether a positive skin punch biopsy is mandatory to conclude IBC diagnosis has been a matter of debate for a long time. Definitely, a negative skin punch biopsy does not exclude the diagnosis if the clinical manifestation is suggestive of IBC.

5) What are the radiographic findings of IBC?

Expert Perspective: Historically, diagnostic mammography is the initial test performed to evaluate breast symptoms including inflammatory changes. Common mammographic findings for IBC include one or multiple breast lesions, skin thickening, nipple retraction, and axillary lymph node enlargement. An ultrasonography is usually performed synchronously with the mammography and can increase the probability to detect axillary lymphadenopathy.

Of note, a mammography may fail to detect the primary breast lesion and the nodal involvement in approximately 40% of newly diagnosed IBC patients. Therefore, a breast magnetic resonance imaging (MRI) scan is required to better assess the inflammatory features and lymph node status. Typical MRI findings for IBC can be breast enlargement, mass and/or diffuse non-mass enhancement, and global skin thickening and enhancement. In addition, MRI has been proven to be more sensitive in detecting lymph node involvement particularly the internal mammary, chest wall, and infraclavicular and supraclavicular lymphadenopathy.

As previously mentioned, IBC has a very fulminant course, impending an increased risk of metastatic spread at the time of diagnosis. Consequently, a detailed staging is required to assess regional and distant metastatic spread. Standard imaging techniques such as computed tomography and nuclear bone scan are commonly utilized by clinicians for staging purposes. The most frequently detected findings are the primary breast lesions, skin thickening, and regional axillary lymphadenopathy and also chest wall and supraclavicular and mediastinal lymphadenopathy.

Several retrospective studies have shown that more advanced imaging techniques such as positron emission tomography (PET/CT) have higher sensitivity to detect nodal involvement and distant lesions compared to standard techniques.

In conclusion, breast MRI and PET/CT are strongly recommended for newly diagnosed IBC patients to support the diagnosis and assess the extent of the disease (Figure 17.2).

6) What are the histopathological findings for IBC?

Expert Perspective: When IBC is suspected, a biopsy of the underlying breast mass if present and/or tissue samples from architecturally distorted areas are required to confirm the malignancy. The majority of IBCs are high-grade invasive ductal carcinomas, but other histologic subtypes such as lobular cancers have also been reported.

With respect to the HR and HER2 status, IBC is less likely to express estrogen (ER) and progesterone (PR) receptors but has higher incidence of HER2 expression, as compared to non-IBC.

An important histological aspect of IBC is the presence of tumor emboli in the dermal lymphatics. A skin punch biopsy, often obtained to confirm the IBC diagnosis, can detect the dermal lymphatic invasion only in 80% of cases. Technically the biopsy should include the area of most intense erythema and multiple samples to increase the detection probability. As mentioned above, a negative skin punch does not exclude the IBC diagnosis.

Another exclusive finding of IBC is the presence CD44/CD49/CD133-positive mammary stem cells and CD68-positive macrophages in the normal breast tissue surrounding the tumor, but these findings are typically not reported in the clinical-pathological assessment and remain an interesting area for future investigation.

7) Does IBC have an exclusive molecular signature?

Expert Perspective: The evolution of next-generation (NGS) techniques enabled a deeper understanding of the underlying tumor biology. Several retrospective studies have demonstrated that IBC has a distinct molecular signature tightly linked with the

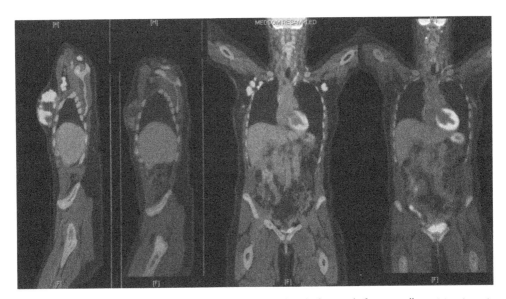

Figure 17.2 PET-CT images in a locally advanced IBC patient before and after neoadjuvant treatment.

clinical diversity and aggressive nature. More specifically, four intrinsic clusters have been described including luminal A, luminal B, HER2-positive, and basal-like. IBC are more likely to be basal-like tumors while non-IBC are primarily luminal subtypes.

IBC appears to have a unique molecular profile characterized by overexpression of the epithelial adhesion protein E-cadherin, overexpression of the RhoC oncogene, and a high frequency of TP53 gene mutations, in addition to a loss of expression of WISP3, which has growth and angiogenesis inhibitory functions.

The most frequently altered genes observed in IBC are *TP53, ERBB2, BRCA, CCDN1, MYC, PIK3CA, NOTCH1, GATA3, FGFR1, JAK2*, and *ARID1A*. Genomic alteration in the DNA repair genes and *ERBB2* amplification are more frequent for IBC while PIK3CA mutations are more frequent for non-IBC.

Interestingly, it is suggested that IBC tumors have significantly reduced transforming growth factor beta (TGF-β) signaling. Inhibition of TGF-β signaling can promote collective-cell migration and lymphatic invasion, which is typical for IBC.

8) How do we treat locally advanced (stage III) IBC?

Expert Perspective: The management of IBC remains a challenge, and a multidisciplinary approach is warranted to improve the outcomes. Treatment for the locally advanced disease, stage III breast cancer is given with curative intent. Expert panels recommend a trimodal approach consisting of preoperative systemic therapy, surgery, and radiation as crucial steps to lower the risk of recurrence.

Efficacy and survival data from large prospective studies that included IBC patients support the application of neoadjuvant systemic therapy.

Neoadjuvant therapy aims to achieve maximal tumor shrinkage, ideally a complete pathological response (pCR). It is well established that IBC patients who achieve a pCR after neoadjuvant therapy have superior survival outcomes compared to those who had residual disease at the time of surgery. Retrospective studies have shown that the pCR rate depends on the tumor subtype. Specifically, HER2+ IBC tumors have the highest pCR rate as compared to HR+/HER2− and triple negative tumors. Escalation strategies should be considered to achieve the best possible response.

The standard of care for neoadjuvant chemotherapy includes anthracycline and/or taxane-based regimens. Anti-HER2-targeted agents and immunotherapy is added for HER2+ and triple negative tumors, respectively.

HER2 positive: Specifically, combination of chemotherapy with trastuzumab and pertuzumab is the preferred regimen for HER2+ tumors. According to the NeoSphere study, which included 29 IBC patients, the cohort treated with neoadjuvant docetaxel plus trastuzumab/pertuzumab followed by adjuvant 5-fluorouracil, epirubicin, and cyclophosphamide and completed one year of trastuzumab had a 45.8% pCR rate and the five-year progression-free survival was 86%.

The subsequent randomized phase II trial TRYPHAENA study compared regimens with or without anthracycline. The subset of patients who received combination of docetaxel, carboplatin plus trastuzumab and pertuzumab had the highest pCR rate. Reported progression-free survival and OS was similar across all cohorts. Although neither of the above studies reported separately IBC patients, other retrospective studies have shown that survival outcomes are similar in IBC and non-IBC patients who achieved a pCR after neoadjuvant treatment.

After completing surgical treatment, patients will continue anti-HER2 treatment with trastuzumab and pertuzumab up to one year. Clinical study data also support the use of trastuzumab emtansine (T-DM1) in the adjuvant setting for patients who did not achieve a pCR. For high-risk patients, extended anti-HER2 treatment beyond one year can also be considered. Neratinib is a pan-HER tyrosine kinase inhibitor, that has received regulatory approval as adjuvant treatment for one year in HER2+ breast cancer patients who completed adjuvant trastuzumab. However, considering the advancement made for the treatment of HER2+ tumors, the role of neratinib in the adjuvant setting is to be defined (see Chapter 13).

Triple negative: In a recently reported study, the addition of immune checkpoint inhibitor pembrolizumab to standard chemotherapy for TNBC including small number of IBC patients increased the pCR rate and improved survival. Patients received paclitaxel plus carboplatin with or without pembrolizumab followed by anthracycline plus cyclophosphamide in combination with pembrolizumab or placebo. Pembrolizumab continued as adjuvant treatment for nine additional cycles. The reported pCR rate in the pembrolizumab arm was 65.8% versus 51.2% for the placebo. The three-year event-free survival rate was 84.5% for the pembrolizumab arm versus 76.8% for the placebo. The benefit from pembrolizumab was irrespective of PD-L1 expression. Following these results, the addition of pembrolizumab to NA platinum-containing chemotherapy followed by adjuvant pembrolizumab became the new standard treatment for TNBC including triple-negative IBC (see Chapter 15).

Hormone receptor positive: HR+/HER2− IBC has the lowest pCR rate, and novel strategies are needed to improve treatment outcomes. In the past few years, enormous progress has been made with the incorporation of CDK4/6 inhibitors in the first-line treatment of advanced HR+/HER2− breast cancer. Subsequently, the efficacy of CDK4/6 inhibitors was also demonstrated in the early stage disease. Today, the combination of endocrine therapy with a CDK4/6 inhibitor is the new standard of care for adjuvant treatment for early stage, high-risk HR+/HER2− breast cancer, including IBC (see Chapter 11).

9) What is the recommended surgical treatment for IBC?

Expert Perspective: Adequate surgical treatment after completing neoadjuvant therapy is fundamental for IBC patients. Because of the diffuse skin and lymphatic involvement, a radical surgical approach is recommended.

Modified radical mastectomy with axillary lymph node dissection remains the standard of care for all IBC patients. It is important for patients who will proceed with surgery to confirm that they had a remarkable response to neoadjuvant treatment. In the situations that swelling and skin erythema persist, additional chemotherapy and/or radiation should be considered to achieve response before proceeding to surgery. Suboptimal surgical treatment and positive margins are associated with a higher rate of locoregional recurrence and poorer survival outcomes.

A large retrospective study showed that breast-conserving strategies or skin sparing mastectomies resulted in worse survival outcomes. There are a few reported studies suggesting that patients who had a good response to neoadjuvant therapy had similar long-term survival outcomes with either radical mastectomy or breast-conserving surgery. However, these are small, single-institution studies, and validation with larger cohorts and prospective studies is needed.

Immediate breast reconstruction is not recommended but can be considered after a substantial recurrence-free interval.

10) How is radiation treatment delivered in IBC patients?

Expert Perspective: Radiation treatment is recommended in all non-metastatic IBC patients.

It usually follows surgery and involves the chest wall and regional lymphatics.

A total dose up to 60–66 Gy is delivered in standard fractions or hypofractionated to the chest wall and internal mammary, ipsilateral axillary, infraclavicular, and supraclavicular lymph nodes.

In patients with poor response to neoadjuvant treatment, radiation can be given preoperatively. In this scenario, there is a higher risk for post-surgical complications.

Currently, efforts are focusing on optimizing radiation treatment for IBC patients. For instance, an ongoing study is evaluating the efficacy of olaparib, a poly(ADP-ribose) polymerase inhibitor (PARPi), administered concurrently with adjuvant radiation in non-metastatic IBC patients. It is suggested that PARPi may have a radiosensitizing effect in certain tumors.

11) What is the treatment for metastatic IBC?

Expert Perspective: The mainstay treatment for *de novo* metastatic or recurrent IBC is systemic chemotherapy. In specific patients with oligometastatic disease and exceptional response to the neoadjuvant therapy, locoregional treatment including modified radical mastectomy with axillary lymph node dissection, and postoperative radiation should be offered. This is supported by small retrospective studies that showed superior locoregional control and survival benefit in carefully selected stage IV IBC patients who received surgery and radiation in addition to systemic therapy.

Hormone receptor positive: Adequate systemic treatment is determined based on the tumor HR and HER2 status. As previously mentioned, HR+ IBC is more aggressive and has worst prognosis compared to HR+ non-IBC. Taxane- and/or anthracycline-based chemotherapy may be considered up front to control the symptoms. After obtaining an optimal response, endocrine therapy in combination with a CDK4/6 inhibitor can be initiated (see Chapter 12).

HER2 positive: Regimens containing anti-HER2-targeted agents are recommended for the HER2+ disease. More recently, newly developed anti-HER2 drugs have expanded the therapeutic choices and significantly improved survival for HER2+ metastatic breast cancer patients.

Dual anti-HER2 regimen, trastuzumab and pertuzumab in combination with chemotherapy is the recommended first-line approach for newly diagnosed, stage IV, HER2+ IBC. After progression to first-line treatment, trastuzumab emtansine (T-DM1) is frequently used.

Tyrosine kinase inhibitor (TKI) tucatinib given in combination with trastuzumab and capecitabine was superior to trastuzumab and capecitabine alone in patients who had progressed to one or more prior anti-HER2 treatments. Of note, a greater benefit was observed in patients with brain metastases. Clinical studies suggest that other TKIs such as neratinib and lapatinib have also shown efficacy in HER2+ patients with brain metastases.

Trastuzumab deruxtecan is an antibody-drug conjugate that has demonstrated durable response in patients with HER2+ metastatic breast cancer who had failed in at least two prior lines of anti-HER2 treatment. Data from the randomized phase III study DESTINY-Breast03 showed that patients who received trastuzumab deruxtecan after progressing to taxane and trastuzumab regimen had an objective response rate 80% compared to 34% in patients who received T-DM1. Subgroup analysis in patients with stable brain metastases showed that objective response rate was 67.4% with trastuzumab deruxtecan versus 20.5% with T-DM1.

Early data also suggest that trastuzumab deruxtecan may be effective in tumors with low HER2 expression that are considered HER2 negative by standard criteria. These results are of great importance and need further investigation in the future (see Chapter 14).

A new anti-HER2 monoclonal antibody, margetuximab, was superior to trastuzumab in heavily pretreated patients (see Chapter 14).

Triple negative: For stage IV triple-negative IBC, chemotherapy with or without immunotherapy is the up-front standard treatment. PD-L1 expression is predictive of response to immunotherapy. Approximately 40% of IBC have high PD-L1 expression indicating potentially increased benefit from immunotherapy. Ongoing studies are further evaluating the efficacy of immunotherapy across all subtypes of IBC.

Antibody-drug conjugate sacituzumab govitecan is a newly developed agent for the treatment of metastatic TNBC composed of a monoclonal antibody targeting the human trophoblast cell-surface antigen 2 (Trop2) linked through a hydrolyzable linker to topoisomerase inhibitor SN-38. The phase III randomized trial ASCENT study investigated the efficacy of sacituzumab govitecan compared to single-agent chemotherapy in advanced TNBC patients who had progressed in prior treatments. The median progression-free survival in patients without brain metastases who received sacituzumab govitecan was 5.6 months versus 1.7 months with chemotherapy while for the entire study population it was 4.8 and 1.7 months, respectively. The median OS was 12.1 months with sacituzumab govitecan versus 6.7 months with chemotherapy (see Chapter 16).

12) What is the focus of prospective research in IBC?

Expert Perspective: To date, IBC remains the most aggressive form of breast malignancies, with very high recurrence and death rates. Future efforts should be focused on identifying novel strategies that will prolong survival for metastatic patients and achieve superior local control and increase the cure rate for locally advanced disease. Several trials are underway investigating new agents and combinatory treatments that will likely expand the therapeutic options for this disease in the future (Table 17.1).

The molecular characterization of IBC in particular is still an area of intensive research, aiming to identify the genomic alterations that drive tumor growth and spread. Gene-expressing profiling of the primary and residual disease can provide valuable information for the primary and acquired mechanism of resistance to treatment. Understanding the biology of this unique disease is fundamental for the implementation of personalized and biologically informed treatment approaches.

Table 17.1 Ongoing clinical trials for IBC.

Clinicaltrials.gov Identifier	Study Design	Setting	Primary Endpoint
NCT03515798	A prospective multicenter open-label, randomized phase II study of pembrolizumab in combination with neoadjuvant (F)EC-paclitaxel regimen in HER2-negative inflammatory breast cancer	NA	pCR
NCT02876302	Phase II study of combination ruxolitinib (INCB018424) with preoperative chemotherapy for triple-negative inflammatory breast cancer	NA	pCR
NCT02623972	A phase II study of eribulin followed by doxorubicin and cyclophosphamide as preoperative therapy for HER2-negative inflammatory breast cancer	NA	pCR
NCT03598257	A phase II randomized trial of olaparib (NSC-747856) administered concurrently with radiotherapy versus radiotherapy alone for inflammatory breast cancer	Adj	IDFS
NCT03202316	A phase II study of triple combination of atezolizumab + cobimetinib + eribulin (ACE) in patients with recurrent/metastatic inflammatory breast cancer	Adv	ORR
NCT02971748	A phase II study of anti-PD-1 (pembrolizumab) in combination with hormonal therapy during or after radiation in patients with hormone receptor (HR)-positive localized inflammatory breast cancer (IBC) who did not achieve a pathological complete response (pCR) to neoadjuvant chemotherapy	Adj	DFS
NCT03742986	Phase II trial of nivolumab with chemotherapy as neoadjuvant treatment in inflammatory breast cancer	NA	pCR
NCT02411656	A phase II study of anti-PD-1 (MK-3475) therapy in patients with metastatic inflammatory breast cancer (IBC) or non-IBC triple-negative breast cancer (TNBC) who have achieved clinical response or stable disease to prior chemotherapy	Adv	iCR/iSD
NCT02876107	A randomized phase II study of neoadjuvant carboplatin/paclitaxel (CT) versus panitumumab/carboplatin/paclitaxel (PaCT) followed by anthracycline-containing regimen for newly diagnosed primary triple-negative inflammatory breast cancer	NA	pCR
NCT03101748	A phase Ib study of neratinib, pertuzumab, and trastuzumab with Taxol (3HT) in primary metastatic and locally advanced breast cancer, and phase II study of 3HT followed by AC in HER2+ primary IBC, and neratinib with Taxol (NT) followed by AC in HR+ / HER2− primary IBC	NA	pCR

NA: neoadjuvant; Adj: adjuvant; Adv: advanced; pCR: pathological complete response; ORR: overall response rate; DFS: disease free survival.

Recommended Readings

Fouad, T.M., Kogawa, T., Liu, D.D., Shen, Y., Masuda, H., El-Zein, R., Woodward, W.A., Chavez-macgregor, M., Alvarez, R.H., Arun, B., Lucci, A., Krishnamurthy, S., Babiera, G., Buchholz, T.A., Valero, V., and Ueno, N.T. (2015 July). Overall survival differences between patients with inflammatory and noninflammatory breast cancer presenting with distant metastasis at diagnosis. *Breast Cancer Res Treat* 152 (2): 407–416. doi:10.1007/s10549-015-3436-x. Epub 2015 May 29. Erratum in: Breast Cancer Res Treat. 2015 Jul;152(2):417.PMID: 26017070; PMCID: PMC4492876.

Cristofanilli, M., Valero, V., Buzdar, A.U., Kau, S.W., Broglio, K.R., Gonzalez-Angulo, A.M., Sneige, N., Islam, R., Ueno, N.T., Buchholz, T.A., Singletary, S.E., and Hortobagyi, G.N. (2007 October 1). Inflammatory breast cancer (IBC) and patterns of recurrence: understanding the biology of a unique disease. *Cancer* 110 (7): 1436–1444. doi: 10.1002/cncr.22927. PMID: 17694554.

Atkinson, R.L., El-Zein, R., Valero, V., Lucci, A., Bevers, T.B., Fouad, T., Liao, W., Ueno, N.T., Woodward, W.A., and Brewster, A.M. (2016 March). Epidemiological risk factors associated with inflammatory breast cancer subtypes. *Cancer Causes Control* 27 (3): 359–366. doi:10.1007/s10552-015-0712-3. Epub 2016 Jan 21. PMID: 26797453; PMCID: PMC4778706.

Luo, R., Chong, W., Wei, Q., Zhang, Z., Wang, C., Ye, Z., Abu-Khalaf, M.M., Silver, D.P., Stapp, R.T., Jiang, W., Myers, R.E., Li, B., Cristofanilli, M., and Yang, H. (2021 June 1). Whole-exome sequencing identifies somatic mutations and intratumor heterogeneity in inflammatory breast cancer. *NPJ Breast Cancer* 7 (1): 72. doi: 10.1038/s41523-021-00278-w. PMID: 34075047; PMCID: PMC8169683.

Matro, J.M., Li, T., Cristofanilli, M., Hughes, M.E., Ottesen, R.A., Weeks, J.C., and Wong, Y.N. (2015 February). Inflammatory breast cancer management in the national comprehensive cancer network: the disease, recurrence pattern, and outcome. *Clin Breast Cancer* 15 (1): 1–7. doi:10.1016/j.clbc.2014.05.005. Epub 2014 Jun 23. PMID: 25034439; PMCID: PMC4422394.

de Bazelaire, C., Groheux, D., Chapellier, M., Sabatier, F., Scémama, A., Pluvinage, A., Albiter, M., and de Kerviler, E. (2012 February). Breast inflammation: indications for MRI and PET-CT. *Diagn Interv Imaging* 93 (2): 104–115. doi:10.1016/j.diii.2011.12.004. Epub 2012 Jan 21. PMID: 22305594.

Resetkova, E. (2008 February). Pathologic aspects of inflammatory breast carcinoma: part 1. Histomorphology and differential diagnosis. *Semin Oncol* 35 (1): 25–32. doi:10.1053/j.seminoncol.2007.11.013. PMID: 18308143.

Liu, J., Chen, K., Jiang, W., Mao, K., Li, S., Kim, M.J., Liu, Q., and Jacobs, L.K. (2017 January). Chemotherapy response and survival of inflammatory breast cancer by hormone receptor- and HER2-defined molecular subtypes approximation: an analysis from the National Cancer Database. *J Cancer Res Clin Oncol* 143 (1): 161–168. doi:10.1007/s00432-016-2281-6. Epub 2016 Oct 4. PMID: 27704268.

Rueth, N.M., Lin, H.Y., Bedrosian, I., Shaitelman, S.F., Ueno, N.T., Shen, Y., and Babiera, G. (2014 July 1). Underuse of trimodality treatment affects survival for patients with inflammatory breast cancer: an analysis of treatment and survival trends from the National Cancer Database. *J Clin Oncol* 32 (19): 2018–2024. doi: 10.1200/JCO.2014.55.1978. Epub 2014 Jun 2. PMID: 24888808; PMCID: PMC4067942.10.

Woodward, W.A. (2015 November). Inflammatory breast cancer: unique biological and therapeutic considerations. *Lancet Oncol* 16 (15): e568–e576. doi:10.1016/S1470-2045(15)00146-1. PMID: 26545845.

Vagia, E., Cristofanilli, M. (2021 April 24). New Treatment strategies for the Inflammatory breast cancer. *Curr Treat Options Oncol* 22 (6): 50. doi: 10.1007/s11864-021-00843-2. PMID: 33893888.

Manai, M., ELBini-Dhouib, I., Finetti, P. et al. (2022 September 19). MARCKS as a Potential Therapeutic Target in Inflammatory Breast Cancer. *Cells* 11 (18): 2926. doi: 10.3390/cells11182926. PMID: 36139501; PMCID: PMC9496908.

18

Male Breast Cancer

Laura A. Huppert[1], Ozge Gumusay[2], Shreya Desai[3], and Hope S. Rugo[1]

[1] *Division of Hematology, Oncology, University of California, San Francisco, CA*
[2] *Acibadem Altunizade Hospital, Breast Health Center, Istanbul, Turkey*
[3] *Rosalind Franklin University of Medicine and Sciences, North Chicago, IL*

Introduction

Male breast cancer accounts for less than 1% of all breast cancers with a rising incidence. In clinical practice, male breast cancer has been relatively understudied because many trials exclude male participants, leading to few prospective studies. Treatment recommendations have largely been extrapolated from data in females. In the last decade, a greater effort has been made to better understand the unique biological and clinical characteristics of male breast cancer. In this chapter, we will summarize the most recent data about the epidemiology of male breast cancer, its pathologic and clinical characteristics, treatment options, and issues related to survivorship.

ER±/HER2− Male Breast Cancer

Case Study 1

A 60-year-old man with a history of type 2 diabetes presents with enlargement of his left breast. Physical examination reveals a firm 1.5 cm mass at six o'clock, one centimeter from the nipple. An enlarged left axillary lymph node is also appreciated. Diagnostic mammogram and ultrasound confirm the presence of a concerning mass at that position, measuring 1.9 cm and a 1.5 cm left axillary lymph node. A core needle biopsy demonstrates grade 3 invasive ductal carcinoma that is ER+ (100%), PR+ (90%), and HER2− (IHC 0), and axillary LN biopsy is positive for metastatic carcinoma. A PET-CT does not show evidence of metastatic disease.

1) What is the incidence and prevalence of male breast cancer?

Expert Perspective: Breast cancer in men accounts for less than 1% of all breast cancers worldwide. There is some geographic variation in incidence, with male breast cancer representing < 0.5% of cases in the United States but up to 6% of cases in Central Africa,

Cancer Consult: Expertise in Clinical Practice, Volume 1: Solid Tumors & Supportive Care,
Second Edition. Edited by Syed A. Abutalib, Maurie Markman, Al B. Benson III, and Hope S. Rugo.
© 2024 John Wiley & Sons Ltd. Published 2024 by John Wiley & Sons Ltd.

likely due to endemic viral hepatitis leading to hyperestrogenism. The lifetime risk of developing breast cancer for a man is approximately 1 in 1,000 compared with 1 in 8 for a woman. Data from the Surveillance, Epidemiology, and End Results (SEER) program indicates that age-adjusted incidence rate has increase from 0.85 cases per 100,000 men in the general population in 1975 to 1.43 cases per 100,000 in 2011. The incidence of male breast cancer rises with advancing age, with the highest incidence seen in men aged 80 years or older; men tend to be about 5–10 years older than women at the time of diagnosis. The incidence of male breast cancer is also high in non-Hispanic black men with an earlier age of diagnosis and inferior outcomes compared with non-Hispanic white men and Hispanic men. Usually, male patients with breast cancer present with more advanced disease compared with females.

2) What are the risk factors?

Expert Perspective: Risk factors for developing male breast cancer include advancing age, family history, certain genetic mutations, excessive estrogen stimulation, and prior radiation or hormonal therapy (Table 18.1). The risk of male breast cancer increases with advancing age. Most cases of male breast cancer are diagnosed after the age of 50 years and carry poor outcomes compared with female breast cancer. Family history of breast cancer increases the risk in men depending on number and degree of family members affected. Men with first-degree relative with breast cancer have a relative risk of 1.9, and men with two affected first-degree relatives have nearly tenfold increased risk, compared with men without family history of breast cancer. Genetic mutations such as *BRCA1* and *BRCA2* also increase the risk. Population

Table 18.1 Risk factors for male breast cancer.

Demographic
Older age
Black race
Environmental
Radiation exposure
Androgen/estrogen imbalances
Obesity
Elevated estrogen levels
External use of estradiol or testosterone
Testicular abnormalities (undescended testis, orchiectomy, testicular injury)
Orchiditis/ epididymitis
Cirrhosis
Gynecomastia
Familial/genetic
Pathogenic mutations in *BRCA1*, *BRCA2*, *PALB2* (partner and localizer of *BRCA2*), *CHEK2*, *PTEN* (Cowden syndrome), *P53* (Li-Fraumeni syndrome)
Klinefelter syndrome (additional X chromosome with high ratio of estrogen/testosterone)
Family history of breast cancer

studies have shown that up to 4% of men with breast cancer have *BRCA1* mutations, and up to 16% of patients have *BRCA2* mutations (see Chapters 45–47). Referral for genetic testing is recommended for male patients with breast cancer because they have increased risk of *BRCA* mutation, particularly *BRCA2*; both genes are inherited in an autosomal-dominant pattern. In one study, a quarter of men reported that they had not been referred for genetic testing. Excessive estrogen stimulation also appears to increase the risk of breast cancer in men. This may be due to previous hormonal therapy, medical comorbidities such as obesity, liver disease, thyroid disorders, or inherited conditions such as Klinefelter syndrome. In particular, Klinefelter syndrome is associated with a 16-to-19-fold increased risk for breast cancer.

3) How should male breast cancer be diagnosed?

Expert Perspective: Most men with breast cancer present with a painless subareolar breast mass. Other symptoms may include skin ulceration, nipple retraction, and/or bleeding from the nipple. The differential diagnosis for a breast mass in a male includes gynecomastia (which is typically bilateral), pseudogynecomastia, infections including breast abscess, lipoma, fibromatosis, and rarely metastatic disease from another primary tumor. If there is concern for breast cancer, breast imaging should be performed. Mammogram remains the diagnostic study of choice and is abnormal in 85–90% of males with breast cancer. After a mass is identified on imaging, a core biopsy should be performed to confirm the diagnosis and determine the receptor status.

Screening mammography is not recommended for the general male population. For men with known *BRCA1* or *BRCA2* mutations, the National Comprehensive Cancer Network (NCCN) recommends annual breast examination, but there is insufficient data to recommend mammographic screening (see Table 18.1 for other genes predisposing risk of male breast cancer).

4) What is the most common male breast cancer receptor subtype?

Expert Perspective: Approximately 95% of breast cancers in men are positive for estrogen receptor (ER) and progesterone receptor (PR) expression and negative for the human epidermal growth factor receptor 2 (HER2). In the International Male Breast Cancer Program, tumors from 1,483 men with breast cancer were analyzed, and 99% were ER+, 82% were PR+, and 97% were positive for androgen receptor. Only 9% of the tumors were HER2+. In this study, 42% were luminal A–like, 49% were luminal B–like, 9% were HER2+, and < 1% were triple-negative breast cancer (TNBC).

The most common histology in male breast cancer is invasive ductal carcinoma (IDC), which occurs in 85–90% of cases. DCIS in men tends to occur at a later age and is often low-grade. Invasive lobular carcinoma (ILC), which accounts for 10% of breast cancers in females, is present in only 1–1.5% of cases in males (see Chapter 10). The lack of lobular carcinomas in males is due to the lack of acini and lobules in the normal male breast. Other uncommon breast cancer subtypes in males include cancers with mucinous and papillary histology.

5) What is the prognosis?

Expert Perspective: Males with breast cancer have lower rates of unadjusted overall survival than females with breast cancer. Much of this may be explained by the older age of diagnosis for men and the shorter life expectancy in general compared to females, but further work is needed to better understand differences in biology and how this contributes to clinical outcomes.

6) How should male breast cancer be managed surgically?

Expert Perspective: Most studies about locoregional therapy for male breast cancer are extrapolated from studies in female patients. Females with early stage breast cancer typically undergo partial mastectomy (a.k.a lumpectomy, breast-conserving therapy) or mastectomy and then sentinel lymph node biopsy or axillary lymph node dissection. Most men undergo mastectomy with either sentinel lymph node biopsy or axillary lymph node dissection. There is no contraindication to breast conserving therapy in male patients, but it is much less common, with only 18% of male patients with T1N0 tumors undergoing breast-conserving surgery according to data from the SEER database. Breast-conserving therapy should be considered because it may improve cosmetic outcomes with no change in survival data according to observational studies. Sentinel lymph node biopsy is the standard of care for females with clinically lymph node negative breast cancer, and the same approach is utilized for male breast cancer.

7) What is the role for radiation therapy in male breast cancer?

Expert Perspective: Adjuvant radiation therapy should be offered to male patients with breast cancer using the same guidelines established for female patients with breast cancer. Data suggests that radiotherapy is often underutilized in males with breast cancer. In data from the SEER database, only 42% of male patients with stage I breast cancer who underwent breast conserving surgery received adjuvant radiation therapy. In male patients undergo breast-conserving therapy, radiation therapy should be recommended in most cases. In men who have node-positive breast cancer and undergo mastectomy, radiation therapy to the axilla should be offered.

8) What is the role of neoadjuvant/adjuvant chemotherapy in male breast cancer?

Expert Perspective: Adjuvant or neoadjuvant chemotherapy should be offered to men with breast cancer who have a high risk of recurrence. Between 1974 and 1988, a single prospective trial evaluated the role of adjuvant chemotherapy in men, enrolling 31 patients with stage II breast cancer including axillary lymph node involvement. All patients underwent mastectomy followed by 12 cycles of cyclophosphamide, methotrexate, and fluorouracil (CMF). With over 20 years of follow-up, the outcomes in this group have been better than historical controls, with 80% survival at 5 years and 42% survival at 20 years. Subsequent observational cohorts have also demonstrated improved survival in men who received adjuvant chemotherapy for high-risk, early stage breast cancer. Genomic tests such as the Oncotype Dx and Mammaprint assays used to help determine the benefit of chemotherapy in female patients are not validated in male patients, as discussed in the next question. It is important to consider the risks and benefits of chemotherapy in each individual patient, keeping in mind that male patients tend to be older at diagnosis and on average have a shorter life expectancy than females.

9) What is the role for Oncotype and Mammaprint in male breast cancer?

Expert Perspective: The role of the Oncotype 21-gene assay recurrence score (RS) and MammaPrint molecular assays are not well studied in male breast cancer and are currently under investigation. Most treatment approaches are extrapolated from data generated in in female patients. However, there are differences in the hormone milieu between males and females that could impact the test results and treatment efficacy, so additional data is needed about how to best utilize these tests in male patients.

Two recent studies demonstrated that Oncotype RS provides prognostic information in men with ER+ breast cancer (Table 18.2). In one study, the role of the Oncotype RS was investigated in 3,806 males and 571,115 females with ER+ breast cancer. Five-year breast cancer specific survival rates were 99.0% and 95.9% for men with an RS of < 18 and an RS between 18 and 31, respectively. Male patients with an RS of ⩾ 31 had an 81% five-year breast

Table 18.2 Selected studies in early stage hormone positive male vs female breast cancer.

Molecular characterization studies

		Oncotype-DX recurrence score (% of patients)		
	n	<18	18–30	⩾31
SEER, male	3,806	58.0	29.6	12.4
SEER, female	571,115	58.2	34.4	7.4
Israeli cohort, male	65	44.6	41.5	13.9
NCDB (2004–2014), male	731	55.1	32.0	9.0
5-year BCSS (%) by Oncotype-DX RS				
SEER, male	322	99.0	95.9	81.0
SEER, female	55,842	99.5	98.6	94.9
Neoadjuvant/adjuvant chemotherapy studies				
	n	Any chemo (%)	Neoadjuvant chemo (%)	5-year OS (%)
NCDB (2004–2016)				
Male	2,017	73.0	26.0	NA
Female	194,010	84.0	45.0	NA
NCDB (2004–2014)				
Male	10,873	45.1	12.6	79.1
Adjuvant endocrine therapy studies				
German population	n	Tamoxifen (%)	AI (%)	Median follow-up: 42.2 months
Male	257	80.5	19.5	17.9% pts died in Tamoxifen arm; 32.2% pts died in AI arm

n, total number of patients; AI, aromatase inhibitors; BCSS, breast cancer–specific survival; chemo, chemotherapy; NA, not available; NCDB, National Cancer Database; pts, patients; OS, overall survival; SEER, Surveillance, Epidemiology, and End Results; #, number of patients.

cancer specific survival, which is lower than the five-year breast cancer specific survival for females (94.9%). In another retrospective study, 10,873 men with stage I–III breast cancer were enrolled in the National Cancer Data Base between 2004 and 2014. An Oncotype RS was sent in 731 patients (34.9%). Among these patients, 403 (55.1%) were found to have a RS of < 18, 234 (32%) had scores between 18 and 31, and 66 (9%) had a score > 31. Chemotherapy was more often administered in patients with Oncotype RS > 31 compared with those with RS < 18 (72.7% vs 4.7%; $P < 0.001$). In summary, there is limited data to guide the use of genomic tests for male patients with breast cancer at present; further studies are needed to better understand the prognostic and predictive value of the Oncotype RS and MammaPrint tests in male patients with breast cancer.

10) What is the role of adjuvant endocrine therapy in male breast cancer?

Expert Perspective: The use of adjuvant endocrine therapy is recommended for all men with hormone receptor positive breast cancer. Men with hormone receptor positive breast cancer who receive adjuvant endocrine therapy have improved overall survival (OS) compared with those who do not receive adjuvant endocrine therapy. However, in historic studies, only 75–80% of male patients with breast cancer received endocrine therapy due it not being offered, it being declined, and/or intolerance.

For male patients with ER+ and/or PR+ breast cancer, tamoxifen is the preferred adjuvant endocrine therapy based on observational studies unless contraindicated. The efficacy of tamoxifen has been demonstrated to be superior to aromatase inhibitors in males in contrast with data for females, and this difference is thought to be due to the fact that testicular production of estrogen is not well inhibited by aromatase inhibitors. There are no prospective randomized trials to evaluate the use of adjuvant tamoxifen in male patients with breast cancer, but several retrospective studies demonstrated that adjuvant endocrine therapy improved recurrence-free survival and overall survival (OS) compared with aromatase inhibitors. Side effects of tamoxifen include hot flashes, weight gain, vision changes, cognitive changes, thromboembolic events, and sexual dysfunction. Despite the potential survival benefit of adjuvant tamoxifen, a large proportion of men with hormone receptor positive breast cancer discontinue tamoxifen due to side effects. For example, in a study of 116 men on tamoxifen, at one year, only 65% continued tamoxifen, and at five years, only 18% continued tamoxifen. Venlafaxine has been shown to be an effective treatment of hot flashes in men with prostate cancer who receive gonadotropin-releasing hormone (GnRH) analogs, and it can also be considered in men with breast cancer treated with tamoxifen or GnRH analogs.

If tamoxifen is contraindicated, such as for patients with a high risk of venous thromboembolism, an alternative option is treatment with a GnRH agonist/antagonist plus an aromatase inhibitor. With aromatase inhibitors alone, it is possible that the hypothalamic-pituitary feedback loop results in an increase substrate for aromatization and prevents complete estrogen suppression. Adding a GnRH analogue is thought to interrupt this negative feedback, and thus complete estrogen suppression may be achieved.

In summary, in male patients with early stage hormone receptor positive breast cancer, we prefer the use of adjuvant tamoxifen, but an aromatase inhibitor (AI) plus a GnRH agonist/antagonist can be used if contraindications.

11) How long should adjuvant endocrine therapy be continued?

Expert Perspective: Adjuvant tamoxifen is recommended for 5–10 years for male patients with hormone receptor positive breast cancer. The decision to extend the duration to 10 years must be individualized based on the risk of recurrence and side effects. Patients who have tolerated therapy and have recurrence risk factors such as nodal status, tumor size, and grade may consider extended endocrine therapy for up to 10 years.

12) What are the role of targeted therapies as adjuvant therapies for early-stage male breast cancer?

Expert Perspective: The monarchE trial randomized individuals with high-risk hormone receptor positive (ER+ and/or PR+) and HER2-negative breast cancer (defined as ≥ 4 positive nodes, 1–3 positive nodes, and tumor size > 5 cm, histologic grade III, or Ki-67 ≥ 20%) to adjuvant endocrine therapy with or without abemaciclib; the addition of two years of adjuvant abemaciclib lead to improvement in disease-free survival, leading to US Food and Drug Administration (FDA) approval (October 2021) of abemaciclib as the first CDK 4/6 inhibitor approved for adjuvant treatment of early stage breast cancer. In patients with *BRCA1* or *BRCA2* germline mutations and high-risk HER2− breast cancer, the phase III OlympiA trial recently demonstrated that one year of adjuvant olaparib can improve three-year invasive, disease-free survival and overall survival. Based on these results, the FDA approved (February 2022) the use of adjuvant olaparib for patients with *BRCA*-mutated, HER2-negative, high-risk early breast cancer who have previously been treated with chemotherapy before or after surgery. We recommend the use of these adjuvant agents in patients with male breast cancer who meet criteria for their use.

13) What is the role of bone-modifying agents in preventing recurrence in patients with early stage hormone receptor positive breast cancer?

Expert Perspective: There is currently no data to support the use of bone-modifying agents to prevent breast cancer recurrence in males, but they can be treated with these agents to prevent or treat osteoporosis.

14) How should hormone receptor positive male breast cancer be treated in the metastatic setting?

Expert Perspective: Treatment of men with metastatic hormone receptor positive breast cancer is similar to the treatment of women with metastatic hormone receptor positive breast cancer. Generally, patients should be treated with endocrine therapy as first-line therapy. Endocrine therapy options in male patients as discussed previously, include tamoxifen, aromatase inhibitor with GnRH analog, or fulvestrant. Although there is limited data for the use of dependent kinase 4/6 (CDK4/6) inhibitors in males, it is recommended that first-line endocrine therapy should be endocrine therapy plus a CDK4/6 inhibitor, similar to use in female patients. Both palbociclib and ribociclib have been approved by the FDA for men with metastatic, hormone receptor–positive breast cancer, in combination with either an aromatase inhibitor or fulvestrant; abemaciclib is also a reasonable off-label substitute. Treatment options in the subsequent line include fulvestrant, the mechanistic target of rapamycin kinase (mTOR) inhibitor everolimus plus tamoxifen or AI, or alpelisib plus fulvestrant if the tumor harbors a *PIK3CA* mutation the gene encoding the p110α catalytic subunit of phosphoinositide 3-kinase. The oral SERD elecestrant was also recently approved for patients with HR+ MBC whose tumors harbor an *ESR1* mutation. After progression on endocrine therapy, chemotherapy and antibody-drug conjugates are utilized.

In summary, for men who present with *de novo* metastatic hormone receptor–positive, HER2-negative breast cancer, we recommend the use of tamoxifen or an aromatase inhibitor with GnRH analog in combination with a CDK4/6 inhibitor. The choice between tamoxifen and aromatase inhibitor/GnRH analog should be driven by patient preferences regarding toxicity given the lack of comparative data regarding efficacy. For men who have previously been treated with adjuvant tamoxifen or who have progressed on tamoxifen in the metastatic setting, we recommend an aromatase inhibitor with GnRH analog plus a CDK 4/6 inhibitor.

15) What is the recommended surveillance for men who have had early stage breast cancer?

Expert Perspective: There are limited data to guide surveillance for men who have had early-stage breast cancer. Physicians should follow patients for symptoms of recurrence, including new lumps, bone pain, chest pain, abdominal pain, or persistent headaches. Continuity of follow-up for patients with breast cancer is recommended and should be performed by a physician experienced in the surveillance of patients with breast cancer and in breast examination including the examination of irradiated breasts. Ipsilateral annual mammogram should be offered to men with a history of breast cancer treated with lumpectomy if technically feasible, regardless of genetic predisposition. Contralateral annual screening mammogram may be offered to men with a history of breast cancer. Breast magnetic resonance imaging is not required after treatment of early stage breast cancer in men. Patients who are treated with GnRH analog therapy should have bone density screening at baseline and every two years. Patients with low bone density should be managed according to guidelines for osteopenia/osteoporosis management.

Case study results: The patient undergoes left breast mastectomy. Pathology demonstrates 2.2 cm of grade 3 IDC that is ER+ (100%), PR+ (90%), and HER2− (IHC 0). Two of four sentinel lymph node were positive. After adjuvant radiation to the axilla, he starts tamoxifen 20 mg daily with plan to continue it for five years.

HER2+ Male Breast Cancer

16) How should early stage HER2+ male breast cancer be managed in the neoadjuvant/adjuvant setting?

Expert Perspective: A high level of HER2 overexpression, as determined by either immunohistochemistry with 3+ staining for the HER2 protein or evidence of HER2 gene amplification by fluorescence *in situ* hybridization (FISH ratio ≥ 2.0 or HER2 copy number ≥ 6.0), is a strong predictive factor for sensitivity to HER2-targeted agents. There are multiple HER2-directed agents that are currently available to treat HER2+ breast cancer, including trastuzumab, which is a monoclonal antibody that binds to the extracellular domain of HER2 and pertuzumab, which is a monoclonal antibody that binds the extracellular dimerization domain of HER2. For patients with stage II or III HER2+ breast cancer for which neoadjuvant chemotherapy is recommended, six cycles of docetaxel, carboplatin, trastuzumab, and pertuzumab (TCHP) is generally recommended. Anthracycline-based regimens are generally avoided for HER2+ breast cancer. The advantage of giving therapy in the neoadjuvant setting is that it allows the provider to assess response to treatment and consider additional adjuvant therapies after surgery if needed.

For patients with HER2+ early-stage breast cancer who proceed directly to surgery without receiving neoadjuvant treatment, adjuvant chemotherapy with HER2-directed therapy is recommended.

17) How should HER2+ male breast cancer be treated in the metastatic setting?

Expert Perspective: Management of metastatic HER2+ breast cancer is the same in males and females. Specifically, for previously untreated patients, treatment with trastuzumab, pertuzumab, and a taxane (either paclitaxel or docetaxel) is recommended based on data from the phase III CLEOPATRA study. Weekly paclitaxel is often preferred as it is better tolerated and has fewer side effects. Subcutaneous formulations of trastuzumab and pertuzumab have received FDA approval and can be considered as alternatives to the IV formulations. In the second line, recent data from DESTINY Breast03 showed that trastuzumab deruxtecan (TDXd) was superior to ado-trastuzumab emtansine (T-DM1) in terms of both PFS and OS. Options for subsequent lines of therapy include T-DM1, tucatinib, trastuzumab, and capecitabine per the HER2 CLIMB study or other anti-HER2 agents.

Triple-Negative Male Breast Cancer

18) How should early-stage triple negative breast cancer in male patients be managed in the neoadjuvant/adjuvant setting?

Expert Perspective: TNBC is defined by the absence of the ER, PR, and HER2 overexpression. It is a very rare entity in males, comprising a small percentage of male breast cancers. In a cohort of 1,054 male patients with breast cancer, TNBC was found in 0.3% of patients. Because there is little data specific to male TNBC, classification and treatment modalities of male breast cancer have largely been extrapolated from female breast cancer.

Prospective studies for male breast cancer in terms of adjuvant and neoadjuvant chemotherapy are lacking. Several observational studies have suggested decreased recurrence and mortality in male patients treated with adjuvant chemotherapy. The best approach for neoadjuvant and adjuvant chemotherapy in TNBC remains anthracycline- and taxane-based regimens. Men with clinically T2 and/or node-positive breast cancer should be evaluated for neoadjuvant chemotherapy and immunotherapy. According to data from the National Cancer Database, males with node positive disease received less neoadjuvant chemotherapy than females (26% males vs 45% females, $P < 0.001$). Response rates after neoadjuvant chemotherapy were generally similar for male (n = 34) and female (n = 15,168) patients with node-positive TNBC (pCR 35.5% in female, pCR 32% in male).

There is an increasing interest in the addition of platinum agents to standard neoadjuvant chemotherapy in females with early-stage TNBC because the addition has shown to improve the pathologic complete response rate (pCR). The addition of pembrolizumab and atezolizumab to neoadjuvant chemotherapy also increased rates of pCR, regardless of programmed death ligand 1 (PD-L1) status in females with breast cancer. In KEYNOTE-522, the addition of pembrolizumab to neoadjuvant chemotherapy improved event-free survival and demonstrated a trend toward increased overall survival. However, there is no data about the role of platinum agents and immune checkpoint inhibitors in men with early stage TNBC.

In summary, male patients with T2 and/or node-positive breast cancer should be considered for neoadjuvant therapy with anthracycline- and taxane-based regimens, with the addition of pembrolizumab regardless of PD-L1 status, identical to the treatment approach for female patients.

19) How should triple-negative male breast cancer be treated in the metastatic setting?

Expert Perspective: Similar to early stage TNBC in males, there is also limited male-specific data for the treatment of metastatic TNBC. Therefore, treatment approaches are extrapolated from data in females. Following is a brief summary of major trials in this setting:

- IMpassion130 was a phase III trial that randomly assigned patients with untreated metastatic TNBC to receive atezolizumab plus nab-paclitaxel or placebo plus nab-paclitaxel. In the intention-to-treat analysis, the median PFS was longer in patients with atezolizumab plus nab-paclitaxel versus placebo plus nab-paclitaxel. There was no significant improvement in OS in the intention to treat population, but the addition of atezolizumab improved OS by 7.5 months in the PD-L1 positive subgroup.
- IMpassion131 was another phase III trial that also assessed the efficacy of atezolizumab in patients with mTNBC, randomizing 651 patients 2:1 to receive atezolizumab or placebo combined with weekly paclitaxel as first line therapy. At the primary PFS analysis, the addition of atezolizumab to paclitaxel did not improve PFS or OS in either the intention-to-treat or PD-L1-positive population.
- KEYNOTE-355 is a phase III trial that randomized 847 patients with mTNBC 2:1 to receive physician's choice of chemotherapy (paclitaxel, nab-paclitaxel, or gemcitabine and carboplatin) with either pembrolizumab or placebo in the first-line setting. The addition of pembrolizumab to chemotherapy improved both PFS and OS in the 38% of patients with tumors that were PD-L1 positive defined as a CPS score of ⩾ 10.

Based on data from KEYNOTE-355, the combination of pembrolizumab with physician's choice chemotherapy of weekly paclitaxel, nab-paclitaxel, or gemcitabine and carboplatin received approval for patients with metastatic PD-L1 plus TNBC defined as a CPS ⩾ 10 (PD-L1 IHC 22C3 pharmDx assay). Given the conflicting data from IMpassion130 and

IMpassion131, Roche withdrew the indication for atezolizumab with nab-paclitaxel as treatment for patients with metastatic TNBC whose tumors express PD-L1 in consultation with the FDA in August 2021, although the combination is still approved in many countries worldwide. It is unclear why differences exist in these study results, but it seems prudent to use nab-paclitaxel as the chemotherapy partner rather than paclitaxel if a taxane is chosen to partner with either pembrolizumab or atezolizumab in patients with PD-L1+ metastatic TNBC.

For male patients with *BRCA1* or *BRCA2* mutations, the PARP inhibitors olaparib and talazoparib are preferred treatment options in the metastatic setting. Antibody-drug conjugates are also a novel treatment strategy. Recently, sacituzumab govitecan, an antibody-drug conjugate targeted to the Trop-2 protein, was approved by the FDA for the treatment of patients with metastatic TNBC who had received at least two prior lines of therapy. Further, a variety of chemotherapy can be given to males with metastatic TNBC, similar to females. Sequential monotherapy is the preferred treatment modality, and combination chemotherapy should be considered in patients with rapid clinical progression and/or a need for rapid symptom and disease control.

Survivorship Issues

20) What important topics in survivorship have been studied in male breast cancer?

Expert Perspective: In the public, breast cancer is often thought as a "female disease," so the diagnosis of male breast cancer brings unique challenges in terms of survivorship issues. Specifically, men diagnosed with breast cancer may have issues with impaired body image, a greater sense of embarrassment/shame, depression/anxiety, and a lack of disease-specific psychosocial support. The unique psychological and physical conditions in male patients with breast cancer is an active area of research. In previous studies, data suggest that sexual dysfunction and hormonal symptoms are common in male breast cancer survivors. Increased rates of depression and anxiety have also been observed. Further studies are needed to evaluate the impact of specific treatments and sociodemographic factors on quality of life in male breast cancer survivors.

Future Direction

Male breast cancer remains an understudied area of breast cancer research, and many gaps remain in our understanding of the biology and optimal treatment choices. It is important to develop a better understanding of the biology of male breast cancer and how it differs from female breast cancer in order to best design and tailor treatment strategies. It is also important to identify barriers to treatment, because research indicates that male patients with breast cancer are often undertreated compared with female patients. There is now an international effort through the International Male Breast Cancer Program to collect tissue samples and follow clinical outcomes of males with breast cancer. Moreover, many clinical trials now allow the enrollment of both male and female patients, thus expanding data to support treatment strategies in male patients with breast cancer. These efforts offer promising opportunities to better understand male breast cancer and hopefully will continue to improve treatment options and outcomes.

Recommended Readings

Cao, L., Hue, J.J., Freyvogel, M. et al. (2021). Despite equivalent outcomes, men receive neoadjuvant chemotherapy less often than women for lymph node-positive breast cancer. *Ann Surg Oncol.* (11):6001-6011.

Cardoso, F., Bartlett, J.M.S., Slaets, L. et al. (2018). Characterization of male breast cancer: Results of the EORTC 10085/TBCRC/BIG/NABCG international male breast cancer program. *Ann Oncol* 29 (2): 405–417. doi:10.1093/annonc/mdx651.

Chavez-Macgregor M., Clarke, C.A., Lichtensztajn, D. et al. (2013). Male breast cancer according to tumor subtype and race: A population-based study. *Cancer* 119 (9): 1611–1617. doi: 10.1002/cncr.27905.

Freedman, B.C., Keto, J., and Rosenbaum Smith, S.M. (2012). Screening mammography in men with BRCA mutations: Is there a role? *Breast J* 18 (1): 73–75. doi: 10.1111/j.1524-4741.2011.01185.x. PMID: 22226069.

Giordano, S.H. (2018). Breast cancer in men. *N Engl J Med* 378 (24): 2311–2320. doi: 10.1056/NEJMra1707939. PMID: 29897847.

Gucalp, A., Traina, T.A., Eisner, J.R. et al. (2019). Male breast cancer: A disease distinct from female breast cancer. *Breast Cancer Res Treat* 173 (1): 37–48.

Hassett, M.J., Somerfield, M.R., Baker, E.R. et al. (2020). Management of male breast cancer: ASCO guideline. *J Clin Oncol* 38 (16): 1849–1863.

Massarweh, S.A., Sledge, G.W., Miller, D.P. et al. (2018). Molecular characterization and mortality from breast cancer in men. *J Clin Oncol* 36 (14): 1396–1404. doi: 10.1200/JCO.2017.76.8861. Epub 2018 Mar 27. PMID: 29584547; PMCID: PMC6075854.

Yadav, S., Karam, D., Bin Riaz, I.et al. (2020). Male breast cancer in the United States: Treatment patterns and prognostic factors in the 21st century. *Cancer* 126 (1): 26–36.

19

Breast Cancer in Pregnancy and Fertility Preservation

Fedro A. Peccatori[1], Hatem Azim[2], and Matteo Lambertini[3,4]

[1] *European Institute of Oncology IRCCS, Milan, Italy*
[2] *Tecnológico de Monterrey, Monterrey, Mexico*
[3] *University of Genova, Genova, Italy*
[4] *IRCCS Ospedale Policlinico San Martino, Genova, Italy*

Introduction

Handling questions and inquiries related to pregnancy and fertility in breast cancer patients comprise one of the most challenging clinical situations for oncologists. Female sex hormones have been long recognized as key drivers for the development and progression of breast cancer. Acknowledging the hormonal surge that occurs during pregnancy and fertility preservation methods, oncologists and fertility specialists have been classically skeptical and uncertain about adequate counseling. In this chapter, we will address two distinct clinical settings. The first is women diagnosed with breast cancer during pregnancy. We will address feasibility and safety of managing cancer during pregnancy, putting into the balance maternal safety and fetal risks. The second is women who are seeking pregnancy following cancer treatment. This entails discussions surrounding feasibility and safety of pregnancy, as well as questions related to methods of fertility preservation that could be safely considered in breast cancer patients and their efficacy.

Case Study 1

A nulliparous 36-year-old patient was diagnosed with a pT1c pN1a infiltrating breast carcinoma. The tumor is ER- and PR-negative but HER2-positive (+3 by immunohistochemistry). She was offered adjuvant treatment with FEC100 (5-fluorouracil 500 mg/m^2, epirubicin 100 mg/m^2, and cyclophosphamide 500 mg/m^2) for three cycles followed by docetaxel (100 mg/m^2) for three cycles. The patient will also receive trastuzumab starting with docetaxel to complete a total duration of one year.

1) **In your opinion, which of the following factors are the most important in determining the risk of chemotherapy-induced amenorrhea in this patient?**
    A) Previous menstrual history.
    B) The sequential use of docetaxel.

Cancer Consult: Expertise in Clinical Practice, Volume 1: Solid Tumors & Supportive Care,
Second Edition. Edited by Syed A. Abutalib, Maurie Markman, Al B. Benson III, and Hope S. Rugo.
© 2024 John Wiley & Sons Ltd. Published 2024 by John Wiley & Sons Ltd.

C) The dose of cyclophosphamide.
D) Concomitant administration of trastuzumab with chemotherapy.

Expert Perspective: The possible impact of chemotherapy on the ovarian function is a frequent concern, particularly for young women who have not started or completed their families.

Age remains the most important determinant of chemotherapy-induced amenorrhea irrespective of the regimen used. At the ages of 37–39 years, there is physiologically accelerated atresia of the oocytes. Hence, chemotherapy-induced amenorrhea rates have been largely variable according to the patient age being above or below 40 years, which coincides with the physiological decline in ovarian reserve. Table 19.1 summarizes the risk of chemotherapy-induced amenorrhea with different regimens according to age.

Alkylating agents are the most gonadotoxic chemotherapeutic agents. Cyclophosphamide has been shown to induce apoptosis of the primordial follicles. The incorporation of taxanes in the adjuvant setting may further increase the risk of chemotherapy-induced amenorrhea associated with classic anthracycline-based regimens. Nevertheless, regimens in which three to four cycles of a taxane are given in sequence to three to four cycles of an anthracycline-based therapy appeared to be less gonadotoxic compared with six to eight cycles of anthracycline- and cyclophosphamide- based regimens. This is believed to be largely related to the cyclophosphamide (albeit lower dose) administered in the sequential regimens. Current available evidence on trastuzumab is limited; however, it does not appear to increase the risk associated with chemotherapy-induced amenorrhea.

Correct Answer: C

Case Study 2

A 39-year-old breast cancer patient who completed five years of adjuvant tamoxifen six months earlier presented to your office pregnant at week eight of gestation. She was worried following her visit to her obstetrician, who recommended an abortion for fear that

Table 19.1 Risk of chemotherapy-induced amenorrhea in %, with different regimens according to age.

Chemotherapy regimen	Age < 30 years	Age 30–40 years	Age > 40 years
AC × 4		13	57–63
CMF × 6	19	31–38	76–96
CAF/CEF × 6	23–47	23–47	80–90
FEC 100 × 6		76.3	
FEC 100 × 3		63.5	
Docetaxel × 3			

AC, adriamycin and cyclophosphamide; CAF, cyclophosphamide, adriamycin, and 5FU; CEF, cyclophosphamide, epirubicin, and 5FU; CMF, cyclophosphamide, methotrexate, and 5FU; FEC, 5FU, epirubicin, and cyclophosphamide.

pregnancy could stimulate breast cancer recurrence. The patient would like to keep her pregnancy but would like to understand whether taking this decision would have a detrimental effect on breast cancer outcome.

2) What would you advise her in this situation?
   A) Pregnancy after ER-positive breast cancer increases the risk of recurrence, but abortion is not recommended because it is not clear that it improves prognosis.
   B) Pregnancy after ER-positive breast cancer increases the risk of recurrence, and hence abortion is preferred because it could reduce such risk.
   C) Pregnancy following breast cancer does not appear to be detrimental irrespective of ER status.
   D) Pregnancy following breast cancer is protective and should be encouraged.

Expert Perspective: Pregnancy following breast cancer, particularly ER-positive disease, represents one of the most controversial issues in managing young breast cancer patients. Despite several studies that have been reported for more than three decades showing that pregnancy after breast cancer is safe, these studies suffered major flaws regarding patient selection, low statistical power, and the lack of information on outcomes according to hormone receptor status.

A multicenter, properly powered study aimed to address many of the limitations highlighted here. This study included more than 1,200 patients, of whom 333 patients became pregnant after breast cancer diagnosis. Importantly, all patients had known ER status. This study showed that pregnancy after ER-positive breast cancer does not increase the risk of breast cancer recurrence at least during the first five years following conception. In the same study, patients who underwent abortion did not appear to have a superior outcome compared with those who continued their pregnancy to term. Hence, women who completed their adjuvant therapy should not be denied the opportunity to become pregnant. Promotion of abortion in these patients for therapeutic reasons remains unjustified in the absence of supporting evidence. A wash-out period of at least three months following tamoxifen completion should be considered before attempting conception. Also, another issue that is seen in clinic is interruption of endocrine therapy to attempt pregnancy. A recent study (POSITIVE; 2023) attempted to answer this question. The investigators reported that among select women with previous HR+ early breast cancer, temporary interruption of endocrine therapy to attempt pregnancy did not confer a greater short-term risk of breast cancer events, including distant recurrence, than that in the external control cohort. However, further follow-up is critical to inform longer-term safety. In the study, eligible women were 42 years of age or younger; had had stage I, II, or III disease; had received adjuvant endocrine therapy for 18 to 30 months; and desired pregnancy. The 3-year incidence of breast cancer events was 8.9% (95% confidence interval [CI], 6.3 to 11.6) in the treatment-interruption group and 9.2% (95% CI, 7.6 to 10.8) in the control cohort.

Correct Answer: C

Case Study 3

A 35-year-old triple-negative breast cancer (TNBC) patient, who is known to be BRCA mutant, was treated with adjuvant chemotherapy AC (adriamycin and cyclophosphamide) regimen for four cycles followed by 12 cycles of weekly paclitaxel. Three years later, she is disease-free and is considering to become pregnant for the first time.

3) **Would you be concerned that the treatment she received could have adverse effects on the fetal outcome?**
   A) No. Significant increase in fetal adverse effects is not foreseen.
   B) Yes. Prior exposure to chemotherapy could increase the risk of fetal anomalies.
   C) This question cannot be answered due to lack of any type of data.

Expert Perspective: There is no evidence that pregnancy in breast cancer survivors is associated with a significant increase in fetal or infant risk of malformations. Recently, a large meta-analysis evaluated the pregnancy outcome of 3,240 women with history of breast cancer and compared them with more than 4 million non–breast cancer patients. No differences were observed between breast cancer patients and women from the general population in terms of completed pregnancies and spontaneous or induced abortions. No differences were also observed in terms of antepartum and/or postpartum hemorrhage. However, offspring of breast cancer patients were at increased risk of low birth weight, preterm birth, and being small for gestational age. No significant increased risk of congenital abnormalities was observed in the offspring of breast cancer patients.

Correct Answer: A

4) **How would you counsel a woman with a *BRCA* pathogenic variant and history of breast cancer who is considering becoming pregnant?**
   A) Pregnancy would increase risk of breast cancer recurrence.
   B) Pregnancy would increase risk of ovarian cancer.
   C) Pregnancy would not worsen maternal prognosis.

Expert Perspective: Approximately 12% of breast malignancies that arise in young women are related to germline deleterious pathogenic variants in the breast cancer susceptibility genes *BRCA1* and/or *BRCA2* (Chapters 45–46). These patients may have a reduced ovarian reserve and fertility potential and are often subjected to risk-reducing bilateral salpingo-oophorectomy by their forties because of increased ovarian cancer risk. Hence, reproductive considerations and family planning may be particularly overwhelming among patients with *BRCA*-mutated breast cancer. Such uncertainty is also shared by the medical community, in which a survey including more than 250 breast cancer specialists showed that almost 50% are concerned about the safety of pregnancy in breast cancer patients harboring a germline *BRCA* pathogenic variant.

A recent study involving more than 1,250 breast cancer patients with *BRCA* pathogenic variants, of whom almost 200 had a subsequent pregnancy provided important insights on this question. The study showed that pregnancy after breast cancer is safe in *BRCA* carriers without apparent worsening of maternal prognosis and is associated with favorable fetal outcomes.

Correct Answer: C

Case Study 4

A 39-year-old old female is diagnosed with a pT2 N1b ER-positive breast cancer. She is planned to start adjuvant chemotherapy. She expressed her concerns regarding the chances for future fertility following chemotherapy.

5) Which of the following option(s) is/are the most reliable to preserve fertility?
   A) Administration of GnRHa with chemotherapy.
   B) Embryo or oocyte cryopreservation.
   C) Ovarian tissue cryopreservation.
   D) Any of the above.

Expert Perspective: The administration of chemotherapy is associated with a risk of permanent and premature amenorrhea, which appears to be related to the patient's age and the cumulative dose of alkylating agents received (see Table 19.1 and Question 1). Although the absolute effect of chemotherapy on ovarian function remains unknown, current evidence points that patients who resume menstruation following chemotherapy administration have poor ovarian reserve. This suggests that the detrimental effect of chemotherapy on ovarian function could be even larger than that on menstrual function. This patient is 39 years old, and thus her chances of developing premature ovarian insufficiency following chemotherapy are not negligible. Hence, she should be counseled upfront on possible strategies to preserve her chances of conceiving.

Embryo cryopreservation has been an established and widely available method in treating infertility since the early 1980s. In the United States, the delivery rate is approximately 30% and 16% per embryo thaw in patients younger than 35 years and older than 40 years of age, respectively. Because patients undergoing ovarian stimulation with embryo cryopreservation are generally not infertile, pregnancy rates might well be higher than those achieved by subfertile couples who might have poor oocytes and sperm quality. The main concern in breast cancer patients remains the potential oncological risk of ovarian stimulation regimens due to significant increase in estradiol levels. However, a series of studies were conducted using letrozole as part of the stimulation protocol and showed similar oocyte yield and low peak estradiol levels with no detrimental effect on breast cancer outcome. Ethical and social considerations of embryo cryopreservation may exist. This procedure requires a partner, and the fate of the cryopreserved embryo, if available, remains a problem in case the patient dies before implantation. These latter two disadvantages to embryo preservation could therefore represent a potential advantage for oocyte cryopreservation, which has gained popularity in recent years because of the better results achieved with ultra-rapid freezing (vitrification).

Ovarian tissue cryopreservation is another possibility to preserve fertility and should be offered only to patients younger than 36 years of age when there is not enough time to undergo ovarian stimulation, which requires at least two weeks.

Use of gonadotropin-releasing hormone agonists (GnRHa) is a reliable method to reduce the risk of chemotherapy-induced premature ovarian insufficiency and the potential increase of chances of future pregnancy. A large meta-analysis showed that the coadministration of GnRHa with chemotherapy reduces the risk of premature ovarian insufficiency by more than 60% and increases the chance of future pregnancy by almost two times. Importantly, no detrimental impact on breast cancer prognosis was observed. Ideally, GnRHa should start at least one week before first chemotherapy treatment and continue until chemotherapy is completed (three–six months). However, for patients interested in fertility preservation, use of GnRHa during chemotherapy should not be considered as an alternative to embryo/oocyte cryopreservation but could be proposed in case the latter is not available or following cryopreservation options.

Correct Answer: B

Case Study 5

A 15 weeks' pregnant patient presents to you with locally advanced breast cancer along with liver metastases. A core biopsy shows grade 3 invasive carcinoma. The tumor is ER and PR negative but is positive for HER2 (+3 by immunohistochemistry). The patient is 40 years old, and this is her first pregnancy after several years of receiving treatment for infertility.

6) The patient comes for a second opinion because her doctor believes that she should proceed for an abortion – an option that she completely refuses. What would you advise her?
   A) Close observation and proceed for delivery once the fetus is viable.
   B) Initiate chemotherapy and anti-HER2 treatment, aiming at delivery once the fetus is viable.
   C) Initiate chemotherapy and anti-HER2 treatment, aiming at delivery as close to term as possible.
   D) Initiate chemotherapy and hold anti-HER2 treatment, aiming at delivery as close to term as possible.

Expert Perspective: This case addresses three key points: (1) the therapeutic role of elective abortion, (2) the safety of chemotherapy and trastuzumab during pregnancy, and (3) the optimal timing of delivery.

Current evidence suggests that induction of abortion in patients diagnosed with breast cancer during pregnancy has no effect on patients' outcome. Hence, abortion should not be promoted for therapeutic reasons.

Delay of therapy could be sometimes considered in case diagnosis is made relatively late during gestation and/or the tumor has favorable features (e.g. grade 1, node negative, and Luminal A-like biology). However, in this patient, treatment should be initiated. The administration of chemotherapy starting in the second trimester is considered safe. Data from large registries suggest that treatment with chemotherapy slightly increases the risk of pregnancy-related complications and premature delivery. However, no increase in malformations or fetal mortality has been observed. Accordingly, chemotherapy should not be denied during the second and third trimesters to patients who require active treatment during pregnancy.

Unlike chemotherapy, anti-HER2 treatment during pregnancy, particularly trastuzumab in the second trimester, has been associated with a high risk of oligohydramnios, resulting in a relatively high rate of fetal prematurity and fetal death. This is believed to be secondary to the inhibitory effect of trastuzumab on HER2, which is expressed on the fetal kidney that is responsible for amniotic fluid production. Based on the limited available data on its administration during pregnancy, it looks clear that trastuzumab should be avoided during gestation.

It is currently recommended to aim for term or near-term delivery in these patients. Early induction of labor does not improve patients' outcome. Standard chemotherapy could be offered to pregnant patients in most cases until week 34 of gestation. More importantly, data from a large prospective study have shown that the long-term intellectual abilities of newborns exposed to chemotherapy in utero and delivered at term are significantly better than those of newborns delivered preterm. Hence, every effort should be made to deliver after the 37th week of pregnancy whenever possible. The only possible exception, which could be relevant for this case, is tumor progression during chemotherapy. In this situation, an early delivery to allow administration of anti-HER2 treatment should be pursued.

Correct Answer: D

Case Study 6

A 33-year-old woman with a viable 12-week pregnancy presented with a suspicious 2.1 cm left breast nodule. Ultrasound guided biopsy was performed, and pathology revealed grade 3 triple-negative invasive breast carcinoma (TNBC). There was no evidence of axillary lymph node involvement on the ultrasound. You propose to the patient an upfront surgery followed by adjuvant chemotherapy. She is inquiring into the feasibility and safety of this strategy during pregnancy.

7) What are the data and consensus of performing sentinel lymph node biopsy in patients diagnosed with breast cancer during pregnancy?

Expert Perspective: Relatively limited clinical data are available on sentinel lymph node biopsy in patients diagnosed with breast cancer during pregnancy. Several simulation studies pointed to the safety of lymphoscintigraphy using Technetium-99. The largest clinical series included 145 patients with clinically node-negative disease. The majority were subjected to Technetium-99 or a combined technique with blue dye. Mapping was successful in all but one patient. The mean number of sentinel lymph nodes was 3.2, and positive sentinel lymph nodes were found in almost 30% of patients. Importantly, at a median follow-up of 48 months, no neonatal adverse events related to sentinel lymph node biopsy were reported, and only one patient experienced isolated axillary recurrence (0.7%).

Recent guidelines are increasingly endorsing the use of sentinel lymph node biopsy during pregnancy yet discouraging the use of blue dye being is associated with risk of allergic reactions, which could be life-threatening.

8) Sentinel lymph node biopsy showed one positive lymph node, which was removed. The patient has a T2N1 disease. What is the systemic therapy that you would consider in this case?
   A) An anthracycline-only based regimen because taxanes are not safe during pregnancy.
   B) A taxane-only based regimen because anthracycline is not safe during pregnancy
   C) An anthracycline-taxane based regimen because both could be given during pregnancy.
   D) None of the above; give postpone adjuvant chemotherapy until after delivery.

Expert Perspective: Administration of chemotherapy should be avoided during the first trimester of pregnancy. Starting from the second trimester, doxorubicin- or epirubicin-based regimens are the most studied during pregnancy. Adriamycin or epirubicin in combination with cyclophosphamide can be used. Studies that evaluated long-term cardiac effects of babies exposed to these regimens during pregnancy did not show a relevant increase in cardiotoxicity secondary to in‐utero exposure, but continuous cardiac monitoring of these children is recommended.

Currently, several reports also endorse the safety of taxanes during pregnancy. Animal models have further suggested minimal transplacental transfer of taxanes being even lower as compared to anthracyclines. Thus, if clinically indicated, taxanes could also be administered during pregnancy. Weekly paclitaxel is preferred given its favorable toxicity profile and no need of prophylactic granulocyte colony stimulating factors. In addition, weekly administration would allow close monitoring of pregnancy.

Correct Answer: C

Recommended Readings

De Haan, J., Verheecke, M., Van Calsteren, K. et al. (2018). Oncological management and obstetric and neonatal outcomes for women diagnosed with cancer during pregnancy: A 20‐year international cohort study of 1170 patients. *Lancet Oncol* 19 (3): 337–346.

Borgers, J.S.W., Heimovaara, J.H., Cardonick, E. et al. (2021).Immunotherapy for cancer treatment during pregnancy. *Lancet Oncol* 22 (12): e550–e561. doi:10.1016/S1470-2045(21)00525-8. PMID: 34856152.

Lambertini, M., Blondeaux, E., Bruzzone, M. et al. (2021). Pregnancy after breast cancer: A systematic review and meta‐analysis. *J Clin Oncol* 39(29): 3293–3305.

Lambertini, M., Ameye, L., Hamy, A.S., et al. (2020). Pregnancy after breast cancer in patients with germline *BRCA* mutations. *J Clin Oncol* 38 (26): 3012–3023. doi:10.1200/JCO.19.02399. Epub 2020 Jul 16. PMID: 32673153.

Lambertini, M., Moore, H.C.F., Leonard, R.C.F. et al. (2018). Gonadotropin‐releasing hormone agonists during chemotherapy for preservation of ovarian function and fertility in premenopausal patients with early breast cancer: A systematic review and meta‐analysis of individual patient‐level data. *J Clin Oncol* 36 (19): 1981–1990.

Lambertini, M., Peccatori, F.A., Demeestere, I. et al. (2020). Fertility preservation and post‐treatment pregnancies in post‐pubertal cancer patients: ESMO clinical practice guidelines. *Ann Oncol* 31 (12): 1664–1678.

Oktay, K., Harvey, B.E., Partridge, A.H. et al. (2018). Fertility preservation in patients with cancer: ASCO clinical practice guidelines update. *J Clin Oncol* 36 (19): 1994–2001.

Partridge, A.H., Niman, S.M., Ruggeri, M. et al. (2023 May 4). Interrupting endocrine therapy to attempt pregnancy after breast cancer. *N Engl J Med* 388 (18): 1645–1656. doi:10.1056/NEJMoa2212856. PMID: 37133584.

Warner, E., Glass, K., Foong, S., and Sandwith, E. (2020). Update on fertility preservation for younger women with breast cancer. *CMAJ* 192 (35): E1003–E1009.

Part 4

Gastrointestinal Cancers

20

Early-Stage Gastroesophageal Cancer and Precursor Lesions

Yixing Jiang and Aaron Ciner

University of Maryland Greenebaum Cancer Center, Baltimore, MD

Introduction

Esophageal cancers exhibit great variation in histology, geographic distribution, and incidence over time. Areas of high incidence include portions of Iran, Russia, and northern China, where squamous cell cancers dominate. In the United States, carcinoma of the esophagus is infrequent, constituting approximately 1% of all cancers and approximately 6% of gastrointestinal malignancies. During the past three decades, the incidence of adenocarcinoma of the distal esophagus and gastroesophageal junction has increased, paralleling the rise of gastroesophageal reflux disease (GERD) in the general population, most notably for patients with a high body mass index (BMI). Squamous cell tumors are more likely to occur in patients who are Black, and these tumors are associated with achalasia, caustic injury, tylosis, Plummer–Vinson syndrome, cigarette smoking, and excessive alcohol consumption. Patients with squamous cell carcinoma of the head and neck are at increased risk of a synchronous or metachronous esophageal cancer of the same histology. Adenocarcinomas of the distal esophagus and gastroesophageal junction more typically arise in Barrett's esophagus. On the other hand, infection with human papillomavirus has been correlated with an increased incidence of squamous cell cancers of the upper esophagus.

In the United States, although the incidence of gastric cancer has decreased approximately 75% during the past few decades, the incidence of gastroesophageal tumors has concomitantly increased. Possible reasons for this rise include the prevalence of obesity, elevated BMI with increased incidence of GERD, and increased calorie consumption. Gastric cancer is seen twice as often in men as in women and more frequently in Black men than in White men. Gastric cancer is a major health issue in both Japan and Korea, and both countries have nationwide screening programs. Cigarette smoking, H. pylori infection, Epstein–Barr virus, radiation exposure, and prior gastric surgery for benign ulcer disease also have been implicated as risk factors. Genetic risk factors include type A blood, pernicious anemia, a family history of gastric cancer, hereditary nonpolyposis colon cancer, Li–Fraumeni syndrome, and hereditary diffuse gastric cancer caused by mutations in the E-cadherin gene, *CDH1* (Chapter 47).

Cancer Consult: Expertise in Clinical Practice, Volume 1: Solid Tumors & Supportive Care,
Second Edition. Edited by Syed A. Abutalib, Maurie Markman, Al B. Benson III, and Hope S. Rugo.
© 2024 John Wiley & Sons Ltd. Published 2024 by John Wiley & Sons Ltd.

Table 20.1 Esophagus and gastroesophageal junction cancers TNM staging AJCC UICC 8th edition.

Tnm And Grade	Description
Tis	High-grade dysplasia, defined as malignant cells confined to the epithelium by the basement membrane
T1	Tumor invades the lamina propria, muscularis mucosae, or submucosa
T2	Tumor invades the muscularis propria
T3	Tumor invades adventitia
T4a	Tumor invades the pleura, pericardium, azygos vein, diaphragm, or peritoneum
T4b	Tumor invades other adjacent structures, such as the aorta, vertebral body, or airway
N1	Metastases in 1 or 2 regional lymph nodes
N2	Metastases in 3 to 6 regional lymph nodes
N3	Metastases in 7 or more regional lymph nodes
M1	Distant metastasis
Grade 1	Well differentiated
Grade 2	Moderately differentiated
Grade 3	Poorly differentiated, undifferentiated

Esophageal and stomach cancers are often diagnosed at an advanced stage (Chapter 21). However, in at least 50% of patients, according to SEER data, the cancer is initially confined to the primary site or regional lymph nodes without distant metastases. The goal of treatment in this setting is curative. In the past decade, multiple therapeutic approaches in early stage gastroesophageal cancer have been validated in rigorous clinical trials. This new data has improved outcomes for patients but also complicated medical decision-making. This chapter reviews the relevant trials in early stage gastroesophageal cancer through clinical vignettes with the aim to provide clinicians with a framework to navigate the complex and changing treatment landscape in this disease setting. Table 20.1 displays staging of esophagus and esophagogastric junction cancers.

Case Study 1

A 65-year-old male presented with progressive dysphagia to solid food. He was evaluated with esophagogastroduodenoscopy (EGD) and endoscopic ultrasound (EUS) by his gastroenterologist. The EGD and EUS showed a mass protruding into the lumen of the distal esophagus and invading into the muscularis propria with no suspicious lymph nodes, clinical stage (c) T2N0 (Table 20.1). He had an esophagectomy with lymph node dissection, R0 resection, but final pathologic stage (p) demonstrated a T3N1 adenocarcinoma. He was referred to you for consideration of adjuvant therapy.

1) What is the best management strategy for this patient?

Expert Perspective: Upfront esophagectomy for clinically staged T2N0 low-risk esophageal adenocarcinoma is a reasonable treatment strategy and consistent with NCCN guidelines. However, discordant pathologic and clinical staging is not uncommon, including the scenario described above. In an analysis of 499 patients with esophageal cancer who underwent primary esophagectomy for cT2N0 disease between 2002 and 2012, under staging of tumor size (pT > 2) or nodal extent (pN > 0) occurred in 32% and 39% of patients respectively (Atay et al. 2019). When pT3–4 or pN1–2 status is detected in a patient who received upfront surgical resection, the potential benefit of adjuvant therapy must be considered.

The three main approaches in this setting are (i) adjuvant chemoradiotherapy, (ii) adjuvant chemotherapy, or (iii) surveillance.

- Support for adjuvant chemoradiotherapy stems from both prospective and retrospective data. A phase 2 study investigated the role of postoperative chemoradiotherapy in patients with resected esophageal or gastroesophageal junction cancer with either T3, N1, or M1a pathologic features. Radiotherapy to a planned dose of 50.4 – 59.4Gy was administered concurrently with two cycles of infusional 5-fluorouracil (5-FU) and cisplatin during the first and fourth weeks of radiation. After a median follow-up of 47 months, the four-year projected survival was 51% and four-year freedom from recurrence was 50% (Adelstein et al. 2009), favourable outcomes compared with historical controls. A preferred alternative regimen is based on the INT-0116 phase 3 trial (Macdonald et al. 2001) and includes an initial two cycles of 5-FU-based chemotherapy, followed by 45 – 50.4Gy radiotherapy concurrent with infusional 5-FU or capecitabine and four additional cycles of 5-FU-based chemotherapy. This large prospective study compared adjuvant chemoradiation to surgery alone in patients with gastric or gastroesophageal junction adenocarcinoma and showed an overall survival benefit with adjuvant therapy.
- Adjuvant chemotherapy alone is an alternative approach in this case. Supportive data is extrapolated from the phase 3 CLASSIC trial in patients with gastric cancer (Bang et al. 2012). After D2 gastrectomy, patients with predominantly node positive disease were randomized to receive six months of adjuvant capecitabine and oxaliplatin (CapeOx) or routine surveillance. After a median of 34 months follow-up, the three-year disease-free survival was 74 versus 59% in favor of the chemotherapy group (HR 0.56; $P < 0.0001$). With this supportive data, the NCCN panel considers either six months of 5-FU and oxaliplatin (FOLFOX) or CapeOx to be a reasonable treatment strategy in patients with esophageal adenocarcinoma who underwent upfront surgical resection and are node positive.
- The trials described above mostly included patients with adenocarcinoma. In patients with squamous cell carcinoma who are discovered to have T3–4 or N+ disease after an R0 resection, the NCCN panel recommends surveillance.

Our Patient: In this case, with pathologic T3N1 disease and a significant risk of recurrence, the preferred approach is adjuvant chemoradiotherapy.

Case Study 2

A 75-year-old female with well-controlled hypertension and type 2 diabetes presented with progressive dysphagia to solid food. She was evaluated with EGD and EUS by her gastroenterologist. EGD and EUS demonstrated an ulcerated mass in the mid-esophagus invading the adventitia and two suspicious lymph nodes, clinical stage T3N1 (Table 20.1). Pathology showed squamous cell carcinoma of the esophagus, and a positron emission tomography–computed tomography (PET–CT) showed no evidence of metastatic disease. She was referred to you for consideration of neoadjuvant therapy.

2) What is the role of neoadjuvant therapy?

Expert Perspective: Since the long-term prognosis is poor with resection alone in patients with clinical T3–T4 or node positive disease, treatment strategies have evolved to improve survival using neoadjuvant therapy (Rice et al. 2009). In patients with localized thoracic esophageal squamous cell carcinoma, multimodal therapy with neoadjuvant chemoradiation followed by surgery is generally recommended. Definitive chemoradiation is an alternative approach in patients who are not candidates for or decline surgery. The landmark phase 3 CROSS trial was conducted in patients with T1N1 or T2–T3N0-1 squamous cell carcinoma or adenocarcinoma of the esophagus or gastroesophageal junction. This trial compared neoadjuvant weekly carboplatin and paclitaxel concurrent with radiotherapy (41.4Gy over five weeks) followed by surgery with surgical resection alone. Overall survival (OS) was significantly increased in the chemoradiation group (median OS 48.6 months vs 24 months, HR 0.68, $P = 0.003$) and importantly the rate of postoperative complications was comparable between arms (van Hagen et al. 2012). Another large phase 3 study, NEOCRTEC5010, evaluated an alternative regimen of vinorelbine and cisplatin with concurrent radiotherapy in a Chinese patient population with resectable non-cervical esophageal squamous cell carcinoma. This study similarly demonstrated a significant improvement in OS (median OS 100 months vs 66.5 months, HR 0.71, $P = 0.025$) (Yang et al. 2018). These data, together with smaller phase two trials and retrospective analyses, established neoadjuvant concurrent chemoradiation as a preferred approach in patients with resectable mid- or distal esophageal squamous cell carcinoma or adenocarcinoma. Ongoing clinical trials, such as PROTECT, look to determine the optimal chemotherapeutic regimen in conjunction with radiotherapy. Other active studies (including NCT03792347, NCT04006041) aim to explore the added benefit of PD-1 or PD-L1 blockade combined with neoadjuvant chemoradiation and may shift the treatment paradigm further.

Case Study 3

A 65-year-old male with a history of heavy alcohol use and cigarette smoking presented with progressive dysphagia to solid food. He was evaluated with EGD and EUS by his gastroenterologist. EGD and EUS showed a mass protruding into the lumen of the mid-esophagus invading the adventitia and two suspicious lymph nodes, clinical stage T3N1 (Table 20.1). A biopsy of the mass showed squamous cell carcinoma of the esophagus. He was treated with weekly carboplatin and paclitaxel concurrent with radiotherapy in the preoperative setting. A repeat PET–CT scan prior to surgical resection showed complete resolution of the fluorodeoxyglucose (FDG)-avid lesion. Endoscopy showed only erythematous mucosa consistent with radiation changes, and random biopsies at the previous tumor site showed no malignancy. You discuss the necessity of surgical resection in the multidisciplinary tumor board.

3) **What is the role of surgery after neoadjuvant chemoradiation in squamous cell carcinoma of the esophagus?**

Expert Perspective: In this case, chemoradiation was administered preoperatively with a resultant complete clinical response. In the CROSS trial (detailed in case #2), pathologic CR occurred in 29% overall and in 49% of patients with squamous cell carcinoma. The necessity of surgical resection in this setting is controversial. Although retrospective database analyses suggest improved survival with tri-modality therapy, two randomized controlled trials, predominantly in patients with squamous cell carcinoma, showed no survival benefit with the addition of surgery. In one study, patients with esophageal squamous cell carcinoma received either induction chemotherapy followed by concurrent chemoradiotherapy and surgery or the same regimen followed by an additional radiation boost. Despite an improvement in local disease control (two-year local progression-free survival of 64 versus 41%), there was no difference in overall survival, and treatment-related mortality was higher in the surgery arm at 13 versus 3.5% (Stahl et al. 2005). In the second trial, FFCD 9102, patients with mostly squamous cell carcinoma received chemoradiotherapy and those with an initial response were randomized to additional chemoradiotherapy or surgery. At a median of 47 months follow-up, there was again improved local control in the surgery arm, but without a significant difference in survival (Bedenne et al. 2007). Of note, no prospective data is available specifically in the patient population with cCR after neoadjuvant chemoradiation. While tri-modality therapy is still the preferred approach in this case, chemoradiotherapy alone may be appropriate in certain circumstances, particularly where patient comorbidities or values support a nonoperative strategy.

Of note, there is potential discordance between clinical complete response and pathologic complete response. In a cohort analysis of patients with predominantly esophageal or gastroesophageal junction adenocarcinoma who received chemoradiation followed by esophagectomy, the sensitivity of clinical complete response for pathologic complete response was 97%, but the specificity was only 30% (Cheedella et al. 2013). Furthermore, there is no prospective data specifically in adenocarcinoma to recommend a nonoperative approach as discussed in patients with squamous cell carcinoma. Therefore, in patients with esophageal or gastroesophageal junction adenocarcinoma who receive initial chemoradiotherapy, surgery is strongly recommended when feasible, even in clinical complete responders.

Case Study 4

A 70-year-old female without comorbidities presented with progressive dysphagia to solid food. She was evaluated with EGD and EUS by her gastroenterologist. EGD and EUS showed a mass protruding into the lumen of the mid-esophagus, invading the muscularis propria and with two suspicious lymph nodes, clinical stage T2N1 (Table 20.1). A biopsy of the mass showed adenocarcinoma of the esophagus. A PET–CT was performed showing no evidence of distant metastatic disease. She was treated with weekly carboplatin and paclitaxel concurrent with radiotherapy in the preoperative setting. Subsequently, she underwent esophagectomy. The final pathology showed a significant amount of residual disease. She was referred to you for discussion of further therapy.

4) **How best to approach residual disease after neoadjuvant chemoradiation and esophagectomy?**

Expert Perspective: Most patients who undergo neoadjuvant chemoradiation and esophagectomy will have residual disease in the surgical specimen. This group has increased risk of recurrence and inferior survival compared to those with pathologic complete response (Scheer et al. 2011). However, the optimal adjuvant strategy to improve outcomes was not previously well-defined and often comprised either active surveillance or additional cytotoxic chemotherapy. In an attempt to address this unmet need, the Checkmate-577 trial randomized patients with stage II or III esophageal or gastroesophageal junction cancer who received neoadjuvant chemoradiation and surgery with residual pathologic disease to 1 year of adjuvant nivolumab or placebo. After a median follow-up of 24.4 months, nivolumab doubled the median disease-free survival from 11 to 22.4 months (HR for disease recurrence or death 0.69, $P < 0.001$). A benefit was seen across demographic and histologic subgroups, and toxicity appeared manageable (Kelly et al. 2021). Even as OS data are anticipated, the magnitude of disease-free survival benefit led to FDA approval and incorporation into NCCN guidelines. In this case therefore, one year of adjuvant nivolumab is recommended.

Going forward, it will be important to identify subgroups who benefit most from checkpoint blockade in early disease and explore the role of immunomodulatory agents in new settings and in rational combinations. More data about biomarkers of response, such as the combined-positive score, in Checkmate-577 are eagerly awaited. Additionally, results from several ongoing studies, including KEYNOTE-975 and NCT03044613, will shed light on the efficacy of PD-1 blockade after definitive chemoradiation and in combination with other agents like LAG-3 inhibitors. These trials may help to broaden the role of immunotherapy in early stage esophageal and gastroesophageal junction cancer.

Case Study 5

A 68-year-old healthy male presented to his gastroenterologist with progressive dysphagia to solids and epigastric discomfort. He was evaluated with EGD and EUS, which showed a mass 1 cm distal to the gastroesophageal junction, clinical T3N0. Biopsy demonstrated adenocarcinoma. Staging workup was negative for evidence of distant metastases. He was referred to you for discussion of the role of chemoradiation or chemotherapy as neoadjuvant therapy prior to surgery.

5) **What is the best approach in newly diagnosed gastroesophageal junction adenocarcinoma?**

Expert Perspective: gastroesophageal junction tumors straddle the border between esophageal and gastric adenocarcinoma. Anatomically, they are divided into three categories, Siewert 1 through 3, based on the location of the tumor epicenter. The AJCC 8th edition staging manual categorizes Siewert types 1 and 2 as esophageal cancer and

Siewert type 3 as gastric cancer. Most prospective trials, however, grouped those with gastroesophageal junction cancer alongside patients with either esophageal or gastric cancer rather than as a distinct entity.

In this case, therefore, two main approaches should be considered. One strategy is to proceed with neoadjuvant chemoradiotherapy based on the CROSS trial described in case #2. Although it predominantly comprised patients with esophageal cancer, patients with gastroesophageal junction tumors represented 24% of the total population in this study. An alternative approach is perioperative chemotherapy, supported by two key studies in patients with gastric and gastroesophageal junction cancer. In the MAGIC trial, patients with stage II or higher gastric, distal esophageal, or gastroesophageal junction adenocarcinoma were randomized to six cycles of perioperative epirubicin, cisplatin, and 5-FU (ECF) or surgery alone. The five-year survival was 36% in the epirubicin, cisplatin, and 5-FU arm, compared with 23% in the control arm (HR for death 0.75, P = 0.009) (Cunningham et al. 2006). Subsequently, the 5-FU, leucovorin, oxaliplatin, and docetaxel regimen of 5-FU, leucovorin, oxaliplatin, and docetaxel was compared with epirubicin, cisplatin, and 5-FU in patients with cT2 or higher or node positive gastric or gastroesophageal junction cancer and demonstrated improved OS (median OS 50 vs 35 months in 5-FU, leucovorin, oxaliplatin, and docetaxel and epirubicin, cisplatin, and 5-FU arms respectively, HR 0.77; P = 0.012) (Al-Batran et al. 2019).

Notwithstanding the pitfalls of cross-trial comparisons, attempts have been made to assess the relative safety and efficacy of neoadjuvant chemoradiotherapy versus perioperative chemotherapy. The adverse event profile differed, with more neutropenia, alopecia, diarrhea, and neuropathy in the FLOT trial and increased risk of esophagitis with the CROSS regimen. However, almost 95% of patients in both studies were able to undergo surgical resection. Although the R0 resection and pathologic complete response rate were numerically higher with the CROSS regimen compared to 5-FU, leucovorin, oxaliplatin, and docetaxel, the median OS and five-year survival rate were nearly identical. Recently, preliminary results of the phase 3 Neo-AEGIS trial, which compared the CROSS regimen with perioperative epirubicin, cisplatin, and 5-FU or 5-FU, leucovorin, oxaliplatin, and docetaxel in patients with esophageal or gastroesophageal junction adenocarcinoma using a non-inferiority statistical design, were reported. At a median follow-up of 24.5 months, there was no difference in estimated three-year survival between arms (56% with CROSS and 57% with epirubicin, cisplatin, and 5-FU /5-FU, leucovorin, oxaliplatin, and docetaxel, HR 1.02), and toxicity was comparable (Reynolds et al. 2021). The ongoing ESOPEC trial (NCT02509286) randomized patients with localized esophageal adenocarcinoma to neoadjuvant chemoradiotherapy per the CROSS protocol or perioperative 5-FU, leucovorin, oxaliplatin, and docetaxel, and results will add further evidence about the comparability of these approaches.

Case Study 6

A 65-year-old male with well-controlled hypertension and type 2 diabetes presented to his gastroenterologist with early satiety and epigastric discomfort. He was evaluated with EGD and EUS, which showed a mass in the body of the stomach and two suspicious lymph nodes, clinical stage T3N1 (Table 20.1) gastric adenocarcinoma. PET-CT showed no distant metastases. He was referred to you for a discussion of neoadjuvant therapy.

6) What is the merit of neoadjuvant therapy in gastric adenocarcinoma?

Expert Perspective: While surgery is the mainstay of treatment in localized gastric cancer, long-term outcomes with resection alone are poor, particularly for patients with ≥ cT2 or node positive disease. As described in Case Study 5, the FLOT4 trial, which compared the 5-FU, leucovorin, oxaliplatin, and docetaxel regimen with epirubicin, cisplatin, and 5-FU, established perioperative 5-FU, leucovorin, oxaliplatin, and docetaxel as an optimal approach for those with a good performance status. More than 75% of patients in this study were cT3–T4 or node positive, and the majority demonstrated an ECOG 0 performance status. Median OS was significantly better in the 5-FU, leucovorin, oxaliplatin, and docetaxel arm, as well as the estimated five-year survival (45% vs 36%). Even as the specific toxicity profile differed between arms, the overall rate of serious adverse events (AE), postoperative complications, and deaths related to chemotherapy were equivalent (Al-Batran et al. 2019). In this case, perioperative chemotherapy with 5-FU, leucovorin, oxaliplatin, and docetaxel is recommended.

Alternative approaches with supportive phase 3 data in gastric cancer include adjuvant chemotherapy or chemoradiotherapy. One concern with these strategies, however, is whether patients will be able to tolerate intensive postoperative treatment. In both MAGIC and FLOT4, for instance, more than 90% of patients received preoperative chemotherapy, while less than 50% completed the entire perioperative regimen. Additionally, neoadjuvant therapy may either facilitate tumor downstaging prior to surgery or allow identification of those who will rapidly progress and not benefit from subsequent gastrectomy.

The KEYNOTE-585 trial (NCT03221426) is an ongoing study designed to improve outcomes further with the addition of pembrolizumab to perioperative chemotherapy in patients with gastric or gastroesophageal junction adenocarcinoma. This combination strategy has demonstrated success in advanced gastroesophageal cancer (Checkmate-649, KEYNOTE-590), and KEYNOTE-585 aims to assess this approach in the early stage setting as well.

Case Study 7

A 75-year-old male with uncontrolled type 2 diabetes and chronic obstructive pulmonary disease, ECOG 2 performance status, presented to his gastroenterologist with early satiety and epigastric discomfort. He was evaluated with EGD and EUS. EGD and EUS showed a mass in the body of the stomach invading the subserosal connective tissue, clinical stage T3N0 gastric adenocarcinoma. A PET scan showed no distant metastases. He was referred to you for a discussion of neoadjuvant therapy.

7) What is the best management strategy for this patient?

Expert Perspective: In patients with significant comorbidities who are still able to undergo surgical resection, triplet combination chemotherapy, such as 5-FU, leucovorin, oxaliplatin, and docetaxel, may be difficult to tolerate, and alternative regimens should be considered. The NCCN panel includes three cycles of neoadjuvant and adjuvant FOLFOX or CapeOx as a preferred perioperative regimen in addition to 5-FU, leucovorin, oxaliplatin, and docetaxel. Support for this perioperative doublet is extrapolated from the CLASSIC trial detailed in Case Study 1. In this study, six months of adjuvant CapeOx improved disease-free survival relative to routine surveillance after D2 gastrectomy in those with mostly T2–3N1 gastric cancer. A follow-up analysis demonstrated an increase in the estimated five-year OS from 69% to 78% with adjuvant therapy as well (Noh et al. 2014). The combination of 5-FU and cisplatin is also efficacious as a perioperative regimen in early stage gastric cancer. The FNCLCC ACCORD phase 3 trial randomized patients with resectable adenocarcinoma of the esophagus, gastroesophageal junction, or stomach to surgery alone or perioperative 5-FU and cisplatin. Patients in the chemotherapy arm had increased survival compared to their counterparts in the surgery alone arm (five-year OS rate 38% vs 24%; HR 0.69; $P = 0.02$) (Ychou et al. 2011).

In this case, a chemotherapy doublet such as FOLFOX or CapeOx is preferred over 5-FU, leucovorin, oxaliplatin, and docetaxel, given the risk of significant toxicity with a triplet regimen. More broadly, the discrepancy between patients enrolled in clinical trials and those frequently seen in practice highlights the need for well-designed prospective studies focusing on frailer adults.

Case Study 8

A 65-year-old male with well-controlled hypertension and type 2 diabetes presented to his gastroenterologist with early satiety and epigastric discomfort. He was evaluated with EGD and EUS. EGD and EUS showed a mass in the body of the stomach invading the muscularis propria, clinical stage T2N0 gastric adenocarcinoma. A PET scan showed no distant metastases. He had subtotal gastrectomy with D2 lymph node dissection. The final pathologic stage is T2N1 with an R0 resection. He was referred to you for a discussion of adjuvant therapy.

8) **What is the role of adjuvant therapy in gastric adenocarcinoma with nodal disease?**

Expert Perspective: This patient received no neoadjuvant therapy, but the pathologic specimen showed N1 disease. The risk of recurrence in this circumstance is high. Two main adjuvant approaches have demonstrated clear benefit in the setting of T3–4 or node positive gastric cancer. The INT-0116 randomized phase 3 trial, described in Case Study 1, showed an OS improvement with adjuvant chemotherapy plus chemoradiotherapy compared to surveillance in patients with resected gastric and gastroesophageal junction adenocarcinoma. The median OS was 27 months in the surveillance group versus 36 months with chemoradiotherapy (HR for death 1.35; $P = 0.005$). Of note, a minority of patients in this trial received D2 resection. Additionally, the benefit of chemoradiotherapy was driven by a significant decrease in local and regional recurrences relative to the surveillance group. The rate of distant recurrences, however, was comparable between arms (Macdonald et al. 2001). Adjuvant chemotherapy alone is an alternative strategy. The CLASSIC study, detailed in Case Study 1, randomized patients to six months of adjuvant CapeOx or surveillance and showed a survival advantage with chemotherapy (Bang et al. 2012).

These two broad adjuvant strategies were compared prospectively in the ARTIST and ARTIST-2 studies. The ARTIST trial randomized patients with prior D2 resection to receive either six cycles of capecitabine and cisplatin (CapeCis) or two cycles of this regimen followed by chemoradiotherapy and two additional cycles of CapeCis. At a median follow-up of 84 months, there was no statistically significant difference in three-year disease-free survival (HR 0.74; $P = 0.092$) or OS (HR 1.13; $P = 0.53$) (Park et al. 2015). Interestingly, an exploratory analysis from ARTIST demonstrated improved disease-free survival in the chemoradiotherapy group in the subset of patients with positive lymph nodes. In light of this finding, the ARTIST-2 trial was designed to compare chemotherapy with chemotherapy plus chemoradiotherapy specifically in those with lymph-node-positive disease. Patients with stage II or III node-positive gastric cancer who underwent D2 resection were randomly assigned to either adjuvant S-1 for one year, S-1 and oxaliplatin (SOX) for six months, or SOX chemotherapy plus chemoradiotherapy. Estimated three-year disease-free survival was nearly identical in the two SOX arms (74% with SOX, 73% with SOX plus chemoradiotherapy) (Park et al. 2021). These data, supported by additional analyses, led the NCCN panel to recommend adjuvant chemoradiotherapy only in cases where R0 resection or D2 lymph node dissection was not achieved.

Our patient: In this patient with T2N1 gastric cancer post-D2 lymph node dissection and R0 resection, chemotherapy with either six months of CapeOx or FOLFOX is recommended.

Case Study 9

A 65-year-old male with well-controlled hypertension presented to his gastroenterologist with early satiety and epigastric discomfort. He was evaluated with EGD and EUS. EGD and EUS showed a mass in the body of the stomach invading the muscularis propria, clinical stage T2N0. A PET scan showed no distant metastases. He had a subtotal gastrectomy with adequate D2 lymph node dissection and R0 resection. The final pathologic stage is T2N0, stage 1b gastric adenocarcinoma. He was referred to you for a discussion of adjuvant therapy.

9) What is the role of adjuvant therapy in gastric adenocarcinoma *without* nodal disease?

Expert Perspective: The key adjuvant studies in gastric cancer predominantly comprised patients with stage II or III disease. The CLASSIC trial, for instance, excluded those with stage 1B cancer, and the INT-0116 study included only 15% with node-negative disease. Moreover, definitions in TNM staging have shifted since landmark trials such as INT-0116, complicating efforts to adduce support from older data. One approach for patients with resected T2N0 gastric cancer is surveillance. An alternative strategy recommended by the NCCN panel is postoperative chemoradiotherapy. An NCDB analysis sheds light on a high-risk subgroup who likely benefit from adjuvant therapy. This retrospective study evaluated outcomes of patients with resected, margin-negative T2N0 gastric cancer between 2003–2011 who received either chemotherapy, chemoradiotherapy, or no treatment postoperatively. Among patients with an inadequate lymph node dissection (< 15 lymph nodes examined), there was an OS benefit in the subgroup who received adjuvant chemoradiotherapy compared to no treatment. In those with ≥ 15 lymph nodes examined during surgery, however, there was no difference in OS between treatment groups (In et al. 2016). In this case, therefore, since the patient had an adequate D2 lymph node dissection and an R0 resection, either surveillance or postoperative chemoradiotherapy is a reasonable approach. In circumstances where either of these surgical endpoints are not achieved, adjuvant chemoradiotherapy is preferred.

Introduction | 245

Case Study 10

A 65-year-old male presented to his gastroenterologist with early satiety and epigastric discomfort. An EGD and EUS showed a mass in the body of the stomach and two suspicious lymph nodes, clinical stage T3N1 gastric adenocarcinoma. PET-CT showed no distant metastases. Immunohistochemistry (IHC) from the biopsy demonstrated 3+ staining for HER-2 expression. He is scheduled to undergo total gastrectomy and perioperative 5-FU, leucovorin, oxaliplatin, and docetaxel but inquired about the role of targeted therapy in early stage gastroesophageal cancer considering his IHC findings.

10) What is the role of targeted therapy in early stage gastroesophageal cancer?

Expert Perspective: Biomarker-based therapies are an important component of treatment in advanced gastric cancer. Trastuzumab is indicated in combination with chemotherapy for HER-2 overexpressing tumors and checkpoint inhibitors are approved in multiple settings based on PD-L1 expression, tumor mutational burden or microsatellite instability. FGFR2b also has demonstrated promise as a relevant and targetable biomarker in metastatic disease (Catenaci et al. 2020; discussed in the next chapter). Translating these targeted approaches into the early stage setting has proved challenging. RTOG-1010, for instance, evaluated standard neoadjuvant chemoradiotherapy in HER-2 positive esophageal or gastroesophageal junction adenocarcinoma with or without trastuzumab. In this study, the trastuzumab arm conferred no survival advantage over chemoradiotherapy alone (median OS 38.9 vs 38.5 months, HR 1.01; CI 0.69–1.47) (Safran et al. 2020). Other studies evaluated HER-2 directed agents in the adjuvant setting in combination with chemoradiotherapy or perioperatively with chemotherapy. Results thus far however have not validated a biomarker-based approach in this subgroup. In this case, therefore, despite strongly positive HER-2 staining in the biopsy specimen, there is insufficient evidence to recommend trastuzumab or other HER-2 targeted agents in addition to standard perioperative 5-FU, leucovorin, oxaliplatin, and docetaxel outside of the context of a clinical trial.

Esophageal dysplasia and Barret's esophagus

11) Which of the following statement(s) about esophageal dysplasia and Barret's esophagus is/are correct?
   A) Incidence of Barret's esophagus is 1 to 5% among symptomatic patients who undergo endoscopy.
   B) Most cases of distal esophageal or gastroesophageal adenocarcinomas have evidence of Barrett's esophagus.
   C) High-grade dysplasia is an indication for more aggressive management.
   D) B and C.

Expert Perspective: The incidence of Barret's esophagus is 10 to 20% among symptomatic patients who undergo endoscopy and 30 to 50% for patients with peptic strictures. Risk factors for Barrett's esophagus include GERD, white or Hispanic race, male gender, advanced age, smoking, and obesity. Approximately 60% of cases of distal esophageal or gastroesophageal adenocarcinomas have evidence of Barrett's esophagus. In a nationwide population study from Denmark, the annual risk of esophageal adenocarcinoma was 0.12% (95% CI 0.09–0.15). Detection of low-grade dysplasia on the index endoscopy was associated with an incidence rate for adenocarcinoma of 5.1 cases per 1,000 person-years. In contrast, the incidence rate among patients without dysplasia was 1.0 case per 1,000 person-years. Risk estimates for patients with high-grade dysplasia were slightly higher. The typical treatment for patients with Barrett's esophagus is surveillance using upper endoscopy and biopsy to examine tissue for evidence of dysplasia. High-grade dysplasia is an indication for more aggressive management, including surgical resection. Tumor markers, such as TP53, may be predictors of potential progression to malignant disease.

Correct Answer: D

Recommended Readings

Adelstein, D.J., Rice, T.W., Rybicki, L.A., Saxton, J.P., et al. (2009). Mature results from a phase II trial of postoperative concurrent chemoradiotherapy for poor prognosis cancer of the esophagus and gastroesophageal junction. *J Thorac Oncol* 4 (10): 1264–1269.

Al-Batran, S.E., Homann, N., Pauligk, C., Goetze, T.O., et al. (2019). Perioperative chemotherapy with fluorouracil plus leucovorin, oxaliplatin, and docetaxel versus fluorouracil or capecitabine plus cisplatin and epirubicin for locally advanced, resectable gastric or gastro-oesophageal junction adenocarcinoma (FLOT4): a randomized, phase 2/3 trial. *Lancet* 393 (10184): 1948–1957.

Atay, S.M., Correa, A., Hofstetter, W.L., Swisher, S.G., et al. (2019). Predictors of staging accuracy, pathologic nodal involvement, and overall survival for cT2N0 carcinoma of the esophagus. *J Thorac Cardiovasc Surg* 157 (3): 1264–1272.

Bang, Y.J., Kim, Y.W., Yang, H.K., Chung, H.C., et al. (2012). Adjuvant capecitabine and oxaliplatin for gastric cancer after D2 gastrectomy (CLASSIC): a phase 3 open-label, randomized controlled trial. *Lancet* 379 (9813): 315–321.

Bedenne, L., Michel, P., Bouche, O., Milan, C., et al. (2007). Chemoradiation followed by surgery compared with chemoradiation alone in squamous cancer of the esophagus: FFCD 9102. *J Clin Oncol* 25 (10): 1160–1168.

Catenacci, D., Rasco, D., Lee, J., et al. (2020). Phase I escalation and expansion study of bemarituzumab (FPA144) in patients with advanced solid tumors and FGFR2b-selected gastroesophageal adenocarcinoma. *J Clin Oncol* 38 (21): 2418–2426.

Cheedella, N.K., Suzuki, A., Xiao, L., Hofstetter, W.L., et al. (2013). Association between clinical complete response and pathological complete response after preoperative chemoradiation in patients with gastroesophageal cancer: analysis in a large cohort. *Ann Oncol* 24 (5): 1262–1266.

Cunningham, D., Allum, W.H., Stenning, S.P., Thompson, J.N., et al. (2006). Perioperative chemotherapy versus surgery alone for resectable gastroesophageal cancer. *N Engl J Med* 355 (1): 11–20.

Hagen, P. van, Hulshof, M.C.C.M., Lanschot, J.J.B. van, et al. (2012). Preoperative chemoradiotherapy for esophageal or junctional cancer. *NEJM* 366 (22): 2074–2084.

In, H., Kantor, O., Sharpe, S.M., Baker, M.S., et al. (2016). Adjuvant therapy improves survival for T2N0 gastric cancer patients with sub-optimal lymphadenectomy. *Ann Surg Oncol* 23 (6): 1956–1962.

Kelly, R.J., Ajani, J.A., Kuzdzal, J., Zander, T., et al. (2021). Adjuvant nivolumab in resected esophageal or gastroesophageal junction. *N Engl J Med* 384 (13): 1191–1203.

Macdonald, J.S., Smalley, S.R., Benedetti, J., Hundahl, S.A., et al. (2001). Chemoradiotherapy after surgery compared with surgery alone for adenocarcinoma of the stomach or gastroesophageal junction. *N Engl J Med* 345 (10): 725–730.

Noh, S.H., Park, S.R., Yang, H.W., Chung, H.C. et al. (2014). Adjuvant capecitabine plus oxaliplatin for gastric cancer after D2 gastrectomy (CLASSIC): 5-year follow-up of an open-label, randomized phase 3 trial. *Lancet Oncol* 15 (12): 1389–1396.

Park, S.H., Lim, D.H., Sohn, T.S., Lee, J. et al. (2021). A randomized phase III trial comparing adjuvant single-agent S1, S-1 with oxaliplatin, and postoperative chemoradiation with S-1 and oxaliplatin in patients with node-positive gastric cancer after D2 resection: the ARTIST 2 trial. *Ann Oncol* 32 (3): 368–374.

Park, S.H., Sohn, T.S., Lee, J., Lim, D.H., et al. (2015). Phase III trial to compare adjuvant chemotherapy with capecitabine and cisplatin versus concurrent chemoradiotherapy in gastric cancer: final report of the adjuvant chemoradiotherapy in stomach tumors trial, including survival and subset analyses. *J Clin Oncol* 33 (28): 3130–3136.

Reynolds, J.V., Preston, S.R., O'Neill, B., Lowery, M.A., et al. (2021). Neo-AEGIS (Neoadjuvant trial in Adenocarcinoma of the Esophagus and Esophago-Gastric Junction International Study): preliminary results of phase III RCT of CROSS versus perioperative chemotherapy (Modified MAGIC or FLOT protocol). *ASCO Virtual Conference* https://ascopubs.org/doi/abs/10.1200/JCO.2021.39.15_suppl.4004.

Rice, T.W., Rusch, V.W., Apperson-Hansen, C., et al. (2009). Worldwide esophageal cancer collaboration. *Diseases of the Esophagus*. 22 (1): 1–8.

Scheer, R., Fakiris, A., and Johnstone, P. (2011). Quantifying the benefit of a pathologic complete response after neoadjuvant chemoradiotherapy in the treatment of esophageal cancer. *Int J Radiat Oncol Biol Phys* 80 (4): 996–1001.

Stahl, M., Stuschke, M., Lehmann, N., et al. (2005). Chemoradiation with and without surgery in patients with locally advanced squamous cell carcinoma of the esophagus. *J Clin Oncol* 23 (10): 2310–2317.

Safran, H., Winter, K.A., Wigle, D.A., DiPetrillo, T.A., et al. (2020). Trastuzumab with trimodality treatment for esophageal adenocarcinoma with HER2 overexpression: NRG Oncology/RTOG 1010. *ASCO Virtual Conference* https://ascopubs.org/doi/abs/10.1200/JCO.2020.38.15_suppl.4500

Yang, H., Liu, H., Chen, Y., et al. (2018). Neoadjuvant chemoradiotherapy followed by surgery versus surgery alone for locally advanced squamous cell carcinoma of the esophagus (NEOCRTEC5010): a phase III multicenter, randomized, open-label clinical trial. *J Clin Oncol* 36 (27): 2796–2803.

Ychou, M., Boige, V., Pignon, J-P., et al. (2011). Perioperative chemotherapy compared with surgery alone for resectable gastroesophageal adenocarcinoma: an FNCLCC and FFCD multicenter phase III trial. *J Clin Oncol* 29 (13): 1715–1721.

21

Metastatic Esophagogastric Cancer

Geoffrey Y. Ku and David H. Ilson

Memorial Sloan Kettering Cancer Center, New York, NY

Introduction

The intent of treatment for metastatic esophagogastric cancer is to control the disease and provide palliation. In this chapter, we discuss recent seminal changes in therapy for metastatic esophagogastric cancer, which involves the addition of immune checkpoint inhibitors to first-line therapy for any cancer of the esophagus, gastroesophageal junction, or stomach. We also discuss the standard-of-care for second-line therapy and focus on emerging targets in this virulent disease. The discussion about early stage esophagogastric cancers is in the preceding chapter. Genetic testing in gastrointestinal tumors is discussed in Chapter 47.

1) What is the optimal first-line regimen for advanced HER2-negative esophagogastric cancer ?

Expert Perspective: The combination of infusional 5FU and cisplatin has been studied extensively since the 1980s, and the doublet of a fluoropyrimidine with a platinum compound remains a reference regimen in many contemporary trials. This doublet is associated with response rates of up to 40%, median progression-free survival of about six months, and median overall survival (OS) of 10 to 12 months. A contemporary and commonly used regimen is the FOLFOX regimen (bolus and infusional 5FU–leucovorin–oxaliplatin).

Little changed over 30 years until the spring of 2021, when immune checkpoint inhibitors were approved in combination with a fluoropyrimidine/platinum doublet. The Checkmate 649 study demonstrated benefit for adding nivolumab, an anti-PD-1 antibody, to FOLFOX or Capeox (capecitabine/oxaliplatin) in patients with esophageal, gastroesophageal junction, or gastric adenocarcinoma. The median OS was 13.8 vs 11.6 months (HR 0.80; $P = 0.0002$) in the intention-to-treat population.

Separately, the KEYNOTE-590 study showed that adding pembrolizumab, another anti-PD-1 antibody, to chemotherapy improved outcomes in patients with esophageal/ gastroesophageal junction adenocarcinoma or squamous cell carcinoma, with a median OS of 12.4 vs 9.8 months (harazd ratio 0.73, $P < 0.0001$).

Although the FDA approved both drugs irrespective of tumor PD-L1 status, subset analyses suggest that the PD-L1 combined positive score (CPS) and histology predict for outcome. As such, the National Comprehensive Cancer Network (NCCN) makes nivolumab/chemotherapy a Category 1 recommendation for tumors with PD-L1 CPS ≥5, whereas it is only a Category 2B recommendation for tumors with PD-L1 CPS 1–4 (with no recommendation for PD-L1 CPS 0 tumors). Similarly, pembrolizumab/chemotherapy is a Category 1 recommendation for esophageal/gastroesophageal junction adenocarcinoma or squamous cell carcinoma with PD-L1 CPS ≥10 but only a Category 2B recommendation for esophageal/gastroesophageal junction adenocarcinoma with PD-L1 CPS 1–9 (with no recommendation for an adenocarcinoma with CPS 0 or SCC with PD-L1 CPS <10).

Our practice is to individualize care based on patient characteristics and the availability of a clinical study. While the FDA approvals above mean that any patient with esophagogastric cancer is now eligible to receive an immune checkpoint inhibitors with chemotherapy, the clinical – and very significant but largely ignored financial – toxicities of these drugs have to be carefully weighed in patients who are less likely to benefit from them and/or to be able to tolerate any immune-related toxicities.

2) What is the optimal first-line regimen for advanced HER2 positive esophagogastric cancer?

Expert Perspective: In 2010, the ToGA study established trastuzumab and chemotherapy as a new standard of care for the approximately 20% of esophagogastric adenocarcinomas that are positive for the HER2 protein. Response rates (47% vs 35%; $P = 0.0017$) and median progression-free survival (6.7 vs 5.5 months; $P = 0.0002$) and OS (13.8 vs 11.1 months; $P = 0.0046$) were all improved with the addition of trastuzumab.

Subsequently, multiple other studies failed to improve upon this standard until spring 2021, when pembrolizumab was approved by the FDA in combination with trastuzumab and a fluoropyrimidine/platinum doublet. Approval was based on the interim analysis of the KEYNOTE-811 study, which showed an improvement in response rates for the addition of pembrolizumab (74.4% vs 51.9%; $P = 0.00006$). At this time, survival outcomes are pending, making the FDA approval on the basis of an improvement in response rates alone notable.

3) Is there benefit for adding a third drug to a fluoropyrimidine/platinum doublet?

Expert Perspective: The only trial that has shown a clear benefit for adding a third drug to the standard fluoropyrimidine–platinum doublet is the V325 study, which randomized patients with gastroesophageal junction and gastric adenocarcinomas to the DCF regimen (docetaxel/cisplatin/5FU) versus 5FU/cisplatin. The addition of docetaxel improved response rates (37% vs 25%; $P = 0.01$) and time to progression (5.6 vs 3.7 months; $P < 0.001$), but OS was only slightly improved (9.2 vs 8.6 months; two-year OS: 18% vs 9%; $P = 0.02$). In addition, the three-drug regimen was associated with significantly more toxicity, including a grade 3/4 neutropenia rate of 82% (vs 57%) and febrile neutropenia in 29% of patients (vs 12%). Despite these significant toxicities, the authors reported a slower decrement in quality-of-life measurements in the DCF arm. On the basis of this study, docetaxel was approved by the US Food and Drug Administration in 2006 for use with 5FU–cisplatin in this context.

Investigators have attempted to modify the regimen to increase tolerability. More contemporary variations included the modified DCF regimen developed at Memorial Sloan

Kettering Cancer Center as well as the FLOT regimen developed in Germany; both involve a one to two day infusional 5-FU regimen given every 14 days. As FLOT has emerged as a standard of- are as peri-operative chemotherapy for locally advanced gastric cancer based on the FLOT4 study, it has also become the preferred docetaxel three-drug regimen in the metastatic setting.

Still, many oncologists reserve three-drug therapy for younger, good-performance-status patients without comorbidities, who accept the risk of greater toxicity of therapy and who have frequent access to toxicity evaluation. A German trial in patients ≥65 years old comparing 5-FU/oxaliplatin (FLO) to FLOT found increased toxicity but no improvement in outcomes in the subgroup with metastatic disease.

It is worth noting that in the United Kingdom, the anthracycline epirubicin was frequently added to the doublet since the 1990s. This regimen was widely used despite the absence of phase III data to suggest a benefit. In recent years, it has largely fallen out of favor globally and is no longer a reference regimen in phase III global studies, in part because the FLOT4 study showed superiority of FLOT vs epirubicin/cisplatin/capecitabine in the peri-operative setting.

Ultimately, the question of a three-drug regimen in the first-line setting has become a less urgent and relevant one, given the benefit noted with adding an immune checkpoint inhibitors to a two-drug regimen.

4) Should first-line chemotherapy be continued until progression or stopped after four to six months?

Expert Perspective: This remains an area of uncertainty, and practice patterns vary widely by geography and physician. No randomized trial has addressed this question. In the United Kingdom, standard practice consists of up to six months of chemotherapy, followed by observation alone even in the absence of progression or serious toxicity. On the other hand, many oncologists in East Asia continue treatment indefinitely until progression or significant toxicity occurs. Similarly, most oncologists in the United States do continue chemotherapy indefinitely.

Our standard practice is to continue first-line chemotherapy until progression. This practice is based on the fact that esophagogastric cancers are moderately chemosensitive; the continuation of chemotherapy may delay tumor progression (radiographically and clinically), and also patients may experience rapid clinical deterioration at the time of radiographic progression that may preclude additional treatment. Because of cumulative toxicity with platinum compounds (especially with oxaliplatin, which is associated with a dose-limiting neuropathy), we do consider maintenance fluoropyrimidine alone after three to four months of chemotherapy. There are no data in esophagogastric cancers to support this, but we do base this strategy partly on the validated strategy of maintenance infusional 5FU alone after initial FOLFOX chemotherapy in advanced colon cancer, as was shown in the OPTIMOX-1 study.

5) Are there data for second-line and beyond chemotherapy?

Expert Perspective: In HER2 negative gastroesophageal junction/gastric adenocarcinoma, the standard second-line regimen since 2014 has been ramucirumab, an anti-vascular endothelial growth factor receptor 2 antibody, with paclitaxel chemotherapy.

The RAINBOW study showed that the addition of ramucirumab to paclitaxel approximately doubled response rates (28% vs 16%; $P = 0.001$) and also led to clinically meaningful improvements in progression-free survival (4.4 vs 2.9 months; HR 0.64; $P < 0.0001$) and OS (9.6 vs 7.4 months; HR 0.81; $P = 0.017$) vs paclitaxel.

In addition to a taxane (either paclitaxel or docetaxel), irinotecan has also been shown to modestly improve survival in the second-line setting (5.3 vs 3.8 months; HR 0.66; $P = 0.007$). Therefore, for patients who receive second-line ramucirumab/paclitaxel, irinotecan is considered as third-line therapy for those patients who maintain a sufficient performance status to receive more treatment.

Finally, trifluridine-tipiracil or TAS-102 was approved in February 2019 as third-line or greater therapy on the basis of the phase 3 TAGS study, which showed a modest improvement in OS vs placebo (5.7 vs 3.6 months; HR 0.69; $P = 0.00058$). As the drug is associated with a minimal response rate (4% vs 2%; $P = 0.28$), cancer-related symptoms are not expected to significantly improve, which limits it use in a patient population that unfortunately often has a considerable disease burden.

For HER2 positive tumors, trastuzumab deruxtecan (T-Dxd), an antibody-drug conjugate of trastuzumab with a potent topoisomerase I inhibitor, was approved by the FDA for patients whose cancer has progressed on prior trastuzumab-based therapy. This approval was based on the DESTINY-Gastric01 study, which was a randomized phase II study of T-Dxd vs physician's choice of irinotecan or paclitaxel as third-line therapy for HER2 positive gastroesophageal junction/gastric cancer patients who had received previous trastuzumab, a fluoropyrimidine, and a platinum drug. The study met its primary endpoint of improving response rates (51% vs 14%; $P < 0.001$) as well as the secondary endpoint of OS (12.5 vs 8.4 months; HR 0.59; $P = 0.01$). A toxicity of T-Dxd that clinicians must be familiar with is pneumonitis, which developed in 10% of patients (none fatal in this study). This FDA approval was also notable as the study enrolled only East Asian patients.

6) Are there data for second-line and beyond immunotherapy?

Expert Perspective: For patients with esophageal squamous cell carcinoma who have not received an immune checkpoint inhibitors in the first-line setting, both pembrolizumab and nivolumab are FDA-approved as second-line therapy. While pembrolizumab is approved for patients whose tumor PD-L1 CPS is ≥10, nivolumab is approved for all patients.

The first approval of an immune checkpoint inhibitor in esophagogastric cancer actually occurred when pembrolizumab received accelerated approval as third-line or greater therapy for gastroesophageal junction/gastric adenocarcinomas whose PD-L1 CPS is ≥1 in September 2017. However, this approval was withdrawn in July 2021 based on re-review of its extremely modest benefit.

7) What new targeted therapies are being evaluated?

Expert Perspective: A novel target that is currently being evaluated in a phase III study is claudin 18.2 (or CLDN18.2), which is a component of the tight junctions between cells that is overexpressed in several cancers, including gastric cancer. In a randomized phase II study, zolbetuximab was evaluated in combination with EOX (epirubicin/oxaliplatin/capecitabine) chemotherapy in gastric cancers that were found to be CLDN18.2 positive by an experimental immunohistochemistry assay. Patients who received zolbetuximab/ chemotherapy had improvements in the primary endpoint of progression-free survival (7.5 vs 5.3 months, harazd ratio 0.44, $P < 0.0005$), as well as improvements in response rates and OS. These data led to the ongoing phase III Spotlight study, which is evaluating FOLFOX with or without zolbetuximab in CLDN18.2-positive gastroesophageal junction/gastric cancers [NCT03504397], and the phase III GLOW study, which is evaluating Capeox with or without zolbetuximab [NCT03653507].

Another promising target is *fibroblast growth factor receptor 2b (FGFR2b)*, which can be overexpressed as a protein or amplified at the gene level. In the randomized phase II FIGHT study, patients with gastroesophageal junction/gastric cancer who had either *FGFR2b* overexpression or *FGFR2b* gene amplification by circulating tumor DNA (ctDNA) were randomized to receive FOLFOX with or without bemarituzumab, an antibody against *FGFR2b*. Of the 910 patients who were screened, 30% were found to be eligible. One hundred and fifty-five patients enrolled; 96% had *FGFR2b* overexpression, 17% had *FGFR2b* ctDNA amplification, and 13% had both. Based on the prespecified statistical plan, the primary endpoint of progression-free survival was met (9.5 vs 7.4 months; HR 0.68; $P = 0.0727$) and there was also an improvement in OS (NR vs 12.9 months; HR 0.58; $P = 0.0268$). The benefit for adding bemarituzumab was greater in tumors with a higher level of *FGFR2b* overexpression and seems to be independent of *FGFR2b* amplification by ctDNA. An unusual adverse event of bemarituzumab is corneal toxicity (26% all grade, 2.6 % grade ≥ 3). Based on these results, a phase III study is planned.

Recommended Readings

Janjigian, Y.Y., Shitara, K., Moehler, M., et al. (2021). First-line nivolumab plus chemotherapy versus chemotherapy alone for advanced gastric, gastro-oesophageal junction, and oesophageal adenocarcinoma (CheckMate 649): a randomised, open-label, phase 3 trial. *Lancet* 398: 27–40.

Kato, K., Cho, B.C., Takahashi, M., et al. (2019). Nivolumab versus chemotherapy in patients with advanced oesophageal squamous cell carcinoma refractory or intolerant to previous chemotherapy (ATTRACTION-3): a multicentre, randomised, open-label, phase 3 trial. *Lancet Oncol* 20: 1506–1517.

Kojima, T., Shah, M.A., Muro, K., et al. (2020). Randomized phase III KEYNOTE-181 study of pembrolizumab versus chemotherapy in advanced esophageal cancer. *J Clin Oncol* 38: 4138–4148.

Shitara, K., Bang, Y.J., Iwasa, S., et al. (2020). Trastuzumab deruxtecan in previously treated HER2-positive gastric cancer. *N Engl J Med* 382: 2419–2430.

Wilke, H., Muro, K., Van Cutsem, E., et al. (2014). Ramucirumab plus paclitaxel versus placebo plus paclitaxel in patients with previously treated advanced gastric or gastro-oesophageal junction adenocarcinoma (RAINBOW): a double-blind, randomised phase 3 trial. *Lancet Oncol* 15: 1224–1235.

22

Early-Stage Colon Cancer

John Krauss[1], Vaibhav Sahai[1], and Al B. Benson III[2]

[1] *University of Michigan, Ann Arbor, MI*
[2] *Northwestern University Feinberg School of Medicine, Chicago, IL*

Introduction

Colorectal cancer is the second most common cause of cancer death after lung cancer. In 2020, approximately 1.93 million cases of colorectal cancer were identified, which led to about 935,000 deaths. Age-standardized incidence of colorectal cancer is reportedly the highest across high-HDI (human development index) regions such as Australia, New Zealand, Europe, North America and Eastern Asia, and lowest in Africa and South-Central Asia. Death rates from colorectal cancer parallel this trend. In the United States, it is predicted there will be approximately 153,020 new cases and 52,550 deaths from colorectal cancer in 2023. Approximately 12% of patients will be younger than 50 years and 11% over the age of 80. Although the incidence is decreasing in elderly patients, it is rising 1 to 3% annually in young adults under 50 years. The lifetime risk of developing colorectal cancer is estimated to be 4.3% for men and 4.0% for women.

The likelihood of survival is dependent on the stage of the colorectal cancer. At diagnosis, 38% of patients have localized disease, 35% have regional involvement, 21% have metastatic cancer, and 7% of patients are unstaged. Based on the SEER database, the five-year survival for colorectal cancer patients with distant metastases is 13%, regional cancer 71%, and 90% in patients with localized colorectal cancer.

The overall incidence and death rates for colorectal cancer have been decreasing over the past 20 years in the United States, a decline largely attributable to screening measures. The incidence and mortality rates have fallen from 57 and 24 per 100,000 people in 1992 to 35 and 13 per 100,000 in 2019, respectively. The five-year relative survival rate of patients with colon cancer has similarly increased from 49% in 1975 to about 63% in 2021.

Cancer Consult: Expertise in Clinical Practice, Volume 1: Solid Tumors & Supportive Care,
Second Edition. Edited by Syed A. Abutalib, Maurie Markman, Al B. Benson III, and Hope S. Rugo.
© 2024 John Wiley & Sons Ltd. Published 2024 by John Wiley & Sons Ltd.

Stage II colon cancer

1) For a patient with completely resected stage II colon cancer, which of the following prognostic features would indicate no benefit from adjuvant chemotherapy?
   A) Lymphatic or vascular invasion.
   B) Deficient mismatch repair (dMMR).
   C) Oncotype DX high recurrence score.
   D) Less than 12 lymph nodes examined in the surgical resection specimen.

Expert Perspective: Stage II colon carcinoma is a biologically heterogeneous entity with a wide range of five-year disease-free survival between 45.7% and 66.7%. Treatment choices as per current National Comprehensive Cancer Network (NCCN) Clinical Practice Guidelines in Oncology for stage II colon cancer include enrollment in a clinical trial, observation, or systemic chemotherapy 5-fluorouracil (5FU)–leucovorin or capecitabine with or without the addition of oxaliplatin, depending on the risk stratification. Traditional high-risk factors for recurrence include T4 disease, poorly differentiated histology, lymphatic, or vascular invasion, perineural invasion, tumor budding, bowel obstruction, less than 12 nodes examined, clinical perforation, or close, indeterminate, or positive margins. While these clinicopathologic risk features offer some overall guidance, they are inadequate in terms of the biologic behavior and risk of recurrence for an individual.

Microsatellite instability high (MSI-H) phenotype, defined as instability in two or more nucleotide markers within the five microsatellite loci, has both predictive and prognostic implications for adjuvant therapy. There is near-complete concordance between an MSI-H phenotype to a deficient mismatch repair (MMR) phenotype.

- A retrospective stratification analysis using MMR status of 1,027 previously randomized patients with stage II and III colon adenocarcinoma to either 5FU with levamisole or leucovorin, or observation, was reported by Sargent et al. (2009, 2010). They showed that patients with deficient mismatch repair (dMMR) have a five-year disease-free survival of 80% compared with 56% for those with proficient MMR or microsatellite stable (MSS) (HR: 0.51; 95% CI: 0.29–0.89; $P = 0.009$). In patients with stage II colon cancer with dMMR or MSI-H who were treated with adjuvant 5FU chemotherapy, there was a statistically decreased overall survival (OS) compared to the surgery alone arm (HR: 2.95; 95% CI: 1.02–8.54; $P = 0.04$).
- An analysis of the ACCENT database reported by Cohen et al. suggests that adding oxaliplatin to fluoropyrimidine adjuvant chemotherapy improved the overall survival of stage III patients (HR 0.52; CI 0.28–0.93). The stage III MSI-H patients did not appear to benefit from 5FU (disease-free survival, HR 1.01; 95% CI: 0.41–2.51; $P = 0.98$), and only the MSS stage III patients obtained any survival advantage from adjuvant 5FU (disease-free survival, HR: 0.64; 95% CI: 0.48–0.84; $P = 0.001$).

Oncotype DX is a gene expression assay that includes seven recurrence risk genes and five reference genes, and it calculates a recurrence score (low, intermediate, or high) predictive of the risk of recurrence of stage II–III colon cancer at three years. Validation studies have shown significant correlation between the risk of recurrence and the recurrence score.

Oncotype DX can serve as important prognostication tool, but studies have not been conducted to determine the ability of the Oncotype DX test to predict a response to adjuvant chemotherapy.

Correct Answer: B

2) **Which of the following management options would you consider for a patient with R0 resected stage II or node-negative colon adenocarcinoma with high-risk features?**
   A) 5FU or capecitabine alone.
   B) 5FU–oxaliplatin or FOLFOX.
   C) Capecitabine–oxaliplatin or CapeOx.
   D) Observation.
   E) All of the above.

Expert Perspective: Although it is universally accepted that most stage III patients should receive adjuvant chemotherapy, there is uncertainty regarding whether stage II patients derive sufficient benefit from chemotherapy to warrant the toxicity. The initial evidence to support the role of adjuvant chemotherapy came from the INT-0035 trial that randomized 325 patients with resected stage II colon cancer to either 5FU–levamisole for one year or observation. At a median follow-up of seven years, 5FU–levamisole yielded a trend toward superior recurrence-free survival (HR: 0.69; 95% CI: 0.44–1.08; $P = 0.10$) over observation. However, there was no improvement noted in OS (72% in each arm; $P = 0.83$). The QUASAR trial also showed benefit in risk of recurrence at two years for 2,146 patients with resected stage II colon cancer who were treated with 5FU–LV compared to patients who received no adjuvant therapy (HR: 0.71; 95% CI: 0.54–0.92; $P = 0.01$), with a trend toward better OS (HR: 0.86; 95% CI: 0.66–1.12). Furthermore, a large pooled analysis of seven randomized controlled trials (NCCTG, ECOG-NCCTG-INT, SWOG-INT0035, Siena, NCIC-CTG, FFCD, and GIVIO) with 1,440 patients with node-negative disease revealed only a 4% absolute benefit in five-year disease-free survival (76% versus 72%; $P = 0.49$), and no benefit in OS (81% versus 80%; $P = 0.11$). In contrast, the ACCENT data set, which included 6,896 patients with resected stage II disease from 18 phase III adjuvant trials, showed an absolute benefit of 5% in eight-year OS (72.2% versus 66.8%; $P = 0.026$). Although probably real, the survival benefit from adjuvant chemotherapy for an average patient with stage II cancer is small and may not justify the cost involved, potential for long-term toxicity, and inconvenience to the patient.

This has prompted researchers to identify high-risk features within stage II disease (as listed in Question 1) that adversely affect the disease-specific survival and predict benefit from adjuvant chemotherapy. However, only a few adjuvant clinical trials have stratified patients according to these risk factors, and certainly did not include all of them.

- A meta-analysis of four sequential NSABP clinical trials that compared adjuvant 5FU-based chemotherapy with each other versus no treatment showed that patients with Dukes B colon cancer ($n = 1565$) who had average-risk features (absence of obstruction, localized bowel perforation, or extension of tumor into adjacent organs) had a 32% reduction in mortality (HR: 0.68; 95% CI: 0.50–0.92; $P = 0.01$), whereas those with high-risk features had a 20% reduction of mortality (HR: 0.80; 95% CI: 0.55–1.17; $P = 0.26$).

This translated into 5% absolute improvement in mortality in each category, thus counteracting the argument that only patients with high-risk features would derive benefit from adjuvant chemotherapy.
- An NCCTG trial restricted eligibility to high-risk stage II (T4 disease and bowel perforation or obstruction) and stage III patients, and randomly assigned 317 patients to either adjuvant 5FU–LV chemotherapy or observation. Overall, there was a clear benefit in OS (74% vs 63%; $P = 0.01$) in the chemotherapy arm, with only a trend toward benefit for patients with stage II cancer ($n = 57$) on exploratory analysis (90% vs 74%; $P = 0.15$).
- Also, a large pooled analysis of seven randomized controlled trials with 1,440 patients with node-negative disease failed to show benefit of chemotherapy in T4 low-grade (69% versus 71%) or high-grade (57% versus 46%) colon cancer compared to surgery alone in an underpowered subset analysis.

Despite the lack of data from randomized clinical trials, the NCCN Clinical Practice Guidelines recommend discussion of adjuvant chemotherapy with medically fit patients with stage II disease with clinicopathologic high-risk features. Furthermore, MSI-low, defined as instability in less than two nucleotide markers within the five microsatellite loci, or MSS stage II colon cancer patients with a clinicopathologic risk factor would be considered potential candidates for 5FU-based chemotherapy after detailed discussion with patients; however, the management of the subset of patients with MSI-H tumors with traditional risk factor(s) is not clear, and they should be enrolled in a clinical trial or observed without adjuvant chemotherapy.

There are minimal data to recommend use of oxaliplatin with 5FU-based therapy in this patient population.

- The MOSAIC trial randomized 2,246 patients, including 899 with stage II disease, to infusion–bolus 5FU–LV versus FOLFOX4, and found no improvement in five-year disease-free survival or six-year OS between the two arms (OS 86.9% vs 86.8%; HR: 1.00; 95% CI: 0.70–1.41; $P = 0.986$). However, a nonsignificant trend toward improved five-year disease-free survival in high- versus average-risk patients was observed with the addition of oxaliplatin (HR: 0.84; 95% CI: 0.50–1.02) in an unplanned analysis. Therefore, the addition of oxaliplatin is considered an appropriate option for stage II patients with high-risk features, but not for those with average-risk features.
- Lastly, the question of chemotherapy duration for stage II patients has been explored in the IDEA collaborative. In a planned subset of stage II patients, FOLFOX was administered to 1,254 patients, and CapeOx was administered to 2019 patients. The five-year disease-free survival rate was 80.7% in the patients who received three months of therapy, and 83.9% for the patients who received six months of therapy ($P = 0.39$ for non-inferiority).

Patients should be encouraged to enroll in clinical trials as efforts continue to compare risk versus benefit from adjuvant therapy.

Correct Answer: E

3) **Which of the following is not a feature of a microsatellite instability high (MSI-H) T3 N0 colon cancer?**
    A) Higher tumor mutation burden, typically over 10 mutations per 10^6 DNA base pairs.
    B) Better prognosis than microsatellite stable T3 colon cancers.

C) Benefit from adjuvant chemotherapy after surgery.
D) Increased infiltration with CD8+ T cells, CD4+ T cells, and macrophages.

Expert Perspective: Patients with MSI-H colorectal tumors have a prognostic advantage regardless of the tumor stage at diagnosis with a hazard ratio of 0.65 for overall survival. Approximately 15% of all colorectal cancers are MSI-H, but only 2 to 4% of them present as stage IV at diagnosis. MSI-H phenotype has a higher prevalence in stage II than stage III colon cancers and has been associated with a decreased risk of nodal and distant metastasis. The precise explanation is not clear, but some of the pathologic differences include significant association of MSI-H tumors with increased intratumoral activated cytotoxic T-lymphocytes, apoptosis to proliferation index, and decreased p53 expression or *KRAS* mutations. Resected T3N0 MSI-H colorectal cancers have been demonstrated to not benefit from adjuvant fluorouracil chemotherapy. Controversy exists as to the benefit of FOLFOX chemotherapy for MSI-H colon cancer with either T4 and/or lymph node positive status. Immune checkpoint inhibition has become the standard of care for MSI-H stage IV unresectable colorectal cancer (Chapter 24). Clinical trials are ongoing to assess the role of the addition of immune checkpoint inhibition to standard chemotherapy for resected stage II and stage III colon cancer. A preliminary study of neoadjuvant therapy with immune checkpoint inhibition in patients with MSI-H resectable colon cancer reported that 12 of 20 patients had a complete pathologic response after treatment with ipilimumab and nivolumab.

Correct Answer: C

Stage III colon cancer

4) Which of the following adjuvant chemotherapy regimens would you not consider for a patient with R0 resected stage III or node-positive colon adenocarcinoma?
   A) 5FU or capecitabine alone.
   B) 5FU–oxaliplatin or FOLFOX.
   C) Capecitabine–oxaliplatin or CapeOx.
   D) 5FU–irinotecan or FOLFIRI.

Expert Perspective: There are several trials to substantiate the role of adjuvant 5FU–LV in patients with node-positive or stage III colon cancer. The Intergroup Trial INT-0035 was the first large randomized study that showed that treatment with 5FU–levamisole in patients with resected Dukes stage C colon cancer ($N = 929$) reduced the risk of cancer recurrence by 41% ($P < 0.0001$) and overall death rate by 33% ($P = 0.006$) compared to observation (the levamisole-alone arm produced no detectable effect) after a median follow-up of three years. The NSABP C-03 trial randomized 1,081 patients with Dukes stage B and C either to MeCCNU, vincristine, and 5FU (MOF) or to 5FU–LV. At three years, the arm with 5FU–LV showed a significant increase in disease-free survival (73% vs 64%; $P = 0.0004$) as well as OS (84% vs 77%; $P = 0.007$) compared to the MOF arm. The benefit was also confirmed by the NCCTG trial and the pooled analysis by IMPACT investigators solidifying the role of adjuvant 5FU–LV. The survival benefit of the addition of oxaliplatin in node-positive disease was evaluated by the MOSAIC trial that randomized 2,246 patients, including 1,347 patients with stage III disease ($n = 672$, and $n = 675$ in mFOLFOX4 and 5FU–LV, respectively). The probabilities of survival at six years were 72.9% and 68.7%, respectively (HR: 0.80; 95% CI: 0.65–0.97; $P = 0.023$), corresponding to a 30% reduction in risk of death in favor of adjuvant FOLFOX4 for six months. The addition of oxaliplatin was also evaluated in the NSABP C-07 trial with 2,407 patients with stage II or III colon cancer randomized to 5FU–LV with or without oxaliplatin. After a median follow-up of 52.5 months, the OS showed improvement with the addition of oxaliplatin (FLOX regimen) (HR: 0.80; 95% CI: 0.69–0.93; $P = < 0.004$), but this improvement was not apparent after eight years of follow-up (HR: 0.88; 95% CI: 0.75–1.02; $P = 0.08$) and did not differ by the stage of disease ($P = 0.38$). However, the FLOX regimen remained superior for disease-free survival (HR: 0.82; 95% CI: 0.75–0.93; $P = 0.002$).

The addition of irinotecan to 5FU–LV is not considered a standard approach for adjuvant chemotherapy for resected stage II or III colon cancer based on no improvement when compared to 5FU–LV, as shown in the CALGB 89803, PETACC-3, and ACCORD-02 trials.

Use of oral fluoropyrimidines, such as capecitabine, has also been studied as both monotherapy and combination therapy for colon cancer. The phase III X-ACT trial randomized 1,987 patients with stage III colon cancer to either capecitabine or bolus 5FU–LV for six months in a non-inferiority trial. After a median follow-up of 6.9 years, capecitabine was at least equivalent to 5FU–LV in terms of both disease-free survival (HR: 0.88; 95% CI: 0.77–1.01) and OS (HR: 0.86; 95% CI: 0.74–1.01). There are no phase III trials comparing CapeOx to FOLFOX in adjuvant therapy for stage III colon cancer. However, a phase III trial compared CapeOx to 5FU–LV alone and reported a superior disease-free survival (70.9% vs 65%; HR: 0.80; 95% CI: 0.69–0.93; $P = 0.0045$) and five-year OS (77.6% vs 74.2%; HR: 0.87; 95% CI: 0.72–1.05; $P = 0.15$). Lastly, the ACCENT database ($n = 11,953$) evaluated whether the addition of oxaliplatin to fluorouracil improved survival in elderly (> 70 years) compared to fluorouracil alone. The statistical analyses suggest no statistically significant interactions between treatment arm and age, although the stratified point estimates suggested that oxaliplatin may provide a short-term reduction in the risk of recurrence in elderly patients (disease-free survival, HR: 0.94; 95% CI: 0.78 to 1.13), but no long-term benefit is achieved (OS, HR: 1.04; 95% CI: 0.85 to 1.27), possibly due to high rate of mortality due to alternative causes.

To summarize, the benefit of addition of oxaliplatin to 5FU or capecitabine in resected stage III colon cancer has been shown across multiple randomized trials and is widely accepted as the first-line standard regimen. If oxaliplatin cannot be administered due to advanced age (>70 years), preexisting neuropathy, or general frailty, then monotherapy with either 5FU–LU or capecitabine is acceptable.

Correct Answer: D

5) **Which of the following management options would you consider for a patient with R0 resected stage III or node-positive colon adenocarcinoma with MSI-H?**
   A) 5FU alone.
   B) CapeOx or FOLFOX.
   C) Immunotherapy with PD-1 blockade.
   D) Observation.

Expert Perspective: Patients with stage III disease have shown survival benefit from adjuvant 5FU-based chemotherapy across multiple trials, including INT-0089, but optimal management of stage III patients with MSI-H is not entirely clear. A retrospective stratification analysis using mismatch repair (MMR) status of previously randomized 1,027 patients with stage II and III colon adenocarcinoma to either 5FU with levamisole or leucovorin, or observation was reported by Sargent et al. They showed that patients with stage III colon cancer and defective MMR (dMMR) derived no benefit in overall survival from 5FU ($n = 39$) compared to surgery alone ($n = 24$) (HR, 1.01; 95% CI: 0.41 to 2.51; $P = 0.98$). Another retrospective study evaluated 32 patients with stage III MSI-H colon cancer treated by 5FU–LV ($n = 20$) or FOLFOX ($n = 12$) and noted improvement in disease-free survival in patients on the FOLFOX arm (HR: 0.17; 95% CI: 0.04 to 0.68; $P = 0.01$) compared to the 5FU-only arm. The MMR proteins do not recognize and therefore do not repair the DNA adducts formed by the oxaliplatin, which may drive the cytotoxic effect. Sinicrope et al. reported a benefit of 5FU treatment for stage III patients with MSI compared with MSS tumors (time to recurrence, $P = 0.016$; disease-free survival, $P = 0.047$; OS, $P = 0.041$). However, the beneficial treatment effect was restricted to MSI tumors with germline defect ($n = 99$) (disease-free survival: HR: 0.26; 95% CI: 0.09–0.77; $P = 0.009$) with no benefit noted in sporadic MSI tumors ($n = 245$) secondary to hypermethylation (disease-free survival: HR: 0.79; 95% CI: 0.35–1.80; $P = 0.577$). This may suggest another subclassification in colon cancer with potential for a predictive role in determining use of adjuvant therapy for stage III disease. The ATOMIC trial (combination chemotherapy with or without atezolizumab in treating patients with stage III colon cancer and deficient mismatch repair) is currently enrolling and testing whether immunotherapy can further improve the cure rate of standard chemotherapy in patients with resected MSI-H colon cancers. Currently, until there are more data evaluating the MSI-H stage III population, all medically fit patients with stage III colon cancer are recommended to receive adjuvant chemotherapy with FOLFOX.

Correct Answer: B

6) **What is the recommended duration of adjuvant chemotherapy with CapeOX in a patient with resected low risk (T3N1) R0 stage III resected colon adenocarcinoma?**
   A) Nine months.
   B) Six months.
   C) Three months.

Expert Perspective: A phase III trial by André et al. in 2003 reported that nine months versus six months of adjuvant therapy with fluorouracil does not lead to an improvement in disease-free survival (HR: 0.94; $P = 0.63$). The International Duration Evaluation of Adjuvant Therapy (IDEA) collaboration was a non-inferiority trial comparing three months to six months of therapy. Six trials, conducted in Europe and the United States, randomized 12,834 patients to three months versus six months of therapy with either CapeOx or FOLFOX. The prospective pooled analysis failed to establish non-inferiority of the three-month chemotherapy arm in patients with stage III colon cancer. However, in an analysis of a subgroup of patients with T1-3N1 cancer ($n = 7471$), the three-year disease-free survival with three months of chemotherapy (83.1%) was non-inferior to six months of chemotherapy (83.3%; HR: 1.01; 95% CI: 0.90 to 1.12). As expected, adherence was lower in the six-month group for both the 5FU/capecitabine and oxaliplatin. For example, oxaliplatin adherence in the FOLFOX arm was 91.4% for the three-month duration, and 72.8% for the six-month duration ($P = <0.001$). Neurotoxicity was significantly lower in the three-month FOLFOX arm (16.6%) than the six-month arm (47.7%). However, there was an unexpected difference in disease-free survival between the FOLFOX and CapeOx arms. Three months of CapeOx was non-inferior to six months of CapeOx in the low-risk group, with a three-year disease-free survival of 85% and 83.1% (HR: 0.85; 95% CI: 0.71 to 1.01), respectively. In contrast, non-inferiority for three versus six months of FOLFOX could not be established, with the three-year disease-free survival of 81.9% and 83.5%, respectively.

The updated OS and disease-free survival rate at five years also rejected non-inferiority between three and six months of chemotherapy in patients with stage III cancer but noted an absolute difference of only 0.4% in OS in favor of the group treated with six months of chemotherapy. Among patients treated with CapeOx, three months of therapy was not significantly non-inferior to six months of therapy for OS, with the five-year OS rate of 82·1% for the three-month group and 81·2% for the six-month group. However, in the low-risk subgroup treated with CapeOx, the point estimates and 95% CIs of the HRs for OS and disease-free survival at five years fell within the prespecified margins of non-inferiority; therefore, three months of CapeOx can be considered the standard of care for this subset.

Correct Answer: C

7) **What is the recommended duration of adjuvant chemotherapy in a patient with resected high-risk (T4, N2, or both) colon adenocarcinoma?**
   A) Nine months.
   B) Six months.
   C) Three months.

Expert Perspective: The International Duration Evaluation of Adjuvant Therapy (IDEA) collaboration was a non-inferiority trial comparing 3 months to 6 months of therapy. Six trials, conducted in Europe and the United States, randomized 12,834 patients to three months versus six months of therapy with either CapeOx or FOLFOX. The prospective pooled analysis failed to establish non-inferiority of the three-month chemotherapy arm in patients with stage III cancer, but in a preplanned analysis of a subgroup of patients with T4 or N2 stage disease or both (n = 5256), the three-year disease-free survival with three months of chemotherapy (62.7%) was inferior to six months of chemotherapy (64.4%; HR 1.12; 95% CI: 1.03–1.23; $P = 0.01$). A predictive tool was developed based on the IDEA collaborative data. The tool predicts a range of disease-free survival benefit based on T stage and N stage. For example, T1N1a patients, with a baseline cure rate of 79.6% with surgery, are predicted to get 5.6% benefit from fluoropyrimidines, plus a 2.3% benefit from three months of oxaliplatin, and an additional 0.8% benefit from six months of oxaliplatin. On the other end of the spectrum, a T4N2b patient is predicted to have a 13.9% cure rate with surgery alone and an added 11.2% benefit with fluoropyrimidines, plus a 6.4% benefit with three months of oxaliplatin and an additional 2.5% benefit from six months of oxaliplatin. This small improvement in the three-year disease-free survival rate with the use of six months versus six months of oxaliplatin along with significantly higher rates of neurotoxicity (as discussed in Q6) should be discussed with the patient.

Correct Answer: B

8) **Which of the following biological agents would you add to the adjuvant chemotherapy regimen for patients with resected stage II and III colon cancer for possible micrometastatic disease?**
   A) Bevacizumab.
   B) Cetuximab.
   C) Panitumumab.
   D) None of the above.

Expert Perspective: Several trials have investigated the use of biological agents targeting anti-VEGF (vascular endothelial growth factor) or anti-EGFR (epidermal growth factor receptor) as potential adjuvant therapy to eradicate micrometastatic disease but have so far yielded disappointing results.

- In the NSABP C-08 phase III trial, 2,672 patients with resected stage II and III colon cancer were randomized to either six months of modified FOLFOX6 or mFOLFOX6 + bevacizumab followed by six months of maintenance bevacizumab. The disease-free survival at 15 months showed benefit for the bevacizumab arm (HR: 0.61; 95% CI: 0.48–0.78; $P < 0.001$); however, after a median follow-up of 55 months, the addition of bevacizumab to mFOLFOX6 did not result in an overall significant increase in disease-free survival (HR: 0.93; 95% CI: 0.81–1.08; $P = 0.34$) or OS (HR: 0.96; 95% CI: 0.79–1.15; $P = 0.64$). The authors proposed several mechanisms for this incongruity, including a pure cytostatic effect of bevacizumab or masking of the recurrence due to decreased permeability that would obscure imaging findings, as well as the potential development of an aggressive phenotype after completion of anti-VEGF therapy based on preclinical murine models.
- The AVANT trial randomized 3,451 patients with resected high-risk stage II and stage III patients with colon cancer to either mFOLFOX4 or mFOLFOX4 + bevacizumab or CapeOx + bevacizumab followed by six months of maintenance bevacizumab for patients in the last two arms. There was no significant difference in disease-free survival (HR: 1.17; 95% CI 0.98–1.39; $P = $ NS for the mFOLFOX6 + bevacizumab arm and HR: 1.07; 95% CI 0.90–1.28; $P = $ NS for the CapeOx + bevacizumab arm) or OS (HR 1.31; 95% CI 1.03–1.67; $P = $ NS for the mFOLFOX6 + bevacizumab arm and HR 1.27; 95% CI 0.99–1.62; $P = $ NS for the CapeOx + bevacizumab arm).
- The phase III QUASAR2 trial (capecitabine versus capecitabine + bevacizumab) in 1,941 patients with high-risk stage II and stage III colon cancer also yielded no benefit with the addition of bevacizumab in the three-year disease-free survival (75.4% vs 78.4%; $P = 0.54$). The results of the ECOG 5202 (FOLFOX vs FOLFOX + bevacizumab in stage II high-risk MSI–L-18q LOH or MSS–18q LOH stage II patients) are pending.
- Anti-EGFR therapy also appeared promising, with the ability to directly target the micrometastatic tumor cells even prior to angiogenesis. However, the NCCTG phase III trial N0147, which randomized 1,847 patients with resected phase III wild-type *KRAS* colon cancer to mFOLFOX6 with or without cetuximab for six months, showed that the three-year disease-free survival favored mFOLFOX6 alone (HR 1.2; 95% CI 0.96–1.50; $P = 0.22$). In fact, the OS showed a trend toward worse survival with addition of cetuximab (HR 1.3; 95% CI 0.96–1.80; $P = 0.13$).
- The interim analysis of the PETACC-8 phase III trial, which randomized 1,602 patients with *KRAS-WT* to mFOLFOX4 with or without cetuximab, has also shown no difference

in disease-free survival (HR 1.05; 95% CI 0.85–1.29; $P = 0.66$) after a median follow-up of 39.6 months.

In summary, to date there are no data to support the use of targeted biological agents in the adjuvant therapy of colon cancer.

Correct Answer: D

Circulating tumor DNA and its implications

9) In a patient with resected low-risk stage II colon adenocarcinoma, circulating tumor DNA (ctDNA) evaluation will impact which of the following?
   A) Consideration for adjuvant chemotherapy.
   B) Duration of adjuvant chemotherapy.
   C) Monitor for relapse in conjunction with symptoms and cross-sectional imaging.
   D) None of the above.

Expert Perspective: There is an urgent need to find new biomarkers to monitor for early metastases and to monitor the efficacy of systemic adjuvant therapy beyond CEA levels. FDA-approved tests are now available to detect ctDNA in blood of patients with resected colon cancer. The Signatera™ test by Natera uses resected tumor tissue to derive a custom panel of 16 mutations for each patient. In a prospective study, 125 patients with stage I, II, and III colon cancer underwent ctDNA measurement before and after surgery. Preoperatively, ctDNA was detected in 89% of patients, while only 10% of patients had detectable ctDNA after definitive surgery. The ctDNA positive patients had a 70% chance of relapse, while the ctDNA negative patients had a 12% chance of relapse (HR: 7.2; 95% CI: 2.7–19.0; $P < 0.001$). Furthermore, ctDNA detection after adjuvant chemotherapy in seven patients was associated with rapid relapse. In contrast, the FDA-approved Guardant Reveal™ ctDNA test does not require the primary tumor for sequencing and evaluates the epigenetic signatures of aberrant DNA methylation in conjunction with tumor-derived genomic alterations. In a prospective study of 103 patients with stage I to IV colorectal cancer treated with curative intent, 84 patients had evaluable plasma drawn for evaluation of ctDNA. Follow-up at a predefined timepoint revealed that all 15 patients who had detectable ctDNA at one month had recurrence, compared to only 12 of 49 patients (24.5%) without detectable ctDNA. The Guardant assay is now being evaluated in a phase II/III COBRA trial (NCT04068103) in patients with resected stage IIA colon cancer to compare the rates of ctDNA clearance in patients with detectable ctDNA treated with or without postoperative adjuvant chemotherapy. In addition, the DYNAMIC (NCT03737539) and the PRODIGE70-CIRCULATE (NCT04120701) trials are underway.

Correct Answer: D

Cancer in a polyp

10) During screening colonoscopy, a polyp was removed from the right colon. Which of the following scenarios has the lowest risk of relapse with serial observation?
    A) A polyp removed in a single specimen with high-grade invasive carcinoma and a negative margin.
    B) A polyp removed in a single specimen with low-grade invasive carcinoma and a negative margin.
    C) A polyp removed piecemeal with low-grade carcinoma and a negative margin
    D) A polyp removed in a single specimen with carcinoma with angiolymphatic invasion.

Expert Perspective: Identification of invasive cancer cells in a polyp is an uncommon but not rare situation, occurring in 2 to 6% of resected polyps. There is controversy as to the ideal management of these, with options including observation with follow-up colonoscopy in low-risk cancers with complete excision and a definitive en bloc resection of the segment of colon and the draining lymph nodes for high-risk polyps. Risk factors for recurrence include sessile polyp growth pattern, positive margin, poor differentiation, and lymphatic or venous invasion. In case series of 114 patients, about half of the polys that contain invasive cancer are sessile and the other half pedunculated. Venous and/or lymphatic invasion occurs only rarely, and histologic grade 3 cancers incidence was about 3%. There is no consensus for the definition of a positive margin of resection. It has variably been defined as either tumor in the transected margin, less than 1 mm from the transected margin, or less than 2 mm from the transected margin. Tumor margin status cannot be reliably determined in polyps resected piecemeal when more than one fragment contains invasive cancer. Thus, patients who have a polyp containing invasive cancer cells that has been resected as a single specimen, and the cancer is identified as low grade, with negative resection margins, have a very low risk of systemic recurrence and can be observed without a definitive cancer operation.

Correct Answer: B

Recommended Readings

Andre, T., Boni, C., Navarro, M., et al. (2009). Improved overall survival with oxaliplatin, fluorouracil, and leucovorin as adjuvant treatment in stage II or III colon cancer in the MOSAIC trial. *J Clin Oncol* 27: 3109–3116.

Andre, T., Meyerhardt, J., Iveson, T., et al. (2020). Effect of duration of adjuvant chemotherapy for patients with stage III colon cancer, (IDEA collaboration): final results from a prospective, pooled analysis of six randomized, phase III trials. *Lancet Oncol* 21: 1620–1629.

Benson, A.B., III, Venook, A.P., Al-Hawary, M.M., et al. NCCN clinical practice guidelines in oncology: colon cancer. Version 2.2021. http://www.nccn.org., accessed September 22, 2022.

Cohen, R., Taieb, J., Fiskum, J., et al. (2020). Microsatellite instability in patients with stage III colon cancer receiving fluoropyrimidine with or without oxaliplatin: anACCENT pooled analysis of 12 adjuvant trials. *J Clin Oncol* 39: 642–651.

Morton, D., Seymour, M., Magill, L. et al. (2023 March 10). Preoperative chemotherapy for operable colon cancer: mature results of an international randomized controlled trial. *J Clin Oncol* 41 (8): 1541–1552. doi:10.1200/JCO.22.00046. Epub 2023 Jan 19. PMID: 36657089; PMCID: PMC10022855.

Park, I.J., You, Y.N., Agarwal, A., et al. (2012). Neoadjuvant treatment response as an early response indicator for patients with rectal cancer. *J Clin Oncol* 30: 1770–1776.

Sargent, D., Sobrero, A., Grothey, A., et al. (2009). Evidence for cure by adjuvant therapy in colon cancer: observations based on individual patient data from 20,898 patients on 18 randomized trials. *J Clin Oncol* 27: 872–877.

Sargent, D.J., Marsoni, S., Monges, G., et al. (2010). Defective mismatch repair as a predictive marker for lack of efficacy of fluorouracil-based adjuvant therapy in colon cancer. *J Clin Oncol* 28: 3219–3226.

Seitz, U., Bohnacker, S., Seewald, S., et al. (2004). Is endoscopy polypectomy an adequate therapy for malignant colorectal adenomas? Presentation of 114 patients and a review of the literature. *Dis Colon Rectum* 47: 1789–1797.

Siegel, R.L., Wagle, N.S., Cercek, A. et al. (2023 May-June). Colorectal cancer statistics, 2023. *CA Cancer J Clin* 73 (3): 233–254. doi:10.3322/caac.21772. Epub 2023 Mar 1. PMID: 36856579.

23

Early-Stage Rectal Cancer

Hannah J. Roberts, Theodore Hong, and Aparna Parikh

Massachusetts General Hospital, Harvard Medical School, Boston, MA

Introduction

Colorectal cancer is the third most common cause of cancer and the second most common cause of cancer deaths in the United States. Rectal cancer comprises nearly one third of all colorectal cancers with approximately 45,000 new cases per year. Risk factors include a personal history of adenomatous polyps greater than 1 cm or polyps with villous or tubulovillous histology, smoking, a high fat diet, a positive family history, and inflammatory bowel disease. Approximately 5% are related to inherited syndromes, such as familial adenomatous polyposis (FAP) or hereditary nonpolyposis colorectal cancer (HNPCC), otherwise known as Lynch syndrome (Chapter 47). Screening recommendations in the US have recently changed for average risk adults to start at age 45, and include colonoscopy every ten years, flexible sigmoidoscopy with fecal occult blood test every three years, or an annual fecal occult blood test. Rectal tumors are distinct from colon tumors with regards to management, primarily because the rectum lies in the narrow bony pelvis, historically making margin-negative resections more difficult to achieve than in the colon. This translates to a higher local failure rate than in colon cancer, necessitating distinct multimodality management strategies. Blood supply and lymphatic drainage are also distinct from colon cancer, leading to differing patterns of metastatic spread. The mainstay of treatment for locally advanced rectal cancers has been a combination of chemoradiotherapy and a total mesorectal excision, followed by adjuvant chemotherapy to address local and distant control. With modern approaches such as total mesorectal excision and chemoradiotherapy the local recurrence rate has improved substantially, leaving the field to entertain if all modalities are necessary for every patient, while also thinking of strategies to mitigate the threat of distant failure.

Cancer Consult: Expertise in Clinical Practice, Volume 1: Solid Tumors & Supportive Care,
Second Edition. Edited by Syed A. Abutalib, Maurie Markman, Al B. Benson III, and Hope S. Rugo.
© 2024 John Wiley & Sons Ltd. Published 2024 by John Wiley & Sons Ltd.

Case Study 1

A 50-year-old woman presents with a partially circumferential nonobstructing mass from 6.0 cm to 10.0 cm from the anal verge found on screening colonoscopy. MRI of the pelvis revealed an enlarged presacral lymph node on the mesorectal fascia. A PET-CT was performed that revealed an FDG-avid primary tumor and avidity in the presacral lymph node.

1) What is the best initial management for this patient?
   A) Preoperative total neoadjuvant therapy with or without adjuvant chemotherapy
   B) Preoperative chemoradiation with capecitabine or 5-FU and adjuvant chemotherapy
   C) Upfront surgery (total mesorectal excision)

Expert Perspective: The treatment of locally advanced rectal cancer has evolved in recent years. While the standard of care included chemoradiation followed by total mesorectal excision followed by adjuvant FOLFOX, this sequence has been challenged by the results of the randomized PRODIGE 23 and RAPIDO trials, which have made total neoadjuvant therapy the current standard of care for locally advanced rectal cancers, particularly tumors (such as in this case) that are T3, T4, or node-positive (Table 23.1).

- PRODIGE 23 looked at clinical T3 or T4 rectal cancers and randomized patients to neoadjuvant chemotherapy and chemoradiation or standard therapy. The neoadjuvant therapy arm received six cycles of mFOLFIRINOX followed by long-course radiotherapy (50.4 Gy in 28 fractions) with concurrent capecitabine, followed by surgery and adjuvant mFOLFOX for six cycles or capecitabine for four cycles. The standard therapy arm received long-course radiotherapy with concurrent capecitabine (50.4 Gy in 28 fractions) followed by total mesorectal excision, followed by adjuvant chemotherapy with 12 cycles of modified FOLFOX or eight cycles of capecitabine. The primary endpoint, three-year disease-free survival, was improved with the neoadjuvant therapy arm at 76% vs 69% in the standard therapy arm. Likewise, the neoadjuvant therapy arm also performed better with distant metastasis-free survival (HR 0.64; 95% CI 0.44–0.93; P = 0.017), and there was a trend towards improved OS (HR 0.65; 95% CI 0.40–1.05; P = 0.0773). The pathologic complete response rate was 30% in the neoadjuvant therapy arm and 12% in the standard arm. There was no difference in adverse events (Conroy et al. 2021). While not purely total neoadjuvant therapy given the use of adjuvant chemotherapy, the results of this trial support the use of upfront chemotherapy and chemoradiation therapy. Following the results of this trial, the neoadjuvant therapy regimen including mFOLFIRINOX for six cycles followed by long-course chemoradiation has become an accepted standard neoadjuvant option for locally advanced rectal cancer.
- The results of the RAPIDO trial also added to this paradigm shift towards total neoadjuvant therapy, although with a different regimen. This trial included patients with clinical T4, N2, involved mesorectal fascia, extramural vascular invasion, or enlarged lymph nodes. The total neoadjuvant therapy arm in this trial used short-course radiation (25 Gy in five fractions), first explored by the Swedish Rectal Trial Group in the context of total mesorectal excision, followed by 18 weeks of chemotherapy (six cycles of CAPOX or nine cycles of FOLFOX), followed by surgery. Adjuvant chemotherapy with CAPOX or FOLFOX was optional per physician discretion or hospital policy. The standard therapy arm received long-course radiation (50.4 Gy in 28 fractions) with concurrent capecitabine, followed by surgery, followed by adjuvant chemotherapy (with eight cycles of CAPOX or 12 cycles of FOLFOX) if stipulated by hospital policy. The primary endpoint, disease-related treatment

Table 23.1 AJCC staging of colorectal cancer.

TNM	Description
Tis	Carcinoma *in situ*, intramucosal carcinoma (involvement of lamina propria with no extension through muscularis mucosae).
T1	Tumor invades the submucosa (through the muscularis mucosa but not into the muscularis propria).
T2	Tumor invades the muscularis propria.
T3	Tumor invades through the muscularis propria into pericolorectal tissues.
T4a	Tumor invades* through the visceral peritoneum (including gross perforation of the bowel through tumor and continuous invasion of tumor through areas of inflammation to the surface of the visceral peritoneum).
T4b	Tumor directly invades* or adheres¶ to adjacent organs or structures.
N1a	One regional lymph node is positive.
N1b	Two or three regional lymph nodes are positive.
N1c	No regional lymph nodes are positive, but there are tumor deposits in the subserosa, mesentery, nonperitonealized pericolic, or perirectal/mesorectal tissues.
N2a	Four to six regional lymph nodes are positive.
N2b	Seven or more regional lymph nodes are positive.
M1a	Metastasis to 1 site or organ is identified without peritoneal metastasis.
M1b	Metastasis to ≥2 sites or organs is identified without peritoneal metastasis.
M1c	Metastasis to the peritoneal surface is identified alone or with other site or organ metastases.

* Direct invasion in T4 includes invasion of other organs or other segments of the colorectum as a result of direct extension through the serosa, as confirmed on microscopic examination or, for cancers in a retroperitoneal or subperitoneal location, direct invasion of other organs or structures by virtue of extension beyond the muscularis propria (i.e., respectively, a tumor on the posterior wall of the descending colon invading the left kidney or lateral abdominal wall; or a mid- or distal rectal cancer with invasion of prostate, seminal vesicles, cervix, or vagina).
A tumor that is adherent to other organs or structures, grossly, is classified cT4b. However, if no tumor is present in the adhesion microscopically, the classification should be pT1-4a, depending on the anatomical depth of wall invasion. The V and L classification should be used to identify the presence or absence of vascular or lymphatic invasion, whereas the PN prognostic factor should be used for perineural invasion.

failure, was 23.7% in the total neoadjuvant therapy arm and 30.4% in the standard arm (HR 0.75, 95% CI 0.60–0.95, P = 0.019). The pathologic complete response rate was improved in the total neoadjuvant therapy arm at 28% versus 14% in the standard arm, with no difference in surgical complications. Although there was an improvement in distant metastasis-free survival, there was no difference in OS. However, these results are somewhat difficult to interpret given the lack of standardization of adjuvant chemotherapy, as half of the patients in the control arm received no chemotherapy (Bahadoer et al. 2021). These results add to the growing body of literature supporting total neoadjuvant therapy.

The outcomes with short-course radiation versus long-course radiation with concurrent chemotherapy were evaluated by the TROG Intergroup trial (Ngan et al. 2012). Short-course radiation was given as 5 Gy × 5 fractions, and long-course was 50.4 Gy in 1.8 Gy fractions with concurrent

225 mg/m² 5FU. The primary endpoint was local recurrence. All patients received MRI of the pelvis or endoscopic ultrasound. There was no difference in local control, overall survival, or late toxicity between the two regimens. Both regimens are therefore considered acceptable.

Although total neoadjuvant therapy is now a generally accepted standard of care, the specific total neoadjuvant therapy regimen varies greatly by practice patterns, given the distinct regimens tested in these trials, and needs to be tailored to each individual patient. The currently accepted total neoadjuvant therapy approaches include short-course radiation or long-course chemoradiation followed by FOLFOX/CAPOX, or FOLFIRINOX, followed by long-course chemoradiation as summarized in Table 23.2. Whether it is safe and effective to mix and match these regimens has not yet been tested in clinical trials. Although it is possible that an upfront chemoradiation approach may lead to more clinical complete responses, this has not been tested with the intensification of chemotherapy with FOLFIRINOX. As such, the use of FOLFIRINOX vs FOLFOX or short- versus long-course radiation and the sequence of these therapies within total neoadjuvant therapy depends on the comfort and joint decision making of the multidisciplinary team, with these major trials to guide specific combinations and sequencing. The OPRA trial, as discussed below, will further inform on the use of induction versus consolidation chemotherapy with rates of clinical complete response following total neoadjuvant therapy. Although pelvic radiation plus sensitizing chemotherapy with a fluoropyrimidine (chemoradiotherapy) before surgery has been standard care for locally advanced rectal cancer in North America. Whether neoadjuvant FOLFOX

Table 23.2 Examples of Total Neoadjuvant Therapy Regimens.

First Therapy	Second Therapy	Adjuvant Therapy	Trial
Chemoradiation: 50.4 Gy IMRT with continuous infusion of fluorouracil 250 mg/m² on days 1 to 14 and 22 to 35 of radiotherapy and oxaliplatin 50 mg/m² on days 1, 8, 22, and 29 of radiotherapy	FOLFOX x 3 cycles (Oxaliplatin 100 mg/m² administered as a 2-hour infusion, followed by a 2-hour infusion of leucovorin 400 mg/m², followed by a continuous 46-hour infusion of fluorouracil 2,400 mg/m², repeated on day 15 for a total of three cycles)	None	CAO/ARO/AIO-13
mFOLFIRINOX x 6 cycles (Oxaliplatin 85 mg/m², irinotecan 180 mg/m², leucovorin 400 mg/m², and fluorouracil 2400 mg/m² continuous infusion every 14 days for 6 cycles	50.4 Gy with concurrent capecitabine 800 mg/m² twice daily orally.	Three months of mFOLFOX or capecitabine (Oxaliplatin 85 mg/m², leucovorin 400 mg/m², and 400 mg/m² fluorouracil bolus followed by 46-hour continuous infusion with 2400 mg/m² every 14 days or capecitabine 1250 mg/m² orally twice daily on days 1–14 every 21 days	PRODIGE

Table 23.2 (Continued)

First Therapy	Second Therapy	Adjuvant Therapy	Trial
25 Gy in five fractions	6 cycles CAPOX or 9 cycles of FOLFOX (Capecitabine 1000 mg/m² orally twice daily on days 1–14, oxaliplatin 130 mg/m² on day 1, every 21 days or FOLFOX4: oxaliplatin 85 mg/m² on day 1, leucovorin 200 mg/m² on days 1 and 2, followed by bolus fluorouracil 400 mg/m² and fluorouracil 600 mg/m² for 22 hours on days 1 and 2, every 14 days)	CAPOX or FOLFOX4 per physician discretion or hospital policy	RAPIDO
FOLFOX4 x two cycles (oxaliplatin 85 mg/m² and fluorouracil 400 mg/m² IV bolus d1 and 600 mg/m² IV continuous infusion with leucovorin 200 mg/m² d1, d15, and every 15 days.)	Chemoradiation: 45–50.4 Gy with oral Tegafur* 1200 mg/day	four to six cycles of bolus 5-FU (425 mg/m²) and leucovorin (200 mg/m²) on days 1–5, every 28 days per physician discretion	Calvo et al. 2006

* Not available in the US.

can be used in lieu of chemoradiotherapy is an alternative approach was reported by investigators of PROSPECT trial. In this trial adults with rectal cancer that had been clinically staged as T2 node-positive, T3 node-negative, or T3 node-positive who were candidates for sphincter-sparing surgery were eligible to participate. The primary end point was disease-free survival. At a median follow-up of 58 months, FOLFOX was non-inferior to chemoradiotherapy for disease-free survival (hazard ratio for disease recurrence or death, 0.92; 90.2% confidence interval [CI], 0.74 to 1.14; P = 0.005 for noninferiority). Five-year disease-free survival was 80.8% (95% CI, 77.9 to 83.7) in the FOLFOX group and 78.6% (95% CI, 75.4 to 81.8) in the chemoradiotherapy group. The groups were similar with respect to overall survival (hazard ratio for death, 1.04; 95% CI, 0.74 to 1.44) and local recurrence (hazard ratio, 1.18; 95% CI, 0.44 to 3.16). In the FOLFOX group, 53 patients (9.1%) received preoperative chemoradiotherapy and 8 (1.4%) received postoperative. The trial will continue to follow the participants and collect additional data on disease-free survival, overall survival, local recurrence-free survival, and other secondary endpoints for 8 years. chemoradiotherapy.

Correct Answer: A

2) What is the historical background of treating rectal cancer with neoadjuvant therapy?

Expert Perspective: The German Rectal Study first published results in 2004 and became the basis for the sequence of rectal cancer therapy for the last 15 years. This trial compared preoperative chemoradiation with postoperative chemoradiation in patients with T3, T4, or node-positive disease. The preoperative treatment included 50.4 Gy with three or four fields in 28 fractions with concurrent 5FU (1000 mg/m^2 over five days during the first and fifth weeks). The postoperative regimen was the same but with an additional 5.4 Gy boost to the tumor bed (55.8 Gy total). Surgery included total mesorectal excision. Adjuvant chemotherapy, which included four cycles of bolus 5FU (500 mg/m^2/d, five times weekly every four weeks), was then given four weeks following total mesorectal excision in the preoperative chemoradiation arm or four weeks following chemoradiation in the postoperative arm. The results of the trial heavily favored the preoperative chemoradiation arm. Compliance of both chemoradiation and adjuvant chemotherapy was improved in the preoperative arm. The rate of sphincter preservation was nearly double in the preoperative arm (39% vs 19%, $P < 0.004$). Local recurrence was 6% in the preoperative chemoradiation arm vs 13% in the postoperative arm ($P = 0.006$). Furthermore, there were fewer grade 3 to 4 side effects. Notably, there was no difference in overall survival (OS), disease-free survival, or the rate of distant metastasis, but distant recurrence was still more common than local recurrence, with rates of 36 to 38% (Sauer et al. 2004). Given the improvements in local control with higher rates of compliance and lower toxicity with improved rates of sphincter preservation, preoperative chemoradiation became the standard of care. This sequence remained standard of care for a long period of time.

The German Rectal Study, when the field started to note that with neoadjuvant treatment up to 36% could achieve a clinical complete response, inspired further study of more intensified preoperative therapy with total neoadjuvant therapy (Cercek et al. 2018, Habr-Gama et al. 1998). The CAO/ARO/AIO-12 trial evaluated pathologic complete response rates in patients with stage II or III rectal cancer following chemoradiation with concurrent fluorouracil/oxaliplatin and either induction or consolidation chemotherapy with three cycles of FOLFOX followed by surgery. The pathologic complete response rate in those treated with induction chemotherapy was 17% and 25% in those who underwent consolidation, and only the consolidation arm met the prespecified endpoint ($P < .001$). They also found better compliance rates with upfront chemoradiation and no difference in surgical morbidity (Fokas et al. 2019). The logic for total neoadjuvant therapy is multifactorial and includes not only an opportunity to decrease distant failure with early systemic treatment but also less toxicity, better compliance, improved R0 resection rates, and increasingly, an opportunity to entertain nonoperative management.

There were many single institution and smaller total neoadjuvant therapy approaches that were evaluated, but ultimately the publication of the randomized PRODIGE 23 and RAPIDO trials began to establish a new standard of care for these patients.

3) The patient undergoes total neoadjuvant therapy with neoadjuvant FOLFIRINOX followed by long-course chemoradiation. What is the most appropriate concurrent chemotherapy regimen?

A) Capecitabine or continuous infusion 5-FU
B) Bolus 5-FU
C) FOLFOX or CAPEOX
D) Any of the above

Expert Perspective: Although 5-FU, capecitabine, and oxaliplatin are all radiosensitizers, the specific concurrent chemotherapy regimen given with radiation may include capecitabine or continuous infusion 5-FU. A US Intergroup study demonstrated superior outcomes in rectal cancer with continuous infusion over bolus 5-FU (O'Connell et al. 1994). Multiple trials in colorectal cancer have demonstrated similar outcomes between 5-FU and orally administered capecitabine. Capecitabine is often more convenient for patients. There is no role for additional concurrent oxaliplatin. NSABP R-04, a phase III randomized trial of 1,608 patients with stage II and III rectal cancer, looked at preoperative continuous infusion 5-FU (225 mg/m^2 day for seven days/week throughout radiotherapy) or capecitabine (825 mg/m^2 orally twice daily throughout the course of radiotherapy) with or without oxaliplatin (50 mg/m^2 intravenously weekly for five days during radiotherapy) with 50.4–55.8 Gy radiation therapy. Of note, total mesorectal excision was not mandated in this trial. There was no difference in the pathologic complete response rate with concurrent capecitabine or 5-FU without oxaliplatin. Although there was no benefit with the addition of oxaliplatin with regards to local-regional failure, disease-free survival, or OS, there was, however, an increase in grade 3–4 diarrhea with its use (Allegra C. et al. 2015). Therefore, the accepted concurrent chemotherapy regimens include either capecitabine or continuous infusion 5-FU.

Correct Answer: A

4) Upon reevaluation with sigmoidoscopy and MRI of the pelvis, the patient is found to have a clinical complete response. What is the next best course of management?
   A) Proceed with total mesorectal excision
   B) Watchful waiting
   C) Give additional chemotherapy

Expert Perspective: Although the correct answer is A, because total mesorectal excision remains the standard of care, there is a growing interest in the potential for nonoperative management of rectal cancer. Surgery with total mesorectal excision includes either a low anterior resection or an abdominoperineal resection, which results in a permanent colostomy. However, even in patients who do not have a permanent colostomy, there is significant morbidity with regards to bowel function related to decreased reservoir capacity, incontinence, and sexual dysfunction.

There have been prospective studies evaluating the possibility of nonoperative management. A Brazilian study by Habr-Gama et al. evaluated 183 patients with clinical stage I to III rectal cancer who underwent chemoradiation with 50.4 Gy and six cycles of 5-FU delivered every 21 days. On endoscopic evaluation, 90 of 183 patients (49%) had a clinical complete response. Of these patients, 28 (31%) eventually developed a recurrence, 17 of which occurred during the first year (Habr-Gama et al. 2014). More recently, the OPRA trial included those with stage II to III rectal cancers randomized to chemoradiation followed by FOLFOX or CAPEOX, versus FOLFOX or CAPEOX followed by chemoradiation. Patients were restaged eight weeks following total neoadjuvant therapy with endoscopy and MRI. Of 304 patients who underwent TNT, 74% (225/304) were offered watchful waiting, and ultimately 53% (95% CI 45–62) in the upfront chemoradiotherapy arm and 41% (95% CI 33–50, $P = 0.01$) in the induction chemotherapy arm achieved organ preservation at three years in intention-to-treat analysis (Garcia-Aguilar et al. 2022). These results are encouraging, suggesting that organ preservation may be feasible in select patients.

Table 23.3 Frequency of follow-up surveillance studies following management (adapted from the OPRA study protocol).

	Year 1	Year 2	Year 3–5	Year >5
Digital rectal exam	4 months	4 months	6 months	12 months
Endoscopy	4 months	4 months	6 months	12 months
CEA	4 months	4 months	6–12 months	12 months
MRI	6 months	6 months	12 months	N/A
CT Imaging	12 months	12 months	12 months	12 months

However, there is good reason to be cautious about organ preservation. Local recurrences can occur beyond five years despite treatment to the primary site. Recurrences may occur in the deep mesorectal fat and can go undetected by endoscopy alone. Therefore, watchful waiting must be wary of late local recurrences with a close follow-up schedule that includes digital rectal exams, endoscopy, and MRI surveillance. Although the optimal timing of follow-up has not yet been determined, the OPRA trial has specified follow-up as summarized in Table 23.3.

In the absence of a clinical trial, organ preservation, though a reasonable option for select patients, should still be viewed as experimental. As total neoadjuvant therapy becomes more common, more clinical complete responses will be observed. At this point in time, it appears feasible that a subset of patients may safely forgo surgery; however, the strategies to optimize and monitor this subset are still being studied. Sequencing may be an important area to address, particularly if organ preservation is the stated goal up front, while being cautious of those patients at highest risk for distant recurrence. Patients with a clinical complete response to total neoadjuvant therapy should be encouraged to explore ongoing nonoperative clinical trials or proceed with surgery, as this remains the most well-studied treatment paradigm.

Correct Answer: A

Case Study 2

A 60-year-old woman presented with a T2N1 rectal cancer detected on screening colonoscopy. The patient underwent neoadjuvant chemoradiation followed by surgery, with pathology showing an ypT2N1 tumor.

5) **What is the next best step?**
    A) Observation
    B) Adjuvant FOLFOX chemotherapy
    C) Both A and B are reasonable options based on patient preference.

Expert Perspective: Adjuvant chemotherapy has been studied in the context of the GITSG7175, NSABP R-01, and NSABP R-02. The OS was improved in both GITSG and NSABP R-01; however, it was not in NSABP R-02. The ADORE study was a randomized phase II study for patients who received chemoradiation therapy and total mesorectal excision with ypT3-4 or node-positive disease. Patients were randomized to receive either 5-FU and leucovorin or FOLFOX for four cycles. There was a disease-free survival benefit with FOLFOX in both pathologic stage II and III patients, but only a survival benefit in stage III patients. Given this patient's pathologic stage III disease, adjuvant chemotherapy should be recommended. Of note, the role of adjuvant therapy in the setting of total neoadjuvant therapy is not well understood, though PRODIGE included three months of adjuvant mFOLFOX or capecitabine and RAPIDO allowed patients to receive adjuvant chemotherapy if specified by physician discretion or hospital policy. It would therefore be reasonable to consider adjuvant chemotherapy in select high-risk patients with persistent pathologic disease.

Correct Answer: B

Case Study 3

A 28-year-old man presented to his primary care physician with two years of rectal bleeding. Digital rectal exam revealed a palpable mass in the rectum. A colonoscopy was performed and was notable for a small sessile mass 6 cm proximal to the anal verge measuring 21 mm. Biopsy showed moderately differentiated adenocarcinoma, microsatellite stable. The CT scan staging was negative for distant metastatic disease. MRI of the pelvis showed a 2 cm mass, about 5.2 cm from the top of the anal sphincter. He was staged as T1/T2 N0 rectal cancer.

6) What is the best management for this patient?
   A) Wide local excision
   B) Transabdominal resection/total mesorectal excision
   C) Total neoadjuvant therapy
   D) A or B

Expert Perspective: Both wide local excision and total mesorectal excision should be discussed with this young patient. Candidates for wide local excision include T1 tumors <3 cm in size within 8 cm of anal verge involving less than 30% of the bowel circumference. Preoperative imaging should show no lymphadenopathy. Histology should be well to moderately differentiated. The patient should be counseled that while there is significantly reduced morbidity with regards to bowel and sexual function with wide local excision, recurrence rates are significantly higher. Furthermore, there is a chance that surgery could reveal high-risk features that would necessitate a completion total mesorectal excision.

Several studies have evaluated recurrence following wide local excision and total mesorectal excision (low anterior resection or abdominoperineal resection) in T1 adenocarcinomas. Recurrence rates are consistently more than double with wide local excision. This has not translated into a survival benefit at five years; however, a ten-year follow-up did find an increased rate of cancer-related death after four years in those who underwent transanal excision. While many argue that these recurrences can be appropriately salvaged with total mesorectal excision, this requires close long-term surveillance so the curative window is not missed. Furthermore, salvage surgery is associated with increased morbidity and lower rates of sphincter preservation compared to upfront total mesorectal excision, highlighting the importance of appropriate patient selection.

Although some patients may opt for the improved quality of life with wide local excision and accept the higher risk of failure, it is crucial that they be willing to undergo close surveillance to monitor for recurrence. Surveillance should include digital rectal exams, proctoscopy, and MRI with contrast or EUS every three to six months for two years and then every six months up to five years. Colonoscopy should be performed one year following surgery, and for advanced adenomas, yearly thereafter. In the absence of an advanced adenoma this may be repeated in three years followed by five-year intervals.

Correct Answer: D

Case Study continued: The patient declined radical surgery due to concerns about the morbidity and opted for wide local excision. Pathology showed a 2.2 cm moderately differentiated adenocarcinoma involving 0/1 lymph node (pT1N0) with lymphovascular invasion and perineural invasion. Margins were negative, with a mucosal margin of 0.6 cm and a radial margin of 0.9 cm.

7) **What is the appropriate management for this patient? What if he continues to refuse invasive surgery?**
   A) Adjuvant chemoradiation
   B) Adjuvant chemotherapy
   C) Adjuvant radiation
   D) Completion total mesorectal excision

Expert Perspective: While the patient's surgery achieved negative margins for his stage I (pT1N0) tumor, the lymphovascular invasion and perineural invasion are considered high-risk features that warrant completion total mesorectal excision. Several studies have shown significantly worse outcomes with perineural invasion and lymphovascular invasion. A multivariate analysis of colorectal cancer patients by Lieberg et al. found perineural invasion to be an independent prognostic factor for poorer outcomes and found that those with perineural invasion had significantly worse five-year OS of 25% vs 72%. Furthermore, patients with node-negative disease with perineural invasion had significantly worse disease-free survival and OS than node-positive patients without perineural invasion, highlighting the importance of this pathologic feature (Liebig et al. 2009). Lymphovascular invasion has also been shown to have high rates of local failure and occult lymph node involvement. Additional high-risk features include positive margins, poorly differentiated tumors, and deep invasion to the lower third of the submucosal layer.

Although less morbid, wide local excision does not adequately stage the nodal basin and has higher rates of failure even in T1 patients. As such, patients with pT1 tumors with any high-risk feature should be counseled regarding additional management. This ideally includes transabdominal resection with total mesorectal excision. Total mesorectal excision is the complete excision of the visceral mesorectum to the level of the levator ani removing the primary tumor and surrounding fatty lymphovascular tissue. Lymph nodes are scattered throughout the mesorectum and are neither palpable nor mappable at < 3 mm. This resection technique allows for en bloc removal of the lymph nodes in this high-risk area.

Patients who are not surgical candidates or who decline surgery should be offered chemoradiation or short-course radiation, with possible adjuvant chemotherapy. Data on adjuvant chemoradiation is relatively scarce. A metanalysis including 4,674 patients evaluated outcomes following pT1-T2 rectal cancer followed by observation, total mesorectal excision, or adjuvant chemoradiation. Among patients with high-risk T1 tumors, recurrence rates were 13.6% with observation, 4.1% (1.7–9.4%) with total mesorectal excision, and 3.9% (2.0–7.5%) with chemoradiation (van Oostendorp et al. 2020). The majority of included studies were retrospective and heterogeneous, limiting a conclusion regarding completion total mesorectal excision versus adjuvant chemoradiation, but the significantly higher rate of failure with no additional treatment is clear. The ongoing multicenter TESAR trial in the Netherlands aims to further study outcomes and quality of life between adjuvant chemoradiation and completion total mesorectal excision. This trial randomizes patients with intermediate risk pT1 and T2 tumors who have undergone local excision to adjuvant chemoradiation versus radical surgery. The primary outcome is three-year local recurrence, while secondary outcomes will evaluate morbidity, disease-free survival, OS, stoma rate, functional outcomes, cost, and health-related quality of life. The results of this non-inferiority trial will hopefully further inform us regarding the potential for organ preservation in high-risk early stage rectal cancers.

In the absence of total mesorectal excision, this high-risk patient should be encouraged to undergo adjuvant chemoradiation to reduce the risk of local recurrence.

Correct Answer: D

Case Study continued: Following adjuvant therapy with chemoradiation and adjuvant capecitabine, the patient declined close follow-up. He ultimately underwent CT staging two years later that showed no evidence of distant metastasis. However, MRI of the pelvis showed a possible 1.9 cm presacral soft tissue recurrence adherent to the posterior wall of the rectum.

8) **What is the next best step in management for the patient's local recurrence?**
    A) Wide local excision and chemotherapy
    B) Total mesorectal excision
    C) Re-irradiation

Expert Perspective: Althoughthe patient's priorities and wishes are of utmost importance, we would continue to recommend a complete surgical resection with total mesorectal excision.

Given the dose constraints with re-irradiation, radiation would only be a palliative measure. We would strongly encourage that this patient with localized disease pursue a more definitive approach. Surgery would entail an LAR, which includes a coloanal anastomosis with a temporary diverting ileostomy.

There is greater morbidity with salvage total mesorectal excision compared to upfront total mesorectal excision. In an effort to maximize quality of life, surgeons have tried sphincter-saving procedures and reservoir techniques to minimize fecal incontinence and urgency, as well as nerve sparing techniques to reduce the risk of sexual dysfunction. The hypogastric nerves, inferior to the hypogastric plexus, presacral nerves, and the splanchnic nerves are most at risk of damage from surgery. However, even with nerve-sparing techniques complete functional preservation may not be maintained. Particularly in this case of recurrent disease, with the additional postradiation scar tissue, tumor removal is the core priority, and nerve sparing may not be possible. The patient must be counseled regarding his risk of bowel and sexual dysfunction. Given his recurrent disease, he should also be advised to undergo adjuvant chemotherapy, though its use in this setting is not well defined.

Correct Answer: B

Case Study 4

A 58-year-old man with a history of well controlled Crohn's disease not on active therapy underwent a screening colonoscopy that revealed an area of ulceration in the rectum that was biopsied, showing adenocarcinoma. MRI of the pelvis showed a 5.1 cm rectal mass with extramural extension and four suspicious mesorectal lymph nodes. CT staging was negative for distant metastases.

9) What is the next best step in management?
A) Neoadjuvant chemotherapy
B) Inflammatory bowel disease with short-course radiation (5 Gy × 5)
C) Inflammatory bowel disease with long-course chemoradiation (45–50.4 Gy)
D) Upfront surgery
E) B or C.

Expert Perspective: Patients with IBD (Crohn's disease or ulcerative colitis) have a higher incidence of colorectal cancer, with one population study from 1998 to 2010 observing this risk to be 60% higher than the general population (Herrinton et al. 2012). This incidence is thought to be lower with Crohn's disease than with ulcerative colitis. However, the treatment for rectal lesions is complicated by the fact that those with inflammatory bowel disease may have higher rates of acute toxicity from radiation, though this risk is diminished in more modern studies.

In one series from Massachusetts General Hospital, 28 patients with inflammatory bowel disease were treated with abdominal or pelvic radiation between 1970 and 1999. The overall incidence of severe toxicity was 46% (13/28 patients), and 21% (6/28) were unable to complete radiotherapy. Late toxicity requiring hospitalization or surgical intervention was 29% (8/28). However, the authors compared those treated with conventional techniques versus more specialized modern techniques and found a significant difference in late toxicity, 73% versus 23% ($P = 0.02$). This highlights the need to consider modern techniques, such as IMRT, as well as the anatomical location of the tumor with regards to the bowel.

Similarly, a more modern series of 19 patients treated at Stanford University from 1997 to 2011 found that acute grade ⩾ 2 toxicity occurred in 28% of patients treated with IMRT versus 100% of patients with more traditional 3D treatment ($P = 0.01$). Acute and late grade ⩾ 3 toxicity occurred acutely in two patients (11%) and one patient (6%), respectively. This more modern series suggests that select patients with inflammatory bowel disease may safely undergo abdominopelvic radiation.

A larger study of 161 patients with inflammatory bowel disease and rectal cancer from the Dutch pathology registry (PALGA) found similar results supporting the safety of radiation in those with inflammatory bowel disease. Of these, 41% (66 of 161) underwent preoperative therapy. Severe acute grade ⩾ 3 toxicity occurred in 0.0% (0 of 32), 7.7% (1 of 13), and 28.6% (6 of 21) in patients who underwent short-course radiation therapy, long-course radiation therapy, or chemoradiation, respectively ($P = 0.004$). The 30-day postoperative complication rate was no different between preoperative therapy groups. This study suggests that preoperative therapy may be safely given and that perhaps short-course treatment is better tolerated; however, this conclusion is limited by small numbers and events. Caution should be taken in patients with active inflammation, as these retrospective studies capture patients with inflammatory bowel disease more broadly.

Patients with high-risk disease and well-controlled inflammatory bowel disease should be considered for preoperative therapy. Patients should be counseled regarding possible increased adverse effects of radiation and chemoradiation; however, they may be reassured that modern radiation techniques have significantly improved the rates of acute and late toxicity. Patients with active inflammation should be treated cautiously, depending on the degree of severity and the patient's anatomy. Well-controlled inflammatory bowel disease should not preclude patients from consideration of total neoadjuvant therapy. In this patient with high-risk disease and well-controlled inflammatory bowel disease, we would recommend consideration of total neoadjuvant therapy with either short-course radiation or long-course chemoradiation.

Correct Answer: E

Case Study 5

A 51-year-old woman presents with a T3N1c rectal cancer that is found to be mismatch repair deficient (dMMR).

10) **What is the next best step?**
   A) Upfront total mesorectal excision
   B) Chemoradiation followed by total mesorectal excision and adjuvant chemotherapy
   C) Neoadjuvant chemotherapy followed by chemoradiation and surgery
   D) Neoadjuvant immunotherapy

Expert Perspective: Mismatch repair (MMR) is the cellular process that corrects mismatched base pairs and small insertion-deletion loops (indels) that form during replication. A deficiency in MMR leads to accumulation of these mutations, creating new satellite DNA sequences that can be measured as microsatellite-high (MSH-H) or microsatellite-intact (MSI-I). MMR mutations may occur either sporadically by epigenetic silencing of the MLH1 promoter region or through a germline mutation in MLH1, MSH2, MSH6, PMS2, or EPCAM such as with Lynch Syndrome. MSI-H/dMMR status impacts a tumor's response to treatment and pattern of metastatic spread, as well as having implications for familial screening. The detection of dMMR/MSH-H tumors is therefore recommended for all colorectal cancers.

dMMR/MSI-H status is both a prognostic and predictive marker, with a more favorable prognosis in early stage tumors but with limited benefit of 5-FU based chemotherapy. Although total neoadjuvant therapy has moved adjuvant chemotherapy to the upfront setting, those with MSI-H tumors may not receive the same benefit as those with tumors that are MSI-I. A retrospective analysis from Memorial Sloan Kettering Cancer Center found that 29% (6 of 21) of patients with dMMR progressed on neoadjuvant chemotherapy, while zero pMMR patients progressed and 89% pMMR had tumor downstaging (3:1 pairing; $P = 0.0001$). Analysis using patient organoids replicated this resistance to FOLFOX chemotherapy. Meanwhile, the pathologic complete response rate of dMMR and pMMR was similar in those receiving upfront chemoradiation (Cercek et al. 2020). This suggests that patients with dMMR have similar response rates to chemoradiation, but more limited responses to chemotherapy. While this study was small and retrospective in design, total neoadjuvant therapy should be undertaken with caution and requires close monitoring for progression during induction chemotherapy.

Recently, checkpoint inhibitors have been shown to be beneficial in patients with metastatic dMMR tumors; however, their use in the localized neoadjuvant setting is not well understood. A recent phase 2 study from Memorial Sloan Kettering Cancer Center evaluated the use of PD-1 blockade with dostarlimab in patients with dMMR stage II or III rectal cancer. Patients were given six months of dostarlimab therapy alone. All 12 patients achieved a clinical complete response with at least six months of follow-up. Although these results are promising, longer follow-up is needed (Cercek et al. 2022). In the recent NICHE study, patients with dMMR and pMMR colon cancer were given combination ipilimumab and nivolumab. After a median follow-up of 25 months, all patients with dMMR tumors (32 of 32) had a pathologic response, including 69% (22 of 32) with a complete response. In those with pMMR tumors, 30% (9 of 30) had a pathologic response, including 10% (3 of 30) complete responses (Verschoor et al. 2022). The ongoing phase II SWOG trial evaluating the use of neoadjuvant nivolumab and ipilimumab combined with short-course radiation in MSI-H/dMMR locally advanced rectal tumors will further inform this question.

Correct Answer: D

Case Study continued: For this patient with a dMMR rectal cancer, an upfront immunotherapy approach may be most advantageous given the promising results above; however, given the short follow- up in available data, this would ideally be done in the setting of a clinical trial. However, given the lack of longer follow-up, it would not be unreasonable to offer neoadjuvant chemoradiation followed by surgery. Additionally, it would be reasonable to consider total neoadjuvant therapy as an alternative option, though the patient should be monitored closely for progression on induction 5-FU based chemotherapy.

Recommended Readings

Allegra, C.J., Yothers, G., O'Connell, M.J., et al. (2015). Neoadjuvant 5-FU or capecitabine plus radiation with or without oxaliplatin in rectal cancer patients: a phase III randomized clinical trial. *J Natl Cancer Inst* 107 (11): 2–9. doi: 10.1093/jnci/djv248.

Bahadoer, R.R., Dijkstra, E.A., van Etten, B., et al. (2021). Short-course radiotherapy followed by chemotherapy before total mesorectal excision (TME) versus preoperative chemoradiotherapy, TME, and optional adjuvant chemotherapy in locally advanced rectal cancer (RAPIDO): a randomised, open-label, phase 3 trial. *Lancet Oncol* 22 (1): 29–42. doi: 10.1016/S1470-2045(20)30555-6.

Basch, E., Dueck, A.C., Mitchell, S.A., et al. (2023). Patient-reported outcomes during and after treatment for locally advanced rectal cancer in the PROSPECT trial (Alliance N1048). *J Clin Oncol* Jun 4: JCO2300903. doi: 10.1200/JCO.23.00903. Epub ahead of print. PMID: 37270691.

Calvo, F.A., Serrano, F.J., Diaz-González, J.A., et al. (2006). Improved incidence of pT0 downstaged surgical specimens in locally advanced rectal cancer (LARC) treated with induction oxaliplatin plus 5-fluorouracil and preoperative chemoradiation. *Ann Oncol* 17 (7): 1103–1110. doi: 10.1093/annonc/mdl085.

Cercek, A., Dos Santos Fernandes, G., Roxburgh, C.S. et al. (2020). Mismatch repair-deficient rectal cancer and resistance to neoadjuvant chemotherapy. *Clin Cancer Res* 26 (13): 3271–3279. doi: 10.1158/1078-0432.CCR-19-3728.

Cercek, A., Lumish, M., Sinopoli, J., et al. (2022 June 23). PD-1 blockade in mismatch repair-deficient, locally advanced rectal cancer. *N Engl J Med* 386 (25): 2363–2376. doi: 10.1056/NEJMoa2201445. Epub 2022 Jun 5.

Cercek, A., Roxburgh, C.S.D., Strombom, P., et al. (2018). Adoption of total neoadjuvant therapy for locally advanced rectal cancer. *JAMA Oncol* 4 (6): e180071. doi: 10.1001/jamaoncol.2018.0071.

Conroy, T., Bosset, J.-F., Etienne, P.-L., et al. (2021). Neoadjuvant chemotherapy with FOLFIRINOX and preoperative chemoradiotherapy for patients with locally advanced rectal cancer (UNICANCER-PRODIGE 23): a multicentre, randomised, open-label, phase 3 trial. *Lancet Oncol* 22 (5): 702–715. doi: 10.1016/s1470-2045(21)00079-6.

Fokas, E., Allgäuer, M., Polat, B., Klautke, G., Grabenbauer, G.G., Fietkau, R., et al. (2019 December 1). German rectal cancer study group. Randomized phase II trial of chemoradiotherapy plus induction or consolidation chemotherapy as total neoadjuvant therapy for locally advanced rectal cancer: CAO/ARO/AIO-12. *J Clin Oncol* 37 (34): 3212–3222. doi: 10.1200/JCO.19.00308. Epub 2019 May 31.

Garcia-Aguilar, J., Patil, S., Gollub, M.J., et al. (2022 April 28). Organ preservation in patients with rectal adenocarcinoma treated with total neoadjuvant therapy. *J Clin Oncol* JCO2200032. doi: 10.1200/JCO.22.00032.

Habr-Gama, A., de Souza, P.M., Ribeiro, U., Jr, Nadalin, W., Gansl, R., Sousa, A.H., Jr, Campos, F.G., and Gama-Rodrigues, J. (1998 September). Low rectal cancer: impact of radiation and chemotherapy on surgical treatment. *Dis Colon Rectum* 41 (9): 1087–1096. doi: 10.1007/BF02239429.

Habr-Gama, A., Gama-Rodrigues, J., São Julião, G.P., et al. (2014). Local recurrence after complete clinical response and watch and wait in rectal cancer after neoadjuvant chemoradiation: impact of salvage therapy on local disease control. *Int J Radiat Oncol Biol Phys* 88 (4): 822–828. doi: 10.1016/j.ijrobp.2013.12.012.

Herrinton LJ, Liu L, Levin TR, et al. Incidence and mortality of colorectal adenocarcinoma in persons with inflammatory bowel disease from 1998 to 2010. *Gastroenterology*. 2012 Aug;143(2):382-9. doi: 10.1053/j.gastro.2012.04.054. Epub 2012 May 15. PMID: 22609382.

Ngan, S. Y., Burmeister, B., Fisher, R. J., et al. (2012). Randomized trial of short-course radiotherapy versus long-course chemoradiation comparing rates of local recurrence in patients with T3 rectal cancer: Trans-Tasman Radiation Oncology Group Trial 01.04. *Journal of Clinical Oncology*, 30(31), 3827–3833. doi: 10.1200/JCO.2012.42.9597

O'Connell, M.J., Martenson, J.A., Wieand, H.S., et al. (1994)Improving adjuvant therapy for rectal cancer by combining protracted infusion fluorouracil with radiation therapy after curative surgery. Improving *N Engl J Med* 331: 502–507.

Sauer, R., Becker, H., Hohenberger, W., et al. (2004). Preoperative versus postoperative chemoradiotherapy for rectal cancer. *N Engl J Med* 351 (17): 1731–1740. doi: 10.1056/nejmoa040694.

Schrag D., Shi, Q., Weiser, M.R, et al. (2023). Preoperative Treatment of Locally Advanced Rectal Cancer. *N Engl J Med* Jun 4. doi: 10.1056/NEJMoa2303269. Epub ahead of print. PMID: 37272534.

van Oostendorp, S.E., Smits, L.J.H., Vroom, Y., et al. (2020). Local recurrence after local excision of early rectal cancer: a meta-analysis of completion TME, adjuvant (chemo) radiation, or no additional treatment. *Br J Surg* 107 (13): 1719–1730. doi: 10.1002/bjs.12040.

Verschoor, Y.L., Berg, J.V.D., Beets, G., et al. (2022). Neoadjuvant nivolumab, ipilimumab, and celecoxib in MMR-proficient and MMR-deficient colon cancers: final clinical analysis of the NICHE study *J Clin Oncol.* 40 (16_suppl): 3511–3511. doi: 10.1200/JCO.2022.40.16_SUPPL.3511.

24

Recurrent and Metastatic Colorectal Cancer

Joseph Heng and Blase Polite

University of Chicago, Chicago, IL

Introduction

The incidence of colorectal cancer steadily increases with age. It affects approximately 135,430 patients in the United States every year. Among all cancers, it is the second leading cause of death in the United States. Colorectal cancer is both sporadic and familial (see Chapter 45). The incidence of colorectal cancer is higher in developed countries than in developing countries. Nearly 60% of cases develop over the age of 65 years; 30% are ≥75 years. The United States Census Bureau projects that by the year 2030, the number of Americans over age 65 will double. Approximately 20 to 25% of newly diagnosed colon cancers are metastatic at presentation. The most common metastatic sites are the regional lymph nodes, liver, lungs, and peritoneum.

The last 10 years have seen major advances in the treatment of metastatic colorectal cancer, resulting in an improvement in median overall survival of almost three years in inoperable metastatic colorectal cancer compared to a historical median of one year at the turn of the millennium. New biologic drugs have been approved that include immune checkpoint inhibitors for tumors that have microsatellite instability, targeted therapies for *BRAF V600E* mutations, and incorporation of HER2-directed therapies for tumors with *ERBB2* amplification. Sequencing and selection of anti-EGFR versus anti-VEGF agents have been clarified. This chapter will use case-based studies to review advancements in the field of metastatic colorectal cancer and apply those to contemporary clinical practice. Unlike a typical board-review-based series, we have chosen many cases where there remains controversy because solid level-one evidence is lacking. In our choices of the best answer, we provide a rationale for our treatment decisions.

Case Study 1

A previously healthy 55-year-old man presented three years ago with abdominal pain and was found to have a large obstructing colon cancer of the ascending colon. It was resected, revealing a T3N0 lesion that was microsatellite stable. He returns three years later after surgery with malaise, weight loss, and abdominal discomfort. Carcinoembryonic agent (CEA) is 15, and a CT scan shows multiple hepatic and pulmonary metastases. Liver biopsy identifies adenocarcinoma, which on special stains is CDX2 and CK20 positive and CK7 negative, consistent with recurrent metastatic colon cancer. Next-generation sequencing reveals *RAS/RAF*-wildtype, MSS, *ERBB2* non-amplified cancer. He returns to discuss medical treatment. You have a discussion regarding life-prolonging combination chemotherapy.

1) **Which chemotherapy combination is most appropriate at this time?**
   A) FOLFOX (5-fluorouracil, leucovorin, and oxaliplatin).
   B) FOLFIRI (5-fluorouracil, leucovorin, and irinotecan).
   C) FOLFOX + bevacizumab.
   D) FOLFOXIRI + bevacizumab.
   E) FOLFOX + cetuximab.

Expert Perspective: In highly fit candidates with minimal comorbidities, combination chemotherapy using a fluoropyrimidine with oxaliplatin and irinotecan is recommended. The Phase III TRIBE study showed a statistically significant four-month overall survival advantage for FOLFOXIRI and bevacizumab over FOLFIRI and bevacizumab. Meta-analyses suggest this benefit is most pronounced for right-sided PAN *RAS/RAF* WT tumors. Although retrospective analyses have shown that overall survival is increased with the use of cetuximab over bevacizumab in *RAS/RAF*-WT left-sided colon cancers, the opposite is true for right-sided tumors in the front-line metastatic setting.

Correct Answer: D

Case Study 2

The patient finishes 12 cycles of chemotherapy, and a restaging CT scan shows significant reduction in tumor burden. However, he now has painful grade 3 neuropathy that is preventing him from buttoning his shirts. He asks what he can do now to prolong his time to disease progression.

2) **Which is the most appropriate step at this time for continuing chemotherapy?**
   A) Capecitabine.
   B) Capecitabine + bevacizumab.
   C) Active surveillance.
   D) Bevacizumab alone.
   E) Continue FOLFOXIRI + bevacizumab.

Expert Perspective: The patient has already finished 12 cycles of FOLFOXIRI + bevacizumab, and he can subsequently transition to maintenance chemotherapy. Maintenance bevacizumab alone is not indicated for metastatic colorectal cancer. Maintenance capecitabine with bevacizumab was shown to prolong progression-free survival in the CAIRO 3 study over active surveillance with a numerical but not statistically significant improvement in overall survival. If the patient develops adverse events or desires a break from therapy, then active surveillance is appropriate. This case also shows the risks of prolonged oxaliplatin therapy and it is our practice to stop the oxaliplatin after eight cycles of therapy.

Correct Answer: B

Case Study 3

The patient continued maintenance capecitabine with bevacizumab for six months, but his restaging CT scan showed growth in his bilateral pulmonary nodules. He remains highly functional and can take care of all activities of daily living. He continues to have difficulty buttoning his shirt and tying his shoes.

3) Which is the most appropriate next treatment at this time?
- A) FOLFIRI.
- B) FOLFOX + bevacizumab.
- C) FOLFIRI + bevacizumab.
- D) Irinotecan + cetuximab.
- E) Triflurudine/tipiracil.

Expert Perspective: With disease progression, restarting irinotecan that demonstrated disease control in his earlier treatment course along with 5-FU and bevacizumab would be the most appropriate step, rather than switching to triflurudine/tipiracil, because the patient's tumor has not demonstrated resistance to irinotecan. There is evidence of improved overall survival in continuing anti-VEGF inhibition with chemotherapy beyond first-line progression compared to chemotherapy alone. While irinotecan and cetuximab could be considered, the PRODIGE 18 showed a numerical if not statistically significant advantage to bevacizumab over cetuximab in this setting, and given this is a right-sided original primary, we would opt for bevacizumab beyond progression. Oxaliplatin is no longer an option given his continued grade 3 neuropathy.

Correct Answer: C

Case Study 4

A 30-year-old steel mill worker presented to the emergency department with abdominal pain. On CT scan, he was found to have thickening of his cecum and bilateral sub-centimeter pulmonary nodules. A colonoscopy was performed, which found a partially obstructing colonic mass, with biopsies positive for poorly differentiated adenocarcinoma. Next-generation sequencing of the tumor revealed an MSI-H tumor with a *BRAF V600E* mutation. The patient was discharged to follow up with an oncologist. The patient's family is seeking aggressive treatment.

4) Which treatment is best at this time?
- A) Pembrolizumab.
- B) FOLFOX + bevacizumab.
- C) Encorafenib + cetuximab.
- D) FOLFOXIRI + bevacizumab.

Expert Perspective: KEYNOTE-177 demonstrated a significantly improved progression-free survival with the use of pembrolizumab in MSI-H/dMMR colorectal cancer over chemotherapy (16.5 vs 8.2 months; also refer to Chapters 45 and 47). A recent survival update shows a numerical but not statistically significant overall survival benefit. This is confounded by significant patient crossover to pembrolizumab. Attention should be paid to the fact that in the first six months of this trial, there was a sharp decrease in the progression-free survival curve of the pembrolizumab arm compared to the chemotherapy arm. This should be taken into consideration for patients with a high burden of disease where rapid response is needed. For these patients, we either start with an aggressive chemotherapy regimen like FOLFOXIRI and bevacizumab and then switch to pembrolizumab after maximal response is achieved or perform a short follow-up CT scan (at six to eight weeks) to confirm response to immunotherapy. There are no data to support the use of encorafenib (ATP-competitive inhibitor of protein kinase B-raf (*BRAF*) that suppresses the *MAPK* pathway) and cetuximab in the frontline setting.

Correct Answer: A

Case Study 5

The patient was started on pembrolizumab, and his restaging CT scan in three months showed disease progression with new bilateral pulmonary nodules and retroperitoneal adenopathy. He has continued to stay active throughout his treatment course and exercises four times a week.

5) Which is the most appropriate next treatment at this time?
  A) Ipilimumab + nivolumab.
  B) Encorafenib + binimetinib + cetuximab.
  C) Encorafenib + cetuximab.
  D) FOLFOXIRI + bevacizumab.

Expert Perspective: The Phase III BEACON study showed an improved OS benefit with the use of BRAF-inhibitor-based therapy over irinotecan + cetuximab in *BRAF V600E*–mutated colorectal cancers. However, there was no difference in benefit between the triplet therapy arm (encorafenib + binimetinib + cetuximab) and the doublet therapy arm (encorafenib + cetuximab), and the triplet therapy resulted in increased toxicity compared to doublet therapy. In a patient with rapid progression on pembrolizumab monotherapy, we would not procced with additional immunotherapy in the second line. Aggressive chemotherapy would not be a wrong choice in this case, but given that patient is asymptomatic and the BEACON data, we would support the less toxic doublet regimen.

Correct Answer: C

Case Study 6

A 65-year-old retired businessman with obesity, diabetes and a possible diagnosis of non-alcoholic fatty liver disease presented with symptoms of abdominal pain, bloating, and hematochezia. He presented to the emergency department, where a CT scan revealed a sigmoid mass and two hypodense lesions in the right lobe of the liver. He was admitted, and colonoscopy confirmed adenocarcinoma of the sigmoid colon arising in an adenoma. His hemoglobin was 6.5 g/dL. On discussion with the colorectal surgeon, he elected to have a laparoscopic low anterior resection. Pathology showed T3, N1 moderately differentiated adenocarcinoma (1 of 22 lymph nodes positive) with negative margins. Extended *RAS* and *RAF* testing showed no mutations. Mismatch repair protein expression was intact by immunohistochemistry. His case was discussed in tumor board, and a hepato-biliary surgeon deemed him to be a candidate for right hepatectomy. The surgeon asks your opinion on the role of chemotherapy in this case.

6) Which is the most appropriate recommendation in this case?
    A) Three months of neoadjuvant FOLFOX.
    B) Three months of neoadjuvant FOLFOX + cetuximab.
    C) Six months of adjuvant FOLFIRI.
    D) Surgical resecton of his hepatic disease.

Expert Perspective: The patient in this case has oligometastatic left-sided colorectal cancer with liver metastases without *RAS/RAF* mutations and has already undergone resection of the primary colon tumor. Although the initial reaction is to want to give chemotherapy to this patient, we would recommend upfront surgical resection for the following reasons. First, we now have a large Phase III trial that shows no overall survival benefit to perioperative FOLFOX chemotherapy (EORTC). Second, given the need for a right hepatectomy and the patient's underlying fatty liver disease, chemotherapy may risk damage to the remnant liver. Regarding the other choices, the NEW EPOC phase 3 trial showed that the addition of cetuximab to chemotherapy worsened the progression-free survival and overall survival of patients with resectable colorectal liver metastases compared to chemotherapy alone. Irinotecan-based therapy has not been shown to improve outcomes in patients with resectable hepatic disease and has not shown an adjuvant benefit in patients with stage II and III colon cancer.

Correct Answer: D

Case Study 7

Unfortunately, six months after surgical resection, restaging CT scans showed multiple hepatic lesions in the remnant liver, and he was not felt to be a candidate for further surgical therapy. Review of NGS from the hepatic resection continued to show the PAN *RAS/RAF* WT tumor but also showed amplification of nonalcoholic fatty liver disease. IHC evaluation showed the tumor to be HER2 3+ by IHC.

7) What is the next best course of treatment?
    A) FOLFIRI and bevacizumab.
    B) FOLFOX and trastuzumab.
    C) Embolization of left hepatic disease with Y-90 with FOLFOX.
    D) FOLFIRI + cetuximab.

Expert Perspective: We would choose FOLFIRI and bevacizumab in this case. As discussed previously, the preponderance of data supports the use of anti-EGFR-based therapy in patients with PAN *RAS/RAF* WT left sided tumors; however, the presence of *ERBB2* amplifications complicates this case. Data from the phase II HERACLES trial showed that none of the evaluable patients in that trial with *ERBB2* amplification responded to previous cetuximab or panitumumab, suggesting that the *ERBB2* amplification may make these tumors resistant to anti-EGFR therapy. Given the crosstalk between the ERBB1 (*EGFR*) and *ERBB2* pathways, this is biologically plausible; therefore, we opt to use a bevacizumab-containing regimen as frontline therapy in this case. The data are simply not available to justify using trastuzumab-based therapy in chemotherapy-naïve metastatic colon cancer patients. The use of liver-directed therapy with selective internal radiotherapy deserves special attention. The SIRFLOX trial compared FOLFOX with or without Y-90-based therapy, and although it showed an improvement in liver progression-free survival, there was no improvement in overall PFS or overall survival. In addition, toxicity was significantly increased in the Y-90 arm.

Correct Answer: A

Case Study 8

The patient subsequently progressed on oxaliplatin- and irinotecan-based regimens. He continues to feel well and has an ECOG PS of 1.

8) What would be your next treatment choice?
   A) Regorafenib.
   B) Trifluridine-tipiracil.
   C) Trastuzumab and pertuzumab.
   D) Trastuzumab deruxtecan.

Expert Perspective: Based on the MyPathway, patients receiving trastuzumab and pertuzumab had an overall response rate of 32% with a median duration of disease response of six months. It should also be noted that these patients had received a median of four prior therapies before entering this trial. Trastuzumab deruxtecan is an antibody drug conjugate that has shown response rates of 45% in the DESTINY-CRC01 trial but comes at the cost of significant toxicity. In addition, this therapy can be given with success in patients who progress on previous trastuzumab therapy. Although there are no head-to-head comparisons between a trastuzumab-containing regimen and either regorafenib (an orally active inhibitor of angiogenic tyrosine kinases [including the VEGF receptors 1 to 3], as well as other membrane and intracellular kinases) or Triflurudine/tipiracil (oral cytotoxic agent that consists of the nucleoside analog trifluridine [a cytotoxic antimetabolite that inhibits thymidylate synthase and, after modification within tumor cells, is incorporated into DNA, causing strand breaks] and tipiracil, a potent thymidine phosphorylase inhibitor, which inhibits trifluridine metabolism and has antiangiogenic properties as wel), the impressive response rate and duration of response for a trastuzumab-containing regimen argue for its use first. The SUNLIGHT study, demonstrated a statistically significant OS improvement in patients randomized to the Triflurudine/tipiracil plus bevacizumab arm compared to those randomized to Triflurudine/tipiracil (Hazard ratio 0.61; 95% CI: 0.49, 0.77; 1-sided p<0.001). This led FDA approval of trifluridine and tipiracil with bevacizumab, for metastatic colorectal cancer previously treated with fluoropyrimidine-, oxaliplatin- and irinotecan-based chemotherapy, an anti-VEGF biological therapy, and if RAS wild-type, an anti-EGFR therapy. Recently, a phase II trial (MOUNTAINEER) of over 80 patients with HER2-positive, RAS wild-type, chemotherapy-refractory metastatic CRC, demonstrated objective response rate of 38% of trastuzumab in combination with tucatinib. Based on these data, the FDA approved trastuzumab in combination with tucatinib in adult patients with RAS wild-type, HER2-positive unresectable or metastatic CRC that has progressed following treatment with fluoropyrimidine-, oxaliplatin-, and irinotecan-based chemotherapy.

Correct Answer: C

Recommended Readings

André, T., Shiu, K.K., Kim, T.W., et al. (2020). Pembrolizumab in microsatellite-instability-high advanced colorectal cancer. *N Engl J Med* 383 (23): 2207–2218.

Bennouna, J., Sastre, J., Arnold, D., et al. (2013 January). ML18147 study investigators. Continuation of bevacizumab after first progression in metastatic colorectal cancer (ML18147): a randomised phase 3 trial. *Lancet Oncol* 14 (1): 29–37. doi: 10.1016/S1470-2045(12)70477-1. Epub 2012 Nov 16. PMID: 23168366.

Bridgewater, J.A., Pugh, S.A., Maishman, T., et al. (2020). Systemic chemotherapy with or without cetuximab in patients with resectable colorectal liver metastasis (New EPOC): long-term results of a multicentre, randomised, controlled, phase 3 trial. *Lancet Oncol* 21 (3): 398–411.

Cremolini, C., Loupakis, F., Antoniotti, C., et al. (2015 October). FOLFOXIRI plus bevacizumab versus FOLFIRI plus bevacizumab as first-line treatment of patients with metastatic colorectal cancer: updated overall survival and molecular subgroup analyses of the open-label, phase 3 TRIBE study. *Lancet Oncol* 16 (13): 1306–1315. doi: 10.1016/S1470-2045(15)00122-9. Epub 2015 Aug 31. PMID: 26338525.

Kanemitsu, Y., Shimizu, Y., Mizusawa, J., et al. (2021 September 14). JCOG colorectal cancer study group. Hepatectomy followed by mFOLFOX6 versus hepatectomy alone for liver-only metastatic colorectal cancer (JCOG0603): a phase II or III randomized controlled trial. *J Clin Oncol* JCO2101032. doi: 10.1200/JCO.21.01032. Epub ahead of print. PMID: 34520230.

Kopetz, S., Grothey, A., Yaeger, R., et al. (2019). Encorafenib, binimetinib, and cetuximab in *BRAF* V600E-mutated colorectal cancer. *N Engl J Med* 381 (17): 1632–1643.

Meric-Bernstam, F., Hurwitz, H., Raghav, K.P.S., et al. (2019 April). Pertuzumab plus trastuzumab for HER2-amplified metastatic colorectal cancer (MyPathway): an updated report from a multicentre, open-label, phase 2a, multiple basket study. *Lancet Oncol* 20 (4): 518–530. doi: 10.1016/S1470-2045(18)30904-5. Epub 2019 Mar 8. PMID: 30857956; PMCID: PMC6781620.

Simkens, L.H., van Tinteren, H., May, A., et al. (2015). Maintenance treatment with capecitabine and bevacizumab in metastatic colorectal cancer (CAIRO3): a phase 3 randomised controlled trial of the Dutch colorectal cancer group. *Lancet* 385 (9980): 1843–1852.

Strickler, J.H., Cercek, A., Siena, S. et al. (2023 May). Tucatinib plus trastuzumab for chemotherapy-refractory, HER2-positive, RAS wild-type unresectable or metastatic colorectal cancer (MOUNTAINEER): a multicentre, open-label, phase 2 study. *Lancet Oncol* 24 (5): 496–508. doi:10.1016/S1470-2045(23)00150-X. PMID: 37142372.

Tejpar, S., Stintzing, S., Ciardiello, F., et al. (2017 February 1). Prognostic and predictive relevance of primary tumor location in patients with RAS wild-type metastatic colorectal cancer: retrospective analyses of the CRYSTAL and FIRE-3 trials. *JAMA Oncol* 3 (2): 194–201. doi: 10.1001/jamaoncol.2016.3797. Erratum in: *JAMA Oncol* (2017 Dec 1) 3(12): 1742.PMID: 27722750; PMCID: PMC7505121.

Van Hazel, G.A., Heinemann, V., Sharma, N.K., et al. (2016 May 20). SIRFLOX: randomized phase III trial comparing first-line mFOLFOX6 (plus or minus bevacizumab) versus mFOLFOX6 (plus or minus bevacizumab) plus selective internal radiation therapy in patients with metastatic colorectal cancer. *J Clin Oncol* 34 (15): 1723–1731. doi: 10.1200/JCO.2015.66.1181. Epub 2016 Feb 22. Erratum in: *J Clin Oncol* (2016 Nov 20) 34(33): 4059. PMID: 26903575.

25

Pancreatic Adenocarcinoma

Evan Walker, Andrew Ko, and Margaret Tempero

University of California, San Francisco, CA

Introduction

Pancreatic ductal adenocarcinoma is diagnosed in >60,000 people and leads to >48,000 deaths annually in the US. Only 10 to 15% of tumors are amenable to surgical resection at diagnosis; therefore the vast majority of pancreatic ductal adenocarcinomas are incurable, leading to an overall five-year survival rate of about 10%. As such, pancreatic ductal adenocarcinoma is currently the third-leading cause of US cancer-related mortality and will rise to the second-leading cause by 2030. Risk factors include increasing age, male gender, family history of pancreatic ductal adenocarcinoma, inherited genetic syndromes increasing risk for cancer, and hereditary pancreatitis. Several modifiable risk factors have also been established, including obesity, tobacco use, and diabetes mellitus.

Treatment of pancreatic ductal adenocarcinoma depends on the stage of disease and, for nonmetastatic tumors, the feasibility of surgical resection. For nonmetastatic resectable pancreatic ductal adenocarcinoma, treatment may consist of a combination of systemic therapy, radiation, and surgery. For unresectable and/or metastatic disease (most cases), cytotoxic chemotherapy is the mainstay of treatment. The increasing prevalence of germline genetic testing and somatic tumor molecular profiling has led to the identification of patient subgroups that may benefit from targeted therapeutics. However, these subgroups encapsulate <10% of patients: additional research is needed to expand therapeutic options for most patients with pancreatic ductal adenocarcinoma. Due to the limited prognosis associated with pancreatic ductal adenocarcinoma, quality of life concerns should be emphasized in treatment-related shared decision making between patients and providers early in the disease course.

25 Pancreatic Adenocarcinoma

Case Study 1

A 72-year-old woman presented to the emergency department with chest pain and shortness of breath for one day. A computed tomography (CT) angiogram of the chest revealed a segmental pulmonary embolism, for which she was started on anticoagulation with low molecular weight heparin (LMWH). Limited imaging of the upper abdomen demonstrated a pancreatic head lesion with mixed cystic and solid components concerning for malignancy. She was clinically stable and was discharged. Several days later, she presents to your office for further evaluation.

1) What do you recommend as the next step in her diagnostic evaluation?
   A) Positron emission tomography (PET)–CT.
   B) CT scan with multiphasic pancreatic protocol.
   C) Endoscopic ultrasound (EUS).
   D) Abdominal magnetic resonance imaging (MRI).
   E) Endoscopic retrograde cholangiopancreatography (ERCP).

Expert Perspective: Cross-sectional abdominal imaging is the appropriate first step in evaluating a suspicious pancreatic mass and should occur prior to any interventional diagnostic procedure. The primary objectives of imaging are to better delineate the extent of a pancreatic mass, visualize the degree to which a tumor involves mesenteric vasculature, and potentially identify evidence of metastatic disease. Togther, this information should be used in multidisciplinary consultation to select patients for whom surgical resection may be feasible.

Optimal multiphase cross-sectional imaging includes a noncontrast phase plus arterial, pancreatic parenchymal, and portal venous phases of contrast enhancement with cuts that are ideally < 1 mm. Multiphasic protocols allow for selective visualization of critical arterial and venous structures to assess for vascular invasion (see Figure 25.1, created with Biorender.com). Contrast enhancement is necessary to distinguish between a hypodense lesion in the pancreas and the surrounding parenchyma. Pancreatic ductal adenocarcinoma is a hypovascular tumor with dense stroma, and it is therefore best detected in the late arterial phase, when pancreatic parenchyma enhances but the hypoperfused tumor does not.

A pancreatic protocol CT scan is the preferred imaging modality for characterizing pancreatic ductal adenocarcinoma. Pancreatic protocol MRI is an acceptable alternative but does not provide superior visualization and is commonly more expensive and less available than a pancreatic protocol CT scan. Abdominal MRI is thus better used to adjudicate indeterminate liver lesions or as an alterative if iodinated contrast is contraindicated.

Endoscopic ultrasound (EUS) is complementary to pancreatic protocol CT as a staging tool for tumors with questionable vascular or lymph node involvement but no definitive evidence of metastatic disease on CT scan. EUS should not be used alone, as the positive predictive value for mesenteric arterial invasion is inferior to that of a pancreatic protocol CT scan. PET-CT is not routinely used in the staging of pancreatic ductal adenocarcinoma but may be considered for patients at high risk of occult metastatic disease (e.g. those with large primary tumors and/or regional lymph nodes and markedly elevated cancer antigen 19–9 (CA 19–9) but no evidence of metastatic disease on CT scan). ERCP is not a

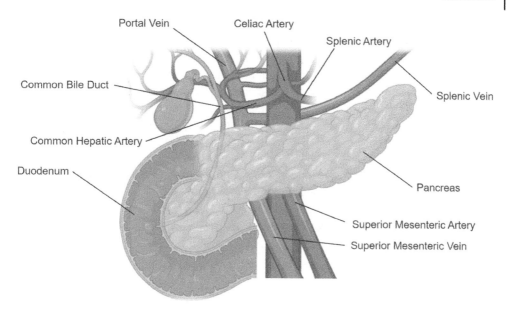

Figure 25.1 Anatomical orientation of pancreas for surgical consideration.

useful staging tool for pancreatic ductal adenocarcinoma, though it can be used for biliary decompression with endobiliary stenting if needed.

Correct Answer: B

A CT scan with pancreatic protocol is performed and demonstrates a 3 cm pancreatic head mass with associated extra-hepatic biliary dilation and pancreatic duct dilation distal to the mass. There is peripancreatic lymphadenopathy and tumor involvement of mesenteric vasculature consistent with unresectable disease, but no evidence of distant metastases. A CT scan of the chest is also negative for metastases. Serologic studies reveal CA 19–9 of 800 U/mL (normal < 37 U/mL) and a total bilirubin of 5.0 mg/dL (normal < 1.2 mg/dL). The patient reports jaundice and generalized pruritis over the past week. A pathologic diagnosis has not yet been confirmed.

2) **What is the best next step?**
    A) CT-guided percutaneous biopsy.
    B) ERCP with biliary stent placement.
    C) EUS with fine-needle aspiration (FNA).
    D) Percutaneous biliary drainage.
    E) B and C.

Expert Perspective: Systemic therapy is the mainstay of treatment for unresectable pancreatic ductal adenocarcinoma, and a pathologic diagnosis is imperative prior to starting treatement. A pancreatic mass biopsy can be obtained by FNA with either EUS guidance or CT guidance. EUS-directed FNA is preferred due to the higher diagnostic yield and safety, as well as the possible risk of peritoneal seeding with a percutaneous approach. In addition to obtaining a biopsy, the patient's cholestasis should be addressed prior to initiation of cytotoxic chemotherapy, both to mitigate the risk of cholangitis in the setting of iatrogenic immunosuppression and because the metabolism of some chemotherapeutic agents is dependent on optimized hepatic function. Endoscopic biliary decompression is preferred over a percutaneous approach for patient comfort; if a percutaneous approach is necessitated, subsequent internalization should be pursued if possible. Of note, cholestasis can cause elevated CA 19–9 independent of tumor expression, so this test should be repeated to redefine a baseline level after biliary decompression.

Correct Answer: E

3) **FNA of the pancreas reveals adenocarcinoma, and treatment with chemotherapy is planned. How should her anticoagulation be managed?**
    A) Stop anticoagulation.
    B) Continue low molecular weight heparin.
    C) Transition to warfarin.
    D) Transition to apixaban.
    E) Transition to rivaroxaban.

Expert Perspective: This patient has an acute venous thromboembolism requiring ongoing anticoagulation, and LMWH is the optimal choice. In the pivotal CLOT trial, the LMWH molecule dalteparin was superior to vitamin K antagonists such as warfarin for preventing recurrent thromboembolism (HR 0.48; 95% CI 0.30–0.77; $P = 0.002$) and did not increase bleeding risk. The direct oral anticoagulant rivaroxaban was compared to LMWH for patients with cancer in the SELECT-D trial, demonstrating six-month thromboembolism recurrence rates of 11% with dalteparin and 4% with rivaroxaban (HR 0.43; 95% CI 0.19–0.99). Rates of major bleeding were similar, but a higher rate of clinically relevant nonmajor bleeding was observed with rivaroxaban (13% vs. 4%). In the CAR-RAVAGIO study, the direct oral anticoagulant apixaban and dalteparin led to similar rates of recurrent thromboembolism and bleeding. It is important to note that higher rates of bleeding with direct oral anticoagulants have been observed, particularly in the SELECT-D trial, for patients with gastrointestinal malignancies. Until there is more safety data in this patient population, LMWH is preferred, especially in the setting of intact intraluminal primary tumors at high risk for bleeding (Chapter 51).

Correct Answer: B

Case Study 2

A 70-year-old woman presented with a pancreatic mass and several peripheral lung nodules. Biopsy of a lung nodule confirmed metastatic pancreatic ductal adenocarcinoma. She is very fatigued, has mild nausea and vomiting, and her Eastern Cooperative Oncology Group (ECOG) performance score is 2. She is interested in starting systemic chemotherapy.

4) **What molecular testing is indicated at this time?**
    A) Tumor molecular profiling.
    B) Germline genetic testing (with referral to a genetic counselor).

C) Both A and B.
D) Neither A nor B.

Expert Perspective: Commensurate with recent advances in pancreatic ductal adenocarcinoma screening and targeted therapeutics, germline and somatic multigene sequencing are now integral components of pancreatic ductal adenocarcinoma care.

Germline genetic testing with concomitant genetic counseling is now universally recommended for patients with pancreatic ductal adenocarcinoma. Test results can inform cancer screening for the proband and family members and can also influence treatment selection, such as use of poly-ADP ribose polymerase (PARP) inhibitors for patients harboring pathogenic *BRCA1/2* mutations. Several recent observational studies have reported significant rates of pathogenic germline mutations in unselected patients. For example, a 2017 study from Johns Hopkins University reported that 4% of all patients with pancreatic ductal adenocarcinoma harbored pathogenic germline alterations, but only 3 of 33 patients with these alterations had a family history of pancreatic ductal adenocarcinoma, and most did not have the canonical features of an inherited cancer syndrome, such as a personal or family history of other cancers. Based on these reports, both the American Society for Clinical Oncology (ASCO) and the NCCN in 2018 broadened their recommendations for germline testing to include all patients with pancreatic ductal adenocarcinoma (see Chapters 45–47).

Somatic tumor molecular profiling can also guide the selection of targeted treatment in later lines of therapy. For example, tumors with high microsatellite instability (MSI-H) or deficient DNA damage mismatch repair due to alterations in MLH1, MSH2, MSH6, or PMS2 can be treated with immunotherapy. Mutations in genes associated with DNA damage homologous recombination repair, such as *BRCA1/2* or *PALB2*, may predict sensitivity to platinum-basd chemotherapies. Other somatic fusions (*ALK, NRG1, NTRK, ROS1*) or mutations (*BRAF, HER2*) can be treated with molecularly targeted therapy or prompt enrollment in clinical trials. Due to the improved outcomes associated with tailored treatment approaches, tumor molecular profiling is recommended for all patients with advanced/metastatic pancreatic ductal adenocarcinoma who are candidates for systemic therapy.

Correct Answer: C

5) Which of the following regimens is the best option for systemic treatment?
   A) FOLFIRINOX.
   B) Gemcitabine/nab-paclitaxel.
   C) Gemcitabine/cisplatin.
   D) Gemcitabine/erlotinib.
   E) Referral to hospice.

Expert Perspective: The mainstay of treatment for metastatic pancreatic ductal adenocarcinoma is systemic cytotoxic chemotherapy. The most robust phase III data support the three-drug regimen FOLFIRINOX (5-fluorouracil (5-FU) with leucovorin, irinotecan, oxaliplatin) or the doublet gemcitabine/nab-paclitaxel in the frontline setting.

In the 2011 PRODIGE 4/ACCORD 11 phase III trial, frontline treatment with FOLFIRINOX improved median overall survival compared to the prior reference standard of gemcitabine, from 6.8 months to 11.1 months (HR 0.57, 95%CI 0.45–0.73, $p < 0.001$). The improvement in efficacy with FOLFIRINOX was accompanied by increased rates of cytopenias, diarrhea, and sensory neuropathy. Based on clinical experience garnered over the subsequent decade, this regimen is best used to treat otherwise healthy patients expected to tolerate this aggressive triplet regimen well. Specifically, FOLFIRNOX should be used for patients with ECOG performance scores of 0–1.

In the 2013 MPACT phase III trial, frontline treatment with gemcitabine/nab-paclitaxel improved median overall survival compared to gemcitabine monotherapy from 6.7 months to 8.5 months (HR 0.72, 95% CI 0.62–0.83, p < 0.001). Neutropenia, fatigue, and neuropathy were more common in the combination arm. Cross-trial numerical comparisons of efficacy are limited by differences in trial design: the MPACT trial enrolled patients globally, including from countries with potentially less access to supportive care, as well as those with poorer peformance status, while the PRODIGE 4/ACCORD 11 trial enrolled exclusively in France and was limited to more robust individuals. Regarding toxicity, however, gemcitabine/nab-paclitaxel is more tolerable than FOLFIRINOX and thus should preferentially be used for patients with ECOG performance scores of 2.

Gemcitabine/cisplatin has been compared to gemcitabine monotherapy in multiple phase II/III trials, but this combination has not demonstrated superior outcomes in unselected patients with pancreatic ductal adenocarcinoma. In the 2007 NCIC-CTG AP.3 trial, gemcitabine/erlotinib statistically significantly improved median overall survival compared to gemcitabine monotherapy from 5.91 to 6.24 months. This is not a clinically significant improvement, and erlotinib is not routinely used to treat pancreatic ductal adenocarcinoma.

In summary, for this patient with an ECOG performance score of 2, gemcitabine/nab-paclitaxel represents the most appropriate frontline regimen among the listed answer choices. Gemcitabine alone could also be considered if the patient is unlikely to tolerate a doublet chemotherapy regimen.

Correct Answer: B

Case Study continued: The patient begins treatment with gemcitabine/nab-paclitaxel. Several weeks later, germline testing results return, revealing no pathogenic mutations, while tumor molecular profiling shows no actionable findings. After five months of treatment, her fatigue has improved and her ECOG performance score is 1, but she has developed painful peripheral neuropathy. Restaging CT scans show progression of lung metastases. She is interested in continuing treatment.

6) What is the best option for second-line therapy?
   A) Nanoliposomal irinotecan/5-FU/leucovorin.
   B) Nanoliposomal irinotecan.
   C) Capecitabine.
   D) Gemcitabine/nab-paclitaxel/cisplatin.
   E) Oxaliplatin/5-FU/leucovorin.

Expert Perspective: There are sparse data to guide optimal second-line treatment for pancreatic ductal adenocarcinoma after progression on frontline therapy. For patients who are candidates for additional treatment, components of frontline regimens not previously received are often repurposed for the second-line setting.

Over the past decade, several phase III trials have been conducted to guide therapeutic selection in the gemcitabine-refractory setting. In the 2014 CONKO-003 trial, the combination of oxaliplatin and 5-FU/leucovorin (OFF) compared to 5-FU/leucovorin alone improved median overall survival from 3.3 months to 5.9 months (HR 0.66, 95% CI 0.48–0.91, p = 0.01) for patients previously treated with gemcitabine monotherapy. However, the 2016 PANCREOX trial, which also compared oxaliplatin and 5-FU/leucovorin (administered as modified FOLFOX6) to 5-FU/leucovorin alone in the post-gemcitabine setting, provided contrasting data. The PANCREOX trial demonstrated no difference in progression-free survival and worse overall survival with the addition of oxaliplatin.

The 2015 NAPOLI-1 trial demonstrated that nanoliposomal irinotecan/5-FU/leucovorin, compared to 5-FU/leucovorin, improved median overall survival from 4.2 to 6.1 months (HR 0.67; 95% CI 0.49–0.92; P = 0.012) for patients previously treated with gemcitabine-based regimens. It should be noted that the comparator arm for this trial (5-FU/leucovorin alone) is not a conventionally utilized second-line therapy, and thus the real-world marginal benefit of the combination regimen compared to other acceptable second-line regimens, such as the standard formulation of irinotecan/5-FU/leucovorin (FOLFIRI), may be more modest or nonexistant. Regardless, the NAPOLI-1 trial established a new evidence base for second-line therapy that avoids exacerbation of treatment-related neuropathy associated with frontline oxaliplatin or nab-paclitaxel. Therefore, this regimen is preferred after progression on gemcitabine-based therapy.

Correct Answer: A

Case Study 3

A 75-year-old man was newly diagnosed with locally advanced unresectable pancreatic ductal adenocarcinoma. He was asymptomatic, and his ECOG performance score was 0. His CA 19–9 was 1500 U/mL. He began systemic therapy with FOLFIRINOX. After six months of treatment, he has developed cumulative fatigue and mild nausea but no other adverse events. His ECOG performance score is 1, and his CA 19–9 has descended to 10 U/mL. Repeat CT scans of the chest, abdomen, and pelvis demonstrate moderate treatment response in the primary tumor and no distant metastases.

7) What is your next step in management?
  A) Stop chemotherapy, continue surveillance imaging.
  B) Multidisciplinary consultation to consider local therapies.
  C) Continue with current treatment.
  D) Refer for surgery.

Expert Perspective: Locally advanced pancreatic cancer is, by definition, unresectable at presentation, and systemic therapy is an appropriate first step in management. In the event of disease control after four to six months of systemic therapy, the next steps are less well defined. The pivotal LAP07 trial randomized 269 patients with progression-free disease after four months of gemcitabine-based chemotherapy to two additional months of chemotherapy vs chemoradiotherapy. With median follow-up of 36.7 months, median overall survival did not statistically significantly differ between groups [chemotherapy

16.5 months (95% CI 14.5–18.5 months); chemoradiotherapy 15.2 months (95% CI 14.5–18.5 months); HR 1.03 (95% CI 0.79–1.34) $P = 0.83$]. Thus, chemoradiation is not the standard of care in this setting and historically has only been used for select cases (e.g. situations in which local disease control may improve quality of life).

However, recent data from the Massachusettes General Hospital and other centers have led to reconsideration of resection for patients who undergo preoperative chemotherapy and chemoradiation in a total neoadjuvant therapy paradigm. In the setting of nonprogressive disease after treatment, restaging CT scans are unable to distinguish posttreatment fibrosis from viable cancer, impeding predictions of which tumors have responded and are now amenable to total (R0) resection. Instead, decreases in CA 19–9 have emerged as a more reliable predictor of tumor resectability. Incorporating these data, some providers advocate treating locally advanced tumors with chemotherapy followed by chemoradiation, and if the patient remains a surgical candidate and either a radiographic response or a decreased CA 19–9 is observed, performing diagnostic laparoscopy followed by potential tumor resection. A crucial aspect of resectability is the posttreatment interface between tumor and vasculature: this should be explored early in the operation, and preoperative planning should include the possible necessity of arterial resection (with or without reconstruction), short-segment venous reconstruction (primary repair, vein patch, or segmental resection with anastomosis) or long-segment venous reconstruction (interposition of an autologous or synthetic graft). Additional data on clinical outcomes are needed before adopting this workflow into routine practice, but multidisciplinary consultation to discuss this option is warranted for patients with locally advanced disease who respond well to initial chemotherapy.

Correct Answer: B

Case Study 4

A 40-year-old woman presented with a pancreatic mass and scattered hepatic lesions. A CT-guided biopsy of one of the liver lesions confirmed a diagnosis of metastatic pancreatic ductal adenocarcinoma. She was otherwise healthy and had no functional limitations. Her mother developed breast cancer at age 52. Due to high suspicion of an inherited cancer syndrome, you ordered expedited germline testing using a multi-gene panel (including *BRCA1*, *BRCA2*, and *PALB2*) while preparing for the start of systemic chemotherapy. This testing reveals a pathogenic *BRCA2* mutation.

8) Which regimen do you recommend?
   A) FOLFIRINOX.
   B) Gemcitabine/nab-paclitaxel.
   C) Gemcitabine/cisplatin.
   D) Gemcitabine.
   E) A or C.

Expert Perspective: The genes *BRCA1/2* and *PALB2* encode key proteins involved with homologous recombination DNA damage repair, and pathogenic germline mutations in these genes cause loss of this DNA repair mechanism. Pancreatic ductal adenocarcinomas arising in patients harboring these mutations are uniquely susceptible to platinum-based chemotherapeutics such as oxaliplatin or cisplatin. Thus, these patients should be treated with either FOLFIRINOX or gemcitabine/cisplatin if they are able to tolerate combination chemotherapy. Of note, while gemcitabine/cisplatin has not demonstrated improved efficacy over gemcitabine monotherapy in randomized trials enrolling unselected patients, a remarkable response rate of 65% has been reported among patients with *BRCA1/2* and *PALB2* mutations treated with this regimen. FOLFIRINOX and gemcitabine/cisplatin have not been directly compared in this setting, but gemcitabine/cisplatin is associated with fewer adverse effects and may be an appropriate choice for patients unlikely to tolerate the toxicity of a triplet regimen. When suspicion of a germline mutation is high and gemcitabine/cisplatin would be preferred (and therefore germline test results would directly influence frontline treatment selection), expedited germline testing for *BRCA1/2* and *PALB2* can be considered before starting treatment if the patient is clinically stable and therapy is not excessively delayed (Chapters 45–47).

Correct Answer: E

Case Study continued: The patient opted for treatment with FOLFIRINOX. After six months of treatment, restaging CT scans showed partial tumor response. She is interested in remaining on active treatment but has developed severe peripheral neuropathy in her hands and feet. She asks to switch to a less aggressive regimen unlikely to worsen her neuropathy.

9) Which maintenance regimen do you recommend?
    A) Continue with FOLFOX (5-FU/leucovorin, oxaliplatin).
    B) Switch to gemcitabine/nab-paclitaxel.
    C) Capecitabine.
    D) Olaparib.
    E) No effective maintenance treatment exists.

Expert Perspective: Peripheral neuropathy and other cumulative treatment-related adverse effects often limit the duration of FOLFIRINOX to six months, even if a tumor remains susceptible to this regimen. At time of intolerance to treatment, options include a chemotherapy break or a switch to maintenance therapy. The rationale for a maintenance approach is to prolong progression-free survival by continuing an active treatment while balancing therapeutic efficacy with quality of life. In the absence of phase III data to guide this decision for unselected patients, conventional practice is to continue the least toxic components of an effective frontline regimen (e.g. reducing FOLFIRINOX to fluoropyrimidine monotherapy, such as 5-FU or capecitabine). Alternatively, patients can begin a treatment holiday with regular surveillance and resumption of therapy when progressive disease is detected.

In 2019, the POLO trial provided the first phase III data to support pancreatic ductal adenocarcinoma maintenance therapy. Among patients with germline *BRCA1/2* mutations and stable or responsive disease after ⩾four months of platinum-based chemotherapy, the PARP-inhibitor olaparib, compared to placebo, prolonged progression-free survival from 3.8 months to 7.4 months (HR 0.53; 95% CI 0.35–0.82; $P = 0.004$). Thus, olaparib is the preferred maintenance option for this patient population. Of note, when offered this treatment, patients should be educated that long-term follow-up from the POLO trial revealed no effect on median overall survival (19.0 months for olaparib and 19.2 months for placebo).

Correct Answer: D

Case Study 5

A 45-year-old previously healthy woman presented with a pancreatic mass. CT scans of the chest, abdomen, and pelvis revealed a 4 × 5 cm hypoattenuating, partially cystic pancreatic head mass that contacted the superior mesenteric artery (SMA) involving 120° of the circumference but did not involve other vascular structures. No distant metastases were detected. CA 19-9 was 2200 U/mL. An EUS-guided biopsy was performed and confirmed a diagnosis of pancreatic ductal adenocarcinoma. Her ECOG performance score is 0.

10) What is your next step in management?
  A) Refer for surgical resection now.
  B) Neoadjuvant FOLFIRINOX, followed by surgical reassessment for resection.
  C) Neoadjuvant FOLFIRINOX, followed by pancreatic stereotactic body radiation therapy (SBRT), followed by surgical reassessment for resection.
  D) SBRT, followed by surgical reassessment for resection.

Expert Perspective: In recent years, a new subclassification of borderline resectable pancreatic ductal adenocarcinoma has gained traction. These are tumors that are considered technically resectable but with a high likelihood of positive margins. Although the precise definition of borderline resectability varies between different consensus guidelines, the NCCN defines this for nonmetastatic pancreatic head tumors as those that contact either (1) the common hepatic artery without extension to the celiac or hepatic artery bifurcation, (2) the SMA involving ≤ 180° of vessel circumference, (3) variant arterial anatomy, (4) the superior mesenteric vein or portal vein involving > 180° of vessel circumference (or ≤ 180° but with contour irregularity or thrombosis not precluding reconstruction), or (5) the inferior vena cava.

The appropriate management of borderline resectable pancreatic ductal adenocarcinoma remains the subject of ongoing investigation. The phase II 4-arm ESPAC-5F trial, reported in 2020, compared immediate surgery vs neoadjuvant gemcitabine/capecitabine vs neoadjuvant FOLFIRINOX versus neoadjuvant capecitabine-based chemoradiation. Rates of surgical resection did not differ between arms; however, one-year survival for patients who received immediate surgery was 40% (95% CI 26%–62%) compared to 77% (95% CI 66–89%) for those who received neoadjuvant therapy (HR 0.27; 95% CI 0.13–0.55; $P < 0.001$). This trial provides strong evidence that some form of neoadjuvant therapy is necessary, though it did not provide support for a specific preferred modality.

The phase II Alliance 021501 trial, initially reported in 2021, compared eight cycles of neoadjuvant FOLFIRINOX vs seven cycles followed by five days of either SBRT or hypofractionated image-guided radiation therapy (HIGRT). At an interim analysis after 30 patients were accrued to each arm, 57% of patients in the FOLFIRINOX arm had been able to receive tumor resection, compared to 33% in the FOLFIRINOX plus radiation group. Thus, the trial was closed due to futility of the combination arm. At follow-up, the

FOLFIRINOX alone group also had numerically superior median overall survival (31.0 vs. 17.1 mo), comparing favorably to historical controls. Thus, FOLFIRINOX represents the reference neoadjuvant standard for borderline resectable pancreatic ductal adenocarcinoma. Additional study is needed to determine if a subset of patients may benefit from radiation or whether extended conventional chemoradiation is more efficacious, as is being studied in the ongoing PANDAS-PRODIGE 44 trial. Results from the PREOPANC-2 trial, comparing neoadjuvant FOLFIRINOX to neoadjuvant gemcitabine-based chemoradiation and adjuvant gemcitabine, will also help elucidate the optimal approach.

Correct Answer: B

Case Study continued: Neoadjuvant FOLFIRINOX was started. After six cycles, her CA 19–9 descended to 25 U/mL. CT scans of the chest, abdomen, and pelvis demonstrated tumor regression and no distant metastases. The tumor was deemed resectable, and she underwent Whipple pancreaticoduodenectomy. Pathologic examination revealed a 2 cm tumor, evidence of treatment effect, negative margins, and two of seven positive lymph nodes. One month postoperatively, she has recovered from surgery. Postoperative CT imaging shows no evidence of disease, and her CA 19–9 is undetectable.

11) **What is your next step in management?**
    A) Start surveillance with serial CA 19–9 and CT chest, abdomen, and pelvis.
    B) Adjuvant FOLFIRINOX for six additional cycles.
    C) Adjuvant gemcitabine for three months.
    D) Adjuvant gemcitabine/capecitabine for three months.
    E) Treat as metastatic disease.

Expert Perspective: There are no definitive data to guide the optimal duration of neoadjuvant chemotherapy, though trials are underway to inform this decision, and clinical practice currently varies among institutions. Conventional practice is to complete up to six total months of perioperative (including bothpreoperative and postoperative) chemotherapy in this setting. Therefore, after surgical resection and postoperative imaging, patients who received <six months of preoperative chemotherapy (e.g. < 12 cycles of FOLFIRINOX) and remain candidates for treatment should be considered for adjuvant chemotherapy. The selection of an optimal adjuvant regimen (i.e. whether to continue with the same preoperative regimen or switch to an alternative) can be informed by the preoperative radiographic and CA 19–9 response, as well as the evidence of treatment effect on the surgical pathology specimen. Regardless of the regimen chosen, the duration of therapy depends on the number of neoadjuvant cycles already completed. In the event of positive surgical resection margins (R1 resection), chemoradiation can also be considered, typically after completion of systemic therapy.

Correct Answer: B

Case Study 6

A 62-year-old man presented with a new diagnosis of pancreatic ductal adenocarcinoma. CT scans of the chest, abdomen, and pelvis ordered in the setting of transient dyspnea and abdominal pain showed a dilated main pancreatic duct. A pancreatic protocol CT scan revealed a 2.4 cm pancreatic head mass but no involvement of the mesenteric vasculature, no suspicious lymphadenopathy, and no distant metastases. An EUS confirmed localized disease, and FNA revealed adenocarcinoma. His symptoms have now resolved, his ECOG performance score is 0, and he is considering surgery. He presents to your clinic to discuss next steps in his management.

12) **What do you recommend as the optimal treatment sequence?**
   A) Surgical resection followed by adjuvant chemotherapy.
   B) Neoadjuvant chemotherapy followed by surgery, followed by adjuvant chemotherapy.
   C) Chemoradiation followed by surgery.
   D) Surgical resection followed by radiation to the resection bed.
   E) Either A or B.

Expert Perspective: Pancreatic ductal adenocarcinoma is characterized by early disease dissemination; even patients with radiographically localized disease should be considered to have micrometastatic spread, and thus all patients should receive systemic therapy as part of their treatment plan. The optimal treatment sequence for radiographically localized disease is still being determined. The longstanding paradigm has been to resect the tumor immediately and, once the patient has recovered, treat with adjuvant systemic therapy. However, this paradigm has recently been challenged, and institutional standards at many medical centers have now shifted to give chemotherapy before surgery, even for resectable disease. Utilization of neoadjuvant therapy immediately addresses occult micrometastatic disease and, by providing a biologic waiting period, can select for indolent disease more likely to be cured by surgery, thereby avoiding a highly morbid operation for treatment-refractory tumors that are unlikely to be cured.

The use of perioperative therapy for resectable disease is supported by the Dutch PREOPANC-1 phase III trial and the Japanese Prep02/JSAP-05 phase II/III trial. The PREOPANC-1 trial randomized patients with resectable or borderline resectable pancreatic ductal adenocarcinoma to preoperative chemoradiotherapy or upfront surgery. Patients randomized to preoperative treatment experienced improved R0 resection rates, disease-free survival, locoregional failure-free survival, and, for those who underwent surgery, improved overall survival. Overall survival in the intention-to-treat population was numerically greater for patients who received neoadjuvant therapy (16.0 vs 14.3 months), but this did not reach statistical significance (HR 0.78; 95% CI 0.58–1.05; $P = 0.096$). The Prep02/JSAP-05 trial randomized patients to neoadjuvant chemotherapy vs upfront surgery and demonstrated improved median overall survival associated with the neoadjuvant approach, from 26.6 months to 36.7 months (HR 0.72; 95% CI 0.55–0.94; $P = 0.015$). However, this trial used a regimen (gemcitabine/S-1) that is not approved for use in the United States.

To better inform the optimal perioperative chemotherapeutic regimen, the SWOG S1505 phase II trial randomized patients to either FOLFIRINOX or gemcitabine/nab-paclitaxel, given for 12 weeks before and 12 weeks after surgery. A pick-the-winner design was utilized, comparing both arms against an a priori efficacy threshold of 40% two-year survival. Two-year survival was 41.6% for the FOLFIRINOX group and 48.8% for the gemcitabine/nab-paclitaxel group, but neither demonstrated statistically significant improvement compared to the reference standard. Thus, the optimal perioperative regimen remains undetermined.

Several active randomized phase II and III trials (Alliance 021806, NorPACT-1, NEONAX, PANACHE01, and PREOPANC-2) seek to further clarify the benefit of perioperative chemotherapy, as well as the optimal regimen, for patients with localized disease.

Correct Answer: E

Case Study 7

A 55-year-old woman with no prior health concerns rapidly developed weight loss and polyuria. Hemoglobin A1c was 8.2%, and she was started on metformin for diabetes mellitus. Six months later, she developed epigastric abdominal pain. A CT scan of the abdomen and pelvis revealed a pancreatic head mass.

13) **For patients >50 years old with incident diagnosis of diabetes mellitus, which of the following statements about for pancreatic ductal adenocarcinoma is correct?**
    A) Pancreatic ductal adenocarcinoma risk is equal to that for the age-adjusted general population.
    B) Pancreatic ductal adenocarcinoma risk is greater than that for the age-adjusted general population and equal to that for patients with longstanding diabetes.
    C) Pancreatic ductal adenocarcinoma risk is greater than that for both the age-adjusted general population and those with longstanding diabetes.
    D) If incident diabetes is accompanied by weight loss, pancreatic ductal adenocarcinoma risk is lowered.

Expert Perspective: Although longstanding diabetes mellitus is a modest pancreatic ductal adenocarcinoma risk factor, new-onset diabetes has been strongly linked to pancreatic ductal adenocarcinoma. In patients >50 years old, incident diabetes is associated with an approximately eight-fold increase in risk over the subsequent three years. This association is indicative of pancreatogenic diabetes (i.e., diabetes that is caused by pancreatic ductal adenocarcinoma but diagnosed prior to the cancer). Pancreatic ductal adenocarcinoma is thought to cause glucose intolerance via a paraneoplastic phenomenon that differs from classic type 2 diabetes in that glucose control paradoxically worsens with weight loss. Beta-cell dysfunction and insulin resistance occur at early stages of pancreatic ductal adenocarcinoma before glandular destruction by local invasion and can be improved by tumor resection. Current research seeks to investigate the utility of incident diabetes or biomarkers of pancreaticogenic diabetes for pancreatic ductal adenocarcinoma screening.

Correct Answer: C

Case Study continued: Despite imaging consistent with a pancreatic tumor, an EUS-guided biopsy was nondiagnostic. A CT scan of the chest revealed no evidence of metastatic disease. She underwent Whipple pancreaticoduodenectomy. Pathology revealed a 2 cm pancreatic ductal adenocarcinoma with negative margins (R0 resection), 0 of 9 involved lymph nodes, and no perineural or lymphovascular invasion. She has recovered well from the surgery, with ECOG performance score 0, and presents to your clinic to discuss further treatment.

14) What do you recommend as the next step in treatment?
   A) Start surveillance with CT chest, abdomen, pelvis every three to six months.
   B) Adjuvant FOLFIRINOX.
   C) Adjuvant gemcitabine.
   D) Adjuvant gemcitabine/capecitabine.
   E) Adjuvant gemcitabine/nab-paclitaxel.

Expert Perspective: Even in the absence of high-risk pathologic features, pancreatic ductal adenocarcinoma is likely to recur after resection. Adjuvant chemotherapy is recommended for up to six months to mitigate this risk. This principle was first established by the phase III ESPAC-1 trial, which demonstrated that 5-FU/leucovorin improved median overall survival compared to observation from 14.0 months to 19.7 months (HR 0.66; 95% CI 0.52–0.83; $P = 0.0005$). The subsequent phase III CONKO-001 trial demonstrated that gemcitabine improved median disease-free survival compared to observation from 6.9 months to 13.4 months, and gemcitabine subsequently became the reference standard.

Despite the routine use of adjuvant chemotherapy, mortality remains high among patients with resected pancreatic ductal adenocarcinoma. Thus, three subsequent randomized phase III trials sought to intensify adjuvant therapy by comparing combination cytotoxic regimens to gemcitabine monotherapy.

The phase III ESPAC-4 trial compared gemcitabine/capecitabine to gemcitabine alone. Median overall survival was improved in the combination arm from 25.5 months to 28.0 months (HR 0.82; 95% CI 0.68–0.98; $P = 0.032$). Soon thereafter, the phase III NCIC-CTG PA.6 trial demonstrated a remarkable benefit associated with FOLFIRINOX; compared to gemcitabine, FOLFIRINOX improved median overall survival from 35.0 months to 54.4 months (HR 0.64; 95% CI 0.48–0.86; $P = 0.003$). The triplet regimen FOLFIRINOX was associated with higher incidence of adverse effects, but FOLFIRINOX has emerged as the standard of care for patients who are able to tolerate this intensive approach.

The combination regimen of gemcitabine/nab-paclitaxel was then evaluated in the phase III APACT trial. The primary endpoint of this trial was disease-free survival as evaluated by blinded independent radiographic review. Although the primary endpoint of extending independently evaluated disease-free survival was not met (18.8 months vs 19.4 months, HR 0.88; 95% CI 0.73–1.06; $P = 0.18$), the combination regimen did improve investigator-assessed median disease-free survival from 13.7 months to 16.6 months (HR 0.82; 95% CI 0.69–0.97; $P = 0.02$) and median overall survival from 37.7 months to 41.8 months (HR 0.80; 95% CI 0.68–0.95; $P = 0.009$). Radiographic evidence of pancreatic ductal adenocarcinoma progression can be difficult to ascertain, and thus independent review may be a less effective metric for progression compared to investigator-assessed outcomes. Therefore, gemcitabine/nab-paclitaxel may represent an effective regimen in this setting, but additional data are necessary to definitively support its use.

Chemoradiation, administered after adjuvant chemotherapy and restaging imaging, can be considered in the event of positive resection margins (R1 resection). Due to conflicting data regarding efficacy in this setting, use of chemoradiation should be guided by multidisciplinary discussion. Additional data are awaited from the phase II/III Radiation Therapy Oncology Group (RTOG) 0848 trial, which randomized resected patients with no evidence of progressive disease after five cycles of adjuvant gemcitabine-based chemotherapy to one additional cycle or one additional cycle followed by fluoropyrimidine-based chemoradiation. Of note, this trial was amended midway through enrollment to allow alternative adjuvant regimens. Regardless of the outcome, systemic chemotherapy should remain the top priority for adjuvant treatment.

Correct Answer: B

Screening for Pancreatic Adenocarcinoma

Case Study 8

You are caring for a 53-year-old man with metastatic pancreatic ductal adenocarcinoma. Germline genetic testing reveals a pathogenic mutation in *ATM*, and cascade genetic testing reveals that his 48-year-old brother also carries the mutation. The patient's brother wishes to discuss screening for pancreatic ductal adenocarcinoma. After an in-depth discussion regarding limitations and cost of screening, the high incidence of detected pancreatic abnormalities, and uncertainties about the potential benefits, he decides to proceed with screening.

15) **Which annual screening modality would you select?**
    A) CT chest, abdomen, and pelvis.
    B) MRI abdomen/MRCP.
    C) EUS.
    D) B and/or C.
    E) There is no effective way to screen for pancreatic ductal adenocarcinoma, even in high-risk individuals.

Expert Perspective: Over 80% of pancreatic ductal adenocarcinoma is diagnosed at an advanced, incurable stage. Early detection of localized pancreatic ductal adenocarcinoma with an effective screening tool could improve curative resection rates and overall survival. However, population-based screening is not feasible given the low incidence and the lack of a noninvasive test with high sensitivity and specificity.

The diagnostic yield of screening high-risk individuals has been investigated in prospective cohort studies. The Cancer of the Pancreas Screening 2 (CAPS2) study used EUS to detect preinvasive pancreatic neoplasms in 10% of patients with Peutz-Jeghers Syndrome or a family history of pancreatic ductal adenocarcinoma. The subsequent multicenter CAPS3 study then compared the sensitivity of various screening modalities. Among 216 high-risk patients, 43% were found to have pancreatic abnormalities. EUS detected 43%, MRI detected 33%, and CT detected 11%. Most abnormalities were confirmed to be intraductal papillary mucinous neoplasms, and high-grade dysplasia was detected in three of five patients who underwent pancreatic resection. Given the poor sensitivity in this study, CT scans are not recommended for pancreatic ductal adenocarcinoma screening.

The utility of EUS and/or MRI for detecting early stage tumors has been further evaluated in recent studies of selected high-risk individuals (those with known pathogenic germline alterations in pancreatic ductal adenocarcinoma susceptibility genes and/or extensive family history of pancreatic ductal adenocarcinoma) and has resulted in resection rates of 75 to 90% for screen-detected pancreatic ductal adenocarcinoma. An analysis of high-risk individuals enrolled in the CAPS1-4 studies detected a remarkable 85% three-year survival for patients with screen-detected pancreatic ductal adenocarcinoma, but these data are susceptible to lead-time bias and represent small numbers; additional research is needed to determine whether early detection leads to decreased mortality. Future screening programs may also incorporate new noninvasive technologies such as circulating tumor cells or cell-free DNA to complement imaging-based protocols.

Current NCCN recommendations emphasize the importance of shared decision-making for high-risk patients considering screening, including education about the risk of false-positive findings, the cost, and the limitations of screening. Annual MRI and/or EUS is the preferred modality, but the recommended age to begin screening depends on individual genetic risk factors. For patients with pathogenic *ATM* muations, pancreatic ductal adenocarcinoma screening should be considered at age 50, or at 10 years younger than the earliest familial pancreatic ductal adenocarcinoma diagnosis, whichever is earlier.

Correct Answer: D

Pain Management

Case Study 9

You are caring for a 72-year-old man with locally advanced pancreatic ductal adenocarcinoma who recently discontinued frontline systemic therapy due to severe fatigue and nausea. His functional status has improved since stopping treatment, but he has developed severe mid-abdominal pain radiating to his back. Recent CT scans show local progression of pancreatic disease without evidence of metastases. He is receiving around-the-clock acetaminophen, gabapentin, and escalating doses of opiate analgesics, but he is starting to experience somnolence and constipation.

16) What are your next steps in pain management?
    A) Increase opiate analgesic doses further.
    B) EUS-guided celiac plexus neurolysis.
    C) Palliative pancreatic radiotherapy.
    D) Refer to hospice.
    E) Either B or C.

Expert Perspective: About 50 to 75% of patients with unresectable pancreatic ductal adenocarcinoma will develop severe abdominal pain during the course of their illness. While mild pain can be treated with acetaminophen or other nonopiate medications, pain intensity can escalate with local disease progression, and the subsequent moderate to severe pain frequently requires opiate analgesia. As opiate requirements escalate, patients can experience adverse effects such as sedation, dizziness, respiratory depression, and constipation, which can worsen abdominal discomfort.

Pancreatic ductal adenocarcinoma–associated pain is largely attributable to tumor infiltration of celiac nerves responsible for abdominal nociception. EUS-guided celiac plexus neurolysis can be an effective tool to palliate these symptoms when around-the-clock analgesic administration is insufficient and/or patients experience adverse analgesic-associated effects. A Cochrane review of randomized controlled studies found that celiac plexus neurolysis statistically significantly improved abdominal pain compared to analgesics alone at four and eight weeks after the procedure. Importantly, opiate use was also significantly reduced for the patients receiving neurolysis (Chapter 52).

Palliative pancreatic radiotherapy can also help control pancreatic ductal adenocarcinoma–associated pain. Radiation should be considered in the setting of large tumors compressing other structures. In such cases, the tumor is likely to be causing pain due to mass effect rather than nerve infiltration, and thus tumor shrinkage with radiation may improve quality of life, though it is unlikely to impact disease-related survival. Decisions to pursue palliative radiation should be made in a multidisciplinary setting.

Correct Answer: E

Future Directions

While cytotoxic chemotherapy remains the primary systemic treatment option for pancreatic cancer to date, future research will hopefully broaden the available options to include targeted agents. For example, over 90% of pancreatic cancers are driven by mutations in the oncogene *KRAS*, which has proven difficult to target thepeutically. However, recent promising results have been obtained with the covalent *KRAS* inhibitors sotorasib and adagrasib specifically for pancreatic cancers harboring a *KRAS G12C* mutation, which occurs at a rate of about 2%. In a recent phase I/II trial among 38 patients with advanced *KRAS G12C*-mutated pancreatic cancer, sotorasib generated a response rate of 21% with encouraging rates of progression-free and overall survival. In another recent phase I/II trial of adagrasib among patients with GI malignancies harboring *KRAS G12C* mutations, partial responses were seen in five of 10 evaluable patients with pancreatic cancer. In addition to *KRAS G12C*, additional rare genomic alterations are currently targetable with small molecules (e.g. gene fusions of *ALK, NRG1, NTRK, ROS1, FGFR2* and *RET*, or mutations in *BRAF*) or immunotherapy (microsatellite instability). Further study is warranted to identify additional genomically-informed therapeutics and to investigate novel promising treatment modalities.

Recommdeded Readings

Bekaii-Saab, T.S., Spira, A.I., Yaeger, R., et al. (2022). KRYSTAL-1: updated activity and safety of adagrasib (MRTX849) in patients (pts) with unresectable or metastatic pancreatic cancer (PDAC) and other gastrointestinal (GI) tumors harboring a KRASG12C mutation. *J Clin Oncol* 40 (suppl 4): 519.

Canto, M.I., Almario, J.A., Schulick, R.D., et al. (2018). Risk of neoplastic progression in individuals at high risk for pancreatic cancer undergoing long-term surveillance. *Gastroenterol* 155 (3): 740–751.

Conroy, T., Desseigne, F., Ychou, M., et al. (2011). FOLFIRINOX versus gemcitabine for metastatic pancreatic cancer. *N Engl J Med* 364 (19): 1817–1825.

Conroy, T., Hammel, P., Hebbar, M., et al. (2018). FOLFIRINOX or gemcitabine as adjuvant therapy for pancreatic cancer. *N Engl J Med* 379 (25): 2395–2406.

Fong, Z.V. and Ferrone, C.R. (2021). Surgery after response to chemotherapy for locally advanced pancreatic ductal adenocarcinoma: a guide for management. *J Natl Compr Canc Netw* 19 (4): 459–467.

Golan, T., Hammel, P., Reni, M., et al. (2019). Maintenance olaparib for germline BRCA-mutated metastatic pancreatic cancer. *N Engl J Med* 381 (4): 317–327.

Hammel, P., Huguet, F., Van Laethem, J.L,. et al. (2016). Effect of chemoradiotherapy vs chemotherapy on survival in patients with locally advanced pancreatic cancer controlled after 4 months of gemcitabine with or without erlotinib: the LAP07 randomized clinical trial. *JAMA* 315 (17): 1844–1853.

Mizrahi, J.D., Surana, R., Valle, J.W., et al. (2020). Pancreatic cancer. *Lancet* 395 (10242): 2008–2020.

O'Reilly, E.M., Lee, J.W., Zalupski, M., et al. (2020). Randomized, multicenter, phase II trial of gemcitabine and cisplatin with or without veliparib in patients with pancreas adenocarcinoma and a germline BRCA/PALB2 mutation. *J Clin Oncol* 38 (13): 1378–1388.

Shindo, K., Yu, J., Suenaga, M., et al. (2017). Deleterious germline mutations in patients with apparently sporadic pancreatic adenocarcinoma. *J Clin Oncol* 35 (30): 3382–3390.

Sohal, D.P.S., Duong, M., Ahmad, S.A., et al. (2021). Efficacy of perioperative chemotherapy for resectable pancreatic adenocarcinoma: a phase 2 randomized clinical trial. *JAMA Oncol* 7 (3): 421–427.

Strickler, J.H., Satake, H., Hollebecque, A., et al. (2022). First data for sotorasib in patients with pancreatic cancer with KRAS p.G12C mutation: a phase I/II study evaluating efficacy and safety. *J Clin Oncol* 40 (suppl36): 360490.

Vasen, H., Ibrahim, I., Ponce, C.G., et al. (2016). Benefit of surveillance for pancreatic cancer in high-risk individuals: outcome of long-term prospective follow-up studies from three European expert centers. *J Clin Oncol* 34 (17): 2010–2019.

Von Hoff, D., Ervin, T., and Arena, F. (2013). Randomized phase III study of weekly nab-paclitaxel plus gemcitabine versus gemcitabine alone in patients with metastatic adenocarcinoma of the pancreas (MPACT). *N Engl J Med* 369 (18): 1691–1703.

Wang-Gillam, A., Li, C., Bodoky, G., et al. (2016). Nanoliposomal irinotecan with fluorouracil and folinic acid in metastatic pancreatic cancer after previous gemcitabine-based therapy (NAPOLI-1): a global, randomised, open-label, phase 3 trial. *Lancet* 387 (10018): 545–557.

26

Hepatocellular Cancer

Pedro Luiz Serrano Uson Junior[1] and Mitesh Borad[2]

[1] Hospital Israelita Albert Einstein, São Paulo, SP
[2] Mayo Clinic, Phoenix, AZ

Introduction

Globally, liver cancer is estimated to be the sixth most commonly diagnosed cancer, with more than 900,000 new cases in 2020. In the same period, it was estimated there were 830,000 deaths related to the disease. Liver cancer is the leading cancer in transitioned countries, including those of eastern Asia, southeastern Asia, and northern and western Africa. In addition, it is the leading cancer cause of death in multiple countries, including Mongolia, Thailand, Egypt, and Guatemala. Hepatocellular carcinoma (HCC) is the histological type of 75 to 85% of primary liver cancer cases. Multiple risk factors are related to the development of the disease, most commonly hepatitis B virus (HBV), hepatitis C virus (HCV), alcohol abuse, and metabolic syndrome (Table 26.1). Around half of the cases of HCC in the world are related to chronic HBV. Patients may present with paraneoplastic syndrome of hypoglycemia, hypercalcemia, erythrocytosis and dermatomyositis.

The incidence of liver cancer is rising, and mortality rates as well. If the disease is diagnosed in early stages, normally it is manageable with local treatments with curative intent, including resection, ablative techniques, and liver transplantation. Cases with localized disease treated with curative intent have a median overall survival of more than five years. However, most cases are diagnosed in advanced stages. The cure rate for patients with early stage disease is about 60 to 70%; however, for patients with more advanced disease, the five-year survival rate is only 10 to 25%. Treatments for those patients with advanced disease include chemoembolization, radioembolization, systemic treatment with immunotherapy, and antiangiogenics, including kinase inhibitors. Most patients with metastatic HCC will die from the disease within one to two years irrespective of treatment received.

Table 26.1 Risk factors for hepatocellular cancer.

Hepatitis B, C, and D
Alcohol-related cirrhosis
Tobacco
Nonalcoholic fatty liver disease
Autoimmune hepatitis
Primary biliary cirrhosis
Hereditary hemochromatosis
Thorotrast
Nitrosylated compounds
Aflatoxin B1
Betel nut chewing
Androgen steroids
Wilson disease
Alpha-1 antitrypsin deficiency
Porphyria
Glycogen storage disease

Screening Methods

1) **What are the risks and benefits of screening methods for hepatocellular carcinoma?**

Expert Perspective: Screening for HCC in patients at high risk of developing the disease is important. The American Association for the Study of Liver diseases (AASLD) recommends that ultrasound (US) should be done every six months in patients at high risk. A large trial from China with more than 18,000 patients evaluated the impact of screening in patients with high risk, including cases of HBV or history of chronic hepatitis. Serum alpha fetoprotein (AFP) and US every six months in this trial resulted in a 37% reduced risk of HCC mortality. Several studies evaluated this common form of screening and found it to be cost-effective.

Studies also evaluated the impact of isolated AFP for screening in high-risk populations. Some limitations of this strategy include multiple cutoffs evaluated in the trials. However, a Chinese study evaluated the impact of AFP and US, both alone and combined, using an AFP cutoff of ≥20 ng/ml. The study demonstrated that the combination of AFP and US has the higher detection rate (92%) and an acceptably low false-positive rate (7.5%).

Populations considered at a high risk for developing HCC include patients with liver cirrhosis induced by viral infections (HBC, HCV) as well as nonviral causes of cirrhosis (alcohol, NASH, autoimmune disorders, and others). In addition, HBV carriers are also considered at a high risk irrespective of underlying liver disease. Based on the AASLD guidelines and Liver Imaging Reporting and Data System (LI-RADS) guidelines, patients with rising serum AFP or identification of liver nodule(s) ≥10 mm on US should undergo additional image exams, including abdominal MRI or CT scans.

Diagnostic Approaches

2) Which imaging characteristics are diagnostic for hepatocellular carcinoma, obviating the need for liver lesion biopsy?

Expert Perspective: Most patients with early disease are asymptomatic. In cases of advanced disease, multiple signs and symptoms can be present, including ascites, fatigue, jaundice, weight loss, and abdominal pain. HCC is characterized by arterial hypervascularity and wash-out on portal venous phases since most of the HCC blood supply originates from the hepatic artery. Optimal imaging used for the diagnosis of HCC includes multiphasic liver CT scan and intravenous contrast-enhanced MRI. The diagnosis is characterized by the intense arterial uptake followed by contrast wash-out, or hypointensity in the delayed nonperipheral venous phase. For patients with cirrhosis, an enhancing capsular appearance and growth between images can be considered as meeting diagnostic criteria. PET scans are variably helpful, as only approximately 65% of HCC lesions accumulate FDG.

For patients with cirrhosis during HCC surveillance, a finding of classical arterial enhancement using a single image technique and liver nodules between 1 to 2 cm can be used for diagnosis of HCC without the need for a confirmatory biopsy. AASLD and LI-RADS guidelines address these considerations. Also, a gadolinium contrast is preferred for MRI. Rising AFP levels can provide supporting diagnostic information during screening. If there is a suspicious finding on ultrasound during surveillance, another imaging method with or without AFP should be considered. For better stratification of suspicious lesions, multidisciplinary discussion is highly recommended. Data have shown that multidisciplinary team management of HCC improves multiple outcomes, including rates of curative treatments and overall survival in advanced stages.

In cases with high certainty of a HCC diagnosis, biopsy could be avoided. The most important pathologic issue is a diagnosis of the fibrolamellar variant, which has a superior prognosis compared to traditional HCC. Additionally, approximately 5% of all liver cancers are combined HCC-cholangiocarcinoma. Complications of biopsy nowadays are relatively rare. Risk of bleeding is about 0.6% and not necessarily related to the degree of hepatic dysfunction, and thrombocytopenia is a relevant risk factor. Tumor seeding along the needle tract has been reported to occur at the rate of approximately 3%. This is probably lower now that a sheath is used to encase the actual biopsy trocar. If a patient is headed towards potential transplantation, percutaneous biopsy is usually avoided because of the theoretical risk of needle tract recurrence enhanced by immunosuppression.

Staging and Initial Workup

3) Which staging system is commonly used in HCC?

Expert Perspective: The initial workup in a patient with newly diagnosed HCC involves a multidisciplinary approach. Investigation of the etiology should include a hepatitis panel and assessment of associated comorbidities and hepatic function. Recommended additional exams for staging include chest CT scan, pelvic CT scan, and bone scans if skeletal symptoms are present. AFP is also recommended. If an active viral infection is detected,

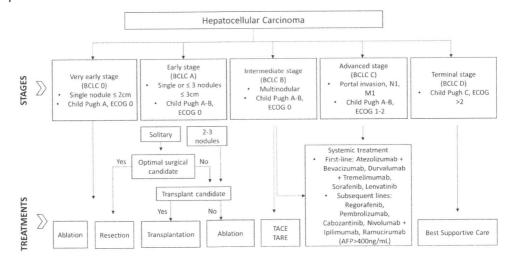

Figure 26.1 BCLC staging system and available treatment strategies. Legend: ECOG: Eastern Cooperative Oncology Group performance status, TACE: transarterial chemoembolization, TARE: Transarterial radioembolization.

patients should be referred to a hepatologist or infectious disease specialist for evaluation for antiviral treatment.

Multiple staging systems can be used to grade and treat HCC. One of the most commonly used systems is the Barcelona Clinic Liver Cancer (BCLC) staging system. This staging system includes not only the anatomical assessment of the tumor but also clinical characteristics of the patients, including liver function (Child-Pugh) and clinical performance status (ECOG) (Figure 26.1). This grading system is also commonly used for treatment assessment and enrolment in trials.

Treatment for Localized Disease

Ablation and Resection

4) **What is the preferred method of treatment for localized HCC in patients with and without cirrhosis?**

Expert Perspective: Patients with a solitary tumor can be managed with resection. Partial hepatectomy can be a curative therapy for most patients with a localized solitary mass of any size. Careful assessment of underlying disease is necessary to address the effectiveness and safety of the procedure. In appropriate patients, five-year survival may be as high as approximately 60%. Future liver remnant evaluation (~20% without cirrhosis and 30 to 40% in Child Pugh class A and adequate vascular and biliary inflow/outflow) should be done with preoperative images, including CT/MRI. Scans can also evaluate satellite nodules and metastatic spread. In cases of successful resection, no adjuvant treatment is recommended to date. However, control of underlying viral hepatitis B whenever present should continue.

Another option of treatment for localized small nodules is ablative procedures including percutaneous, laparoscopic, and open procedures. Radiofrequency ablation (RFA), microwave ablation (MWA), and percutaneous ethanol injection (PEI) are the methods most commonly used. Multiple studies have evaluated the efficacy of RFA and PEI in solitary tumors ≤ 5 cm or up to three tumors ≤ 3 cm. RFA in those studies seems to be superior in efficacy and rates of recurrence when compared to PEI. Due to these observations, RFA and MWA are replacing PEI as the most used ablation techniques. Studies comparing RFA with resection suggest that both treatments are equally effective. The choice of which treatment to apply for localized solitary tumors should include a careful evaluation of tumor location and liver function. The best outcomes for ablative therapies are observed in solitary tumors < 2 cm.

Liver Transplantation

For patients with localized disease and moderate to severe cirrhosis, liver transplantation is an alternative to resection in the absence of portal hypertension. It is an attractive option due to treatment of the underlying liver disease, cirrhosis, and potentially avoids complications related to future liver remnant. The Milan criteria were proposed for unresectable HCC and cirrhosis, for patients with single tumors ≤5 cm, or no more than three tumors ≤3 cm, and no macrovascular invasion. UNOS criteria are based on this, including transplantation as an alternative for patients with single tumors ≥2 cm and ≤5 cm, or two to three esions ≥1 cm and ≤3 cm and no macrovascular invasion or extrahepatic spread. The MELD score includes parameters such as INR, serum creatinine, sodium, and bilirubin levels to assess the severity of liver disease and allocate priority to transplantation. Recurrence rates after transplantation are around 15%. Complications of the procedure and immunosuppression have dropped since the early years of liver transplants, because of improvements in preoperative screening and imaging, better patient selection, and newer immunosuppressive regimens. Multiple studies have evaluated transplantation beyond the standard criteria. As an example, for tumors ≥5 cm, the University of California, San Francisco (UCSF) criteria have been used (size limit of 6.5 cm). Contradictory outcome results from these studies make this a subject in need of ongoing investigation.

Transarterial Treatments

5) What are the utilities of transarterial approaches in the treatment of HCC?

Expert Perspective: Transarterial treatments, including transarterial chemoembolization (TACE) and radioembolization (TARE), are methods of treatment used in tumors staged as BCLC B, intermediate (Figure 26.1). TACE involves intra-arterial administration of chemotherapy (frequently doxorubicin) along with embolic material such as ethiodide oil or, more recently, polyvinyl alcohol drug-eluting beads. This method achieves very high intratumoral drug concentrations while causing local ischemia simultaneously. Side effects may range from pain, nausea, fever, and fatigue to gallbladder ischemia, abscess, and hepatic failure (although the latter is very uncommon). This modality has the advantage of potentially being able to treat multiple tumours simultaneously, since the arterial supply is used as the delivery system. TARE also employs the arterial system, to deliver microscopic glass or resin beads (microspheres) coated with Yttrium-90 to the tumour. Rather than the larger 300 μm drug-eluting beads used for chemoembolization, the beads for radioembolization are approximately

32 μm. This means that they do not actually cause significant ischemia by blocking arterioles and are only trapped as they traverse the capillaries. Beta-particle emission will then cause DNA damage in tumour cells within an approximately 2.5 mm radius. The lack of overt ischemia allows this method to be used for patients who have portal vein thrombosis.

Both strategies can also be used as a bridge therapy for transplantation. Transarterial treatments can reduce the dropout rates for patients on liver transplantation waiting lists and decrease the risk of tumor progression. Furthermore, no evidence of higher complications on post transplantation outcomes were observed in these studies. Transarterial treatments improve overall survival when compared to best supportive care in unresectable HCC. In this group of patients and those with more advanced HCC, TACE and TARE were evaluated with systemic antiangiogenics including sorafenib and lenvatinib in multiple studies, with contradictory outcomes. In the phase III LAUNCH trial, which enrolled predominantly patients with hepatitis B-related HCC and advanced disease (portal vein tumor thrombus, a large intrahepatic tumor burden, or extrahepatic spread), the combination of lenvatinib plus TACE in the first-line setting improved survival and more than doubled the response rate compared with lenvatinib alone, but grade III or IV adverse events were also more common. Multivariable analysis revealed that portal vein tumor thrombus and treatment allocation were independent risk factors for OS. Additional experience with lenvatinib plus TACE is needed in Western populations, where HCC is more often alcohol-related, before it can be concluded that this is a preferred approach over systemic therapy alone (especially immunotherapy-based approaches) for frontline therapy of advanced HCC. Bland transarterial embolization (TAE) is another technique evaluated as an alternative to resection. Studies have shown that TAE with microspheres alone is non-inferior to TACE in response rate and other disease outcomes. Transarterial treatments should not be used in patients with Child Pugh C score. Other contraindications may include bilirubin > 3mg/dL and patients with renal insufficiency.

Radiotherapy

6) **Is there a role for radiotherapy in the treatment of HCC?**

Expert Perspective: Radiotherapy can be used as an alternative strategy for cases where ablative and embolization techniques are unavailable, contraindicated, or have failed. External beam radiotherapy may be used for symptom palliation.

Treatment for Advanced and Metastatic Disease

7) **What are some of the considerations in selection of systemic therapy in advance HCC?**

Expert Perspective: The effectiveness of systemic chemotherapy alone in advanced cancers is poor. Sorafenib was the treatment of choice for advanced HCC for several years.

Recently, sorafenib was surpassed in efficacy by several combinations including immunotherapeutic drugs (Table 26.2). The combination of the anti-PDL1 inhibitor, atezolizumab plus the anti-VEGF bevacizumab is now considered the standard of care for the treatment of patients with metastatic HCC based on a randomized clinical trial. All patients eligible for this regimen were evaluated and if necessary, treated for esophageal varices, so an upper endoscopy before starting the treatment is mandatory. Patients with underlying autoimmune disease (e.g. rheumatoid arthritis) are also excluded from an immunotherapy regimen. The response rate with this combination is about 30%, which is higher than previously observed with single tyrosine kinase inhibitors including sorafenib. For most patients with advanced or unresectable HCC, including elderly patients, the combination would be the best choice. Some exceptions should be made; the study only included patients with Child Pugh A (score of 5 to 6; Tables 26.2 and 26.3), The trial also excluded patients who had a myocardial infarction or stroke within the previous three months, were on therapeutic anticoagulation, or had coinfection with HCV or HBV. The combination appears to be active and safe in this subgroup of patients. For patients with Child Pugh B score, sorafenib or nivolumab could be used, based on data from a cohort in this subgroup of patients in the CheckMate-040 study. Furthermore, atezolizumab or other immunotherapy should not be routinely used in organ-transplanted patients. Immunotherapy in this group of patients is associated to organ rejection. For patients who have undergone organ transplantation, preferred first-line treatment includes sorafenib or lenvatinib. Lenvatinib is non-inferior to sorafenib on first-line treatment for patients with advanced HCC. NCCN suggests limiting use of lenvatinib to individuals with no worse than Child Pugh A.

Most currently approved regimens for second-line treatment, including regorafenib, pembrolizumab, nivolumab plus ipilimumab, and ramucirumab, were evaluated after sorafenib failure. Interestingly, in patients from Asia with previously treated advanced HCC, pembrolizumab (KEYNOTE-394) significantly prolonged overall survival (median 15 versus 13 months) and PFS, and ORR was greater versus placebo. Except for cabozantinib (Child Pugh A), most patients were previously treated with sorafenib. In the CELESTIAL trial a small proportion of the patients received third-line systemic treatment, including previous treatment with chemotherapy and immunotherapy.

No randomized prospective data have shown efficacy of a regimen after the combination of atezolizumab and bevacizumab. The consensus from most experts is to use a tyrosine kinase inhibitor including cabozantinib or regorafenib, or even sorafenib or lenvatinib, after atezolizumab and bevacizumab failure. For patients with alpha fetoprotein above 400 ng/mL, ramucirumab could also be an option considering the safety profile and rates of adverse events compared to the other drugs. However, ramucirumab was also not evaluated after atezolizumab and bevacizumab in the trial. Multiple other combinations of immunotherapy with antiangiogenics are being evaluated and in the future may expand the arsenal of treatment of advanced HCC (i.e., pembrolizumab and lenvatinib, nivolumab and regorafenib, atezolizumab and cabozantinib). More recently, sorafenib was surpassed in efficacy by a regimen without an antiangiogenic using a combination of durvalumab and tremelimumab in the HIMALAYA trial (Table 26.2). This regimen would be an excellent option for patients with contraindications to antiangiogenics.

Table 26.2 Randomized trials evaluating immunotherapy versus sorafenib in first-line treatment for advanced hepatocellular carcinoma.

Study	Design	Drug	N°	Characteristics	ORR	DCR	mPFS (mo)	mOS (mo)
Yau et al. 2022 Checkmate 459	Phase III	Nivolumab	371	Child-Pugh A	15%	55%	3.7	16.4
		Sorafenib	372	Treatment naïve	7%	58%	3.8	14.7
Finn et al. 2020 IMBRAVE150	Phase III	Atezolizumab + Bevacizumab	336	Child-Pugh A	27.3%	73.6%	6.8	19.2
		Sorafenib	165	Treatment naïve	11.9%	55.3%	4.3	13.4
Kelley et al. 2022 COSMIC 312	Phase III	Atezolizumab + Cabozantinib	432	Child-Pugh A	11%	78%	6.8	15.4
		Sorafenib	217	Treatment naïve	3.7%	65%	4.2	15.5
		Cabozantinib	188		6.4%	84%	5.8	NP
Ren et al. 2021 ORIENT-32	Phase II/III	Sintilimab + IBI305	380	Child-Pugh ≤ B7	24%	73%	4.6	NR
		Sorafenib	191	Treatment naïve	8%	63%	2.8	10.4
Abou-Alfa et al. 2022 HIMALAYA	Phase III	Durvalumab	389	Child-Pugh A	17%	54.8%	3.7	16.6
		Durvalumab + Tremelimumab	393	Treatment naïve	20.1%	60.1%	3.8	16.4
		Sorafenib	389		5.1%	60.7%	4.1	13.8

NR: Not reached, NP: Not presented
Anti-PD1: Nivolumab, Sintilimab
Anti-PD-L1: Atezolizumab, Durvalumab
Anti-CTLA-4: Tremelimumab
Anti-VEGF: Bevacizumab, IBI305
Tyrosine kinase inhibitors: Sorafenib, Cabozantinib

Table 26.3 Modified Child-Pugh classification for severity of cirrhosis.

Parameter	1 point	2 points	3 points
1. Ascites	Absent	Slight	Moderate
2. Encephalopathy	None	Grade 1–2	Grade 3–4
3. INR or PT (seconds over control)	< 1.7 < 4	1.7–2.3 4 to 6	> 2.3 > 6
4. Albumin	> 3.5 g/dL	2.8 to 3.5 g/dL	< 2.8 g/dL
5. Bilirubin	< 2 mg/dL	2 to 3 mg/dL	> 3 mg/dL

INR: international normalized ratio; PT: prothrombin time.
Modified Child-Pugh classification of the severity of liver disease according to the degree of ascites, the serum concentrations of bilirubin and albumin, the prothrombin time, and the degree of encephalopathy. A total Child-Turcotte-Pugh score of 5 to 6 is considered Child-Pugh class A (good operative risk), 7 to 9 is class B (moderate operative risk), and 10 to 15 is class C (poor operative risk).

Recommended Readings

Abou-Alfa, G. K. et al. (2022). Tremelimumab plus Durvalumab in Unresectable Hepatocellular Carcinoma. *NEJM Evidence*: EVIDoa2100070.

Finn, R.S. et al. (2020). Atezolizumab plus bevacizumab in unresectable hepatocellular carcinoma. *N Engl J Med* 382 (20): 1894–1905.

Heimbach, J.K., Kulik, L.M., Finn, R.S., Sirlin, C.B., Abecassis, M.M., Roberts, L.R., et al. (2018). AASLD guidelines for the treatment of hepatocellular carcinoma. *Hepatology* 67 (1): 358–380.

Kelley, R. K. et al. (2022). Cabozantinib plus atezolizumab versus sorafenib for advanced hepatocellular carcinoma (COSMIC-312): a multicentre, open-label, randomised, phase 3 trial. *Lancet Oncol* 23(8): 995–1008.

Liver Imaging reporting and data system. Available at: http://www.acr.org/quality-safety/resources/LIRADS. (Accessed February 2022).

Mehta, N. and Yao, F.Y. (2019). What are the optimal liver transplantation criteria for hepatocellular carcinoma? *Clin Liver Dis* 13 (1): 20.

Qin, S., Chen, Z., Fang, W. et al. (2023 March 1). Pembrolizumab versus placebo as second-line therapy in patients from Asia with advanced hepatocellular carcinoma: a randomized, double-blind, phase III trial. *J Clin Oncol* 41 (7): 1434–1443.

Ren, Z. et al. (2021) Sintilimab plus a bevacizumab biosimilar (IBI305) versus sorafenib in unresectable hepatocellular carcinoma (ORIENT-32): a randomised, open-label, phase 2–3 study. *Lancet Oncol* 22(7): 977–990.

Sonbol, M.B. et al. (2020). Systemic therapy and sequencing options in advanced hepatocellular carcinoma: a systematic review and network meta-analysis. *JAMA Oncol* 6 (12): e204930.

Sung, H. et al. (2021). Global cancer statistics 2020: GLOBOCAN estimates of incidence and mortality worldwide for 36 cancers in 185 countries. *CA: A Cancer J Clini* 71 (3): 209–249.

Uson, Junior, P.L.S. et al. (2021). Immunotherapy and chimeric antigen receptor T-cell therapy in hepatocellular carcinoma. *Chin Clin Oncol* 10 (1): 11.

Yau, T. et al. (2022). Nivolumab versus sorafenib in advanced hepatocellular carcinoma (CheckMate 459): a randomised, multicentre, open-label, phase 3 trial. *Lancet Oncol* 23 (1): 77–90.

Peng Z, Fan W, Zhu B, et al. Lenvatinib Combined With Transarterial Chemoembolization as First-Line Treatment for Advanced Hepatocellular Carcinoma: A Phase III, Randomized Clinical Trial (LAUNCH). J Clin Oncol. 2022 Aug 3:JCO2200392. doi: 10.1200/JCO.22.00392. Epub ahead of print. PMID: 35921605.

27

Biliary Tract Cancers

David B. Zhen[1] and Vaibhav Sahai[2]

[1] University of Washington/Fred Hutchinson Cancer Center, Seattle, WA
[2] University of Michigan, Ann Arbor, MI

Introduction

Biliary tract cancer encompasses bile duct cancer, also known as cholangiocarcinoma (intrahepatic, hilar, and extrahepatic), and gallbladder cancer. It is categorized as a rare cancer per the National Institute of Health definition and represents only about 3–5% of all gastrointestinal malignancies. The estimated age-standardized incidences of cholangiocarcinoma and gallbladder cancer are 1.6 and 1.13 cases, respectively, per 100,000 people per year in the United States. Worldwide, the incidence varies significantly depending on the region, increasing to 40-fold higher in endemic regions such as Thailand. Globally and in the United States, the incidence and mortality of biliary tract cancer, specifically intrahepatic cholangiocarcinoma, has risen over the past several decades, some of which may be related to recent changes in the International Classification of Disease (ICD) classification, but also due to improved diagnostic procedures and increase in risk factors such as cirrhosis, alcoholic liver disease, and hepatitis C. The incidence increases with age, with most patients being diagnosed between 50 and 70 years of age, although cholangiocarcinoma arising in the context of primary sclerosing cholangitis or choledochal cysts may present nearly two decades earlier. There is a gender disparity in gallbladder cancer with slightly higher incidence in women. In Asia, particularly Thailand, infection with hepatobiliary flukes of the genera Clonorchis and Opisthorchis is associated with 40-fold higher risk of intrahepatic cholangiocarcinoma. At least two genetic disorders are associated with an increased risk of cholangiocarcinoma: Lynch syndrome (hereditary nonpolyposis colorectal cancer) and a rare inherited disorder called multiple biliary papillomatosis (see Chapters 45 and 47). High rates of gallbladder cancer are seen in South American countries, particularly Chile, Bolivia, and Ecuador, as well as some areas of northern India, Pakistan, Japan, Korea, and Poland. These populations all share a high prevalence of gallstones and/or salmonella infection, both recognized risk factors for gallbladder cancer. In addition, obesity, tobacco, alcohol, and workers in the oil, paper, chemical, shoe, textile, and cellulose acetate fiber manufacturing industries have high risk of these cancers.

The likelihood of survival is dependent on the stage with five-year survival rates for localized cholangiocarcinoma and gallbladder cancer is as high as 15–25% and 65%,

Cancer Consult: Expertise in Clinical Practice, Volume 1: Solid Tumors & Supportive Care,
Second Edition. Edited by Syed A. Abutalib, Maurie Markman, Al B. Benson III, and Hope S. Rugo.
© 2024 John Wiley & Sons Ltd. Published 2024 by John Wiley & Sons Ltd.

respectively, but less than 3% for those diagnosed with metastatic disease. Moreover, the anatomic location of cholangiocarcinoma influences survival, with poorer outcomes with hilar and extrahepatic disease as opposed to intrahepatic subtype.

1) **For a patient with a solitary resectable intrahepatic cholangiocarcinoma, which of the following treatment options would be recommended?**

    A) Neoadjuvant chemotherapy followed by surgical resection.
    B) Up-front surgical resection followed by adjuvant chemotherapy.
    C) Ablation.
    D) Neoadjuvant chemotherapy followed by surgery and adjuvant chemotherapy.

Expert Perspective: Up-front surgical resection followed by adjuvant chemotherapy is currently considered the standard for solitary, resectable intrahepatic cholangiocarcinoma. Prognostic factors associated with improved outcomes after surgical resection include achieving complete, margin-negative (R0) resection and lower nodal disease burden. The data for neoadjuvant chemotherapy is from retrospective, single-institution studies in locally advanced patients, wherein rates for tumor downstaging with gemcitabine and cisplatin of 20–36% correlated with improved overall survival. However, the use of neoadjuvant therapy in patients with resectable disease has not been well studied, and retrospective studies in this setting show conflicting results on improved outcomes. More studies are needed to determine the role of neoadjuvant chemotherapy in resectable intrahepatic cholangiocarcinoma.

Similarly, prospective data are also lacking on the use of ablation for solitary intrahepatic cholangiocarcinoma. Unlike the frequent use of ablation in hepatocellular carcinoma less than 3 cm, surgical resection remains the mainstay of therapy for cholangiocarcinoma given its more aggressive disease biology and higher likelihood of a healthier, non-cirrhotic liver remnant (Chapter 26). However, there are a few single institutional series that suggest benefit of this approach, particularly for patients who may not be optimal surgical candidates or those with a high likelihood of recurrence.

Correct Answer: B

2) **Which of the following would you recommend to a patient diagnosed with an incidental T1b (muscle) invasive gallbladder adenocarcinoma after a simple laparoscopic cholecystectomy?**

    A) Capecitabine.
    B) Gemcitabine-capecitabine.
    C) Extended cholecystectomy followed by observation.
    D) Extended cholecystectomy followed by chemotherapy.

Expert Perspective: Patients with T1b invasive (muscle layer) gallbladder carcinoma have a 15% risk of lymph node metastasis, with the risk of lymph node metastases increasing to > 70% with T4 disease. In patients with ≥T1b disease, extended or radical cholecystectomy with resection of adjacent liver tissue from segments IVb and V along with lymph node dissection should be performed for medically fit patients as extended resection has shown to improve survival outcomes in retrospective studies. Based on the current NCCN guidelines, adjuvant chemotherapy is preferred for all patients with ≥T1b disease regardless of nodal status, although larger studies are needed to determine the relative absolute benefit of adjuvant chemotherapy in those without nodal involvement and lower T stage (i.e. T1/2N0 vs T3/4N0). Capecitabine monotherapy for six months is considered the standard-of-care adjuvant therapy for patients with resected biliary tract cancer based on the BILCAP trial. The BILCAP study was a phase III, open-label trial that randomized patients to either capecitabine 1,250 mg/m^2 twice a day administered on days 1 through 14 on every 21-day cycles for eight cycles or observation. While not statistically significant, the intention-to-treat analysis showed a trend toward improvement in the primary endpoint of median OS in the group who received adjuvant capecitabine (53 months vs 36 months; HR 0.81; 95% CI 0.63–1.04; $P = 0.097$). However, a statistically significant difference in OS was observed in the prespecified per-protocol analysis whereby 17 ineligible patients (progression of disease before starting adjuvant therapy, no surgical intervention pursued, and prolonged surgical wound healing preventing/delaying initiation of adjuvant therapy) were removed from the overall analysis, favoring adjuvant capecitabine over observation (HR 0.75; 95% CI 0.58–0.97; $P = 0.028$). The median recurrence-free survival was 25.9 months vs 18.5 months in favor of the capecitabine group.

A single-arm phase II trial, SWOG S0809, explored the role for adjuvant gemcitabine and capecitabine given on 21-day cycles followed by capecitabine-radiation (45 Gy to regional lymphatics; 54–59.4 Gy to tumor bed) in resected extrahepatic biliary tract and gallbladder cancer. This demonstrated a median overall survival of 34 months with a two-year disease-free survival of 54% and 11% local relapse rate. The generalizability of these results is limited by the single-arm design and exclusion of patients with intrahepatic cholangiocarcinoma. The ongoing ACTICCA-1 trial (NCT02170090) is a phase III trial evaluating gemcitabine and cisplatin in the adjuvant setting for biliary tract cancer. The control arm was initially observation but later revised to capecitabine after results of the BILCAP study. Recently, the phase II STAMP trial conducted in Asia randomized patients with resected lymph node positive extrahepatic cholangiocarcinoma to either gemcitabine and cisplatin or capecitabine, and failed to demonstrate a difference in overall survival between the two arms. The phase II/III OPT-IN trial (NCT04559139), which is currently enrolling patients with gallbladder cancer (stages II–III), incidentally identified on simple cholecystectomy to determine the difference in overall survival for patients given neoadjuvant gemcitabine and cisplatin prior to extended cholecystectomy followed by adjuvant gemcitabine and cisplatin compared to patients who receive only adjuvant gemcitabine and cisplatin after extended resection.

Correct Answer: D

3) Which of the following management options would you consider for a patient with R1 resected stage IIIB or node-positive gallbladder adenocarcinoma with MSI-H?
   A) Capecitabine.
   B) Chemoradiation.
   C) Gemcitabine-capecitabine.
   D) Gemcitabine-cisplatin.
   E) Immunotherapy with PD-1 blockade.

Expert Perspective: Please refer to the answer for Question 2 to review the data for options A, C, and D. The randomized phase III trial PRODIGE12/ACCORD18, comparing adjuvant gemcitabine plus oxaliplatin (GEMOX) for six months and observation, showed no significant differences in recurrence-free and overall survival. While adjuvant radiation for margin-positive disease is reasonable given the relative high risk of locoregional relapse in this setting, the benefit of adjuvant radiation for node-positive disease is still debatable given the concern that nodal involvement is more a surrogate for distant metastatic relapse, thus emphasizing the importance of systemic chemotherapy in these patients. A meta-analysis of 21 clinical trials involving 1,465 patients with extrahepatic cholangiocarcinoma or gallbladder carcinoma reported significantly higher five-year overall survival rate in patients with adjuvant radiotherapy versus no radiotherapy if they had positive lymph nodes (odds ratio 0.15; $P < 0.0001$) or margins (odds ratio 0.40; $P = 0.02$), but no difference if they had margin-negative disease (odd ratio 0.57; $P = 0.08$). Pembrolizumab is an FDA approved therapy for patients with unresectable or metastatic solid tumors with high microsatellite instability or deficient mismatch repair that have progressed following prior treatment and who have no satisfactory alternative treatment options, and thus would not be a suitable option for adjuvant therapy.

Correct Answer: A

4) **Which of the following management options would you consider (outside of a trial) in a patient with extrahepatic distal cholangiocarcinoma with metastases to the liver with no prior therapy?**
   A) Gemcitabine-cisplatin.
   B) Gemcitabine-nab-paclitaxel.
   C) Gemcitabine-cisplatin plus nab-paclitaxel.
   D) Gemcitabine-cisplatin plus durvalumab.
   E) FOLFIRINOX.

Expert Perspective: The landmark ABC-02 phase III trial demonstrated significant improvement in median overall survival with gemcitabine and cisplatin compared to gemcitabine alone (11.7 months vs 8.1 months, respectively; HR 0.64; 95% CI: 0.52–0.80; $P < 0.001$) in patients with advanced biliary tract cancer with no prior systemic therapy. The gemcitabine and cisplatin arm also demonstrated an improvement in median progression-free survival (8.0 months vs 5.0 months), objective response rate (26.1% vs 15.5%), and disease control rate (81.4% vs 71.8%) compared to gemcitabine alone. The combination of gemcitabine and nab-paclitaxel was evaluated in a similar patient population (n = 74) in a phase II single-arm trial. The median progression-free and overall survival estimates were 7.7 months and 12.4 months, respectively, while the objective response rate was reported as 30%. More recently, another single-arm phase II trial of gemcitabine, nab-paclitaxel, and cisplatin in a similar patient population (n = 60) reported a median progression-free survival of 11.8 months, median overall survival of 19.2 months, and an objective response rate of 45%. These results led to a phase III trial, SWOG S1815, which randomized 441 patients to gemcitabine, cisplatin, and nab-paclitaxel versus gemcitabine and cisplatin. Unfortunately, the gemcitabine, cisplatin and nab-paclitaxel arm did not lead to an improved response rate, progression-free survival or overall survival compared to gemcitabine and cisplatin. A phase II/III trial, PRODIGE 38 AMEBICA, compared modified FOLFIRINOX (5-fluorouracil, leucovorin, irinotecan, and oxaliplatin) to gemcitabine plus cisplatin in 191 patients with treatment-naive advanced biliary tract cancer. The study failed to meet its primary endpoint of improvement in the six-month progression-free survival rate (44.6% vs 47.3%) after completion of the phase II portion. Additionally, there was no significant difference in median progression-free survival (6.2 months vs 7.4 months) or overall survival (11.7 months vs 13.8 months). Most recently the results of phase III randomized TOPAZ-1 (global) trial evaluating gemcitabine and cisplatin +/− durvalumab in untreated advanced or metastatic biliary tract cancer were reported. Overall, 685 patients were randomly assigned to durvalumab (n = 341) or placebo (n = 344). The durvalumab plus gemcitabine and cisplatin demonstrated statistically significant prolonged overall survival versus placebo plus gemcitabine and cisplatin regardless of PD-L1 or MSI status. The hazard ratio for overall survival was 0.80 (95% CI 0.66–0.97; $P = 0.021$). The estimated 24-month overall survival rate was 24.9% (95% CI 17.9–32.5) for durvalumab and 10.4% (95% CI 4.7–18.8) for placebo. The hazard ratio for progression-free survival was 0.75 (95% CI 0.63–0.89; $P = 0.001$). Objective response rates were 26.7% with durvalumab and 18.7% with placebo. The incidences of grade 3 or 4 adverse events were 75.7% and 77.8% with durvalumab and placebo, respectively. A trend toward overall and progression-free survival benefit with durvalumab and chemotherapy was observed across all subgroups analyzed. Based on these data, durvalumab was FDA approved in the first-line setting for advanced biliary tract cancer in combination with gemcitabine and cisplatin on September 2022 and is considered a new standard of care for up-front treatment of unresectable and metastatic disease. In another placebo-controlled phase III trial (KEYNOTE-966) of over 1000 patients with treatment-naïve, locally advanced or metastatic biliary tract cancers, the addition of pembrolizumab to gemcitabine plus cisplatin improved overall survival (median 13 versus 11 months) with an acceptable toxicity profile.

Correct Answer: D

5) **Which of the following systemic therapeutic(s) would you consider for a patient with metastatic intrahepatic cholangiocarcinoma with *IDH1* mutation after progression on first-line chemotherapy with gemcitabine-cisplatin?**
   A) FOLFOX.
   B) FOLFIRI.
   C) Liposomal irinotecan, 5-fluorouracil, leucovorin.
   D) Ivosidenib.
   E) Enasidenib.
   F) A, B, and D.

Expert Perspective: The phase III ABC-06 trial enrolled 162 patients with advanced biliary tract cancer after progression on gemcitabine-cisplatin chemotherapy and randomized them to either active symptom control plus 5-fluorouracil, leucovorin, and oxaliplatin (FOLFOX), or active symptom control alone. The study met its primary endpoint of improvement in median overall survival (6.2 months vs 5.3 months; adjusted HR 0.69; 95%

CI 0.50–0.97; $P = 0.031$) in favor of the chemotherapy-containing arm. In addition, the objective response rate was 5%, and median-progression-free survival 4.0 months on the FOLFOX arm. A phase II trial conducted in South Korea randomized 120 patients to either modified FOLFOX or modified FOLFIRI (plus 5-fluorouracil, leucovorin, and irinotecan). Of the 101 evaluable patients, there was no significant difference in the median overall survival (6.3 months and 5.7 months), progression-free survival (2.8 months and 2.1 months), and objective response rates (5.9% vs 4.0%), respectively. In another phase IIb trial (NIFTY) conducted in South Korea, 174 patients were randomized to either 5-fluorouracil, leucovorin, and liposomal irinotecan regimen or 5-fluorouracil/leucovorin alone. The primary endpoint of median progression-free survival was significantly longer in the liposomal irinotecan containing arm (7.1 months vs 1.4 months; HR 0.56; 95% CI 0.39–0.81; $P = 0.0019$). In addition, the median overall survival was 8.6 months versus 5.5 months (HR 0.68; 95% CI 0.48–0.98; $P = 0.035$) in favor of the liposomal irinotecan-containing arm.

The phase III ClarIDHy trial randomized 187 patients with previously treated advanced cholangiocarcinoma harboring *IDH1* mutations to either an oral *IDH1* inhibitor ivosidenib 500 mg once daily or placebo. The ivosidenib arm demonstrated significant improvement in the primary endpoint of median progression-free survival (2.7 months vs 1.4 months; HR 0.37; 95% CI 0.25–0.54; one-sided $P < 0.0001$). The median overall survival was 10.8 months with ivosidenib and 9.7 months on the placebo arm (HR 0.69; 95% CI 0.44–1.10; $P = 0.06$); however, when adjusted for crossover (N = 43), the median overall survival for the placebo arm was 6.0 months (HR 0.46; 95% CI 0.28–0.75; one-sided $P = 0.008$). The objective response rate with ivosidenib was 2%. These results led to the FDA approval in August 2021. Enasidenib is an oral targeted inhibitor of IDH2 and has not been evaluated in a clinical trial likely due to the rarity of these mutations in cholangiocarcinoma.

Correct Answer: F

6) **Based on which of the following molecular alteration(s) reported on next-generation sequencing analysis of tumor for your patient with intrahepatic cholangiocarcinoma would you consider the use of an *FGFR* inhibitor?**
   A) *FGFR2* amplification.
   B) *FGFR2* point mutation.
   C) *FGFR2* rearrangement or fusion.
   D) None.

Expert Perspective: Fibroblast growth factor receptor (*FGFR*) signaling drives tumorigenesis through cellular proliferation, migration, survival, invasion, and angiogenesis. Pemigatinib, a selective, potent, oral inhibitor of FGFR1, 2, and 3 was evaluated in 146 patients with previously treated, advanced biliary tract cancer in the phase II FIGHT-202 study. Patients were enrolled into one of three cohorts based on their underlying FGFR alteration: (i) *FGFR2* fusions or rearrangements, (ii) other *FGFR* alterations (e.g. amplification or point mutations), or (iii) no FGF/FGFR alterations. Oral pemigatinib was administered at a starting dose of 13.5 mg once daily for 14 days of every 21-day cycle. Patients (n = 107) harboring *FGFR2* fusions or rearrangements showed an objective response rate of 35.5% with a disease control rate of 82.2%. Median progression-free survival was 6.9 months, and median overall survival was 21.1 months. Another oral *FGFR1-3*inhibitor, infigratinib, was similarly evaluated in a phase II trial in 122 patients with advanced biliary tract cancer previously treated with at least once gemcitabine-containing regimen. Infigratinib is dosed 125 mg once daily for 21 days on every 28-day cycle. In 108 patients with FGFR2 fusions or rearrangements, an objective response rate of 23.1% and disease control rate of 84.3% was reported with median progression-free and overall survival of 7.3 months and 12.2 months, respectively. Futibatinib, a highly selective inhibitor of *FGFR1-4* was tested in a pahse II FOENIX-CCA2 study. There was an objective response rate of 42% (95% CI 32–52) with a mean duration of response of 9.7 months (95% CI 7.6–17.0). Oral futibatinib is administered at a dose of 20 mg once daily. Based on these data, the Federal Drug Administration (FDA) granted accelerated approval to pemigatinib, infigratinib and futibatinib for previously treated patients with advanced biliary tract cancer harboring *FGFR2* fusions or rearrangements. Recently, the new drug application for infigratinib was withdrawn by the pharmaceutical company.

In comparison, 20 patients with other *FGF/FGFR* alterations, including *FGFR2* amplifications and point mutations on the phase II FIGHT-202 trial showed no partial response, and the median progression-free and overall survival estimates were 2.1 months and 6.7 months, respectively. However, there is ongoing investigation into whether some of these activating *FGFR2* mutations and amplifications may actually benefit from pan-FGFR inhibitors.

Correct Answer: C

Recommended Readings

Abou-Alfa, G.K., Macarulla, T., Javle MM et al. (2020 June). Ivosidenib in IDH1-mutant, chemotherapy-refractory cholangiocarcinoma (ClarIDHy): a multicentre, randomised, double-blind, placebo-controlled, phase 3 study. *Lancet Oncol* 21 (6): 796–807.

Abou-Alfa, G.K., Sahai, V., Hollebecque A et al. (2020 May). Pemigatinib for previously treated, locally advanced or metastatic cholangiocarcinoma: a multicentre, open-label, phase 2 study. *Lancet Oncol* 21 (5): 671–684.

Benson, A.B., D'Angelica, M.I., Abbott DE et al. (2022 May 1). Hepatobiliary cancers, version 2.2022, NCCN clinical practice guidelines in oncology. *J Natl Compr Canc Netw* 19 (5): 541–565.

Goyal, L., Meric-Bernstam, F., Hollebecque, A. et al. (January 2023). Futibatinib for FGFR-Rearranged Intrahepatic Cholangiocarcinoma. NEJM 388 (3): 228–239.

Kelley, R.K., Ueno, M., Yoo, C. et al. (2023 June 3). Pembrolizumab in combination with gemcitabine and cisplatin compared with gemcitabine and cisplatin alone for patients with advanced biliary tract cancer (KEYNOTE-966): a randomised, double-blind, placebocontrolled, phase 3 trial. *Lancet* 401 (10391): 1853–1865. doi:10.1016/S0140-6736(23)00727-4. Epub 2023 Apr 16. PMID: 37075781.

Oh, D-Y., He, A.R., Qin, S. et al. (2022 2022). Durvalumab plus gemcitabine and cisplatin in advanced biliary tract cancer. *NEJM Evid* 1(8) DOI:https://doi.org/10.1056/EVIDoa2200015.

Lamarca, A., Palmer, D.H., Wasan HS et al. (2021 May). Second-line FOLFOX chemotherapy versus active symptom control for advanced biliary tract cancer (ABC-06): a phase 3, open-label, randomised, controlled trial. *Lancet Oncol* 22 (5): 690–701.

Primrose, J.N., Fox, R.P., Palmer DH et al. (2019 May). Capecitabine compared with observation in resected biliary tract cancer (BILCAP): a randomised, controlled, multicentre, phase 3 study. *Lancet Oncol* 20 (5): 663–673.

Valle, J., Wasan, H., Palmer DH et al. (2010 April 8). Cisplatin plus gemcitabine versus gemcitabine for biliary tract cancer. *N Engl J Med* 362 (14): 1273–1281.

28

Carcinoid and Neuroendocrine Tumors

Mintallah Haider and Jonathan Strosberg

Moffitt Cancer Center, Tampa, FL

Introduction

Neuroendocrine tumors (NETs) are a diverse group of neoplasms encompassing different biochemical and clinical behavior. This variability leads to differences in prognosis and treatment, with the opportunity to personalize recommendations to each tumor in an individual. While NETs can arise from several sites of origin, gastrointestinal tract and bronchial primaries are the most common. Partially due to advancements in diagnostic evaluations and imaging, the incidence of NETs has steadily increased over the past five decades, more recently nearing seven new cases per 100,000 per year. A potential for tumors to have indolent biology contributes to a higher prevalence. The pathologic classification of NETs is complex and evolving. Tumor differentiation and proliferation rate categorize tumors and contribute to diagnostic evaluations and treatment formulation. The majority of NETs are well differentiated, and most are grade 1 and 2 (Ki67 index less than 20% and mitotic count less than 20 HPFs). The more recently defined entity of well differentiated grade 3 NETs harbors a proliferation index > 20 and is now included in the 5th edition of the WHO Classification of Tumors of the Digestive System. The site of origin coupled with an expert assessment of differentiation and grading contribute to an understanding of tumor biology and anticipated behavior within a disease spectrum. Through this, the appropriate diagnostics and multidisciplinary treatment can be designed, encompassing active surveillance, surgical treatment, cytotoxic interventions and theranostics.

Case Study 1

Treatment of incidental appendix NET: Which patients have an indication for oncologic surgical resection?

A 31-year-old woman presents with progressive right lower quadrant pain associated with anorexia and nausea. CT demonstrates findings consistent with appendicitis, and she undergoes appendectomy. Pathology reports a 1.4 cm well-differentiated grade 1 NET.

1) **What is the next best step in management?**
   A) Annual surveillance colonoscopy.
   B) Obtain a PET scan.
   C) Annual surveillance CT.
   D) Right hemicolectomy.
   E) No further assessments indicated.

Expert Perspective: Neuroendocrine tumors are the most frequent appendiceal neoplasms and are typically found incidentally at appendectomy. When considering incidental localized appendiceal NETs in adults, tumor size is the primary factor determining need for additional surgical management (Figure 28.1). Tumors measuring less than 1 cm with negative margins and less than 3 mm of infiltration of the mesoappendix have a low potential for regional and distant metastatic disease and portend an excellent prognosis. These cases are adequately served with simple appendectomy. Tumors measuring greater than 2 cm carry up to a 40% risk of metastatic disease and are best served with complete oncologic right hemicolectomy.

The treatment challenge is found in tumors measuring between 1 and 2 cm (AJCC T1b): consideration of a small risk of metastatic disease has to be balanced with surgical risk. Potential features of increased risk include intermediate (as opposed to low) tumor grade, positive margins on appendectomy, lymphovascular invasion, tumor location in appendiceal

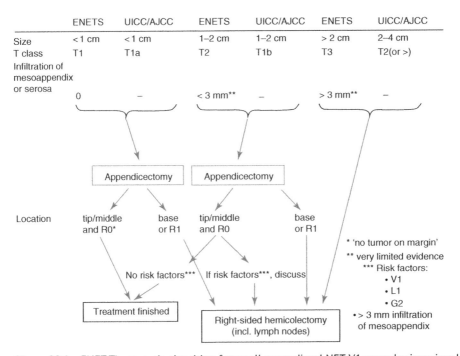

Figure 28.1 ENET Therapeutic algorithm for small appendiceal NET. V1: vascular invasion; L1: lymphatic invasion; G2: grade 2 tumor (Ki-67: 3–20%). Pape UF, Niederle B, Costa F, et al. ENETS Consensus Guidelines for Neuroendocrine Neoplasms of the Appendix (Excluding Goblet Cell Carcinomas). *Neuroendocrinology.* 2016; 103(2): 144–152. doi:10.1159/000443165.

base (as opposed to tip), greater than 3 mm mesoappendix invasion (AJCC T3 disease), or invasion into surrounding organs (AJCC T4 disease). Presence of one or more factors may contribute to a surgical decision of right hemicolectomy if the patient is deemed a surgical candidate. (Table 28.1) The main reason for controversy is that tumors 1–2 cm in size are associated with a risk of locoregional lymph node involvement; however, risk of distant metastatic disease appears to be negligible, even with long-term surveillance.

There is no role for adjuvant systemic therapy after surgical management of localized disease, including node-positive disease. There is no recommendation for surveillance of tumors less than 1cm treated with R0 appendectomy. Likewise, there is no surveillance recommendation for tumors greater than 1 cm treated with R0 hemicolectomy without nodal disease. Surveillance recommendations are consensus driven and recommended in particular circumstances: (i) patients with tumors measuring greater than 2 cm, (ii) smaller tumors in the presence of high-risk features outlined above who are not deemed candidates for oncologic resection, and (iii) patients treated with hemicolectomy and found to have nodal disease. Surveillance should include a history and physical as well as conventional imaging at 6–12 months post surgery and then every 1–2 years for up to 10 years. MRI may be preferred in young patients of childbearing age to reduce radiation exposure.

It is important to note that mixed adenocarcinoid tumors, while demonstrating neuroendocrine features, carry a higher risk of metastasis and compromised prognosis. These tumors are treated as appendix adenocarcinomas, and simple appendectomy is not sufficient.

Correct Answer: E

Table 28.1 AJCC 8th Ed. Appendix NET Staging.

T category		N category		M category	
Tx	Cannot be assessed	Nx	Cannot be assessed	M0	None
T0	No evidence of tumor	N0	Negative	M1	Metastases present
T1	< 2 cm	N1	Regional lymph nodes involved	M1a	Limited to liver
T2	> 2 to ≤ 4 cm			M1b	≥ 1 extrahepatic site
T3	> 4 cm or Subserosal invasion or mesoappendix involvement			M1c	Hepatic and extra hepatic sites
T4	Perforates into peritoneum or invades adjacent organs/structures (excluding subserosa of adjacent bowel)				

Case Study 2

What is the best way to evaluate incidental rectal NET?

A healthy 30-year-old man undergoes a screening colonoscopy due to a family history of colon adenocarcinoma. A solitary 1.2 cm polyp identified in the mid-rectum is removed with hot snare. Margins are positive. Pathology reports a T1 1.2 cm well-differentiated NET, Ki67 1%.

2) What is the next appropriate evaluation?
   A) Referral to surgery.
   B) Somatostatin analogue.
   C) EUS with endoscopic mucosal resection.
   D) Repeat colonoscopy in five years.
   E) Somatostatin receptor imaging.

Expert Perspective: Rectal NETs are often identified on screening endoscopy and low-grade tumors measuring less than 2 cm have an excellent prognosis. Tumor size is the primary guide in management after colonoscopy. The risk of regional lymph node involvement and metastatic disease for tumors less than 1cm is 1–10% and increases to 60–80% with lesions greater than 2 cm.

Per consensus guidelines, endoscopic management is preferred for superficial lesions measuring less than 1 cm. Surgery is advised for tumors greater than 2 cm or those with associated lymph node metastases.

Controversy lies in the management of rectal NETs between 1 cm and 2 cm, where the metastatic risk is 10–15%. Though data is mixed regarding surgical management, tumors with relatively high mitotic rate / ki-67 index (intermediate grade) and invasion of the muscularis propria can be counseled regarding surgery, while low-grade tumors without invasion of muscularis propria can be addressed with local resection. (Figure 28.2).

There is no recommendation for adjuvant treatment, except in the case of adjuvant chemotherapy for poorly differentiated neuroendocrine carcinomas.

In terms of surveillance after surgery, for grade 1–2 tumors measuring less than 1 cm without lymph node involvement, there is no surveillance recommendation, though these data are based on grade 1 tumors and may not apply to tumors with higher Ki67 index. Grade 1–2 tumors between 1 cm and 2 cm should undergo multiphase CT or MRI within the first year and then annually thereafter. For grade 1–2 tumors measuring greater than 2 cm, multiphase CT or MRI should be completed within the first year and then annually thereafter for 10 years. Routine chromogranin A levels are not recommended (see also Chapter 23).

Correct Answer: C

Case Study 3

Comparing MIBG and peptide receptor radiotherapy for metastatic unresectable paraganglioma and pheochromocytoma

A 69-year-old man with a history of resected right-sided pheochromocytoma eight years prior presents with multiple sites of back pain, hip pain, and hypertension. CT revealed right

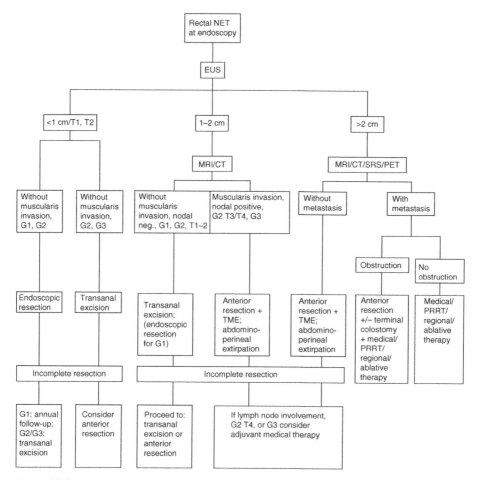

Figure 28.2 ENET Rectal NET Management. Adapted from Ramage JK, De Herder WW, Delle Fave G, et al. ENETS Consensus Guidelines Update for Colorectal Neuroendocrine Neoplasms. *Neuroendocrinology.* 2016; 103(2): 139–143. doi:10.1159/000443166.

suprarenal tumors and multiple lytic bone lesions. Bone biopsy reported metastatic pheochromocytoma, Ki67 10%.

3) What staging study do you recommend?
　A) I MIBG scintigraphy.
　B) ^{68}Ga-DOTATATE PET-CT.
　C) Octreoscan.
　D) FDG PET.
　E) A and B.

Expert Perspective: All patients with pheo/paraganglioma should be staged by cross-sectional imaging while functional imaging is indicated to evaluate metastatic disease. Iodine 123 meta-iodobenzylguanidine (^{123}I-MIBG) was most commonly used previously but has poor resolution and a lower detection rate compared to PET-based nuclear imaging modalities. Specifically, there is increasing experience with ^{68}Ga- or ^{64}Cu-labeled somatostatin receptor analog PET-CT (somatostatin receptors inhibitor) in detecting pheo/paraganglioma and determining receptor expression for treatment modalities. In a recent meta-analysis, the pooled detection rate of ^{68}Ga-DOTATATE PET/CT was 93%, compared to 74% for FDG-PET and 38% for I-MIBG scintigraphy (Han et al. 2018). In another study, ^{68}Ga-DOTATATE PET was evaluated for initial staging and restaging in paragangliomas and demonstrated a sensitivity of 84% for pheochromocytoma and 100% for paragangliomas. Additionally, the radiographic findings contributed to changes in management in 50% of pheochromocytoma and 44% of paraganglioma cases (Gild et al.).

Correct Answer: E

4) **The I MIBG scintigraphy demonstrates avid disease, and ^{68}Ga-PET-CT has heterogeneous uptake. What treatment would you consider next?**
   A) ^{131}I-MIBG.
   B) Somatostatin analog.
   C) Peptide receptor radiotherapy with ^{177}Lu- DOTA-TATE.
   D) Capecitabine.
   E) Radiation to painful metastatic sites.

Expert Perspective: ^{131}I-MIBG is a well-established treatment for unresectable paragangliomas, following ^{123}I-MIBG scintigraphy demonstrating the presence of cell membrane norepinephrine transporter system. A meta-analysis of 243 pooled patients treated with ^{131}I-MIBG reported a 3% complete and 27% partial response and stable disease in 52% (van Hulsteign et al.). Toxicities include myelotoxicity, hypothyroidism, hypogonadism, acute respiratory distress syndrome (ARDS), and hypertension. High specific activity (HSA) ^{131}I-MIBG received FDA approval after demonstrating partial response or stable disease in 92% of patients with metastatic paragangliomas. Although this product may be less toxic than conventional ^{131}I-MIBG, side effects remain a concern, with 90% of patients experiencing grade 3 or higher hematologic adverse events and 72% of patients experiencing other severe events (Pryma et al.).

The utility of peptide receptor radiotherapy in paragangliomas is described in small-volume retrospective data and case reports. In a pooled cohort, peptide receptor radiotherapy achieved partial response or stable disease in 89.9% of patients, with acceptable toxicity (Table 28.2). In a particular study, ^{131}I-MIBG, ^{90}-Y-DOTATATE, ^{177}Lu-DOTA-TATE, and combination ^{131}I-MIBG with ^{90}Y-DOTATATE were compared in progressive metastatic paragangliomas (Nastos et al.). Peptide receptor radiotherapy demonstrated superior OS, progression-free survival, and treatment response when compared to ^{131}I-MIBG.

The decision to proceed with systemic therapy is based on disease progression and/or presence of symptoms related to hormonal syndrome such as uncontrolled hypertension, arrhythmias, psychiatric symptoms as opposed to indolent disease that can be monitored over time. A second decision point compares MIBG versus functional PET, with the treatment targeting the modality with higher uptake. The challenge is encountered when uptake is equivocal, in which case toxicity and predisposition are considered. For younger patients without prior myelotoxic treatments and fewer bone metastases, MIBG is a better clinical fit, while older patients with compromised marrow reserve

Table 28.2 PRRT in PGGL in 2006–2019, adapted from *Endocrine-Related Cancer*, 26(11), R627-R652.

Authors	Radiopharmaceutical	N	% of responders	Median PFS (months)	Median OS (months)
van Essen et al.	^{177}Lu-DOTA-TATE	12	25%	NA	NA
Forrer et al.	^{177}Lu-DOTA-TATE	28	18%	NA	NA
Imhof et al.*	^{90}Y-DOTATOC	39	18%	NA	NA
Zovata et al.**	^{177}Lu-DOTA-TATE	4	50%	NA	NA
Puranik et al.	^{177}Lu-DOTA-TATE/^{90}Y-DOTATOC**	9	44%	NA	NA
Estevao et al.*	^{177}Lu-DOTA-TATE	14	71%	NA	NA
Pinato et al.**	^{177}Lu-DOTA-TATE	5	20%	17	NA
Nastos et al. 2017	^{177}Lu-DOTA-TATE/^{90}Y-DOTATOC**	13	100%	38.5	60.8
Kong et al.	^{177}Lu-DOTA-TATE	20	47%	39	NA
Yadav et al. 2019	^{177}Lu-DOTA-TATE	25	84%%	32	NA
Zandee et al.	^{177}Lu-DOTA-TATE	30	23%	30	NA
Vyakaranam et al. 2019	^{177}Lu-DOTA-TATE	22	9	21.6	49.6
Kolasinska*	^{177}Lu-DOTA-TATE	13	8	35	68

All studies retrospective unless otherwise indicated.
* prospective
** case series

should be considered for peptide receptor radiotherapy. End organ function can also offer guidance; HSA-^{131}I-MIBG tends to be associated with less catecholamine release compared to peptide receptor radiotherapy, and this is favorable in patients with cardiovascular disease. There are no particular differences when considering renal and hepatic function, though both should be monitored closely with either treatment. Other important factors to consider are insurance coverage and distance to treatment in the patient's community (Pacak et al.).

Correct Answer: A

Case Study 4

What is the appropriate assessment of type 1 gastric NET?

A 52-year-old is referred to evaluate a history of gastric neuroendocrine tumor. An EGD demonstrated a gastric polyp that was resected, and pathology noted a 2 mm NET, Ki-67 2%.

28 Carcinoid and Neuroendocrine Tumors

Table 28.3 Gastric NET.

	Type I	Type II	Type III
Frequency	70–80%	5%	20%
Gastric pH	Basic	Acidic	Normal
Gastrin level	High	High	Normal
Clinical scenario	Hypergastrinemic state secondary to atrophic gastritis	Zollinger-Ellison Syndrome, MEN-I (gastrin producing tumor duodenum or pancreas)	often solitary, aggressive, often metastatic to lymph nodes and/or liver

5) What is the next step in evaluation?
   A) Gastrin level.
   B) CT abdomen and pelvis with contrast.
   C) Referral to surgery for gastrectomy.
   D) DOTATATE PET.

Expert Perspective: Well-differentiated gastric NETs are divided into three categories (Table 28.3) with type 1 being related to elevated gastrin in the setting of atrophic gastritis, type 2 being related to elevated gastrin in the setting of a gastrinoma, and type 3 being sporadic. Measurement of gastrin level (ideally off PPI) is therefore typically the first step in evaluation of gastric NETs. Type 3 NETs are often malignant; however, type 1 gastric NETs very rarely metastasize. Conventional imaging with CT or MRI has a limited role in type 1 gastric NETs but are important in type 2 to rule out gastrinoma. Similarly, somatostatin receptor imaging is unlikely to be of benefit in type 1 due to the rarity of metastatic disease unless a gastric tumor is large (> 2cm). Pathological evaluation of the stomach for evidence of atrophic gastritis can also help confirm type 1 gastric NET. Laboratory evaluation should also include complete blood count and B_{12} level since B_{12} deficiency is very common with atrophic gastritis.

Most type 1 gastric NETs are small and multifocal. They are typically managed with endoscopic surveillance, often once a year, and endoscopic resection of tumors. Advanced endoscopic resection techniques such as endomucosal resection (EMR) can be considered for relatively large tumors. Type 3 (sporadic) gastric NETs are often managed with formal gastrectomy, although small, low-grade T1 tumors can sometimes be managed endoscopically.

Surveillance recommendations are based on consensus, and EGD is recommended every two years, though this timeline can be structured based on findings of number, size, and growth pattern of new lesions.

Correct Answer: A

Case Study 5

Is a well-differentiated grade 3 neuroendocrine tumor different from neuroendocrine carcinoma?

A 79-year-old man with history of CAD presents with unintentional 15 lbs weight loss over the course of three months and is found to have a 2.5 cm tail of pancreas mass and multifocal liver metastases. He has progressive anorexia and fatigue as well as right upper quadrant discomfort. A liver biopsy identifies well-differentiated grade 3 NET, Ki67 30%. His performance status is ECOG 1.

6) Which of the following statements about this patient's disease is correct?
   A) Well-differentiated grade 3 NETs have less aggressive behavior.
   B) Well-differentiated grade 3 NETs carry mutations in genes such as MEN1, DAXX, or ATRX.
   C) Distinguishing between grade 3 NET and neuroendocrine carcinoma can be a diagnostic challenge.
   D) All of the above.

Expert Perspective: The PRONET group evaluated an epidemiological study of 778 newly diagnosed neuroendocrine neoplasms. Of the 85% well-differentiated cases, 20% were grade 3 (defined as Ki67 greater than 20%). Poorly differentiated neuroendocrine carcinomas are highly aggressive and almost always presenting with Ki67 greater than 50% and associated with *TP53* and *RB1* mutations. Standard first-line treatment consists of a platinum-based regimen (carboplatin-etoposide). In contrast, well-differentiated grade 3 NETs harbor less aggressive behavior with Ki67 typically less than 50–60% and carry mutations in genes such as *MEN1, DAXX, or ATRX*, similarly to grade 1 and 2 NETs. Distinguishing between grade 3 NET and neuroendocrine carcinoma can be a diagnostic challenge. In a pathology evaluation of 33 cases, only one of three of the cases achieved consensus based on morphology, with 61% rendered ambiguous (Tang et al.) Of note, large cell neuroendocrine carcinoma (LCNEC) was especially challenging and overlapped greatly with well-differentiated grade 3 based on morphology. In this particular study, Ki67 was also not definitive. Ancillary immunohistochemistry was contributory: well-differentiated grade 3 NET lacked immunohistochemistry evidence of *TP53, RB1*, or *SMAD4* mutations, which were found in neuroendocrine carcinoma while loss of DAXX and ATRX was exclusive to well-differentiated grade 3 NET. Of interest, disease-specific medial survival was 75 months for well-differentiated grade 3 and 11 months for neuroendocrine carcinoma, confirming the clinical importance of distinguishing between the two entities.

Correct Answer: D

7) In addition to CT or MRI, what is an appropriate staging PET for well-differentiated grade 3 NET?
   A) FDG PET-CT.
   B) Ga68 PET-CT.
   C) MIBG.
   D) A and B.

Expert Perspective: Functional imaging is uniquely applicable in NET management and informs staging as well as treatment. The majority of grades 1 and 2 NET express somatostatin receptors that can be identified on somatostatin receptor imaging. While the primary site is known in a majority of cases, in those cases with unknown primary, a DOTATATE PET can be informative. A meta-analysis including 1,143 patients with pancreas NET, grades 1–3, reported a pooled detection rate of 81% for the primary lesion, with a sensitivity of 79.6% and specificity of 95% (Bauckneht et al.). The positive correlation between Ki67 and FDG-PET avidity is well described. In a study of pancreas NET, FDG-PET demonstrated 40%, 60%, and 95% sensitivity in grade 1, grade 2, and grade 3 NETs, respectively (Lieu et al.). For well-differentiated grade 3 NET, dual modality PET may also be informative, and this approach is described in the NETPET score (Chan et al.). The scoring system differentiates between five categories based on number of lesions avid on each PET type, and the score was the only variable significant on multivariate analysis in association with tumor grade and OS. Data specific to well-differentiated grade 3 NET is not robust; however, heterogeneity can be better evaluated with dual PET and guide treatment decisions. Though these data are intriguing, dual PET imaging is not a standard approach and is not within NCCN guidelines.

Correct Answer: D

8) **The patient's Ga-68 PET is avid in the pancreas primary, liver metastases, and demonstrates bone metastases that were not avid on FDG PET. What is the recommended first-line treatment?**
   A) Carboplatin plus etoposide.
   B) Capecitabine plus temozolomide.
   C) Peptide receptor radiotherapy.
   D) Single agent somatostatin analogue.
   E) B or C per physician/patient discussion.

Expert Perspective: The treatment approach for metastatic well-differentiated grade 3 NET is more aligned with lower grade NET rather than neuroendocrine carcinoma, particularly with Ki67 less than 50%. In a retrospective study of 204 patients with well-differentiated grade 3 NET and neuroendocrine carcinoma treated with platinum-based chemotherapy, disease control rate and progression-free survival were significantly higher in neuroendocrine carcinoma while OS was significantly longer in well-differentiated grade 3 NET, demonstrating lower efficacy of platinum-based chemotherapy in well-differentiated grade 3 NET (Heetfeld et al.). Furthermore, in the NORDIC trial, Ki-67 with a cutoff for response was identified at Ki67 of 55%.

There are limited data to guide treatments for well-differentiated grade 3 NET, although temozolomide-based regimens, peptide receptor radiotherapy, and other treatments used in grade 1 and 2 NETs can be considered in the first-line setting. While PROMID and CLARINET demonstrated the efficacy of somatostatin analogs in NET, nearly all patients on PROMID were low grade and the CLARINET study limited Ki67 at < 10%. For well-differentiated grade 3 NET, single-agent somatostatin analog could be considered in patients who are relatively asymptomatic with low volume disease. More aggressive therapy is appropriate for patients with grade 3 tumors and symptoms related to tumor growth.

A retrospective study from Mayo Clinic evaluated clinical outcomes in 30 evaluable patients with grade 3 NET, with Ki67 index ranging from 20.4 to 90% (Liu et al.). Primary sites included midgut, esophagus, lung, and unknown primary. The most common treatment modality was capecitabine combined with temozolomide (CAPTEM), followed by ^{177}Lu-DOTA-TATE (peptide receptor radiotherapy), platinum-etoposide, FOLFOX, and everolimus. The majority of patients had somatostatin receptor imaging–positive disease. CAPTEM (capecitabine and temozolomide) regimen achieved overall response rate of 35%, disease control rates of 65%, and median progression-free survival was 9.4 months; however, all values were higher when capecitabine combined with temozolomide was used as first-line when compared to second-line setting. Overall response rate was 28.6% with FOLFOX, 25% with platinum-etoposide, and 20% with peptide receptor radiotherapy. FOLFOX achieved the longest median progression-free survival of 13.4 months compared to 2.94 months with platinum-etoposide.

CAPTEM regimen (capecitabine combined with temozolomide) was evaluated in a phase II study that included 30 patients with grade 3 NET/ neuroendocrine carcinoma, with Ki67 index greater than 20% but less than 55% (Jeong et al.). Lung primaries were not included, though five patients had unknown primary sites. Overall response rate was 30%, and disease control rate was 76.7%; however, when evaluating patients with Ki67 less than 55%, overall response rate was 36%, and disease control rate was 84%. There was no difference between pancreas versus non-pancreas primaries.

The role of Ki67 as a biomarker for treatment response with CAPTEM regimen (capecitabine combined with temozolomide) was evaluated in 151 patients (Wang et al.). The overall response rate was 26.5%, and disease control rate was 76.2%; however, patients with Ki67 index ranging from 10 to 40% had a significantly higher overall response rate when compared to those with Ki67 greater than 40% and those with Ki67 less than 10%.

Peptide receptor radiotherapy may also play a role in treatment of metastatic well-differentiated grade 3 NET. A review of studies evaluating peptide receptor radiotherapy in grade 3 neuroendocrine neoplasms identified three articles, with a majority of patients having pancreas primaries and receiving peptide receptor radiotherapy as second line or subsequent treatment. Response rate ranged from 31 to 42% and disease control rates ranged from 69 to 78% (Sorbye et al.). The authors evaluated progression-free survival and OS in two groups, with lower Ki67 being less than or equal to 55% and higher Ki67 being more than 55%. Progression-free survival in the lower Ki67 group ranged from 11 to 16 months compared to 4–6 months in the higher Ki67 group. The OS ranged from 31 to 46 months in the lower Ki67 group compared to 7–9 months in the higher. Toxicity did not differ from that reported with peptide receptor radiotherapy in grade 1–2 NET. The NETTER 2 trial is evaluating peptide receptor radiotherapy in gastroenteropancreatic grade 2–3 NET as a first-line treatment (NCT03972488).

Correct Answer: E

Case Study 6

What is the role of peptide receptor radiotherapy in bronchial NET?

A 54-year-old woman with well-differentiated lung NET metastatic to bone and liver progressed on octreotide LAR and everolimus. She does not have respiratory symptoms but does have back pain associated with bone metastases. Her Octreoscan at diagnosis was positive, and a subsequent Ga68 DOTATATE PET confirms avid lung, liver, and bone disease. CT scan shows growth of liver metastases and increasing number of bone metastases.

9) **What is the next best treatment?**
   A) Capecitabine and temozolomide.
   B) Change octreotide to lanreotide and continue everolimus.

C) Peptide receptor radiotherapy.
D) Add external beam radiation to palliate painful metastases and continue current treatment.
E) A or C.

Expert Perspective: Lung NETs (typical or atypical carcinoid tumors) are relatively poorly studied. Somatostatin analogs have not been evaluated in a randomized, controlled fashion but can be considered in patients with relatively indolent somatostatin-receptor-positive metastatic tumors.

Everolimus has been shown to delay progression versus placebo in the RADIANT-4 trial and is the only FDA approved treatment for progressive lung NET. In a subgroup analysis of 90 lung NET patients, those treated with everolimus experienced a median progression-free survival of 9.2 months compared to 3.6 months with placebo (Fazio et al.). CAPTEM was evaluated as a second line or beyond treatment in 20 patients with lung NET (Al-Toubah et al.). Disease control rate was 85%, median progression-free survival was 13 months, and median OS was 68 months, with the majority of adverse events being grade 1.

Naraev et al. conducted a large literature review to report on the accumulating experience of peptide receptor radiotherapy in lung NET. When comparing outcomes of lung NET with pancreas or midgut primaries treated with peptide receptor radiotherapy, lung NET has a shorter median progression-free survival and OS. In addition, pooled data suggest similar outcomes for typical and atypical carcinoids though higher chromogranin A levels and higher hepatic tumor burden are reported negative risk factors (Sabet et al.). In this retrospective evaluation of 22 patients with progressive/metastatic grade 1–2 lung NET treated with ^{177}Lu-DOTA-TATEE, progression-free survival was 27 months and OS was 42 months.

A retrospective assessment of 22 patients with symptomatic metastatic/advanced lung NET treated with ^{177}Lu-DOTA-TATE were assessed for response, mortality, and OS (Parghane et al.). Of 19 evaluable patients, 79% reported symptomatic response, and overall response rate was 63%. Of interest, all of the nonresponses had moderate to intense FDG-avid lung or metastatic lesions, highlighting the importance of careful selection of patients for peptide receptor radiotherapy due to tumor heterogeneity. Median OS was 40 months, and no major adverse events were reported.

Another retrospective analysis reported efficacy and tolerability in 94 evaluable patients with lung NET who received peptide receptor radiotherapy with three protocols ^{90}Y-DOTATOC, ^{177}Lu-DOTA-TATE, and combination (Mariniello et al.). The overall response rate was 30%, and disease control rate was 76%. Median OS was 58.8 months, and median progression-free survival was 28 months. ^{177}Lu-DOTA-TATE achieved the highest five-year survival (61.4%) while the combination approach achieved the highest RR (38.1%). Adverse events included nausea and mild myelosuppression and nephrotoxicity, without grade 3 or 4 nephrotoxic events reported and no grade 4 myelotoxicity reported.

The data remain mostly retrospective but are sufficiently encouraging to justify higher-quality trials for peptide receptor radiotherapy in lung NET (NCT04276597).

Correct Answer: E

Case Study 7

What is the appropriate first-line treatment for metastatic pancreatic NET?

A 57-year-old man with history of well-differentiated grade 2 nonfunctional pancreas NET (ki-67 8%) is on surveillance. He is now found to have new bilobar liver lesions, largest measuring 1.5 cm and three bone lesions on restaging CT compared to prior CT eight months earlier, which showed no evidence of disease. A PET DOTATATE is positive in all areas. He is asymptomatic. A biopsy of a liver mass confirms recurrence.

10) **What is the initial treatment recommendation?**
    A) Somatostatin analog.
    B) Everolimus.
    C) Carboplatin-etoposide.
    D) Sunitinib.
    E) Continue observation as he remains asymptomatic.

Expert Perspective: The treatment landscape for metastatic pancreatic NET includes several options and though sequencing is not well defined, the approach can be personalized to somatostatin receptors expression, burden of disease, and functionality.

In the setting of asymptomatic low volume disease with indolent biology, monitoring with cross-sectional imaging at 3–4-month intervals is reasonable.

A general approach for initial treatment can be aided by somatostatin receptor imaging. The utility of somatostatin analog in somatostatin receptors–positive disease was described in CLARINET, which included 45% pancreatic NETs, and lanreotide demonstrated 42% improvement in progression-free survival, and this can be broadened to include all somatostatin analogue as first-line treatment. In addition, somatostatin analogue can address secretory tumors with palliation of symptoms (Caplin et al.).

For somatostatin receptor imaging–negative disease, it is important to note two concepts: (i) SRI (somatostatin receptor imaging)-PET is the preferred modality to establish somatostatin receptors disease as SRI-SPECT is more likely to produce false-negative results, and (ii) a negative SRI-PET should prompt close evaluation of pathology to exclude higher-grade disease. In the setting of somatostatin receptors–negative disease, the role of somatostatin analogue is less certain, and targeted therapies may be more appropriate. RADIANT 3 evaluated everolimus versus placebo in progressive grade 1–2 pancreatic NET; the overall response rate was 5%, and the median progression-free survival was 11 months with everolimus compared to 4.6 months with placebo. Notable adverse effects included mucositis, hyperglycemia, ash, diarrhea, myelosuppression, and pneumonitis (Yao et al.). Similarly, sunitinib was compared to placebo in progressive grade 1–2 pancreatic NETs; overall response rate was 9%, and sunitinib improved progression-free survival from 5.5 months to 11.4 months. Common adverse effects were hypertension, palmar-plantar erythrodysesthesia, diarrhea, fatigue, and myelosuppression (Raymond et al.). There are no data comparing somatostatin analogue to targeted therapies or comparing each targeted therapy, and the decision of first-line treatment can be guided by functional imaging, with the goal of tumor control rather that cytoreduction with these treatments.

Another factor that guides treatment sequencing is large volume of disease, which is defined as liver tumor volume > 25–50% in some studies, and wherein the treatment goal is cytoreduction. In this setting, chemotherapy, liver-directed therapies, and peptide receptor radiotherapy are first-line considerations. Streptozocin-based regimens demonstrate mixed results and have an unfavorable toxicity profile, yielding way to temozolomide-based regimens (Kunz et al.). Capecitabine and temozolomide has reported overall response rate ranging from 30 to 70% in pancreatic NET with good tolerability. Response predictors such as alternative lengthening of telomeres (as it relates to chromosomal instability), O(6)-methylguanine DNA methyltransferase deficiency, and proliferative activity have not been confirmed, and there are no biomarker selection criteria to guide the treatment decision with capecitabine and temozolomide (Cives et al.). Peptide receptor radiotherapy is an established treatment for somatostatin receptors positive midgut NET, and though phase III data are lacking for pancreatic NET, there is concrete evidence of efficacy. For example, phase II data in 60 patients with progressive pancreatic NET reported disease control rate of 81.7% and median progression-free survival of 28.7 months. Another prospective trial of 95 pancreatic NET patients reported 42.9% partial response and 49% stable disease (Sansovini et al.; Garske-Roman et al.).

For liver-dominant disease, intra-arterial hepatic therapy achieves response rates ranging from 40 to 70% though phase III data are lacking and preferred modality of treatment is under investigation (NCT02724540), though drug eluting bead have demonstrated unfavorable toxicity and are not recommended. Liver-directed therapies are also helpful in palliating secretory syndromes in functional tumors.

Prospective comparative studies focused on pancreatic NET are lacking resulting in variations of clinical practice and ongoing debates regarding sequence of treatment. Nevertheless, there are multiple treatment options with proven efficacy and tolerability, and treatment can be personalized. Large volume centers with multidisciplinary care offer consensus and comprehensive care.

Correct Answer: A

Case Study 8

Is there a role for immune therapy in treating poorly differentiated neuroendocrine carcinoma?

A 63-year-old woman with metastatic poorly differentiated neuroendocrine carcinoma of the stomach received treatment with two cycles of carboplatin-etoposide. Restaging CT reveals progression in the primary mass as well as liver and bone metastases. PET is avid in the primary and metastatic sites. ECOG performance status is 1.

11) **What is the next best treatment recommendation?**
    A) Peptide receptor radiotherapy.
    B) Capecitabine and temozolomide.
    C) Ipilimumab plus nivolumab.
    D) TACE to treat the liver and continue with another two cycles of current regimen.

Expert Perspective: Poorly differentiated extrapulmonary neuroendocrine carcinomas have a poor prognosis, and trial data are limited due to disease rarity and difficulty in classification. Metastatic neuroendocrine carcinoma should be treated quickly with first-line chemotherapy, often similar to the treatment paradigm of small-cell lung cancer. The NORDIC NEC study reported the experience of 252 patients treated with platinum-based chemotherapy, and the median OS was 11 months compared to 1 month in 53 patients treated with best supportive care. Response rate was 31% and 33% achieved disease stability. Poor functional status, primary colorectal tumors, thrombocytosis, and elevated LDH were identified as poor prognostic factors. Tumors with Ki-67 greater than 55% had higher response to platinum chemotherapy, although overall survival was shorter compared to tumors with Ki67 less than 55% (Sorbye et al.).

There are few standard treatment options for platinum-resistant neuroendocrine carcinoma (defined as progression within 3–6 months of treatment). Studies evaluating combination immunotherapy with ipilimumab/nivolumab have shown some activity, although response rates have varied. There are data to support consideration of immunotherapy, particularly as a second-line treatment, in neuroendocrine carcinoma though still requiring further evaluation. CA209-538 evaluated combination ipilimumab and nivolumab in rare cancers and included 29 patients with NET: 10% with low grade, 45% with intermediate grade, and 45% with high-grade disease (Klein et al.). The response rate in the high-grade cohort was 31%. The highest response was found in pancreas primary and atypical lung NET. In assessing toxicity, 66% of patients experienced immune-related events, 34% of which were grade 3 or 4.

SWOG S1609 evaluated a combination of ipilimumab and nivolumab in 19 patients with high-grade neuroendocrine neoplasms and reported a response rate of 26%. The larger NIPINEC study evaluated the same immunotherapy combination. In a cohort of 43 patients poorly differentiated gastroenteropancreatic neuroendocrine carcinoma patients, the objective response rate was 12%. Given the absence of any other standard treatments for platinum-refractory patients and the potential for long-term remission with immunotherapy, ipilimumab/nivolumab can be considered (Girard, Patel). Clinical trials are recommended in this setting.

Correct Answer: C

Recommended Readings

Coriat, R., Walter, T., Terris, B., Couvelard, A., Ruszniewski, P. (2016). Gastroenteropancreatic well-differentiated grade 3 neuroendocrine tumors: review and position statement. *Oncologist* 21 (10): 1191–1199. doi: 10.1634/theoncologist.2015-0476.

Delle fan. et al. (2016). ENETS consensus guidelines update for gastroduodenal neuroendocrine neoplasms. *Neuroendocrinology* 103: 119–124. doi: 10.1159/000443168.

Jha, A, Taïeb, D, Carrasquillo, JA, et al. (2021). High-specific-activity-131I-MIBG versus 177Lu-DOTATATE targeted radionuclide therapy for metastatic pheochromocytoma and paraganglioma. *Clin Cancer Res* 27 (11): 2989–2995. doi: 10.1158/1078-0432.CCR-20-3703.

Krug, S., Damm, M., Garbe, J. et al. (2021). Finding the appropriate therapeutic strategy in patients with neuroendocrine tumors of the pancreas: guideline recommendations meet the clinical reality. *J Clin Med* 10 (14): 3023. Published 2021 July 7. doi: 10.3390/jcm10143023.

Naraev, B.G., Ramirez, R.A., Kendi, A.T., Halfdanarson, T.R. (2019). Peptide receptor radionuclide therapy for patients with advanced lung carcinoids. *Clin Lung Cancer* 20 (3): e376-e392. doi: 10.1016/j.cllc.2019.02.007.

Pape, U.F., Niederle, B., Costa, F. et al. (2016). ENETS Consensus guidelines for neuroendocrine neoplasms of the appendix (Excluding Goblet Cell Carcinomas). *Neuroendocrinology* 103 (2): 144–152. doi: 10.1159/000443165.

Park, S.S., Kim, B.C., Lee, D.E. et al. (2021). Comparison of endoscopic submucosal dissection and transanal endoscopic microsurgery for T1 rectal neuroendocrine tumors: a propensity score-matched study. *Gastrointest Endosc* 94 (2): 408–415.e2. doi: 10.1016/j.gie.2021.02.012.

Singh. et al. (2021). Commonwealth Neuroendocrine Tumour Research Collaboration and the North American Neuroendocrine Tumor Society Guidelines for the Diagnosis and Management of Patients with Lung Neuroendocrine Tumors: An International Collaborative Endorsement and Update of the 2015 European Neuroendocrine Tumor Society Expert Consensus Guidelines.

Taïeb, D., Jha, A., Treglia, G., and Pacak, K. (2019). Molecular imaging and radionuclide therapy of pheochromocytoma and paraganglioma in the era of genomic characterization of disease subgroups. *Endocrine-Related Cancer* 26 (11): R627-R652.

29

Anal Cancer

Asad Mahmood and Rob Glynne-Jones

Mount Vernon Cancer Centre, Northwood, UK

Introduction

Squamous cell cancer of the anus is a rare disease that makes up approximately 2% of all cancers in the lower alimentary tract. The incidence is increasing in several countries, particularly in women and among patients aged ≥50 years. Estimates for anal cancer in the United States for 2021 point to 9,090 new cases (6,070 in women and 3,020 in men), Squamous cell carcinoma of anus is commonly associated with human papilloma virus (HPV) infection (usually HPV16 or HPV18). Other risk factors include cigarette smoking, a history of receptive anal intercourse, a history of other HPV-related cancers, human immunodeficiency virus (HIV) infection, and long-term immunosuppressive treatments.

Squamous cell cancer of the anus usually presents as and remains a loco-regional disease. Most patients have symptoms for long periods of time before diagnosis, which are frequently attributed to hemorrhoids. Non-surgical treatment with radical chemoradiation is highly effective while preserving the anal sphincter and represents the standard of care in most cases. Few develop distant metastases unless there is failure of chemoradiation treatment or recurrence at the primary site. Local control without the recourse to a colostomy and enjoyment of an optimal quality of life are the primary aims of treatment.

Three phase III trials showed that radiotherapy with concurrent 5-fluorouracil (5-FU) and mitomycin C achieves better outcomes in terms of local control and recurrence- or disease-free survival (relapse-free survival and disease-free survival, respectively) compared to radiation therapy alone, or radiation therapy combined with 5-FU alone. Phase III trials by the Radiotherapy Therapy Oncology Group RTOG 98–11 and the Action Clinique Coordonees en Cancerologie Digestive ACCORD-03 failed to show benefit for the addition of cisplatin-based neoadjuvant chemotherapy before chemoradiation therapy in terms of colostomy-free survival. In the RTOG 9811 trial, the cisplatin arm confers a worse disease-free survival and a higher colostomy rate. The ACCORD-03 trial also failed to show a benefit in colostomy-free survival from an increase in the radiotherapy boost dose. Adenocarcinomas arising from glandular elements within the anal canal are rare and

Cancer Consult: Expertise in Clinical Practice, Volume 1: Solid Tumors & Supportive Care,
Second Edition. Edited by Syed A. Abutalib, Maurie Markman, Al B. Benson III, and Hope S. Rugo.
© 2024 John Wiley & Sons Ltd. Published 2024 by John Wiley & Sons Ltd.

29 Anal Cancer

usually are more aggressive than squamous cell carcinomas; these cases are treated along the lines of rectal cancer paradigm, which includes surgery with either neoadjuvant or adjuvant chemotherapy. Primary rectal squamous cell carcinomas, which are also very rare, can be difficult to distinguish from anal cancers, but they are treated according to the same approach as anal cancer.

Results of the United Kingdom National Anal Cancer Trial (ACT II) confirm the standard of 5-FU and mitomycin C plus concurrent radiotherapy. Results show three-year relapse-free survival rates of 73% (75% in T1/T2 tumors and 68% for more advanced T3/T4 tumors (Figures 29.1–29.3)). The dose and treatment schedule used in the ACT II trial are now the current standard of care in the United Kingdom for intermediate risk cancers. However, the rarity and the different behavior and natural history (depending on whether

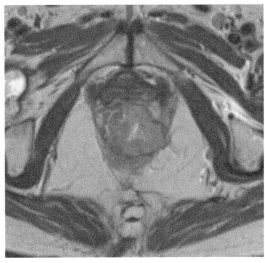

Axial T2-weighted MRI

T2: 2-5cm

Involving external sphincter

Figure 29.1

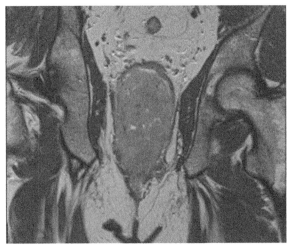

Coronal T2-weighted MRI

T3 >5cm

Figure 29.2

Introduction

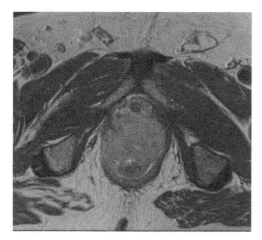

Axial T2-weighted MRI

T4

Involving anterior urogenital structures

Figure 29.3

squamous cell cancer of the anus originates predominantly at the anal margin, at the anal canal, or above the dentate line) provide limited experience for any individual oncologist.

There have been some recent developments in our understanding of the molecular biology, the immune environment, and processes that lead to anal cancer. There have also been some notable successes in prevention with vaccination, imaging, and treatment. The authors hope to provide some information from the randomized and retrospective trials that can assist the medical and radiation oncologist in the practical management of this unusual cancer.

Case Study

A 50-year-old woman presents with a six-month history of pain on defecation and rectal bleeding; she was prompted to seek medical advice by a UK television advertisement. There is no significant past medical history, but the patient is a cigarette smoker. On digital rectal examination (DRE), an anterior mass is palpable extending from 11 to 3 o'clock in the anal canal, and from 1 cm within the anal verge to approximately 4.5 cm superiorly (i.e. measuring approximately 2 × 3.5 cm). No enlargement of the inguinal nodes is palpable. Colonoscopy reveals a mass in the anal canal but no other proximal lesions. Biopsy of the mass shows a poorly differentiated squamous cell carcinoma. The patient is therefore clinically staged as having a cT2N0 squamous cell carcinoma of the anal canal (Figure 29.1).

1) **Should everyone with anal cancer, especially the young patients, be tested for HPV/p16?**

Expert Perspective: HPV infection is closely correlated with squamous cell carcinoma. The presence of the HPV genome has been identified in 80–85% of cases and is like that seen in cervical and vulval carcinoma in women. HPV16 is the most common high-risk HPV genotype found in anal cancer. Exposure to HPV infection is common, almost endemic, in the population who are sexually active and have not been vaccinated. The majority of individuals clear the virus spontaneously within months; however, infection persists in up to 10% and leads to cancer initiation in 1% of infected subjects. It is likely, however, that over time this pattern will change with vaccination, as has been the case in Australia. In the UK since 2008 girls and boys aged 12 to 13 years have been offered vaccination against HPV genotypes 6, 11, 16, and 18, although uptake has been lower than hoped and varies from 60 to 80% each year. In HPV-positive human cancers, two viral oncoproteins, E6 and E7 (which target cellular tumor suppressors), are preferentially expressed via integration of the viral genome into the host DNA. E6 binds to p53, leading to deregulation of DNA damage and apoptotic pathways. E7 targets pRb for degradation, leading to an increase in cell proliferation and genomic instability. The cell cycle regulator p16 is overexpressed in HPV-related anal cancers, which may represent a simple surrogate biomarker for identifying squamous cell carcinoma harboring HPV DNA. A UK study examined samples from 153 patients with anal cancer, treated with radical chemoradiation therapy, for p16 with immunohistochemistry, and found 37 of 137 patients (27%) with moderate or strong p16 staining subsequently relapsed. In contrast, 10 out of 16 (63%) patients with absent or weak staining relapsed. A Danish study supported these finding suggesting p16 positivity to be prognostic for survival, as did a subsequent meta-analysis.

HPV-positive and HPV-negative cancers have a distinct molecular landscape with a different natural history. HPV/p16-positive tumors seem to have better outcomes and are more responsive to conventional chemoradiation therapy than HPV/p16-negative tumors, which are characterized by common *CDKN2A* and *TP53* gene mutations. A Dutch study found a three-year locoregional control rate of 15% and three-year OS of 35% in HPV/p16-negative tumors compared to 82% and 87%, respectively, in HPV/p16-positive tumors. *TP53* gene mutations were detected in 80% of negative tumors versus 6% in positive tumors.

HPV circulating tumor DNA (ctDNA) is sensitive and specific in identifying HPV16 using droplet digital polymerase chain reaction and in the future might be utilized in screening trials and in disease response monitoring as described below. There may also be a role for calculating the HPV viral load for stratifying HPV-positive patients.

2) Do HPV vaccines improve outcomes in invasive squamous cell carcinoma of anus?

Expert Perspective: Safe and effective vaccines are commercially available for the prevention of HPV infection. The bivalent Cervarix vaccine prevents HPV16 and HPV18 infection, the most common cancer-causing HPV genotypes, and the quadrivalent Gardasil vaccine additionally prevents HPV6 and HPV11; the latter is currently used in the NHS HPV vaccination program but will be replaced by the nine-valent Gardasil 9 vaccine during 2021–2022 for both adolescents from 12–13 years (up to 25 years) and MSM (men who have sex with men) up to 45 years. Evidence suggests that the efficacy of these vaccines against oncogenic HPV is more than 90% for anal intraepithelial neoplasia. However, prophylactic vaccines do not prevent anal cancers in patients already infected with high-risk HPVs or they do not add value in individuals who already have anal cancer. Hence HPV vaccines will not improve outcomes at this stage. In these groups, novel therapeutic vaccines to target the HPV oncogenes or the cellular pathways they affect rather than HPV are under investigation. These vaccines potentially could improve clinical outcome for patients with anal cancer, as with other HPV-associated cancers.

3) Should cancers of the anal margin, anal canal, and rectum be treated differently or the same?

Expert Perspective: The definitions of the anal canal and anal margin used by the National Comprehensive Cancer Network (NCCN) separate the anal canal from the rectum with the landmark of the upper border of the anal sphincter and puborectalis muscles. The anal canal extends 3–5 cm in length to the anal verge. The anal margin includes the perianal skin over a 5 cm radius from the anal verge. In practice, at diagnosis most anal carcinomas have extended such that their point of origin is uncertain, and the distinction between anal canal and anal margin tumor is, therefore, often impossible. The natural history and patterns of lymphatic spread are slightly different for these three sites. Local excision of anal margin cancers is possible for small lesions (usually < 1 cm) allowing surgical clearance with safe margins, but it should be performed by specialist surgeons (see Question 6, this chapter).

4) Are there any biomarkers in anal cancer?

Expert Perspective: For more advanced stages of anal cancer, there remains considerable heterogeneity in terms of outcomes. Biomarkers that affect these outcomes would be useful to provide predictive and prognostic information and, in turn, inform individualized therapies. However, most studies have focused on the identification of factors that predict cytotoxic drug response and/or radiosensitivity. These studies have invariably analyzed only a limited number of markers in small numbers of patients, with a variety of treatment regimes, and their results can be considered preliminary. So further refinement is needed in this field.

A recent systematic review examined 29 different biomarkers belonging to nine different functional classes: tumor suppressors, epidermal growth factor receptor (*EGFR*), apoptosis regulation, proliferation index, angiogenesis, tumor-specific markers (e.g. SCCAg and CEA), Hedgehog signaling, and telomerase. Tumor suppressor genes p53 and p21 were the only biomarkers that were prognostic in more than one study. In anal cancer, p53 protein function may be modified either by mutations in its gene or by E6 viral oncoprotein of the HPV. In an analysis of 240 patients randomized in the UKCCR ACT I anal cancer trial, the presence of mutated p53 predicted for a poorer cause-specific survival. Recent data regarding p16 and serum squamous cell cancer antigen are promising, but in summary, there are no current biomarkers that consistently predict sensitivity to chemoradiation.

Regular testing of circulating HPV-DNA (cHPV DNA) in plasma is a promising tool for assessment. In baseline samples, this test showed 100% sensitivity and specificity for HPV-associated squamous cell carcinoma. cHPV-DNA levels post chemoradiation therapy appear to correlate with disease response, since cHPV-DNA was only detectable at 12 weeks post chemoradiation therapy in 2 of 17 patients, both of whom subsequently relapsed.

5) What is the role for sentinel lymph node biopsy in staging anal cancers?

Expert Perspective: Sentinel lymph node biopsy is validated in lymph node staging of small breast tumors with the aim of avoiding a formal axillary dissection. In anal cancer, the rationale for sentinel lymph node biopsy is to spare the patient formal inguinal irradiation and to avoid the skin morbidity associated and the potential for high-radiation doses to the femoral heads. An early systematic review of five published series (only 83 patients) evaluated the outcome of sentinel lymph node biopsy of non-enlarged inguinal nodes in patients with anal cancer. Only 21% of sentinel nodes contained tumor. However, there remain enthusiasts who have refined the technique but with similar histological confirmation of nodal metastasis in the sentinel lymph node in 28 of 123 patients (22.8%).

Because the initial treatment has been nonsurgical for the past 30 years, we do not know the true lymph node status of anal cancer. Currently, in the patient with clinically impalpable nodes, we rely on computed tomography (CT) and magnetic resonance imaging (MRI) in T1 or T2, where the risks of nodal involvement are low (Figure 29.1). Conventionally, routine biopsy is only performed for clinically palpable nodes or those enlarged greater than 10 mm on CT or MRI.

Sentinel lymph node biopsy has not achieved its initial potential in anal cancer, partly because MRI and positron-emission tomography (PET) are increasingly in the routine diagnostic workup. Also, acute morbidity is less with more conformal radiation therapy techniques (e.g. intensity-modulated radiation therapy [IMRT] currently being used). Formal biopsy or sentinel lymph node biopsy can reveal micrometastatic spread of disease compared with the spatial resolution of CT and PET, typically in the range of 5–10 mm. A substantial proportion of involved nodes are < 5 mm in size, but micro-metastatic involvement may not be relevant if the patient is going to receive low-dose elective inguinal irradiation. Also, there are no validated management strategies to stratify treatment for the findings of macroscopic nodal involvement, microscopic involvement, and the presence of a few isolated cells in the light of sentinel lymph node biopsy.

There are also concerns that sentinel lymph node biopsy could prejudice the effectiveness of chemoradiation therapy because radiotherapy may require delay until healing is achieved. In one study of sentinel lymph node biopsy, 24% of patients had a postoperative complication in the groin. Sentinel lymph node biopsy may also compromise the lymphatic drainage, and it may provoke lymphoedema if subsequent high-dose radiation therapy is required following a positive nodal finding on sentinel lymph node biopsy, compared to the low doses necessary for clinically uninvolved nodes. Current prophylactic doses are relatively low—in the region 30–36 Gy. Isolated inguinal failures in the ACT II study were very low for uninvolved nodes treated to 30.6 Gy, and late morbidity was slight for these patients. In contrast, we do not know the morbidity of irradiating to 50.4 Gy after a positive finding on sentinel lymph node biopsy, particularly as with some midline cancers some sentinel lymph node biopsy will require bilateral nodes to be removed.

In summary, intensity-modulated radiation therapy techniques have substantially reduced grades 3 and 4 toxicities when patients receive groin irradiation. Sentinel lymph node biopsy may be more helpful where there is discordance between clinical evidence and imaging features or in the setting of loco-regional recurrence after chemoradiation therapy to decide whether a radical inguinal dissection should be performed, when radical surgical salvage is envisaged.

6) After a local excision, what are acceptable surgical margins, whereby chemoradiation does not need to be administered?

Expert Perspective: Small, early cancers are sometimes diagnosed serendipitously following the removal of anal tags. Often piecemeal resection with numerous fragments makes this unevaluable. At other times, small lesions at the anal margin are subjected to excisional biopsy. Local excision may be considered for well-differentiated small tumors at or outside the anal margin that are less than 2 cm (preferably < 1cm) in size superficially invasive tumors that are completely excised and have ≤ 3 mm of basement membrane invasion and a maximal horizontal spread of ≤ 7 mm, are clinically and radiologically lymph node negative, and can be removed with a surgical clearance of greater than 5 mm. If attempted by surgeons less familiar with anal cancer pathology, a piecemeal resection or a positive margin may result. In summary, assessment of the integrity of the biopsy specimen should be documented. The size of the tumor in terms of the largest dimension, and the resection margins (specified in millimeters), both deep and at the periphery, are required to decide if local excision is adequate or further treatment is advisable. Hence, all the relevant resection margins should ideally be inked.

The ACT3 component of PLATO investigates outcomes for such early, small tumors in patients, who have undergone surgery (local excision). The aim of this non-randomized phase II trial is to determine whether a treatment strategy of surgery alone is safe if surgical margins are >1 mm, and whether low-dose chemoradiotherapy in the case of close margins ≤ 1mm, offers low rates of recurrence.

7) Is there a size criterion for identifying involvement of lymph nodes?

Expert Perspective: Involved nodes are often enlarged, hard, and palpable if superficial, but historical pathology studies, using a "clearing" technique, demonstrated that almost half of all involved pelvic lymph nodes were smaller than 5 mm in diameter. Suspicious perirectal and internal iliac nodes on imaging are rarely biopsied, so there is a significant risk of false positives. Historically, a diameter ranging from 6 to 15 mm has been used, with 10 mm being the most used criterion for the upper limit of a normal lymph node, and this is supported by recent studies. The size criterion should be modified based on the site of the nodes. Historical studies on healthy volunteers suggested that the 95th percentile for the diameter of normal nodes on CT was 7 mm for internal iliac nodes, 8 mm for obturator nodes, and 10 mm for external iliac nodes. A similar study with MRI suggested normal pelvic nodes were even smaller. In contrast, the normal size of benign inguinal lymph nodes is highly variable, often measuring up to 15 mm. Some recommend a size threshold of 8 mm (short-axis diameter) for pelvic nodes and 10 mm for abdominal retroperitoneal nodes.

RTOG 0529 described nodes > 3 cm in size as large-volume macroscopic involvement and treated these to a higher radiotherapy dose (i.e. nodes up to 3 cm maximum in any direction received 50.4 Gy, but for involved nodes > 3 cm the dose was 54 Gy). Other criteria such as shape, central necrosis, and the degree of contrast enhancement in pelvic nodes are often useful, but they have not been completely validated. In addition, normal-sized but potentially involved nodes can be imaged on diffusion MRI. The signal intensity on MRI within a given node can be graded as hypo-intense, isointense, or hyperintense relative to muscle. Note may also be made of the pattern of signal intensity—homogeneous or mixed on the T1- and T2-weighted sequences. In practical terms, given the limited accuracy of relying on a single criterion alone, it seems sensible to use a combination of all of these. We therefore carefully palpate the groins and perform a pelvic CT and MRI (using Royal College of Radiologist guidelines), that is, if the short axis diameter is greater than 15 mm for inguinal, and 10 mm for external iliac, 9 mm for common iliac, 8 mm for obturator, 7 mm for internal iliac, and 5 mm for perirectal nodes. Additional criteria as above contribute to the radiological diagnosis. Clearly abnormal nodes are assumed to be involved and treated to a high-radiation dose. Equivocal nodes are either biopsied or subjected to fine-needle aspiration cytology if accessible, and PET–CT to clarify (Figure 29.4). If nodes are still equivocal, our anal radiology and radiotherapy team decide together.

8) What are the ideal planning target volumes in anal cancer?

Expert Perspective: It is beyond the scope of this chapter to provide a comprehensive clear practical guide to target delineation for every patient with anal cancer. There are several planning guidelines showing anatomical borders to define the clinical target volumes for anal cancer, which include the Radiation Therapy Oncology Group (RTOG) elective nodal anorectal atlas as well as the Australian recommendations. The most current guidelines are the UK consensus guidance (which have been published, validated, and used as the basis for the radiotherapy planning in the PLATO [PersonaLising Anal cancer radio-Therapy dOse] portfolio of studies. This data complements these published contouring atlases RTOG, AGITG, PLATO) all underscore the poor evidence base, since none of the randomized phase III trials have actually reported clear data on the location of recurrences according to the dose received. Historically, anal cancer has been treated in all randomized trials with doses of 1.80 Gy per day, using a shrinking-field technique over the course of treatment covering much of the pelvis, but total doses vary from 50.4 Gy to 64 Gy.

9) Do we always have to include the groins during surgical procedure of anal cancer?

Expert Perspective: For early T1N0 ($\leq$ 2 cm without node involvement) cancers, particularly in patients with major comorbidities, we often omit the inguinal nodes since there is a low risk of failure (possibly < 5%). PET scans and possibly sentinel lymph node biopsy may make this decision more robust.

10) In giving radical chemoradiotherapy for anal cancer, what is the optimal radiation dose?

Expert Perspective: The optimal dose of radiation therapy for anal canal carcinoma is unknown. Norman Nigro (1984) originally utilized 30 Gy in his study. The randomized

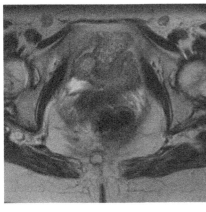
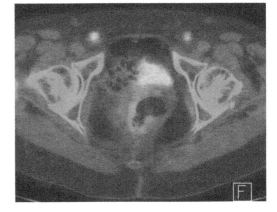

N1: N1a inguinal nodes

Figure 29.4

controlled trials provide information on loco-regional control, relapse-free survival, and colostomy-free survival but have not generated quality-of-life data. Also critically, in these trials there are major differences in the treatment schedules (planning volumes and doses), not only between but also within the individual randomized controlled trials, partly because of a reliance of early response—either histopathogical or clinical—to decide the appropriate total radiation dose.

The RTOG 9811 required clinically positive inguinal nodes to be biopsied by either needle aspiration biopsy or excisional biopsy of a node if needle aspiration was negative. In contrast, pelvic nodes seen on CT scan did not require biopsy. All patients were intended to be treated with a daily dose of 1.8 Gy, five days per week, to a dose of at least 45 Gy in 25 fractions over 5 to 6.5 weeks (a ≤ 10-day break, as indicated, was permitted for skin intolerance). T1 cancers were excluded, but patients with T3 (> 5 cm), T4 (tumor of any size invading adjacent organ(s), such as the vagina, urethra, or bladder), or N + lesions or T2 (> 2 cm but ≤ 5 cm) lesions with residual disease after 45 Gy should receive an additional 10–14 Gy (2 Gy per fraction) to a reduced field, hence radiation doses of up to 59 Gy, depending on the burden of primary and nodal disease.

The ACCORD-03 (only 307 patients randomized in four arms) also explored using initial neoadjuvant chemotherapy with 5-FU–cisplatin and a higher radiation therapy dose in a second randomization where the dose administered reflected the degree of response observed. Thus, the ACCORD 03 trial did not use a mitomycin C, 5-FU chemoradiation control arm. Several possible radiation doses were, therefore, administered according to response. The trial failed to show a benefit in colostomy-free survival from an increase in the radiotherapy boost dose from 15 to 25 Gy.

Also, varying compliance with the planned treatment as defined by protocolized dose reductions of chemotherapy for toxicity, and the potential confounding by subsequent treatment and the availability and accessibility of timely salvage surgery, may also affect some of the observed treatment effects.

In addition, no randomized study clearly reports the site of local failure (in or out of field), or within the planning target volume (PTV), clinical target volume (CTV), or gross tumor volume (GTV). The total dose of radiation therapy for anal cancer continues to be evaluated. Although the total radiation dose is known to affect local control, the benefit of a high dose over 60 Gy may be doubtful, and a high-radiation dose may be associated with complications.

An RTOG pilot study (RTOG 92–08) tested radiation dose escalation within chemoradiation with 5-FU—mitomycin C escalating to 59.4 Gy in 1.8 Gy fractions over 9 weeks with a two-week mandatory rest. The results were compared to the RTOG 87–04 trial in which patients were treated with 45 Gy in a continuous schedule plus the same chemotherapy regimen. This schedule with 59.4 Gy and a two-week break led to a higher colostomy rate than expected (30% vs 9%). There are no data on late effects.

For all these reasons, it is extremely difficult to generate dose-response curves for local control against poor function for the anal canal-sphincter mechanism from randomized control trials. So, it is not possible to assess whether loco-regional failures represent inadequate clinical target volumes or insufficient doses or efficacy of treatment.

- The ACT4 component of PLATO investigates intermediate-risk disease in a randomized phase II trial. The aim of this study is to compare standard doses of chemoradiotherapy

(50.4 Gy in 28 fractions) with a reduced dose (41.4 Gy in 23 fractions), to examine whether the reduced dose can maintain similar local control, while reducing the acute and late side effects of treatment.
- The ACT5 component of PLATO investigates more advanced cT3/T4 tumors in a randomized sequential pilot/phase II/phase III trial. The aim is to compare standard-dose chemoradiotherapy (53.2 Gy in 28 fractions) with two higher doses of chemoradiotherapy (58.8 Gy and 61.6 Gy, both in 28 fractions), to examine whether higher doses of radiotherapy reduce recurrence rates without excess morbidity.

Macroscopic Disease

- Although the total radiation dose is known to affect local control, the benefit of a high dose over 60 Gy is unproven, and a high-radiation dose may be associated with complications. We consider the primary gross tumor volume (which includes the anal canal) should be treated to a maximum of 54 Gy over 30 fractions if concurrent chemotherapy is used. However, for T1 (≤ 2 cm) and non-bulky T2 tumors < 4 cm, a dose of 50.4 Gy in 28 fractions is appropriate according to ACT II data. Doses to involved nodes or regions should depend on the size of nodes. Some have suggested that involved nodes should receive 50.4 Gy if < 3 cm, increasing to 54 Gy if ≥ 3 cm in any one diameter.

Microscopic Disease

- In the MD Anderson Cancer Center series, no patients who were initially node negative in the inguinal area and treated prophylactically to a prescribed dose of 30.6 Gy developed subsequent inguinal disease. In the ACT II study, only 7 of 940 patients developed an isolated inguinal recurrence, 16 of 940 an isolated pelvic nodal recurrence, and a further 5 of 940 developed synchronous inguinal and pelvic nodal recurrence, although it is unclear how many of these patients initially had palpable or involved nodes on imaging and were treated to full dose, and how many were uninvolved and treated prophylactically with a prescribed dose of 30.6 Gy.

Ongoing randomized phase II EA2182 DECREASE (De-Intensified ChemoRadiation for Early Stage Anal Squamous Cell Carcinoma) study is based on the hypothesis that lower chemoradiation doses will be able to effectively treat early stage (T1-2N0) anal squamous cell carcinoma while improving patient-reported health-related quality of life related to anorectal dysfunction, erectile dysfunction, dyspareunia, and vaginal stenosis.

11) **Is there a role for neoadjuvant chemotherapy prior to chemoradiation in anal cancer?**

Expert Perspective: Randomized trial evidence from the RTOG 98–11 and ACCORD-03 phase III trials failed to show a benefit for neoadjuvant cisplatin-based chemotherapy strategies. Induction cisplatin and 5-FU, despite high observed response rates, failed to improve local control, progression-free survival, and colostomy-free survival. In theory this may be because cisplatin-based neoadjuvant chemotherapy prolonged total treatment time and radiobiological repopulation occurred; however, even maintenance chemotherapy after chemoradiation therapy has shown no benefit. Moreover, the colostomy rate appears higher with the use of neoadjuvant chemotherapy cisplatin–5-FU for patients with tumors 5 cm or more, and more mature data suggest that local control and disease-free survival are also worse. Based on data from squamous cell cancer of the head and neck (Chapters 2 and 3), future studies aiming to preserve anal function could assess whether induction chemotherapy with docetaxel, cisplatin, and 5-FU (DCF) followed by chemoradiation therapy in responders improves loco-regional control and colostomy-free survival compared with an unselected approach of high-dose primary chemoradiation therapy in all eligible patients with bulky T3–T4 squamous cell carcinoma. Cisplatin-based neoadjuvant chemotherapy might also be able to identify patients who are less likely to respond to chemoradiation therapy and instead need salvage APR.

12) Is chemoradiotherapy indicated in T1 (≤ 2 cm) anal cancers?

Expert Perspective: According to population data a substantial number of patients present with stage I squamous cell carcinoma of anus, but the evidence base is weak, because patients with T1N0 disease form only a tiny proportion of patients treated within the major randomized phase III studies of squamous cell carcinoma of anus. Hence, the optimal treatment for stage I remains undefined. Options include chemoradiotherapy, radiation alone (often to higher doses), or local excision. While highly effective, chemoradiotherapy is not without its long-term sequalae. Late skin, intestinal, urinary, and sexual toxicities permanently affect patients' lives. There is, therefore, considerable interest in strategies that could omit concurrent chemotherapy or utilize local excision in lieu of radiation entirely.

Some have argued that a pooled analysis did not show a benefit for mitomycin C in T1 tumors and criticize the control arm in the ACT I study as being inadequate in terms of radiation dose. Several National Cancer Database population studies have provided conflicting results, but overall survival appears similar whether chemoradiation therapy or radiation therapy alone is delivered—highlighting the fact that surgical salvage with APR may be easier for small early tumours if recurrent.

There is an innate bias in retrospective and population-derived data. The surgeon is the gatekeeper and even within an MDT (multidisciplinary team meeting) the surgeon will select small superficial well-defined lesions with easy access and an expectation of achieving clear margins for surgery with local excision—and decline/refer those lesions that do not fit these criteria for chemoradiation therapy. Hence surgeons perform an excision biopsy on small lesions that if margin free, is called a local excision and if not, it is called a biopsy and referred for chemoradiation therapy.

Thus, there remains debate as to whether chemoradiation therapy is the optimal management for patients with early stage T1 N0 disease. Many Europeans, therefore, continue to treat small T1 tumors in the anal canal with radiation alone, or even very occasionally brachytherapy alone, and the NCCN guidelines also endorse radiation therapy alone. While overall survival may not differ with an up-front non-chemoradiation approach for T1 tumors this must be weighed up against potential increased long-term side effects from having both initial radiotherapy and then salvage APR.

13) What is the ideal chemotherapy partner for concurrent 5-FU-based chemoradiotherapy in anal cancer: mitomycin C or cisplatin?

Expert Perspective: Chemoradiotherapy is considered the standard of care in anal cancer, and all the phase III trials used a continuous four- or five-day infusion of 5-FU in the first and fifth weeks of radiotherapy in combination with either mitomycin C or cisplatin. None have used a prolonged venous infusion or an oral fluoropyrimidine during the radiotherapy phase as in rectal cancer. Current guidelines (European Society for Medical Oncology and NCCN) recommend 5-FU and mitomycin C in patients with anal cancer.

14) Are there new developments to integrate different chemotherapy agents?

Expert Perspective: Several studies have confirmed safety and efficacy of oral capecitabine at 825 mg/m^2 twice a day, and retrospective comparisons of capecitabine and infusional 5-FU with mature follow-up show a trend toward lower recurrence rates with capecitabine. A systematic review and meta-analysis examined the substitution of capecitabine for infusional 5-FU. Despite the lack of a phase III randomized trial in anal cancer, the pooled analysis showed a complete clinical response at six months of 88% for patients treated with capecitabine. A United Kingdom audit of 242 patients managed with intensity-modulated radiation therapy and a single dose of mitomycin C with either 5-FU (5-FU-mitomycin C) or capecitabine (capecitabine-mitomycin C) showed similar grade 3 or 4 toxicity as well as oncological outcomes at one year. For this reason, capecitabine is recommended as a suitable alternative to 5-FU by NCCN, ESMO-ESSO-ESTRO, and recent UK intensity-modulated radiation therapy guidelines.

Other combinations with platinum drugs have been investigated. A phase II trial at the MD Anderson Cancer Center has explored the combination of capecitabine and oxaliplatin with concomitant radiotherapy. Preliminary results suggest response rates of 91–100% and colostomy-free survival of 100%. A small Chinese study has successfully explored the integration of capecitabine and cisplatin into chemoradiotherapy schedules.

The EORTC 22011–40014 randomized phase I/II study (78 eligible patients) compared 5-FU and mitomycin C in combination with radiation versus mitomycin C and cisplatin with radiation. The mitomycin C–cisplatin arm used a schedule more associated with cervical cancer—25 mg/m^2 per week—giving a total of (25 mg/m^2 × 7 =) 175/mg/m^2. With a median follow-up of two years, the one-year progression-free survival was 76.3% in the control versus 94.2% in the mitomycin C–cisplatin arm, and one-year event-free survival was 74.4% versus 89.2%, respectively. This combination of mitomycin C and cisplatin could be further evaluated, but it might be difficult to take into a phase III setting because of its limited compliance. Promising results have been reported in esophageal cancer in phase III trials using carboplatin/paclitaxel in chemoradiation therapy (Chapter 20). A recent Russian phase I trial of intensity-modulated radiation therapy and concurrent chemotherapy using paclitaxel, capecitabine, and mitomycin C for squamous cell carcinoma of anus reported that 33 of 38 (86.8%) patients achieved a complete clinical response at 26 weeks. Based on these results a phase III clinical trial is currently recruiting in Russia comparing paclitaxel, capecitabine, and mitomycin C combined with intensity-modulated radiation therapy against the standard capecitabine and mitomycin C (NCT02526953).

15) What assessments should be performed following radical chemoradiation therapy to confirm that the treatment has been successful, and when are they ideally performed?

Expert Perspective: Following radical chemoradiation therapy, clinical regression is often slow. Follow-up to assess response should start 6 to 12 weeks after the completion of chemoradiation therapy, but the ACT II trial demonstrated that time to achieve a complete clinical response is often longer than the historically recommended decision-making at 6–8 weeks and up to 26 weeks in some cases. Provided the trajectory of response is favorable, continued surveillance for a persistent abnormality is reasonable.

Recommended methods of assessment include DRE, inguinal lymph node palpation, anoscopy, endoscopic ultrasound, MRI, and thoraco-abdominal CT scan, especially for more advanced disease. There may be a role for PET-CT assessment. In practice, slow healing and persistent ulceration can cause concerns. Routine biopsy of any residual abnormality to confirm complete response is discouraged due to the high risk of ulceration and risk of poor wound healing following chemoradiation therapy.

Early unequivocal detection of recurrence/lack of response to chemoradiotherapy with limited loco-regional disease may offer a better opportunity for long-term disease control with abdominoperineal resection (APR).This, however, creates a tension between defining an early recurrence, which is amenable to surgical salvage, and not allowing sufficient time to elapse for a complete clinical response to be achieved. Only 64% of evaluable patients in the ACT II trial achieved a complete clinical response at the initial 11-week evaluation, compared with 80% at assessment 2 (18 weeks), and 85% at assessment 3 (26 weeks).

Early assessment of response using MRI at 6–8 weeks is not a robust method to predict future clinical outcome but proactive use of the MRI tumor regression grading (mrTRG) system at three and six months and a novel post-treatment "tram-track" sign for anal canal tumors (but not anal margin) may help assess local response and guide further management—although this has not been validated by other series. Alternatively, the use of PET might help to discriminate poor responders and also select patients who have not developed metastatic disease if salvage surgery is considered. Once complete clinical response is achieved, patients should be evaluated for recurrence every three months in the first year, every six months in the second year for a period of two years, and subsequently every 6–12 months until five years with clinical examination including DRE and palpation of the inguinal lymph nodes. Patients tend to relapse loco-regionally rather than at distant sites and within the first 2–3 years—with less than 1% of patients and less than 7% of all relapses after three years. Hence, some have argued for regular pelvic MRI surveillance in the first three years. Because of the rarity of metastatic disease, regular CT scans for metastatic surveillance outside trials remain controversial.

Monitoring of circulating tumor DNA in HPV-positive squamous cell carcinoma of anus may offer a novel additional means of assessing response without recourse to biopsy, particularly in situations when imaging and clinical examination are equivocal. Its utility in the early detection of recurrence during follow-up is to be investigated in a Nordic phase III trial (NOAC-9).

16) Are there newer targets and ongoing or anticipated trials?

Expert Perspective: Some have advocated the integration of biologically targeted agents. Squamous cell carcinoma of the anus commonly overexpresses *EGFR*, and *KRAS* and *BRAF* mutations appear rare. Partial remissions have been observed in patients with wild-type *KRAS* with relapsed anal cancer using cetuximab as a single agent or cetuximab in combination with irinotecan, some of whom had been heavily pretreated.

Based on these observations a Brazilian study integrating cetuximab into chemoradiation therapy, showed a response rate of 95% but the study closed early because of excess toxicity. Similarly, the ACCORD 16 trial showed high levels of toxicity and inferior outcomes with low compliance to treatment. A Scandinavian phase I study employed intensity-modulated radiotherapy (IMRT) or volumetric modulated arc therapy (VMAT) with a simultaneous integrated boost (SIB) to a dose of 57.5/54.0/48.6 Gy in 27 fractions and reported acceptable toxicity and two-year relapse-free survival (RFS) and OS as 73% and 88%, respectively. Two subsequent phase II studies for immunocompetent patients (ECOG 3205) and for HIV-positive patients (AMC045) showed acceptable toxicity and clinical outcomes for patients treated with cetuximab with 5-FU and cisplatin concurrently with radiation—although there were 4–5% treatment-related deaths.

A similar phase II trial in the Grupo Español Multidisciplinar en Cáncer Digestivo (GEMCAD) with panitumumab, mitomycin C, 5-FU, and radiotherapy (NCT01285778), reported that 33/36 (92%) patients developed G3/4 adverse events and outcomes were similarly poor. The French phase I–II FFCD-0904 trial added the anti-EGFR panitumumab, to standard chemoradiation therapy, but expected short-term response endpoints were not achieved. For these reasons, the authors do not believe that these data support further investigation of chemoradiation therapy with *EGFR* inhibitors in squamous cell carcinoma of anus. Like other HPV-driven cancers, squamous cell carcinoma of anus carries potential targets for immunotherapy with checkpoint inhibitors, even though it has a low tumor mutational burden (TMB), due to its inflammatory tumor microenvironment. Surprisingly, non-HPV-driven tumors also have a low TMB. Immune checkpoint inhibitors, mainly anti-PD-1 monoclonal antibodies, such as retifanlimab, nivolumab, and pembrolizumab, have been studied. Early phase studies have shown responses in subsets of patients, but predictive biomarkers for response are needed. In a phase II trial (NCI-9673) in patients with previously treated metastatic squamous cell carcinoma of anus, nivolumab showed a partial response in 19% (7/37) and a complete response in 5% (2/37). In a phase Ib basket trial of pembrolizumab (KEYNOTE-028) 17% (4/24) of patients showed a partial response, with all 24 patients having PDL1 positive ($\geq 1\%$) tumors. The anti-PD-1 monoclonal antibody retifanlimab (INCMGA0012) was evaluated in a phase II study POD1UM-202, in patients with advanced squamous cell carcinoma of anus after platinum failure. The overall response rate was 13.8%, with a median duration of response of 9.5 months. The median progression-free survival and OS were 2.3 months and 10.1 months, respectively. The combination of nivolumab with ipilimumab (NCT-02314169) is being investigated in a previously treated population and, in the first-line setting, the combination of chemotherapy with nivolumab (NCT-04444921) or retifanlimab (POD1UM-303 / InterAACT-2). Results in the metastatic setting have driven phase Ib/II trials integrating checkpoint inhibitors alongside radical chemoradiation and/or as consolidation following chemoradiation therapy in several different trials (EA-2165, RADIANCE, and CORINTH). (Refer to Chapter 50 for immunotherapy-related issues.) Adoptive T-cell therapy is a personalized cancer treatment delivering infusions of tumor-targeted T cells (tumor infiltrating lymphocytes, or TILs). Durable, complete responses have been observed in hematological malignancies, and ongoing studies are underway in patients with solid malignancies. HPV-targeted tumor infiltrating lymphocytes may be effective in HPV-associated cancers, increasing response rates.

17) Is there a standard for palliative chemotherapy in the case of metastatic disease?

Expert Perspective: Approximately 10–20% of patients relapse with distant metastases. Chemotherapy can achieve responses, but complete remission has been reported in < 5% of cases, and hence palliation is the intended outcome. Prognosis is relatively poor with only 10% of patients with distant disease surviving two years or more. Fit patients with metastatic or recurrent disease not amenable to surgery or radiofrequency ablation should receive chemotherapy, but there is no international standard. The choice of chemotherapy is usually influenced by the patient's previous chemotherapy received for early disease, the disease-free interval, and performance status. Current NCCN guidelines recommend the use of carboplatin and paclitaxel chemotherapy as first-line treatment, which offers approximately a 50% response rate. This is based on the recent phase II InterAACT trial, which compared this regimen versus cisplatin and infusional fluorouracil, finding a comparable response rate (59% vs 57%) and median progression-free survival (8.1 months vs 5.7 months; $P = 0.375$) but with higher median OS (20 months vs 12.3 months; HR 2.0; CI 1.15–3.47; $P = 0.014$) and fewer serious adverse events (36% vs 62%; $P = 0.016$).

The triplet regimen of a taxane (docetaxel), platin (cisplatin), and fluoropyrimidine (fluorouracil), i.e. DCF, is an attractive alternative first-line option with potentially higher response rates and some long-term complete remissions (Epitopes-HPV01) but at the cost of great toxicity. An updated analysis reports 25% of the patients treated with DCF remained free of progression. A modified two-weekly DCF regimen (Epitopes-HPV02), with lower doses is still effective with a response rate of 83% and median progression-free survival of 11 months but with fewer grade 3–4 adverse events (53% vs 70%) compared to standard DCF doses.

Conclusion

Despite vaccination programs, HPV-driven anal cancer is likely to remain an ongoing challenge worldwide. A multidisciplinary approach to management is essential with close cooperation and communication required between the surgeon, radiologist, medical oncologist, radiation oncologist, pathologist, and nursing specialists. The results of six randomized phase III trials in anal cancer confirm that the paradigm of external beam radiation therapy with concurrent 5-FU and mitomycin remains the standard of care. However, we need much more data regarding severe complication rates and the proportion of patients who maintain a functioning anus. Liquid biopsies offer promising methods of assessment and surveillance in future, and advances in immunotherapy offer tantalizing hopes of long-term remissions even in metastatic disease.

Recommended Readings

Ajani, J.A., Winter, K.A., Gunderson, L.L. et al. (2008). Fluorouracil, mitomycin and radiotherapy vs fluorouracil, cisplatin and radiotherapy for carcinoma of the anal canal: a randomised controlled trial. *JAMA* 199: 1914–1921.

Glynne-Jones, R., Meadows, H.M., Lopes, A., Muirhead, R., Sebag-Montefiore, D., and Adams, R. (2020 October). ACTII study group. impact of compliance to chemoradiation on long-term outcomes in squamous cell carcinoma of the anus: results of a post hoc analysis from the randomised phase III ACT II trial. *Ann Oncol* 31 (10): 1376–1385.

Glynne-Jones, R., Sebag-Montefiore, D., Adams, R. et al. (2013 February 15). Prognostic factors for recurrence and survival in anal cancer: generating hypotheses from the mature outcomes of the first United Kingdom coordinating committee on cancer research anal cancer trial (ACT I). *Cancer* 119 (4): 748–755.

Glynne-Jones, R., Sebag-Montefiore, D., Meadows, H.M., Cunningham, D., Begum, R., Adab, F. et al. (2017 March). ACT II study group. best time to assess complete clinical response after chemoradiotherapy in squamous cell carcinoma of the anus (ACT II): a post-hoc analysis of randomised controlled phase 3 trial. *Lancet Oncol* 18 (3): 347–356.

Gunderson, L.L., Gunderson, L.L., Winter, K.A. et al. (2012 December 10). Long-term update of US GI intergroup RTOG 98-11 phase iii trial for anal carcinoma: survival, relapse, and colostomy failure with concurrent chemoradiation involving fluorouracil/mitomycin versus fluorouracil/cisplatin. *J Clin Oncol* 30 (35): 4344–4351.

Gunderson, L.L., Moughan, J., Ajani, J.A., Pedersen, J.E., Winter, K.A., Benson, A.B., 3rd, et al. (2013 November 15). Anal carcinoma: impact of TN category of disease on survival, disease relapse, and colostomy failure in US gastrointestinal intergroup RTOG 98-11 phase 3 trial. *Int J Radiat Oncol Biol Phys* 87 (4): 638–645.

Kochhar, R., Renehan, A.G., Mullan, D., Chakrabarty, B., Saunders, M.P., and Carrington, B.M. (2017 February). The assessment of local response using magnetic resonance imaging at 3- and 6-month post chemoradiotherapy in patients with anal cancer. *Eur Radiol* 27 (2): 607–617.

Peiffert, D., Tournier-Rangeard, L., Gerald, J.P., Lemanski, C., Francois, E., Giovannini, M. et al. (2012). Induction chemotherapy and dose intensification of the radiation boost in locally advanced anal canal carcinoma: final analysis of the randomized UNICANCER ACCORD 03 trial. *J Clin Oncol* 30: 1941–1944.

Rao, S., Sclafani, F., Eng, C. et al. (2018). InterAACT: a multicentre open label randomised phase II advanced anal cancer trial of cisplatin (CDDP) plus 5-fluorouracil (5-FU) vs carboplatin (C) plus weekly paclitaxel (P) in patients (pts) with inoperable locally recurrent (ILR) or metastatic treatment naïve disease – an international rare cancers initiative (IRCI) trial. *Ann Oncol* 29 (S8): 715–716.

Werner, R.N., Gaskins, M., Avila Valle, G., Budach, V., Koswig, S., Mosthaf, F.A. et al. (2021 April). State of the art treatment for stage I to III anal squamous cell carcinoma: a systematic review and meta-analysis. *Radiother Oncol* 157: 188–196.

Part 5

Genitourinary Cancers

30

Renal Cancer

James L. Coggan, Alan Tan, and Timothy M. Kuzel

Department of Medicine, Rush University Medical Center, Chicago, IL

Introduction

Kidney cancer is the eighth most common cancer in the United States, with approximately 73,750 new cases diagnosed and 14,830 deaths in 2020. The median age at diagnosis is 64, with up to 16% of cases being distant or metastatic at the time of diagnosis. The disease is more common in men, with higher rates of incidence and death in African American, Hispanic American, and American Indian/Alaska Native populations. By far the biggest risk factor for developing the disease is smoking, followed by poorly controlled hypertension, and obesity. Clear cell histology makes up 75% of cases, with papillary, chromophobe, and medullary making up much of the remainder of cases.

Case Study 1

A 53-year-old man with metastatic clear cell renal cell carcinoma (RCC) diagnosed one week ago presents for evaluation. He is asymptomatic and has an excellent performance status. On imaging, a large, right renal mass and pulmonary nodules are identified. His blood work is notable for hemoglobin of 11 g/dL, while his platelet count, neutrophil count, lactate dehydrogenase (LDH), and calcium are normal. He asks about his long-term prognosis.

1) **Which risk group best predicts the overall survival in patients treated with systemic therapy?**
   A) International Metastatic RCC Database Consortium (IMDC) intermediate-risk group.
   B) IMDC favorable-risk group.
   C) IMDC poor-risk group.
   D) I would utilize the Memorial Sloan Kettering Cancer Center (MSKCC) model.

Expert Perspective: There are two main clinical risk models used to direct treatment in metastatic RCC: the MSKCC and the IMDC models. Analysis of patients treated at the Memorial Sloan Kettering Cancer Center (MSKCC) identified the clinical characteristics of patients that are predictive of shortened survival. Five risk factors predict worse

Cancer Consult: Expertise in Clinical Practice, Volume 1: Solid Tumors & Supportive Care,
Second Edition. Edited by Syed A. Abutalib, Maurie Markman, Al B. Benson III, and Hope S. Rugo.
© 2024 John Wiley & Sons Ltd. Published 2024 by John Wiley & Sons Ltd.

outcomes: low Karnofsky performance status (< 80%), elevated LDH, low hemoglobin, elevated serum calcium, and time from initial diagnosis of RCC to initiation of interferon-α therapy of less than one year. Patients were assigned to three risk groups: favorable (zero risk factors), intermediate (one to two risk factors), and poor risk (three or more risk factors); with median overall survival (OS) of 30 months, 14 months, and 5 months, respectively. The model has been externally validated and remains in use in clinical practice, but its role has been reexamined in the era of targeted therapy and newer immuno-oncology agents (Table 30.1).

IMDC model evaluates prognostic factors in patients treated with front-line vascular endothelial growth factor (VEGF) targeted therapy for metastatic RCC. Like the MSKCC model, low Karnofsky performance status, low hemoglobin, elevated serum calcium, and less than one year from time of diagnosis to treatment all predicted worse outcomes; but this model also includes elevated platelet count and elevated neutrophil count. Patients are again stratified into three risk groups: favorable, intermediate, and poor risk, with median OS of 43 months, 23 months, and 8 months, respectively. The model was externally validated in a study of 1,028 patients at 13 international centers. More recently it demonstrated predictive capacity in modern era of immunotherapy use with the phase III trial comparing first-line combination ipilimumab/nivolumab vs sunitinib (CheckMate 214). Patients in the intermediate- and poor-risk groups had improved outcomes and OS (HR 0.63; $P < 0.01$) in the immunotherapy group, while those in the favorable risk group had improved response rates and progression-free survival had superior outcomes with the tyrosine kinase inhibitor sunitinib. Owing to these factors, the IMDC can be thought of as the preferred prognostic model to guide treatment (Table 30.2).

The authors believe the ability to stratify patients by prognostic category is important for several reasons. Determining prognosis has value academically in terms of trial design. More practically, identifying prognostic variables assists us in our discussions with individual patients in our clinics regarding expected disease course. We also utilize risk category in part to determine choice of therapy.

Correct Answer: A

Table 30.1 Characteristics of patients predictive of shortened survival.

Prognostic Factors	Risk Group	Number of Factors	Median Survival (months)
• Karnofsky PS < 80%	Favorable risk	0	30
• LDH > 1.5 × ULN	Intermediate risk	1 or 2	14
• Hemoglobin < LLN	Poor risk	≥ 3	5
• Corrected calcium > 10 mg/dL			
• Time from original diagnosis to treatment < 1 year			

LDH: lactate dehydrogenase; LLN: lower limit of normal; PS: performance status; ULN: upper limit of normal.

Table 30.2 Additional characteristics of patients predictive of shortened survival.

Prognostic Factor	Risk Group	Number of Factors	Median Survival (months)
• Karnofsky PS < 80%	Favorable risk	0	43 months
• Time from original diagnosis to treatment < 1 year	Intermediate risk	1 or 2	23 months
• Hemoglobin < LLN	Poor risk	≥3	8 months
• Serum calcium > ULN			
• Neutrophil count > ULN			
• Platelet count > ULN			

LLN: lower limit of normal; PS: performance status; ULN: upper limit of normal.

Case Study 2

A 55-year-old woman undergoes a right nephrectomy for a 10 cm renal mass. Pathology is consistent with a T3b (extends into the vena cava below the diaphragm), grade 3 clear cell renal cell carcinoma (Table 30.3 for TNM staging). She presents for follow-up post nephrectomy and is feeling well other than slight fatigue and incisional pain, consistent with postoperative recovery. Based on examination, laboratory studies, and postoperative imaging, she is without evidence of recurrent disease.

2) **What would be appropriate adjuvant therapy?**
   A) Adjuvant sunitinib.
   B) Adjuvant IL-2.
   C) Adjuvant pembrolizumab.
   D) None of the above.

Expert Perspective: While nephrectomy is curative for the majority of patients with clinically localized renal cell carcinoma, approximately 20–40% of patients will subsequently develop metastatic disease. The risk of recurrence appears to increase with advancing stage and increasing grade, and other factors potentially associated with risk of recurrence include histologic subtype, presence of sarcomatoid features, collecting system invasion, and performance status. Several studies have evaluated the utility of adjuvant therapy to reduce the risk of recurrence following nephrectomy, and these have included cytokines, vaccines, targeted therapies, and more recently, immune checkpoint inhibitors. Studies comparing IL-2 and interferon-α (alone or in combination), in addition to vaccines concluded that adjuvant therapy provided no benefit in terms of overall survival or disease-free survival (when compared to no treatment).

Based on favorable outcomes with targeted agents in metastatic populations, multiple phase III trials have been conducted to evaluate their utility in the adjuvant setting. The ASSURE trial randomized patients' post nephrectomy to single-agent sorafenib, sunitinib, or placebo. There was no difference in disease-free survival, and the treatment arms were associated with significant toxicity and dose reductions. Similar negative results were seen in two other large phase III trials comparing pazopanib (PROTECT) and axitinib (ATLAS). To date the only trial demonstrating clinical benefit of TKI in the adjuvant setting is the S-TRAC trial, which compared sunitinib vs placebo. There was a one-year improvement in disease-free survival in the sunitinib arm (HR 0.76), particularly in higher-risk groups, but no benefit was seen in OS, and treatment was associated with significant toxicity and treatment discontinuation.

Owing to their response rates in the metastatic setting, multiple immune checkpoint inhibitors are being evaluated in phase III trials in the adjuvant setting or combined neo-adjuvant and adjuvant setting. The KEYNOTE-564 trial randomized 994 patients with intermediate-high, high risk, or M1 no evidence of disease clear cell RCC to receive one year of either adjuvant pembrolizumab or placebo. The study met its primary endpoint by demonstrating improved disease-free survival at a median follow-up of 24.1 months (HR 0.68; $P = 0.0010$), and improved 12-month disease-free survival (85.7% vs 76.2%) and 24-month disease-free survival (77.3% vs 68.1%, respectively), with results favoring the pembrolizumab arm across all subgroups. Based on these data, the FDA approved adjuvant pembrolizumab in patients with RCC at intermediate-high- or high-risk of disease recurrence following nephrectomy. Additionally, no new safety signals were detected. For those patients who are not candidates for immunotherapy therapy, enrollment in a clinical trial should be considered. If a trial is not available, or if patients are ineligible (e.g. patient with autoimmune disease) or decline participation, then we recommend observation only. Nivolumab (NCT03055013), atezolizumab (NCT 03024996), ipilimumab/nivolumab (NCT03138512), and durvalumab with or without tremelimumab (NCT03288532) are all actively being studied or are recruiting patients.

Correct Answer: C

Case Study 3

A 58-year-old man with metastatic clear cell renal cell carcinoma presents for a second opinion. He is asymptomatic and has an excellent performance status. On imaging, a large, right renal mass and pulmonary nodules are identified. His blood work is only notable for hemoglobin of 11 g/dL.

3) **He asks whether there is a role for nephrectomy in his treatment plan. How do you respond?**
   A) No data support the role of nephrectomy.
   B) Nephrectomy should be considered only for patients with symptoms.
   C) He should be referred to a urologic oncologist for consideration of nephrectomy.
   D) Surgery should only be considered if he responds to systemic therapy first.

Expert Perspective: Resection of a primary renal lesion in the setting of metastatic disease is referred to as a cytoreductive or debulking nephrectomy. Its role in the management of metastatic RCC is under continued investigation and subject to debate. During the cytokine therapy era, cytoreductive nephrectomy was considered standard of care. This was based on the results of the phase III SWOG 8949 trial, which randomized 241 patients to interferon-α alone or in combination with cytoreductive nephrectomy. Patients in the cytoreductive nephrectomy arm had improved OS (11.1 months vs 8.1 months; $P = 0.05$). This was later confirmed by the EORTC 30947 trial.

The role of cytoreductive nephrectomy was reexamined with the approval of targeted therapies for RCC. In the initial trials of many of the targeted agents, most patients had undergone nephrectomy before enrollment. In a retrospective analysis of patients who received vascular endothelial growth factor (VEGF)-targeted therapies, those who underwent cytoreductive nephrectomy appeared to experience an improvement in overall survival (19.8 months vs 9.4 months for those treated with systemic therapy alone; HR 0.44; 95% CI 0.32–0.59; $P < 0.01$). In subgroup analyses, those patients with poor-risk disease or a Karnofsky performance status of < 80% did not appear to benefit. These results led to two phase III clinical trials evaluating VEGF-inhibitors with cytoreductive nephrectomy, although both studies suffered from incomplete enrollment.

- The CARMENA trial evaluated the non-inferiority of sunitinib alone vs cytoreductive nephrectomy followed by sunitinib in the front-line setting for metastatic RCC. In all, 450 patients were randomized, with a hazard ratio for death 0.89 (95% CI 0.71–1.10, with upper boundary of the 95% CI interval not exceeding the fixed noninferiority limit [1.20], confirming non-inferiority of sunitinib alone). Similar response rates and progression-free survival rates were noted between the two arms, with a 1.9% 30-day mortality noted in the cytoreductive nephrectomy arm.
- The SURTIME trial evaluated immediate cytoreductive nephrectomy followed by sunitinib vs delayed cytoreductive nephrectomy following initial treatment with three cycles of sunitinib. The intention to treat progression-free rate was similar (42 vs 43%; HR 0.88), and although there was improved OS in the deferred cytoreductive nephrectomy arm (32.4 months vs 15 months) this was confounded by almost 20% of patients not receiving the assigned treatment, leading the study's authors to conclude that deferred cytoreductive nephrectomy did not improve progression-free survival.

Results from these studies suggest that immediate cytoreductive nephrectomy in the metastatic RCC setting may not be appropriate in most scenarios and warrant a patient-specific multidisciplinary approach. As we have reached the era of widespread use of immune checkpoint inhibitors in metastatic RCC, the question of who truly benefits from cytoreductive nephrectomy (either up front or delayed) has been further examined. Recent published data by the IMDC evaluated 4,639 patients with metastatic RCC who received front-line targeted therapy or immune checkpoint inhibitor. Using multivariate analysis, they sought to determine which patients benefit from cytoreductive nephrectomy if any. The authors suggest that cytoreductive nephrectomy should be avoided in patients with poor-risk disease or in those with rapidly progressive disease. Delayed cytoreductive nephrectomy can be considered in patients with favorable/intermediate disease, those with oligometastatic disease, and those with symptomatic renal masses especially if the patient had a good response to systemic therapy. Given the limitations of available data, patient selection for cytoreductive nephrectomy is critical. Proposed selection criteria have included greater than 75% debulking of tumor burden possible; no central nervous system, bone, or liver metastases; adequate pulmonary and cardiac function; an Eastern Cooperative Oncology Group (ECOG) performance status of 0 or 1; and predominantly clear cell

Table 30.3 Kidney cancer simplified TNM staging AJCC UICC 8th edition.

TNM	DESCRIPTION
T1	Tumor ≤ 7 cm in greatest dimension, limited to the kidney
T2	Tumor >7 cm in greatest dimension, limited to the kidney
T3	Tumor extends into major veins or perinephric tissues but not into the ipsilateral adrenal gland and not beyond Gerota's fascia
N1	Metastasis in regional lymph node(s)
M1	Distant metastasis

histology. A retrospective analysis identified the following characteristics to be predictors of an inferior overall survival with nephrectomy prior to systemic therapy: elevated LDH, hypoalbuminemia, symptoms at presentation due to a metastatic site, liver metastases, retroperitoneal lymphadenopathy, supradiaphragmatic adenopathy, and clinical tumor classification as T3 or greater (Table 10.3). Inferior overall survival and increased risk of death correlated with the number of risk factors, and patients with four or more risk factors did not appear to benefit from cytoreductive nephrectomy.

Furthermore, there are several prospective, randomized trials evaluating the role of cytoreductive nephrectomy after up-front immunotherapy ipilimumab/nivolumab (NCT03977571), peri-operative nivolumab PROSPER RCC (NCT03055013), and most recently SWOG1931 PROBE (NCT04510597) investigating deferred cytoreductive nephrectomy after currently approved IO combinations for RCC.

Correct Answer: C

Case Study 4

A 69-year-old woman was recently diagnosed with metastatic clear cell renal cell carcinoma after biopsy of a liver lesion, two years after nephrectomy for stage III RCC. She has good performance status. She has no history of autoimmune disease. Blood work demonstrates normal complete blood count with differential, LDH, and calcium. She presents to discuss further recommendations.

4) What therapy do you offer this patient?
   A) Sunitinib.
   B) High-dose IL-2.
   C) Lenvatinib + pembrolizumab.
   D) Ipilimumab + nivolumab.

Expert Perspective: The patient has favorable-risk disease by both the IMDC and MSKCC risk models. Before the approval of targeted therapies, the mainstay of front-line treatment for metastatic RCC was cytokine therapy. Sorafenib was first approved in 2006, and sunitinib, which has been utilized as a standard-of-care / control arm in various studies, was approved in 2007 based on the results of a phase III study comparing sunitinib vs interferon-α. Patients in the sunitinib arm demonstrated improved overall-response rate, progression-free survival, and OS rates compared to interferon-alpha, regardless of prognostic group.

But even as checkpoint inhibitors have become more widely used for metastatic RCC, there continues to be a role for targeted therapies, particularly in patients with favorable-risk disease. Owing to their activity in metastatic RCC, several studies were conducted to evaluate checkpoint inhibitors in combination with VEGF-inhibitors. KEYNOTE-426 was a phase III study comparing pembrolizumab-axitinib vs sunitinib, with the combination arm demonstrating improved overall-response rate, median progression-free survival, and median OS (HR for disease progression of death 0.69; $P < 0.001$) for the entire cohort and the intermediate/poor prognostic risk groups. Similarly, the phase III CheckMate 9ER evaluated 651 patients with metastatic RCC who were randomized to either receive the multikinase inhibitor cabozantinib + nivolumab vs sunitinib. At median follow-up of 18.1 months, the cabozantinib + nivolumab arm had improved median progression-free survival (16.6 months vs 8.3 months), 12-month survival (85.7% vs 75.6%; HR 0.60; $P = 0.001$), and overall-response rate (55.7% vs 27.1%; $P < 0.001$). For both above combination therapies the improved outcomes were seen in the study group with statistically significant differences in intermediate/poor prognostic groups, but only favoring, albeit quite substantially, the study arm in favorable-risk groups. Most recently the results of the CLEAR trial were published. This was a phase III study comparing lenvatinib + pembrolizumab vs sunitinib vs lenvatinib + everolimus in front-line metastatic RCC. As with similar combination studies, the lenvatinib + pembrolizumab arm demonstrated improved (with impressive hazard ratios) median progression-free survival, median OS, and overall-response rate relative to sunitinib seen in the entire study population and in the intermediate/poor prognostic risk groups. Notably, CLEAR trial was the first study to demonstrate a statistically significant median progression-free survival benefit in the IMDC favorable-risk group (HR for disease progression or death 0.36), although it should be noted that this regimen did come with an increased side effect profile.

For patients with favorable prognostic risk metastatic RCC we recommend combination therapy with checkpoint inhibitor and tyrosine kinase inhibitors (TKI) over single agent TKI therapy or checkpoint inhibitor therapy without TKI. The NCCN guidelines consider the FDA approved combinations of either lenvatinib + pembrolizumab or cabozantinib + nivolumab as category 1 for favorable-risk RCC.

Correct Answer: C

Case Study 5

A 62-year-old man was recently diagnosed with metastatic clear cell renal cell carcinoma after biopsy of a liver lesion; lung metastases are also noted on imaging. He has a good performance status and no history of autoimmune disease. Blood work is significant for a Hgb 10.2 g/dL, calcium of 11.1, and elevated LDH and platelet count. He presents for initial oncologic evaluation.

5) What is the most appropriate treatment option currently?
   A) Axitinib + pembrolizumab.
   B) Ipilimumab + nivolumab.

C) Lenvatinib + pembrolizumab.
D) Any of the above.

Expert Perspective: The patient has poor prognostic risk disease. Renal cell carcinoma is an immuno-responsive disease that does not typically respond to cytotoxic chemotherapy. Before the era of targeted therapy, cytokines were the mainstay of treatment. With the advent of modern immunotherapy therapy came the use of checkpoint inhibitors in RCC. Nivolumab was approved based on the results of the CheckMate 025 study, which compared nivolumab vs everolimus in patients with metastatic RCC who had received prior treatment. At a median follow-up of 25.0 months in 821 patients, patients in the nivolumab arm had improved median OS (25.0 months vs 19.6 months; HR death 0.73; $P = 0.002$) and overall-response rate (25% vs 5%), with lower rates of grade 3 or 4 toxicity. This led to evaluation of combination immunotherapy therapy in the front-line setting. In 2018, CheckMate 214 was published, which was a large, multicenter international phase III trial comparing ipilimumab + nivolumab vs sunitinib in newly diagnosed metastatic RCC. The primary endpoints specifically evaluated patients with intermediate or poor prognostic risk, although roughly 20% of the almost 1,100 patients had favorable risk disease. At a median follow-up of 25.2 months in patients with intermediate or poor prognostic risk, those in the ipilimumab + nivolumab arm demonstrated improved 18-month survival (75% vs 60%), improved OS (not reached vs 26.0 months; HR 0.63; $P < 0.001$), overall-response rate (42% vs 27%; $P < 0.001$), and complete response rates (9% vs 1%). Conversely, exploratory analysis of patients with favorable prognostic risk demonstrated improved median OS, median progression-free survival, and overall-response rate in the sunitinib arm. This led to the approval of combination ipilimumab + nivolumab for intermediate/poor-risk disease in the front-line setting.

As discussed earlier, several combination therapies are recommended on national guidelines for metastatic RCC. Axitinib + pembrolizumab, cabozantinib + nivolumab, and lenvatinib + pembrolizumab all demonstrated improved overall-response rate, median progression-free survival, and survival rates compared to sunitinib and were specifically studied in the intermediate/poor prognostic risk groups. Also, most recently, results of COSMIC-313 were reported. Among patients with previously untreated, advanced renal-cell carcinoma who had intermediate or poor prognostic risk, treatment with cabozantinib plus nivolumab and ipilimumab resulted in significantly longer progression-free survival than treatment with nivolumab and ipilimumab alone. Grade 3 or 4 adverse events were more common in the experimental group than in the control group. Follow-up for overall survival is ongoing.

In summary, patients with intermediate/poor-risk disease benefit from immunotherapy with a checkpoint inhibitor either in combination with another immunotherapy agent or a targeted agent.

Correct Answer: D

Case Study 6

A 52-year-old man with a history of a kidney transplant who is currently on immunosuppressive therapy presents with a renal mass and pulmonary nodules on imaging. You send him for a needle biopsy of a pulmonary nodule, and pathology is consistent with metastatic papillary renal cell carcinoma.

6) Which of the following is the preferred treatment option?
   A) Cabozantinib.
   B) Nivolumab.
   C) Sunitinib.
   D) Gemcitabine.

Expert Perspective: On the order of 75–85% of renal cell carcinomas are clear cell carcinomas, and the remaining portion, deemed non-clear cell RCC, are composed of several histologic variants. The most common of these subtypes is papillary RCC, which makes up roughly 10–15% of RCC cases. Papillary RCC is a rare and heterogeneous disease and is further differentiated into types 1 and 2. Type 1 papillary RCC is associated with *MET* mutations and the hereditary papillary renal carcinoma syndrome, and type 2 papillary RCC is often associated with mutations in the *FH* gene and the hereditary leiomyomatosis and RCC syndrome (Chapters 45–47). Patients who have undergone kidney transplant are at a higher risk of developing RCC, particularly papillary subtypes.

Due to its relative rarity, data from large prospective trials are lacking, and no standard of care exists. Like most other RCC, papillary RCC does not respond to cytotoxic chemotherapy, but unlike clear cell RCC it is not particularly responsive to single agent immunotherapy, with limited responses to immune checkpoint inhibitors noted. Thus, targeted therapies are currently the mainstay of treatment for papillary RCC.

Prospective phase II studies have demonstrated improved median progression-free survival with sunitinib compared to the mammalian target of rapamycin (mTOR)-inhibitors everolimus and temsirolimus with metastatic non-clear cell RCC. These studies were not specific to papillary RCC, demonstrate only modest improvement, and are further limited by larger *P*-values and wide confidence intervals. Nevertheless, sunitinib has long been considered the preferred agent for metastatic papillary RCC.

More recently, emerging data suggests an increased role for cabozantinib, considering a large majority of papillary RCC contain mutations in the *MET* gene. A small single-arm study of cabozantib in non-clear cell RCC showed improved outcomes in patients with papillary subtype. The SWOG 1500 study was a prospective phase II study at 65 centers across North America comparing sunitinib to three different *MET* inhibitors (cabozantinib, crizotinib, and savolitinib) in the front-line setting for metastatic papillary RCC. After randomization, assignment to the crizotinib and savolitinib arms was halted due to prespecified futility analysis, but 46 patients were randomized to the sunitinib arm and 44 to the cabozantinib arm. Patients in the cabozantinib arm had improved median progression-free survival (9.0 months vs 5.6 months; HR 0.60; $P = 0.01$) and overall-response rate (23% vs 4%; $P = 0.01$) compared to sunitinib, with similar adverse event rates. Another randomized phase II study comparing cabozantinib vs sunitinib for front-line metastatic papillary RCC is currently recruiting patients (NCT035411902).

As papillary RCC is a rare disease, enrollment in clinical trial is preferred, but for those patients unable or unwilling to enroll in a clinical trial we recommend treating with cabozantinib based on the available prospective data.

Correct Answer: A

Case Study 7

A 66-year-old woman presents with shortness of breath, flank pain, and weight loss. Imaging reveals a left kidney mass and multiple lung nodules. Biopsy of a lung lesion reveals metastatic clear cell renal cell carcinoma with sarcomatoid de-differentiation. She has excellent performance status. She presents for initial evaluation.

7) **What therapy do you recommend for her?**
   A) Sunitinib.
   B) Lenvatinib + everolimus.
   C) Ipilimumab + nivolumab.
   D) Sunitinib + gemcitabine.

Expert Perspective: Sarcomatoid or rhabdoid de-differentiation is a relatively rare feature of RCC, occurring in roughly 4% of tumors. It is not considered to be a distinct subtype of RCC but occurs in both clear cell RCC and non-clear cell RCC. Its presence is associated with a more aggressive disease course as it is seen in 15–20% of patients with metastatic RCC, and portends worse outcomes compared to conventional clear cell RCC. Owing to the rarity of this entity, large prospective trials are absent, and most of the available prospective data is taken from subgroup analyses.

Compared to clear cell RCC, sarcomatoid or rhabdoid de-differentiation RCC typically demonstrates lower response rates to single-agent targeted therapy. A retrospective analysis of 43 patients with sarcomatoid RCC treated with anti-VEGF therapy demonstrated a partial response rate of 19%, with no patients achieving a complete response and 33% of patient with PD, while the sarcomatoid RCC group had lower progression-free survival and OS rates compared to non-sarcomatoid RCC patients. A larger retrospective study from the IMDC of 230 patients who received either VEGF- or mTOR-inhibitor therapy (93% received anti-VEGF therapy) demonstrated lower overall-response rate, higher rates of primary refractory disease, and lower progression-free survival and OS rates compared to those with non-sarcomatoid RCC. As with most other RCC, the role of cytotoxic chemotherapy is limited. The phase II ECOG 8802 evaluating doxorubicin and gemcitabine demonstrated 16% overall-response rates (6 of 38), although at the expense of significant toxicity; a separate phase II trial of 32 patients receiving sunitinib in combination with gemcitabine demonstrated overall-response rates of 26%. Sarcomatoid or rhabdoid de-differentiation RCC tumors tend to have increased numbers of tumor-infiltrating lymphocytes and higher PD-L1 expression, making modern immunotherapy therapy a potential treatment option. Subset analysis from several of the pivotal phase III trials leading to the approval of checkpoint inhibitors have demonstrated significantly improved outcomes for patients with sarcomatoid or rhabdoid de-differentiation RCC. In all, 89 of the 425 patients had sarcomatoid or rhabdoid de-differentiation RCC in the CheckMate 214 trial comparing ipilimumab + nivolumab vs sunitinib and demonstrated improved overall-response rates (56.7% vs 19.25) and complete response rates (18.3% vs 0%), as well as progression-free survival (HR 0.61) and OS (HR 0.55) in the immunotherapy arm. Fifty-one of the 432 patients had sarcomatoid or rhabdoid de-differentiation RCC in the KEYNOTE-426 study comparing pembrolizumab + axitinib vs sunitinib and demonstrated improved overall-response rates (58.8% vs 31.5%) and complete response rates (13% vs 2%), as well as progression-free survival (HR 0.54) and OS (HR 0.58) also favoring the inclusion of immunotherapy. Similar improvements were seen in the IMmotion 151 trial comparing atezolizumab + bevacizumab vs sunitinib and the JAVELIN Renal 101 trial comparing avelumab + axitinib vs sunitinib. Furthermore, retrospective data from cohort studies evaluating real-world outcomes from the Harvard group (79 patients) and the IMDC (89 patients) showed improved overall-response rates, progression-free survival, and OS. It should be noted that in all these studies, while patients had improved outcomes with immunotherapy compared to targeted agents, they still had worse outcomes compared to patients with clear cell RCC.

For patients with sarcomatoid or rhabdoid de-differentiation, we recommend treatment with immune checkpoint inhibitors in combination with another immunotherapy agent or a targeted agent if no contraindication to immunotherapy exists.

Correct Answer: C

Case Study 8

A 27-year-old African American man with a past medical history of sickle cell trait presents with right-side flank and back pain. Imaging reveals a 6 cm right kidney mass, multiple lung nodules, and an enlarged supraclavicular lymph node. Biopsy of this lymph node reveals metastatic renal medullary carcinoma.

8) The most appropriate management consists of which of the following?
- A) Nephrectomy alone.
- B) Carboplatin + paclitaxel.
- C) Sunitinib.
- D) Bevacizumab.
- E) Belzutifan.

Expert Perspective: Renal medullary carcinoma (RMC) is a rare subtype of RCC constituting < 1% of cases. It is typically an aggressive disease with a poor prognosis and predominantly affects young African American men. There is an association with sickle cell trait and other hemoglobinopathies, and tumors uniformly contain loss of the *SMARCB1* gene, which plays a role in response to DNA replication stress.

Renal medullary carcinoma typically does not respond to targeted therapy with TKI. A prospective phase II study of 55 patients with non-clear cell RCC were treated with sunitinib, and of the six patients with either RMC or collecting duct tumors, zero had a response with two patients developing progressive disease. Unlike other RCC subtypes, cytotoxic chemotherapy is considered the standard of care, with cytoreductive nephrectomy playing an important role in those who respond to treatment. No prospective data exists to suggest one chemotherapy regimen is preferable over another, but platinum-containing regimens are typically preferred. In a retrospective study of 52 patients with renal medullary carcinoma treated with systemic therapy over the course of 15 years, the overall-response rate to cytotoxic chemotherapy was 29%, with two patients achieving a complete response after receiving carboplatin + paclitaxel. Of note, patients who underwent nephrectomy had improved OS, with improved outcomes for patients who had at least stable disease after neoadjuvant chemotherapy.

There are clinical trials currently recruiting patients with renal medullary carcinoma: a phase II study evaluating nivolumab + ipilimumab (NCT03274258) and another phase II study comparing the proteasome inhibitor ixazomib with gemcitabine + doxorubicin (NCT03587662). Enrollment in clinical trial is preferred, but for patients who do not qualify or wish to enroll, we recommend combination platinum-based cytotoxic chemotherapy.

Belzutifan, a hypoxia-inducible factor inhibitor, was FDA approved for adult patients with von Hippel-Lindau (VHL) disease who require therapy for associated RCC, central nervous system (CNS) hemangioblastomas, or pancreatic neuroendocrine tumors not requiring immediate surgery (Chapters 1 and 28).

Correct Answer: B

Recommended Readings

Blum, K.A., Gupta, S., Tickoo, S.K. et al. (2020). Sarcomatoid renal cell carcinoma: biology, natural history and management. *Nat Rev Urol* 17: 659–678.

Choueiri, T.K., Powles, T., Albiges, L. et al. (2023 May 11). COSMIC-313 Investigators. Cabozantinib plus Nivolumab and Ipilimumab in renal-cell carcinoma. *N Engl J Med* 388 (19): 1767–1778.

Choueiri, T.K., Tomczak, P., Park, S.H., Venugopal, B., Ferguson, T., Chang, Y.H. et al. (2021 August 19). KEYNOTE-564 investigators. adjuvant pembrolizumab after nephrectomy in renal-cell carcinoma. *N Engl J Med* 385 (8): 683–694. doi: 10.1056/NEJMoa2106391. PMID: 34407342.

Graham, J., Dudani, S., and Heng, D.Y.C. (2018). Prognostication in kidney cancer: recent advances and future directions. *J Clin Oncol* 36 (36): 3567–3573.

Gul, A. and Rini, B.I. (2019). Adjuvant therapy in renal cell carcinoma. *Cancer* 125: 2935–2944.

Lee, C.H., Voss, M.H., Carlo, M.I. et al. (2022 March 17). Phase II trial of cabozantinib plus nivolumab in patients with non-clear-cell renal cell carcinoma and genomic correlates. *J Clin Oncol* JCO2101944. doi: 10.1200/JCO.21.01944. Epub ahead of print. PMID: 35298296.

Motzer, R., Alekseev, B., Rha, S.-Y. et al. (2021 February 13). Lenvatinib plus pembrolizumab or everolimus for advanced renal-cell carcinoma. *N Engl J Med* 384: 1289–1300. doi: 10.1056/NEJMoa2035716.

Motzer, R.J., Powles, T., Atkins, M.B. et al. (2022). Final overall survival and molecular analysis in IMmotion151, a phase 3 trial comparing atezolizumab plus bevacizumab vs sunitinib in patients with previously untreated metastatic renal cell carcinoma. *JAMA Oncol* 8: 275–280.

Msaouel, P., Hong, A.L., Mullen, E.A. et al. (2019 February). Updated recommendations on the diagnosis, management, and clinical trial eligibility criteria for patients with renal medullary carcinoma. *Clin Genitourin Cancer* 17 (1): 1–6.

National Comprehensive Cancer Network (NCCN) (2022). NCCN clinical practice guidelines in oncology kidney cancer, version 4.2021.

Pal, S.K., Tangen, C., Thompson, I.M., Jr, Balzer-Haas, N. et al. (2021 February 20). A comparison of sunitinib with cabozantinib, crizotinib, and savolitinib for treatment of advanced papillary renal cell carcinoma: a randomised, open-label, phase 2 trial. *Lancet* 397 (10275): 695–703.

Psutka, S.P., Chang, S.L., Cahn, D. et al. (2019). Reassessing the role of cytoreductive nephrectomy for metastatic renal cell carcinoma in 2019. *Am Soc Clin Oncol Educl Book* 39: 276–283.

Sheng, I.Y. and Ornstein, M.C. (2020). Ipilimumab and nivolumab as first-line treatment of patients with renal cell carcinoma: the evidence to date. *Cancer Manag Res* 12: 4871–4881.

Vano, Y.A., Elaidi, R., Bennamoun, M. et al. (2022 May). Nivolumab, nivolumab-ipilimumab, and VEGFR-tyrosine kinase inhibitors as first-line treatment for metastatic clear-cell renal cell carcinoma (BIONIKK): a biomarker-driven, open-label, non-comparative, randomised, phase 2 trial. *Lancet Oncol* 23 (5): 612–624. doi:10.1016/S1470-2045(22)00128-0. Epub 2022 Apr 4. PMID: 35390339.

Zoumpourlis, P., Genovese, G., Tannir, N., and Msaouel, P. (2020 December 2). Systemic therapies for the management of non-clear cell renal cell carcinoma: what works, what doesn't, and what the future holds. *Clin Genitourin Cancer* S1558-7673 (20): 30266–4.

31

Bladder Cancer

Revathi Kollipara, Alan Tan, and Timothy M. Kuzel

Rush University Medical Center, Chicago, IL

Introduction

In the US, bladder cancer is the most common genitourinary malignancy, and there will be an estimated 83,730 new cases of bladder cancer with 17,200 deaths in 2021. It is the fourth most common type of cancer in men. The five-year relative survival is 76.9%. However, with advanced urothelial bladder cancer, the five-year survival rate is only 35%. All patients must be clinically staged prior to initiation of treatment for bladder cancer. Table 31.1 displays a simplified version of bladder cancer staging. For patients with disease limited to the bladder, the depth of invasion of the primary tumor is the most important prognostic variable in determining the risk of recurrence or progression. The majority (over 70%) of bladder cancer patients are older than 65 at diagnosis. The median age for diagnosis is 72 years in men and 75 years for women. It is two times more common in Caucasians than in African Americans, but the latter population have a higher mortality.

Urothelial carcinoma is the most common histology in bladder cancer and accounts for 95% of bladder cancers. Other variant and less common histologies include squamous (infection/inflammation), small cell (treated with neoadjuvant cisplatin etoposide followed by radiation or cystectomy), adenocarcinoma, and plasmacytoid (aggressive variant and associated with *CDH1* mutations). Common risk factors include environmental and occupational exposures with smoking being the most common risk factor. Smoking cessation can lead to a decreased risk of recurrent cancer. The primary carcinogens in the smoking population are aromatic amines. Occupational exposures to carcinogens such as polycyclic aromatic hydrocarbons and chlorinated hydrocarbons account for up to 20% of cases. Infections such as chronic urinary tract infections (UTIs), chronic self-catheterization and schistosomiasis (more common outside of the US) are also risk factors but for squamous cell carcinoma of the bladder.

Cancer Consult: Expertise in Clinical Practice, Volume 1: Solid Tumors & Supportive Care,
Second Edition. Edited by Syed A. Abutalib, Maurie Markman, Al B. Benson III, and Hope S. Rugo.
© 2024 John Wiley & Sons Ltd. Published 2024 by John Wiley & Sons Ltd.

Table 31.1 Bladder cancer simplified TNM staging, AJCC UICC 8th edition.

TNM	Description
Ta	Noninvasive papillary carcinoma
Tis	Urothelial carcinoma *in situ*: "Flat tumor"
T1	Tumor invades lamina propria (subepithelial connective tissue)
T2	Tumor invades muscularis propria
T3	Tumor invades perivesical soft tissue
T4	Extravesical tumor directly invades any of the following: prostatic stroma, seminal vesicles, uterus, vagina, pelvic wall, abdominal wall
N1	Single regional lymph node metastasis in the true pelvis (perivesical, obturator, internal and external iliac, or sacral lymph node)
N2	Multiple regional lymph node metastasis in the true pelvis (perivesical, obturator, internal and external iliac, or sacral lymph node metastasis)
N3	Lymph node metastasis to the common iliac lymph nodes
M1a	Distant metastasis limited to lymph nodes beyond the common iliacs
M1b	Non-lymph-node distant metastases

Case Study 1

An 83-year-old female presents with hematuria. She undergoes cystoscopy/transurethral resection of a bladder tumor (TURBT) revealing multiple erythematous patches. She receives single-dose intravesical chemotherapy with gemcitabine within 24 hours of the procedure. Pathology reveals a low-grade tumor with concurrent high-grade carcinoma *in situ* (CIS) urothelial carcinoma non-muscle-invasive bladder cancer. She undergoes adjuvant induction BCG therapy for six doses without maintenance. She is then found to have recurrence of non-muscle-invasive bladder cancer five months after completing BCG therapy. She is deemed a poor surgical candidate due to her history of coronary artery disease.

1) **What therapy do you offer next?**
    A) Repeat BCG (bacillus Calmette-Guérin).
    B) Pembrolizumab.
    C) Doxorubicin.
    D) Carboplatin.

Expert Perspective: In this case, the patient is high risk as she has a high-grade CIS urothelial carcinoma. Other high-risk factors include a T1 tumor, tumors > 3 cm in size, or multifocal cancer (Table 31.2). Very-high risk features include patients who are BCG unresponsive or have variant histologies, lympho-vascular invasion, or prostatic urethral invasion. Those with high-risk non-muscle-invasive bladder cancer who are naive to BCG and do not have very high-risk features preferably should start BCG therapy. Those with very-high risk features are recommended to undergo cystectomy. However, cystectomy is a procedure with risk of complications and inferior quality of life especially in the patient presented in the clinical vignette.

Table 31.2 Risk stratification in non-muscle invasive bladder cancer and preferred management.

Risk	Definition	Preferred management
Low	Solitary, low-grade Ta (papillary [exophytic] lesions) primary tumor, < 3 cm in diameter, absence of carcinoma *in situ*	TURBT[†] followed by surveillance cystoscopy
Intermediate	Neither low- or high- risk	TURBT[†] + single intravesical chemotherapy (gemcitabine [preferred] or mitomycin-C) or BCG within 24 hours of TURBT and surveillance cystoscopies
High	High-grade, multiple lesions, or > 3 cm, recurrent lesions, T1 (invasion of submucosa or lamina propria) or carcinoma *in situ*	TURBT[†] + single intravesical chemotherapy (gemcitabine [preferred] or mitomycin-C) within 24 hours + BCG (induction and maintenance) followed by surveillance cystoscopies
Very high risk	Variant histologies, lympho-vascular invasion, or prostatic urethral invasion or BCG unresponsive	Cystectomy

TURBT – Transurethral resection of bladder tumor
[†]The bladder tissue must have muscle presence for accurate histopathology assessment.

When patients are not cystectomy candidates or they elect not to undergo cystectomy, pembrolizumab is an option based on the results of the phase II KEYNOTE-057 trial. The trial, which consisted of 96 patients with BCG-unresponsive high-risk non-muscle-invasive bladder cancer CIS with or without papillary tumors, showed a complete response rate of 41% with a median duration of response of 16.2 months. Pembrolizumab was given 200 mg every three weeks until disease progression or acceptable toxicity for up to two years. Of note, 46% of patients who achieved a complete response had a duration of response of one year or more. The most common adverse events were fatigue, pruritus, and diarrhea with immune-mediated events consisting of about a fifth of the group. About 37% of the patients eventually underwent radical cystectomy. Pembrolizumab is the preferred option in patients who are not surgical candidates or elect not to undergo cystectomy.

Valrubicin is currently FDA approved for BCG-refractory CIS based on the results of a phase II single-arm trial. The complete response rate was 21% with disease-free survival of only 8% at 30 months. In addition, 50% of the patients eventually required cystectomy. While this is currently approved, it is not used frequently in this setting.

Vicineum, an epithelial cell adhesion molecule (EpCAM)-specific antibody fragment fused to Pseudomonas Exotoxin A has shown promise for treating BCG-unresponsive non-muscle invasive bladder cancer. In the phase III VISTA trial, Vicineum was instilled in the bladder two times per week for 6 weeks during the induction phase and then weekly for 6 weeks followed by every 2 weeks for up to 2 years as maintenance. The 3-month complete response rate was 42%. A key secondary endpoint of the trial was "time to cystectomy" and at 3 years, more than 75% of the patients treated with Vicineum remained cystectomy free. Overall, the drug was well tolerated. Recently, another intravesical drug, nadofaragene firadenovec (also known as rAd-IFNa/Syn3) was approved for patients with BCG-unresponsive non-muscle invasive bladder cancer. It has demonstrated promising efficacy for patients with high-risk non-muscle invasive bladder cancer (CIS- with or without papillary tumors) after BCG therapy who were unable or unwilling to undergo radical cystectomy.

Correct Answer: B

Case Study 2

A 77-year-old woman with multiple medical problems presents to you for a second opinion regarding management of her high-grade, muscle-invasive urothelial carcinoma of the bladder. On a CT scan, asymmetric thickening of the bladder wall is noted, but no lymphadenopathy, hydronephrosis, or evidence of visceral metastases is identified. Her urologist is recommending surgery, but she is refusing. While she states that she is appalled at the idea of not having a bladder, she desires active treatment for her cancer. You worry about her ability to tolerate surgery given her multiple comorbidities, including coronary artery disease and diabetes mellitus. She asks if she has options other than surgery.

2) What would you recommend this patient?
   A) Reassuring her and sending her back to her urologist for cystectomy.
   B) Offering her MVAC (methotrexate, vinblastine, adriamycin, and cisplatin) in place of surgery.
   C) Considering a bladder-sparing or trimodality treatment strategy.
   D) Referring for radiation alone.

Expert Perspective: Concurrent chemoradiotherapy following the TURBT ("trimodality therapy") is an NCCN category 1 option for treatment of stage II muscle-invasive bladder cancer, especially in patients judged to not be candidates for radical cystectomy. Often, comorbidities or less than optimal performance status may preclude cystectomy, and sometimes patients may refuse surgery. Pathologic complete response rates after neoadjuvant therapy range from 20 to 40% making chemotherapy without definitive treatment with either surgery or radiation a suboptimal option if a patient is surgical candidate. Definitive radiation has been utilized instead of surgery, but as a single modality it may be inferior to surgery as up to 70% of patients may experience a local recurrence and five-year survival rates are generally suboptimal.

Bladder-sparing or trimodality approaches involve a maximum TURBT followed by bladder irradiation concurrent with radiosensitizing chemotherapy. Ideal patients have undergone a complete TURBT as this is a prognostic factor for long-term survival with this approach. Other clinical patient factors to consider include the ability to tolerate platinum-based chemotherapy, urothelial carcinoma histology, and early stage as opposed to bulky disease. Periodic imaging studies and cystoscopies are performed to monitor for recurrence, and if disease is noted, patients undergo salvage radical cystectomy.

There has not been a randomized trial to compare bladder preservation versus neoadjuvant chemotherapy followed by cystectomy. A study at Massachusetts General Hospital evaluated more than 300 patients with muscle-invasive bladder carcinoma who underwent combined-modality therapy with concurrent cisplatin-based chemotherapy with radiation therapy after maximal TURBT plus neoadjuvant or adjuvant chemotherapy. In this single-institution study, combined-modality therapy achieved a complete remission and bladder preservation in > 70% of the patients.

A phase III trial randomized patients who had undergone a complete TURBT to radiation alone or to radiation in combination with mitomycin C and fluorouracil; the two-year loco-regional disease-free survival was improved from 54% with radiation alone to 67% with combination therapy. However, the difference in overall survival at five years and the rate of cystectomy at two years did not reach statistical significance. Except for gastrointestinal toxicity, which increased from 3% with radiation alone to 10% with the addition of chemotherapy, toxicity was similar in the two arms of the study. Recent phase II studies have showed promise using chemoimmunotherapy such as nivolumab with gemcitabine and cisplatin or pembrolizumab plus gemcitabine with concurrent hypo-fractionated radiotherapy as bladder-sparing treatment regimens.

Correct Answer: C

Our Patient: Trimodality approach is the best option given she has substantial risk for poor outcomes with cystectomy. In our practice, we do utilize a trimodality approach but only for select patients who are poor cystectomy candidates due to either advanced age or comorbidities or for patients who refuse cystectomy. Otherwise, neoadjuvant chemotherapy followed by cystectomy is our preferred treatment strategy for non-metastatic muscle-invasive bladder cancer.

Case Study 3

A 68-year-old man with muscle-invasive bladder cancer undergoes a radical cystectomy

3) **Which of the following statements regarding a lymph node dissection is correct?**
   A) The extent of pelvic lymph node dissection affects survival outcomes post cystectomy.
   B) Pelvic lymph node dissection is only necessary for patients with nodal involvement.
   C) Pelvic lymph node dissection is unnecessary in patients who have received neoadjuvant chemotherapy.
   D) Lymph node dissection only benefits patients with negative surgical margins.

Expert Perspective: A radical cystectomy is an extensive operation. In men, the urinary bladder is removed along with the prostate and seminal vesicles. In women, en bloc resection of the uterus, cervix, ovaries, and anterior vagina is performed. A lymph node dissection is also undertaken in all patients and entails at least a bilateral pelvic lymphadenectomy, which includes the external and internal iliac and obturator nodes, with removal of a minimum of 10–12 lymph nodes and a urinary diversion, typically an ileal conduit (monitor B_{12} levels) or orthotopic neobladder, is created.

At the completion of neoadjuvant chemotherapy, patients should proceed with radical cystectomy regardless of the clinical response, unless there is the development of biopsy-proven metastatic disease. The extent of pelvic lymph node dissection for optimal oncologic control continues to be a debated topic. Multiple groups have published outcomes on series of patients who have undergone cystectomy, and primary T stage and lymph node involvement appear to be predictive of outcomes. A meta-analysis showed that up to 25% of organ-confined muscle-invasive bladder cancer had lymph node metastasis at the time of radial cystectomy. Higher lymph node density was associated with poorer survival outcomes suggesting that identifying pathologic lymph node involvement is crucial in predicting survival as well as driving treatment decisions. The five-year recurrence-free survival rates range from 70 to 80% for patients with organ-confined disease and absence of nodal involvement to as low as 30–35% for those with positive nodes. Patients with extension through the bladder wall (pT3b) and negative nodes have a five-year recurrence-free rate of 50% to 60%. The median time to recurrence in one series was 12 months.

There have been several non-randomized studies and meta-analyses studying extended vs standard pelvic lymph node dissection, but there is limited data in terms of prospective randomized trials. The LEA AUO AB 25/02 phase III trial in 2018 compared super-extended vs standard pelvic lymph node dissection in patients with confirmed T1 grade 2 or muscle-invasive bladder cancer undergoing radial cystectomy. The difference in recurrence-free survival between the super-extended pelvic lymph node dissection group and standard group was not as significant as expected with a recurrence-free survival of 65% vs 59% (HR 0.84; $P = 0.36$). Extended pelvic lymph node dissection does carry a higher risk of complications with uncertain survival benefit, so the risks and benefits must be weighed carefully by the surgical team. SWOG S1011 is another randomized clinical trial that is currently awaiting final analysis. The S1011 trial enrolled > 600 patients with the aim of detecting a 10% improvement in three-year recurrence-free survival between the extended and standard pelvic lymph node dissection.

Correct Answer: A

Case Study 4

A 72-year-old man with muscle-invasive bladder cancer presents to you for a second opinion. Aside from hypertension, he has no significant past medical history or comorbidities. He states that although he is reluctant to undergo cystectomy as recommended to him by his urologist, he wishes to be aggressive with his treatment plan, taking advantage of any possibility to improve his outcome.

4) You realize that his urologist has not discussed neoadjuvant chemotherapy, and you discuss it with the patient, stating that it has which of the following advantages?
   A) An improvement in overall survival.
   B) An increase in pathologic complete response rate.
   C) No increase in surgical complication rates compared with cystectomy alone.
   D) All of the above.

Expert Perspective: Long-term survival following surgery has been evaluated in multiple surgical series, and the five-year survival for patients with pathologically organ-confined bladder cancer (pT2—muscle invasive) is 68%, while those with extravesicular extension or lymph node involvement have a five-year survival rates in the range of 25 to 30%. The goal of neoadjuvant chemotherapy in muscle-invasive transitional cell bladder cancer is to eradicate micrometastatic disease and improve survival. Advantages to neoadjuvant chemotherapy approach include potential downstaging of disease, being able to monitor an intact bladder lesion for response, and avoiding potential postoperative issues or complications that may complicate the delivery of chemotherapy. However, opponents argue that patients may progress such that they become inoperable, losing an opportunity for cure. Further, given the inaccuracies of clinical staging, some patients may be exposed to chemotherapy unnecessarily.

- The benefit of neoadjuvant chemotherapy is supported by clinical trial data. An Intergroup-sponsored study, INT-0080, randomized patients with T2 to T4a urothelial carcinoma to either neoadjuvant MVAC (methotrexate, vinblastine, adriamycin, and cisplatin) followed by radical cystectomy or to surgery alone. Neoadjuvant chemotherapy increased the pathologic complete response rate significantly from 15% with surgery alone to 38% with neoadjuvant MVAC. Further, 85% of patients with a pathologic complete response were alive at five years. Median OS also was greater with neoadjuvant chemotherapy at 77 months vs 46 months with cystectomy alone, but this difference was not statistically significant. While increased toxicity was observed with the addition of MVAC, no chemotherapy-related deaths occurred, and surgical complication rates did not differ between the two arms. A phase II study with a dose-dense version of MVAC (ddMVAC) given in two-week cycles with growth factor support yielded a similar pathologic complete response rate, and the regimen was well tolerated. Five-year OS rate of ddMVAC was 63%. Gemcitabine and cisplatin have only been studied retrospectively as neoadjuvant chemotherapy, but reports suggest similar pathologic complete response rates and survival data. A meta-analysis including 3,005 patients with T2 to T4a urothelial carcinoma from 11 trials reported a significant survival benefit for patients treated with neoadjuvant platinum-based combination chemotherapy equivalent to a 5% absolute improvement in survival at five years.
- However, not all patients are fit for cisplatin-based therapy. Of note, in the curative setting, carboplatin is an inadequate substitute for cisplatin. Patients are deemed unfit if they have one or more of the following criteria: CrCl <60 mL/min, ECOG ⩾2 or KPS 60–70%, grade ⩾2 hearing loss, grade ⩾2 neuropathy, and/or NYHA Class III heart failure. Patients with CrCl between 50 and 60 mL/min may be offered split-dose cisplatin with gemcitabine.
- In the future, pembrolizumab may be an alternative option for neoadjuvant therapy in cisplatin-ineligible patients as the results from the phase II PURE-01 trial which showed a pathological complete response rate of 42% in all patients and 54.3% of patients with a PD-L1 combined positive score (CPS) of >10. KEYNOTE-905/EV303 is an ongoing phase III trial evaluating perioperative pembrolizumab or pembrolizumab plus enfortumab vedotin and cystectomy compared to cystectomy alone in cisplatin-ineligible patients with muscle-invasive bladder cancer.
- Interestingly, few studies have utilized immunotherapy in combination with chemotherapy in the neoadjuvant setting. In the phase II trial, the addition of pembrolizumab to neoadjuvant gemcitabine and split-dose cisplatin resulted in a pathologic complete response rate of 36%. In preliminary results from a separate phase II trial (BLASST-1), the addition of nivolumab to neoadjuvant gemcitabine plus cisplatin resulted in a pathologic complete response rate of 50%.

We typically recommend neoadjuvant chemotherapy for all patients with muscle-invasive urothelial carcinoma who are undergoing radical cystectomy and are appropriate for cisplatin-based chemotherapy.

Correct Answer: D

Case Study continued: The patient opts to undergo cystectomy and declined neoadjuvant chemotherapy. His radical cystectomy pathology is notable for extension through the bladder wall, and two lymph nodes are positive for malignancy. His urologist now refers him back to you for consideration of adjuvant chemotherapy. His postoperative course was complicated by pneumonia, and as a result he became deconditioned and required a stay in an extended care facility.

5) Which of the following statements regarding adjuvant chemotherapy is correct?
    A) Immunotherapy in the adjuvant setting improves outcomes.
    B) Postoperative complications do not interfere with its administration.
    C) Only patients with p53-expressing tumors benefit from adjuvant chemotherapy.
    D) It should be considered in all patients who did not receive neoadjuvant therapy.
    E) A and D.

Expert Perspective: This patient is at particularly elevated risk for developing recurrent bladder cancer. Patients with extravesicular extension or positive nodes have a five-year survival on the order of 25–30%. Adjuvant therapy can be considered when no neoadjuvant therapy was given and for selected patients with pT3-4 or node-positive bladder cancer.

- The EORTC 30994 trial is the largest phase III trial to date studying adjuvant therapy. Inclusion criteria included patients with pT3-T4 or node-positive disease after definitive radial cystectomy and bilateral lymphadenectomy. Patients were randomly assigned 1:1 to adjuvant chemotherapy (gemcitabine and cisplatin for four cycles, high-dose MVAC, or MVAC) or no further therapy until relapse (deferred treatment). There was no significant improvement in OS in the adjuvant therapy group vs deferred treatment group, but progression-free survival was significantly prolonged with a five-year progression-free survival of 47.6% vs 31.8% (HR 0.54; $P < 0.0001$).
- Recent data now suggests that adjuvant immunotherapy may be beneficial in muscle-invasive bladder cancer after radical surgery. The phase III CheckMate 274 trial assigned patients with muscle-invasive bladder cancer to adjuvant nivolumab 240 mg every two weeks vs placebo. Patients who received previous neoadjuvant cisplatin-based therapy were included in the trial as well. The two primary endpoints were disease-free survival in all patients and those with PD-L1 expression > 1%. The latter cohort consisted of 140 patients in the nivolumab arm. The disease-free survival was prolonged in the nivolumab arm compared to the placebo arm (20.8 months vs 10.8 months) and was even more pronounced in the PD-L1 high group. Secondary endpoints including survival free from recurrence outside of the urothelial tract and distant metastasis-free survival also favored the nivolumab arm. Treatment-related side effects were more common in the nivolumab group and similar to previously reported side effects. Quality of life questionnaires completed showed there was not a significant deterioration in quality of life in those that received nivolumab compared to those that received placebo.

While we favor neoadjuvant chemotherapy for patients with muscle-invasive disease undergoing cystectomy, we will consider adjuvant therapy for patients at high risk for recurrence such as those with pathologic T3 or T4 disease or node-positive disease, and typically we give four cycles of cisplatin-based chemotherapy. This is consistent with

NCCN guidelines as of now. In patient ineligible for adjuvant cisplatin-based chemotherapy, we suggest one year of adjuvant nivolumab rather than observation. In addition, data of CheckMate 274 trial in patients who received cisplatin-based neoadjuvant therapy might also be practice-changing, especially for high-risk disease patients.

Atezolizumab was tested as well in the adjuvant setting (IMvigor010), but the trial did not meet its primary endpoint of improved disease-free survival. The phase III study evaluated adjuvant atezolizumab vs observation after radical cystectomy in patients with muscle-invasive bladder cancer. An analysis from the IMvigor010 trial demonstrated that circulating tumor DNA (ctDNA) positivity post cystectomy in muscle-invasive bladder cancer patients was associated with poor prognosis for both disease-free survival and OS. Those patients that were ctDNA positive after surgery had an 80% likelihood of relapse. Additionally, those that were ctDNA positive but cleared ctDNA with treatment of atezolizumab had improved outcomes compared to those that did not clear ctDNA. Though it was a negative trial, it did identify ctDNA as a clinically significant prognostic marker. It is unclear why these two trials of similar design yielded different results. A third trial, Alliance A031501, is an ongoing phase III study evaluating pembrolizumab vs observation in the adjuvant setting in a similar population to CheckMate 274. In a prespecified interim analysis review, the investigators found that pembrolizumab demonstrated a statistically significant and clinically meaningful improvement in disease-free survival compared with observation following surgery.

Correct Answer: A

Case Study 5

A 60-year-old woman who underwent a radical cystectomy 12 months ago presents with new back pain and fatigue. Laboratory studies reveal a hemoglobin level of 10.5 g/dL and an elevated alkaline phosphatase. Her renal function, hepatic function, and serum calcium are all normal. She is noted on CT scan to have retroperitoneal lymphadenopathy, pulmonary nodules, and vertebral lesions, and the bone lesions have uptake on a bone scan. She recognizes that treatment involves chemotherapy, but she is very concerned about toxicity because of multiple side effects that her sister experienced when treated for breast cancer.

6) You recommend which of the following regimens?
    A) MVAC (methotrexate, vinblastine, adriamycin, and cisplatin).
    B) Gemcitabine and cisplatin.
    C) Gemcitabine and carboplatin.
    D) Gemcitabine, cisplatin, and bevacizumab.

Expert Perspective: MVAC (methotrexate, vinblastine, adriamycin, and cisplatin) has long been a standard first-line regimen for patients with metastatic urothelial carcinoma. Two randomized phase III studies established MVAC as the standard first-line regimen. The first was a US Intergroup study randomizing 269 patients with advanced urothelial carcinoma to either single-agent cisplatin or to MVAC. Response rates (39% vs 12%), progression-free survival (10.0 months vs 4.3 months), and overall survival (12.5 months vs 8.2 months; $P = 0.0002$) favored combination chemotherapy significantly. The second study randomized 110 patients with metastatic transitional cell carcinoma either to a regimen consisting of cisplatin, cyclophosphamide, and doxorubicin or to MVAC. A significantly higher response rate (65% vs 46%; $P < 0.05$) and median survival (48.3 weeks vs 36.1 weeks) were observed with MVAC versus cisplatin, cyclophosphamide, and doxorubicin.

In hopes of improving outcomes, a high-dose intensity MVAC regimen given in two-week cycles with growth factor support was compared to standard MVAC given in four-week cycles. In the initial report by EORTC, the overall response rate (63% vs 50%), complete response rate (21% vs 9%), and progression-free survival (9.1 months vs 8.2 months) favored the high-dose arm significantly. The primary endpoint of the study, median OS, was not significantly different, with a median survival of 15.5 months in the high-dose arm and 14.1 months in the standard-dose arm. A subsequent report with a median follow-up of over seven years revealed similar median survival outcomes, but high dose intensity MVAC produced a borderline statistically significant relative reduction in the risk of progression and death compared to MVAC. While this regimen is reasonable to use to increase the likelihood of a response, perhaps in a symptomatic patient, its significant non-hematologic toxicity and lack of a clinically significant improvement in survival may limit the use to more physically robust patients.

Toxicity is a serious consideration with MVAC as the typical bladder cancer patient is elderly or has multiple comorbidities, making them less resilient to aggressive treatment. Myelosuppression, neutropenic fever, sepsis, mucositis, and nausea and vomiting are all common, and patients in some MVAC trials were routinely hospitalized due to toxicity. Furthermore, toxicity-related deaths of advanced patients are reproducibly reported; typically, less than 5% but up to 9% have been observed.

A phase III study randomized 405 patients with advanced urothelial carcinoma to either gemcitabine and cisplatin or MVAC, both administered over 28-day cycles. The overall response rate (49% for gemcitabine and cisplatin vs 46% for MVAC), time to progression (7.4 months for both gemcitabine and cisplatin and MVAC), and median survival (13.8 months for gemcitabine and cisplatin vs 14.8 months for MVAC) were similar between the two arms. However, the toxicity profile favored gemcitabine and cisplatin in terms of rates of grade 3 or 4 neutropenia, neutropenic sepsis, and grade 3 or 4 mucositis. This study was not powered to determine equivalency between the two regimens, but an updated analysis of long-term follow-up continued to show similar outcomes between the two arms. The OS at five years was 13% with GC and 15% with MVAC, a difference that was not statistically significant. Based on these results demonstrating similar efficacy between the two regimens but a superior toxicity profile with gemcitabine and cisplatin, many consider gemcitabine and cisplatin to be the standard first-line regimen for patients with advanced urothelial carcinoma of the bladder.

Limited studies have compared cisplatin and carboplatin. A phase II study randomizing patients to gemcitabine with either cisplatin or carboplatin demonstrated similar overall response rate, time to progression, and survival. However, another small phase II study randomized patients to MVAC or to the triplet methotrexate, carboplatin, and vinblastine (M-CAVI). The two were similar in terms of response rates, but MVAC yielded a superior overall survival of 16 months compared with 9 months in the methotrexate, carboplatin, and vinblastine arm ($P = 0.03$). The lack of adriamycin with methotrexate, carboplatin, and vinblastine and possible underdosing of carboplatin were possible explanations for the difference in survival suggested by the investigators. A phase II comparison of MVEC (methotrexate, vinblastine, epirubicin, and cisplatin) to MVECa (methotrexate, vinblastine, epirubicin, and carboplatin) favored the cisplatin arm significantly in terms of response rates. While an exact comparison of carboplatin and cisplatin cannot be obtained from these data, most prefer cisplatin given the hint of increased activity.

Many patients with advanced bladder cancer are not appropriate for cisplatin-based regimens, often due to advanced age, impaired performance status, or renal insufficiency. A phase III study in Europe (EORTC 30986) randomized patients with impaired renal function, poor performance status, or both to either gemcitabine and carboplatin or to methotrexate, carboplatin, and vinblastine. No differences in overall response rate, progression-free survival, or OS were noted between the two regimens. For patients who are not considered appropriate for cisplatin-based chemotherapy, we typically utilize gemcitabine and carboplatin or single-agent therapy.

Correct Answer: B

Our patient: She is a candidate for cisplatin. Gemcitabine and cisplatin regimen is an acceptable option for front-line standard of care therapy for metastatic bladder cancer. Of note, gemcitabine and cisplatin have similar efficacy and less toxicity compared with MVAC in this particular setting.

Case Study 6

A 74-year-old male with a 50-pack a year smoking history was recently diagnosed with urothelial bladder cancer. CT scans of chest, abdomen and pelvis was notable for numerous liver lesions concerning for metastases. Labs showed normal renal and hepatic function. He completed six cycles of gemcitabine + cisplatin, and repeat CT shows stable disease.

7) What would be considered as appropriate maintenance therapy?
   A) Cisplatin.
   B) Avelumab.
   C) Enfortumab vedotin.
   D) Best supportive care.

Expert Perspective: The patient above has metastatic urothelial cancer with stable disease after first-line combination platinum-based chemotherapy. The phase III trial JAVELIN Bladder 100 trial evaluated the use of avelumab, an anti-PD-L1 antibody, as maintenance therapy. In the trial, patients with either unresectable locally advanced or metastatic urothelial carcinoma were randomized to receive maintenance therapy with avelumab plus best supportive care or best supportive care alone. The primary endpoint was OS, which was significantly longer in the avelumab group than in the control group (one-year survival: 73% vs 58.4%; median OS: 21.4 months vs 14.3 months). The avelumab group also had longer progression-free survival than the control group (median progression-free survival of 3.7 months vs 2 months, respectively). In the PD-L1-positive population, OS was also significantly longer in the avelumab group compared to the control group. This was also the case with the PD-L1-positive patients in the control arm. Adverse events were more common in the avelumab group than the control group with fatigue, pruritus, and urinary tract infections being the most common. In regard to immune-related events, 29.4% (101) of the patients had an event. There was no grade 4 or fatal events (see Chapter 50).

Correct Answer: B

Case Study 7

A 76-year-old male is diagnosed with stage IV unresectable bladder cancer. He has a history of grade 4 chronic kidney disease and ECOG performance status is 2. PD-L1 expression was positive with a CPS ⩾ 10.

8) What therapy do you offer him?
   A) No treatment.
   B) Erdafitinib.
   C) Pembrolizumab plus enfortumab vedotin.
   D) Carboplatin.

Expert Perspective: In patients with advanced/metastatic bladder cancer, first line of therapy should ideally be combination therapy with cisplatin or carboplatin for patients with renal impairment (see Question 6). However, in those patients who are not chemotherapy eligible, PD-1/PD-L1 inhibitor therapy with enfortumab vedotin is option.

- **Pembrolizumab** was approved in the first-line setting based on the KEYNOTE-052 study, which was a phase II trial evaluating first-line pembrolizumab in patients who are cisplatin-ineligible with locally advanced or metastatic urothelial carcinoma. Patients were deemed cisplatin-ineligible if they had one or more of the following: CrCl < 60 mL/min, ECOG performance status of 2, neuropathy grade ⩾ 2, or NYHA class III CHF. Patients received pembrolizumab 200 mg every three weeks for up to 24 months. Results from a five-year follow-up of the study showed an overall response rate of 28.9% for all patients with a median duration of response of 33.4 months and a median OS of 11.3 months. In the group with PD-L1 CPS ⩾ 10, the overall response rate was higher compared to those with PD-L1 CPS < 10 (47.3% vs 20.7%).
- **Enfortumab vedotin with pembrolizumab:** This regimen was granted accelerated FDA approval for patients with locally advanced or metastatic urothelial carcinoma who are ineligible for cisplatin-containing chemotherapy. Efficacy was evaluated in EV-103/KEYNOTE-869 (NCT03288545), a multi-cohort (dose escalation cohort, Cohort A, Cohort K) study. The dose escalation cohort and Cohort A were single-arm cohorts treating patients with enfortumab vedotin-ejfv plus pembrolizumab while patients on Cohort K were randomized to either the combination or to enfortumab vedotin-ejfv alone. Patients had not received prior systemic therapy for locally advanced or metastatic disease and were ineligible for cisplatin-containing chemotherapy. A total of 121 patients received enfortumab vedotin plus pembrolizumab.

The major efficacy outcome measures were objective response rate and duration of response. The confirmed overall response rate in 121 patients was 68% (95% CI: 59, 76), including 12% with complete responses. The median duration of response for the dose escalation cohort + cohort A was 22 months (range: 1+ to 46+) and for Cohort K was not reached (range: 1 to 24+).

The most common adverse reactions (>20%), including laboratory abnormalities, were increased glucose, increased aspartate aminotransferase, rash, decreased hemoglobin, increased creatinine, peripheral neuropathy, decreased lymphocytes, fatigue, increased alanine aminotransferase, decreased sodium, increased lipase, decreased albumin, alopecia, decreased phosphate, decreased weight, diarrhea, pruritus, decreased appetite, nausea, dysgeusia, decreased potassium, decreased neutrophils, urinary tract infection, constipation, potassium increased, calcium increased, peripheral edema, dry eye, dizziness, arthralgia, and dry skin.

The ongoing phase III EV-302 study is evaluating enfortumab vedotin + pembrolizumab with standard-of-care platinum and gemcitabine therapy for patients with previously untreated locally advanced/metastatic bladder cancer regardless of platinum eligibility.

Correct Answer: C

Case Study continued: The patient is started on pembrolizumab plus enfortumab vedotin as he is not a candidate for chemotherapy. Repeat staging scans are consistent with progression. Next-generation sequencing reveals a *FGFR2* mutation.

9) **What therapy do you consider next?**
   A) Gemcitabine.
   B) Enfortumab vedotin.
   C) Erdafitinib.
   D) Atezolizumab.

Expert Perspective: In patients who are platinum-eligible who progress on first-line therapy, PD-1/PD-L1 inhibitor therapy is now considered standard of care second-line therapy. Second-line therapy after progression on pembrolizumab and enfortumab vedotin is less defined. It is essential to test for genetic mutations specifically *fibroblast growth factor receptor (FGFR)* mutational status as well as taking into consideration the adverse effects of therapies and comorbidities.

- **Erdafitinib** is a pan *FGFR* kinase inhibitor that binds to and inhibits *FGFR1, FGFR2, FGFR3,* and *FGFR4* enzyme activity. Erdafitinib also binds to *RET, CSF1R, PDGFRA, PDGFRB, FLT4, KIT,* and *VEGFR2*. Erdafitinib was approved in 2019 based on the results of the phase II BLC2001 trial, which included patients with locally advanced or metastatic urothelial cancer with a *FGFR3* or *FGFR2* alteration who progressed on systemic therapy. The objective response rate was 40% (complete response rate of 3% and partial response rate of 37%) with a median duration of response of 5.5 months and OS of 13.8 months. Most common adverse effects (reported in > 20% of patients) included hyperphosphatemia, stomatitis, dry skin, and fatigue. There is a potential risk of central serous retinopathy, so patients should have a baseline ophthalmology evaluation. In the THOR study, eye disorders other than central serous retinopathy occurred in 42.2% of the patients in the erdafitinib group, with the most frequent being dry eye and conjunctivitis; the percentages of patients with these conditions were similar to those observed in the BLC2001 study. With regards to efficacy the median overall survival was significantly longer with erdafitinib than with chemotherapy (12.1 months vs. 7.8 months; HR for death, 0.64; 95% CI, 0.47 to 0.88; P=0.005). The median PFSl was also longer with erdafitinib than with chemotherapy (5.6 months vs. 2.7 months; hazard ratio for progression or death, 0.58; 95% CI, 0.44 to 0.78; P<0.001).

- **Sacituzumab govitecan**, an antibody-drug conjugate targeting the human trophoblast cell-surface antigen 2 (Trop-2), is another option approved for patients with locally advanced or metastatic urothelial cancer who previously have received platinum therapy and a PD-1/PD-L1 inhibitor. The phase II TROPHY-U-01 trial showed an overall response rate of 27.7% and median duration of response of 7.2 months. This is a reasonable option in the third- or fourth-line setting.

Correct Answer: C

Recommended Readings

Bajorin, D.F., Witjes, J.A., Gschwend, J.E. et al. (2021). Adjuvant Nivolumab versus placebo in muscle-invasive urothelial carcinoma. *N Engl J Med* 384 (22): 2102–2114. doi: 10.1056/NEJMoa2034442.

Bellmunt, J., Hussain, M., Gschwend, J.E. et al. (2021). Adjuvant atezolizumab versus observation in muscle-invasive urothelial carcinoma (IMvigor010): a multicentre, open-label, randomised, phase 3 trial. *Lancet Oncol* 22 (4): 525–537. doi: 10.1016/S1470-2045(21)00004-8.

James, N.D., Hussain, S.A., Hall, E. et al. (2012). Radiotherapy with or without chemotherapy in muscle-invasive bladder cancer. *N Engl J Med* 366 (16): 1477–1488. doi: 10.1056/NEJMoa1106106.

Powles, T., Park, S.H., Voog, E. et al. (2020). Avelumab Maintenance therapy for advanced or metastatic urothelial carcinoma. *N Engl J Med* 383 (13): 1218–1230. doi: 10.1056/NEJMoa2002788.

Powles, T., Rosenberg, J.E., Sonpavde, G.P. et al. (2021). Enfortumab vedotin in previously treated advanced urothelial carcinoma. *N Engl J Med* 384 (12): 1125–1135. doi: 10.1056/NEJMoa2035807.

Yeshchina, O., Badalato, G.M., Wosnitzer, M.S. et al. (2012). Relative efficacy of perioperative gemcitabine and cisplatin versus methotrexate, vinblastine, adriamycin, and cisplatin in the management of locally advanced urothelial carcinoma of the bladder. *Urology* 79 (2): 384–390. doi: 10.1016/j.urology.2011.10.050.

32

Prostate Cancer: Screening, Surveillance, Prognostic Algorithms, and Independent Pathologic Predictive Parameters

Eduardo Benzi and Thomas M. Wheeler

Baylor College of Medicine, Houston, TX

Introduction

Worldwide, there are an estimated 1,400,000 new cases of prostate cancer annually, making it the second most diagnosed cancer in men. Prostate cancer represents 21% of all newly diagnosed cancers in males and 8% of cancer-related deaths. Autopsy series show that nearly 70% of men older than age 80 have occult prostate cancer. Individuals with one first-degree relative diagnosed with prostate cancer have a twofold increased lifetime risk, which increases to fourfold if two or more relatives are affected before age 70. Current estimates suggest that 5–10% of all cases of prostate cancer are hereditary. According to the SEER model (Surveillance, Epidemiology and End Results), the lifelong probability of an American developing an invasive prostate cancer is 11.6% (1 in 9). The incidence of prostate cancer is strongly correlated to the changes in medical practice and PSA monitoring programs. Prostate cancer survival is related to many factors, especially the extent of tumor at the time of diagnosis. Matched for age, Black men have larger tumors as compared with White men. The five-year relative survival among men with cancer localized to the prostate or with regional spread is 100%, compared with 31% among those diagnosed with distant metastases. Prostate cancer mortality rates have declined in the United States between 1992 and 2017, decreasing from 39 to 19 per 100,000 persons. Simulation models suggest that prostate-specific antigen (PSA) screening could account for 45–70% of the decline, mainly by decreasing the incidence of distant-stage disease. Other factors that may explain the decline in mortality rates include advances in treatments for men with localized prostate cancer as well as for those with distant-stage disease. In this chapter we discuss the value of prostate cancer screening programs, prostate cancer prognostic algorithms, and independent pathologic predictive parameters including controversies surrounding these important areas.

Cancer Consult: Expertise in Clinical Practice, Volume 1: Solid Tumors & Supportive Care,
Second Edition. Edited by Syed A. Abutalib, Maurie Markman, Al B. Benson III, and Hope S. Rugo.
© 2024 John Wiley & Sons Ltd. Published 2024 by John Wiley & Sons Ltd.

Case Study 1

A 56-year-old White male with no past medical history presents to his primary care physician for his yearly physical. His exam and laboratory results are all negative except for an elevated prostate serum antigen (PSA) level at 8 ng/mL (normal < 4 ng/mL). Prostate biopsy is scheduled.

1) **In an asymptomatic patient with a normal digital rectal exam, should PSA screening be a standard?**

Expert Perspective: Since the introduction of the PSA test for early detection of prostate cancer in 1987, its use has steadily increased with an estimated 47–58% of all new prostate cancers being screen-detected in the year 2000. This, in turn, has led to an increased incidence with a corresponding decreased proportion of metastatic or locally advanced–stage disease at diagnosis. Interestingly, the declining incidence rate for low-risk disease was temporally associated with decreased prostate cancer screening following the 2012 US Preventive Services Task Force (USPSTF) recommendation against prostate cancer screening.

The primary goal of PSA-based screening is to find men in whom treatment would reduce morbidity and mortality. Although the risk of prostate cancer varies with the PSA level in the serum, the PSA level is not specific to prostate cancer, and most men with an increased PSA do not have cancer. However, in the context of an elevated PSA, a similarly high percent free PSA does lend specificity to a diagnosis of benign prostatic hyperplasia as a cause of increased PSA.

PSA screening has been a persistently controversial topic. The prevalence of clinically insignificant prostate cancer detected by screening, as reported by Draisma et al., is much higher than its incidence in the absence of screening. The possibility of causing harm from overdiagnosis and treatment in patients whose cancer would otherwise have remained latent has many physicians asking if screening is appropriate or even beneficial in some patient populations.

In 2018, the US Preventive Services Task Force (USPSTF) updated its previous recommendations on the use of PSA screening. As mentioned earlier, in 2012, the task force warned against routine PSA screening, citing several studies that found no benefit in overall, or all-cause, mortality; it now recommends screening on an individual basis for men between the ages of 55 and 69 years, based on joint patient and clinician decision. This change, though not quite a reversal, comes as a result of multiple studies showing at least a small reduction in the cancer-related mortality and the long-term risk of metastatic prostate cancer among screened men when compared to their unscreened counterparts. The 2018 USPSTF guidelines still recommend against PSA screening of patients 70 and older based on inadequate evidence of benefit on clinical trials and a low likelihood of benefit given the patient's life expectancy.

In contrast, the American Society of Clinical Oncology (ASCO) recommends testing for asymptomatic men with a life expectancy of 10 years or greater. It emphasizes the findings of the European Randomized Study of Screening for Prostate Cancer (ERSPC) and other studies including the Goteborg trial, which demonstrated a decrease in prostate cancer–related death of 20–44% with the use of screening in men 55–69 years, indicating that in some studies the benefits of screening validate its continued use. These findings were echoed by a recent study that integrated data from both the ERSPC and the Prostate, Lung, Colorectal and Ovarian (PLCO) screening trials, suggesting PSA screening reduced cancer mortality by approximately 30%.

Most recently, the National Comprehensive Cancer Network (NCCN) has released recommendations to begin PSA screening, which include screening for all men starting at 45 years, and for select men as young as 40 years with specific risk factors, namely: (i) Black/African American individuals, (ii) positive family history, and (iii) select germline mutations associated with increased prostate cancer risk (BRCA1, BRCA2, ATM, HOXB13, mismatch repair genes; also refer to Chapters 34, 46, 47). In addition, the NCCN counsels clinicians to discuss increased risk of prostate cancer in patients with history of exposure to Agent Orange, though the exposure itself is not an absolute indication for early screening. These guidelines are based on studies suggesting higher and earlier incidences and mortality of prostate cancer among the selected populations. Testing frequency is also based on risk stratification according to age- and risk factor-specific PSA levels released by the NCCN. Patients aged 45–75 (or 40–75 if risk factors are present) would undergo annual to biennial follow-up if their PSA is between 1 and 3 ng/dL. Patients in this age group with PSA greater than 3 should be evaluated for possible biopsy.

A good medical history is also important in stratifying patient risk for prostate cancer. 5-alpha-reductase inhibitors like finasteride and dutasteride, commonly used in clinical practice, are known to approximately halve the PSA of patients taking them, and clinicians should interpret values accordingly.

The NCCN has also updated its guidance on the use of the digital rectal examination (DRE) for the screening and diagnosis of prostate cancer. According to the NCCN, DRE is not sufficient on its own but can be used as an adjunct baseline test in addition to serum PSA, and though it is most useful in patients with an elevated PSA, it may be performed on all patients. Screening with PSA and DRE is indicated for all patients up to age 75 but should not be performed widely in older men due to the risk of overdiagnosis, particularly in those with a life expectancy of less than 10 years.

PSA screening has been shown consistently in multiple studies across different populations to be associated with lower overall prostate cancer–associated mortality and should therefore be encouraged among both clinicians and patients. The option not to screen must be weighed against the increased incidence of metastatic prostate cancer, the rate of which has risen in the USA following publication of the 2012 USPSTF guidelines recommending against PSA screening.

Ancillary diagnostic testing is also recommended when available. Specifically, multiparametric MRI has emerged as one of the foremost adjuncts to the diagnosis and management of prostate cancer, as it is excellent at characterizing suspicious lesions. These images can be used to identify and stage disease and may serve to guide biopsies. There is still debate whether MRI-characterized lesions should undergo only targeted biopsies, or whether systematic biopsies still offer superior diagnostic yield. This is highlighted by (i) the relatively low sensitivity of MRI (45–78%) for the detection of prostate cancer, and (ii) its tendency to miss small, low-grade tumors with low PSA density, according to at least one study. Perhaps counterintuitively, this latter tendency to miss low-grade carcinomas is considered a distinct advantage by certain experts, as it acts as a hurdle to overtreatment. Interobserver variability among radiologists also plays a role in the performance metrics of multiparametric MRI, with specialist genitourinary radiologists outperforming their generalist counterparts. High-definition scanners and access to high-quality multiparametric MRI biopsy protocols are also key, and patients should be referred to a center with a robust prostate cancer service with experience in the treatment and diagnosis of the disease. Some benefit has been shown from combining risk calculator-derived scores with multiparametric MRI results to decide whether the patient should undergo biopsy, but no consensus has been reached.

MRI-ultrasound image fusion biopsy is a recently developed technique, which, as its name implies, merges stored MRI and real-time ultrasound data to construct a three-dimensional model of the prostate. This model can then be used to guide biopsies to regions of interest or to store systematic biopsy site data, which can be retrieved if a re-biopsy is indicated. Recent reports have shown MRI-US fusion biopsies to have good concordance with final pathology on radical prostatectomy, suggesting it may be a valuable diagnostic modality for prostate cancer.

Both the NCCN and the American Urological Association (AUA) recommend some modality of MRI to help stratify prostate cancer risk, but there are no definitive answers about who and under what diagnostic circumstances would benefit from imaging and imaging-guided biopsy. Any decision to that effect must be made by the clinician and the patient, weighing the benefits and risks of each approach based on their needs and preferences.

Our Patients: The patient underwent a 12-core prostate biopsy, and pathology results are adenocarcinoma, Gleason score 3 + 3 = 6, involving two cores (40% of one and 20% of the second core).

2) Does this patient qualify for active surveillance?

Expert Perspective: Active surveillance is a well-established clinical follow-up method for specific risk strata of prostate cancer. It relies on the principle that less aggressive forms of the disease are less likely to invade and metastasize, thereby causing death. The aim of active surveillance is, ultimately, to treat disease that is likely to progress while affording patients with prostate cancer a longer morbidity-free period, given all current forms of therapy for prostate cancer show relatively high rates of adverse quality-of-life outcomes.

The original active surveillance criteria (Epstein criteria), lists very specific (and restrictive) circumstances that a patient must meet to qualify for active surveillance and define these cases as low risk. They are as follows:

a) Two or fewer cores with cancer and no more than 50% involvement in any one core.
b) PSA density < 0.15%.
c) Gleason score ⩽ 6 (i.e. grade-group 1; absence of Gleason pattern 4 or 5).
d) PSA < 10 ng/mL.
e) Clinical stage T1 (clinically inapparent tumor that is not palpable).

Recently, different reference centers have published their own, less restrictive set of criteria for active surveillance. There has been marked liberalization of the criteria, with most guidelines now allowing for non-interventional follow-up of disease up to T2a (tumor involves one-half of one side or less). The most liberal of these allows for active surveillance in patients with clinical stage as advanced as T2b (tumor involves more than one-half of one side but not both sides), Gleason 3 + 4, and PSA as high as 20 ng/mL in selected cases. Crucially, 15-year cancer-related mortality for this liberal follow-up group did not exceed 1.5%. More restrictive criteria shrink that mortality to no more than 0.5% at 15 years.

In the recent past it was standard practice to use PSA kinetics (i.e. the rate of change in the concentration of PSA), or "PSA velocity," to trigger treatment. While it still sees use as an adjunct surveillance method, it has largely fallen out of favor due to its poor specificity (high rates of false negative) for diagnosis of progression of prostate cancer and thanks to the development of superior diagnostic and follow-up methods. The digital rectal exam has followed a course similar to PSA velocity, as it does not appear to be any better at detecting progression than PSA alone.

Our patient meets these most restrictive criteria and therefore qualifies for active surveillance.

The natural concern associated with active surveillance is increased risk of metastases. While a valid concern, recent data from large retrospective radical prostatectomy studies suggests that lower grade disease, specifically Gleason 3 + 3 (grade group 1), has an essentially zero rate of metastasis and is, therefore, safe for active surveillance. Yearly case-progression risk while on active surveillance has also been widely characterized and is thought to be low, at about 1%. The main risk of active surveillance lies in misattribution of grade due to sampling error, i.e. missing higher-grade disease on the initial biopsy, which is known to occur in 25–30% of systematic biopsies (also refer to Chapter 33).

The patient's PSA level continues to increase over the next several years, and a second prostate biopsy is performed. His pathology report now describes a Gleason pattern 4 in one of two involved cores. The patient undergoes radical prostatectomy.

3) Can the patient's disease-free survival rate be estimated preoperatively?

Expert Perspective: The Kattan preoperative nomogram may be used to determine the patient's disease-free outcome post surgery. Although, in the beginning, radical prostatectomy resulted in nearly 100% occurrence of impotence (and, rarely, incontinence), the advent of "anatomical" radical prostatectomy with sparing of the postero-lateral nerve bundle has been far more successful with less morbidity to the patient. The risk of mortality from surgery is also relatively low (it is currently at < 0.5%), making radical prostatectomy a viable treatment option. Radical prostatectomy is associated with excellent long-term cancer control, with a 40% decrease in the risk of death from prostate cancer in comparison to watchful waiting in some series in a selected subset of patients. Relapse of disease, however, has been reported to be as high as 15–53%. However, the PIVOT trial in the United States failed to show a difference in cancer-specific all-cause mortality in those treated with radical prostatectomy versus observation, although, there was a trend for better outcome in those patients with high-risk disease treated surgically. This high level of variability has led to the advent of nomograms to delineate patient-specific outcomes.

The preoperative Kattan nomogram using preoperative PSA levels, clinical staging, and Gleason scoring from the biopsy specimen are currently used by some clinicians. However, final pathologic staging determined from a radical prostatectomy specimen is far more accurate in recurrence prediction. The Kattan postoperative nomogram, first described by Kattan et al. in 1998, is a postoperative nomogram that relies heavily on the pathologic information from analysis of the radical prostatectomy specimen. It uses several parameters that are well understood to be important prognostic factors to calculate disease-free survival. The independent predictive parameters (preoperative PSA, Gleason score, extraprostatic extension, seminal vesicle invasion, surgical margin, and lymph node status) are each assigned a numerical value according to the nomogram. The sum is then used to predict the likelihood of an 84-month disease-free survival.

The Gleason score of a radical prostatectomy specimen is far more accurate than that of the biopsy due to the significant probability of a higher Gleason–grade cancer being present adjacent to the biopsied tumor. The presence of any Gleason 4 or 5 is an indicator of worse prognosis.

Extraprostatic extension is the extension of tumor into adjacent tissues beyond the prostate capsule, commonly the peri-prostatic adipose tissue. This is not equivalent to positive surgical margins, which means tumor present at the inked margin. Although some institutions report the quantity of capsular invasion, most only report the presence or absence of extraprostatic extension, which is qualified as "focal" for minimal extraprostatic extension and "nonfocal," or "established," for greater amounts of extraprostatic extension. Interestingly, metastasis almost never occurs in prostate cancer without invasion outside the prostatic stroma.

Seminal vesicle involvement by tumor can occur by three pathways. It can occur by tumor expansion along the ejaculatory duct complex and, less commonly, across the base of the prostate. The least common mechanism is by isolated deposits (metastasis) without contiguous tumor. Eggener et al. (2011) argue that seminal vesicle involvement is one of the most important predictors of poor prognosis.

Positive surgical margin is defined as tumor cells at the inked margin. Before processing, the specimen is inked entirely, with different colors used to designate right from left. The apical and bladder base margins are shaved off first and may be submitted in two ways depending on the institution: "en face" or "on edge". If submitted en face, any tumor cells present in the stained section indicate positive surgical margin. Some institutions prefer the "on edge" approach, where the margins are cut into pie-shaped pieces perpendicular to the prostatic urethra. The latter approach allows for better differentiation between near-surgical margins and positive surgical margin. The remainder of the prostate is sliced from apex to base (i.e. superior to inferior) perpendicular to the prostatic urethra to assess surgical margins and extraprostatic extension.

Positive bladder neck margins were historically regarded as T4. However, recent studies have shown microscopic bladder neck invasion tumors to behave more like T3 prostate cancer, and these are now classified as T3a (extraprostatic extension [unilateral or bilateral] or microscopic invasion of bladder neck).

Perineural invasion is present in 75–84% of cases. It is not a reliable indicator of prognosis and is not included in the Kattan nomogram. The assessment of perineural invasion with relevance to prognosis is not approved by the Cancer Committee of the College of American Pathologists. Studies, however, have shown an association with volume of perineural invasion as a predictor of tumor recurrence and progression. Maru et al. (2001) showed an association between the maximum diameter of perineural invasion and adverse pathologic features. A large focus of perineural invasion (≥ 0.25 mm) is also

Introduction

associated with higher rates of progression. More studies will be necessary to validate these findings.

Prostate cancer biomarkers beyond PSA may also have a role in determining the overall disease-free survival pre- and even postoperatively. These tests, available from multiple vendors, employ molecular assays and proprietary calculators to stratify long-term metastasis- and disease-free survival risks based on biopsy or prostatectomy tissue. The NCCN advocates for the use of these tests if they are considered likely to imrpove the specificity of diagnostic screening. There is still debate, however, on their usefulness as adjuncts to MpMRI in the diagnostic evaluation of prostate cancer.

While currently not recommended for routine use by ASCO or the NCCN, molecular biomarker assays can be requested on an individual basis to inform patient and clinician decisions about the risk category of a patient's given cancer. A decision may be made, for example, to assign a patient with Gleason $3 + 4 = 7$ who is hesitant about radical prostatectomy to active surveillance instead, if the molecular profile of his tumor is favorable.

High-intensity focused ultrasound (HIFU) and cryoablation have also emerged as less invasive therapies for prostate cancer versus radical prostatectomy. These treatment modalities use image-guided thermal ablation aimed at lesional tissue and involve less operative risk, more comfortable post-procedural course, and better preservation of noncancerous tissue than both radiation and surgery. While much maligned for its complication rates at inception, cryoablation has been suggested to match disease-free and overall survival with a comparable advantage in biochemical relapse versus external beam radiation. Compared to radical prostatectomy, HIFU has shown significantly lower rates of impairment of both erectile and urinary function in the treatment of primary disease, albeit with a comparatively higher risk of recurrence or persistence—particularly in higher Gleason score cancers and in the setting of limited apical therapy. Primarily as a function of their novelty and limited outcomes data, neither of these treatment modalities are incorporated into AUA, ASCO, or Society for Urologic Oncology (SUO) recommendations for treatment of localized prostate cancer. 2023 NCCN guidelines currently only recommend HIFU or cryosurgery locally in cases of recurrence following radiation therapy in patients without evidence of metastatic disease (NCCN 2023).

Several years after his radical prostatectomy, the patient's nonexistent level of PSA begins to rise from undetectable to 0.1 ng/mL to 0.2 ng/mL to 0.4 ng/mL over an eight-month period. The digital rectal exam is normal postoperatively.

4) Should you proceed to biopsy the prostate bed or give local radiotherapy?

Expert Perspective: Our patient has biochemical recurrence after radical prostatectomy defined as an increase in serum PSA in consecutive measurement. PSA level of ≥ 0.4 ng/mL after successful radical prostatectomy is highly concerning for recurrent disease. According to AUA guidelines, a biochemical recurrence is defined as a serum PSA ≥ 0.2 ng/mL, which is confirmed by a second determination with a PSA ≥ 0.2 ng/mL. Phoenix criteria are used to define biochemical recurrence after external beam radiation therapy. The definition includes a rise of PSA ≥ 2 ng/mL, with a repeat confirmation. It is important to recognize that biochemical recurrence implies absence of detectable disease on a scan. However, in the presence of biochemical recurrence, efforts should include finding metastatic disease. Conventional imaging in biochemical recurrence has historically included CT and NM bone scans; however, these imaging modalities have limited sensitivity at PSA levels < 10–20 ng/mL. Routine staging using PET-CT is not currently recommended due to a paucity of useful data and the considerable expense of the procedure. The value of F-18 fluciclovine and prostate-specific membrane antigen (PSMA) PET-CT scans is discussed in Chapters 33 and 34.

Kundel et al. (2004) determined salvage radiation therapy following RP with biochemical failure to be a safe and effective treatment option. In their study, 66% of patients were disease free and biochemical-failure free at 34.3 months. The therapeutic benefit of salvage radiation therapy, however, is most evident in the presence of a low serum PSA level (< 0.5 ng/mL). HIFU and cryotherapy have also been proposed as radiation alternatives, and the former has been endorsed by the European Society of Medical Oncology, while the latter lacks high-quality data on efficacy and complications.

Other systemic therapies, including chemotherapy, hormonal therapy, and androgen deprivation, may be considered in cases with metastatic disease (Chapter 84).

Our patient is treated with radiotherapy to the prostatic bed, and the PSA becomes undetectable.

Recommended Readings

Autran-Gomez, A.M., Scarpa, R.M., and Chin, J. (2012). High-intensity focused ultrasound and cryotherapy as salvage treatment in local radio-recurrent prostate cancer. *Urol Int* 89 (4): 373–379.

Bekelman, J.E., Rumble, R.B., Chen, R.C., Pisansky, T.M., Finelli, A., Feifer, A. et al. (2018). Clinically localized prostate cancer: ASCO clinical practice guideline endorsement of an American urological Association/American Society for radiation Oncology/Society of urologic oncology guideline. *J Clin Oncol* 36 (32): 3251–3258.

Carlsson, S. Screening and prevention of prostate cancer 2021 (Part 1): evidence for PSA screening May 2021. https://grandroundsinurology.com/screening-and-prevention-of-prostate-cancer-2021-part-1-evidence-for-psa-screening (accessed Jun 2021).

Eggener, S.E., Scott, E., Scardino, P.T. et al. (2011). Predicting 15-year prostate cancer specific mortality after radical prostatectomy. *J Urol* 185: 869–875.

Epstein, J.I., Feng, Z., Trock, B.J. et al. (2012). Upgrading and downgrading of prostate cancer from biopsy to radical prostatectomy: incidence and predictive factors using the modified gleason grading system and factoring in tertiary grades. *Euro Urol* 61: 1019–1024.

Kundel, Y., Pfeffer, R., Lauffer, M., Ramon, J., Catane, R., & Symon, Z. (2004). Salvage prostatic fossa radiation therapy for biochemical failure after radical prostatectomy: the Sheba experience. *The Israel Medical Association journal: IMAJ*, 6(6), 329–331.

Lawrentschuk, N. and Laurence, K. (2011). Active surveillance for low-risk prostate cancer: an update. *Nature* 8: 310–320.

Lilja, H., Ulmert, D., and Vickers, A.J. (2008). Prostate-specific antigen and prostate cancer: prediction, detection and monitoring. *Nature* 8: 268–279.

Maru, N., Ohori, M., Kattan, M.W., Scardino, P.T., Wheeler T.M. (2001). Prognostic significance of the diameter of perineural invasion in radical prostatectomy specimens. *Hum Pathol* 32 (8): 828–833.

Ohori, M., Kattan, M., Scardino, P.T. et al. (2004). Radical prostatectomy for carcinoma of the prostate. *Mod Pathol* 17: 349–359.

Parker, C., Castro, E., Fizazi, K., Heidenreich, A., Ost, P., Procopio, G. et al. (2020). Prostate cancer: ESMO Clinical Practice Guidelines for diagnosis, treatment and follow-up. *Ann Oncol* 31 (9): 1119–1134.

Sklinda, K., Mruk, B., and Walecki, J. (2020). Active surveillance of prostate cancer using multiparametric magnetic resonance imaging: a review of the current role and future perspectives. *Med Sci Monit Int Med J Exp Clin Res* 26: e920252-1.

Tsodikov, A., Gulati, R., Heijnsdijk, E.A., Pinsky, P.F., Moss, S.M., Qiu, S. et al. (2017). Reconciling the effects of screening on prostate cancer mortality in the ERSPC and PLCO trials. *Ann Int Med* 167 (7): 449–455.

33

Early and Locally Advanced Prostate Cancer

James Randall*, Mohammad R. Siddiqui*, Ashley Ross, and Sean Sachdev

Northwestern Memorial Hospital, Chicago, IL
* Contributed equally

Introduction

Prostate cancer is the second most commonly diagnosed malignancy in the United States behind breast cancer with 224,733 new cases diagnosed in 2019, and an estimated 268,490 cases to be diagnosed in 2022 according to the National Cancer Institute's Surveillance, Epidemiology, and End Results Program. Among those diagnoses, approximately 74% of cases will be localized to the prostate or adjacent structures only. Median age at time of diagnosis is 67 years old, with prevalence highest in African Americans at 175.8 cases per 100,000 men per year. Mortality remains low due to improved screening and treatment of the disease; five-year relative survival for localized prostate cancer is now at 100%. However, due to the disease's prevalence it remains the fifth leading cause of cancer-related death. Current areas of focus include improved screening using newer imaging modalities, identification of patients eligible for surveillance, tighter control of recurrent or persistent disease, and extension of treatment options in the metastatic setting.

Multiparametric MRI in Prostate Cancer

1) **What is the role of multiparametric imaging and what does Prostate Imaging Reporting and Data System (PI-RADS) score implies?**

Expert Perspective: The role of magnetic resonance imaging (MRI) in prostate cancer is threefold: providing additional information regarding risk of harboring disease and serving as a tool for lesion localization during biopsy, informing prognosis, and improving nodal staging.

Tiered prostate cancer screening with prostate specific antigen (PSA)-based testing followed by more specific tests and MRI to guide decisions regarding biopsy and biopsy technique is now being implemented. The above strategy allows for detection of localized, clinically significant prostate cancer while limiting unnecessary biopsies. Regardless, many men will be diagnosed with very low-risk or low-risk disease after biopsy and should undergo active surveillance. Advances in MRI technology help produce better and more detailed

Cancer Consult: Expertise in Clinical Practice, Volume 1: Solid Tumors & Supportive Care,
Second Edition. Edited by Syed A. Abutalib, Maurie Markman, Al B. Benson III, and Hope S. Rugo.
© 2024 John Wiley & Sons Ltd. Published 2024 by John Wiley & Sons Ltd.

information regarding disease location and burden and thus help assess risk of progression. Moreover, accurate disease localization has sparked interest in subtotal glandular therapy for prostate cancer, which might spare men from morbidities of whole gland therapy.

Acquisition of multiple MRI sequences during the assessment of prostate cancer, termed "multiparametric imaging," is considered standard of care (Table 33.1). These sequences typically include diffusion weight imaging (DWI) that produces an apparent diffusion coefficient (ADC) map, dynamic intravenous contrast–enhanced (DCE) imaging, and more conventional T2 weighted imaging. Biparametric MRI with DWI and T2 imaging may suffice for some indications such as prostate cancer screening. Together, measurements on these sequences are compiled to produce a Prostate Imaging Reporting and Data System (PI-RADS) score that assesses the likelihood of clinically significant prostate cancer in a prostatic nodule. This system was validated in multiple trials. Information from MRI, such as location relative to the neurovascular bundles, can also guide surgical decision-making that follows diagnosis (Table 33.2).

Table 33.1 Multi-parametric MRI of prostate (mpMRI).

Indications:
- Elevated PSA before initial biopsy
- Continued concern for cancer after negative prostate biopsy
- Prior to repeat biopsy if atypia or high-grade prostatic intraepithelial neoplasia (HGPIN) found on initial biopsy
- Before confirmatory biopsy for those considering active surveillance
- Staging before local intervention (primary or recurrence settings)

Requirements:
- 3 tesla (with or without coil) or 1.5 tesla with coil

Reporting:
- Prostate Imaging Reporting and Data System (PIRADS) V2

High negative predictive value:
- About 90% for PIRADS 1–2
- About 30% of men can avoid biopsy

Superior cancer detection:
- About 12% increase in clinically significant cancer detection

Table 33.2 PI-RADS score system and probability of prostate cancer.

Pi-rads score	Description	Probability of prostate cancer
1	Clinically significant cancer is highly unlikely to be present	2%
2	Clinically significant cancer is unlikely to be present	10%
3	The presence of clinically significant cancer is equivocal	30%
4	Clinically significant cancer is likely to be present	50%
5	Clinically significant cancer is highly likely to be present	80%

Prostatic MRI also serves to provide localization for subsequent biopsy of suspected lesions. Images from the pre-biopsy MRI are used to assist ultrasound-guided biopsy. This is typically done using an ultrasound system that is registered and fused to data from the MRI to accurately target specific portions of the prostate. However, targeted biopsy alone may under-sample the prostate, and thus targeted biopsy is typically done in combination with systematic biopsy.

Prostatic MRI can provide staging information regarding extraprostatic extension as well as invasion of seminal vesicles. MRI of the prostatic fossa can also play a role in detection and localization of recurrent or progressive disease following local management with prostatectomy. This is usually first detected via PSA surveillance and biochemical failure. Information from these studies can then be used to plan salvage radiotherapy. This must be combined with systemic imaging such as bone scan or positron-emission tomography to rule out metastatic disease.

Overall, recent advances in the delivery of MRI as well as the technology behind the scans has allowed for further implementation in the workup and management of prostate cancer. Specifically, magnetic resonance imaging plays a critical role in initial detection of malignancy, localization for biopsy, and staging information in both initial management and recurrent or persistent disease.

Screening

2) Should routine prostate cancer screening be offered to men?

Expert Perspective: Prostate cancer screening was revolutionized in the late 1980s and early 1990s by the implementation of serum testing with prostate specific antigen (PSA). Using PSA as a screening tool significantly improved diagnosis of prostate cancer at an earlier stage. However, PSA-based prostate cancer screening has several limitations. Foremost among these is that it is a nonspecific marker of architectural disruption in the prostate. Without being specific for clinically significant prostate cancer (at least at levels of PSA below 10 ng/mL), reliance on solely elevated PSA to trigger prostate biopsy can lead to the overdiagnosis and often subsequent overtreatment of otherwise benign disease (low risk disease).

The European Randomized Study of Screening of Prostate Cancer (ERSPC) trial was an international, randomized trial studying the effects of PSA-based prostate cancer screening. With a 16-year follow-up, the trial demonstrated a 20% risk reduction in prostate cancer–specific mortality among PSA-screened men with a number needed to invite to screening of 547 and the number needed to diagnose of 18 to prevent a prostate cancer–specific death. The core group of this trial included men ages 55–69 years. Of note, clinically significant prostate cancer is exceedingly rare among men under the age of 40 years. In addition, treatment of PSA screening–detected localized prostate cancer has limited benefit in men with life expectancies of under 10 years.

In the decades following FDA approval of PSA testing, investigators have developed and established testing modalities with greater specificity for clinically significant prostate cancer. As such, elevated PSA levels alone (i.e. those in the range 2.5–10 ng/mL) should seldom lead to immediate prostate biopsy.

Case Study 1

A 56-year-old male initially referred to your clinic to discuss PSA screening decides to get PSA testing, which comes back at 8 ng/mL.

3) The patient is hesitant about pursuing prostate biopsy and asks if there are other tests available to determine his risk of prostate cancer.
   A) Serum- and urine-based tests, which more accurately predict the risk of clinically significant prostate cancer.
   B) Multiparametric MRI (mpMRI) of prostate.
   C) None of the above.

Expert Perspective: Recognizing that PSA is a nonspecific marker of prostate cancer, advanced screening methods have been developed to improve detection of clinically significant (Gleason Grade Group 2–5) prostate cancer. This includes biomarker tests such as prostate health index (PHI), ExoDX Prostate Test, SelectDx, 4Kscore, MyProstate Score test, and imaging with mpMRI of the prostate. Among a PSA-screened population, these tests are most important for their negative predictive value. Use of serum-based tests such as PHI or 4Kscore, urine-based tests such as ExoDx or SelectDx, tests combining urine and serum biomarkers such as MiPS, or imaging tests such as mpMRI can all decrease the rate of biopsy by approximately 30% while missing the diagnosis of less than 5% of potentially clinically significant prostate cancers (the majority of which are of intermediate risk).

Among these screening tests, prostate mpMRI is the only test that allows for determination of a patient's risk of harboring prostate cancer while also localizing potentially significant disease to help guide biopsy. Randomized clinical trials utilizing mpMRI before prostate biopsy and subsequently utilizing the MRI for biopsy targeting have demonstrated non-inferiority and in some cases superiority for the detection of clinically significant prostate cancer while substantially decreasing the number of biopsies performed. They have also reduced the detection of low-grade prostate cancers.

In our practice, we currently employ a tiered approach to prostate cancer screening. For patients such as this, with elevated PSA in the range 2–10 ng/mL, we first order a prostate health index as a cost-effective strategy to eliminate further workup in roughly 30% of men. For most men where prostate health index demonstrates a moderate to high potential risk of prostate cancer, we then offer mpMRI to further risk-stratify and guide management.

Correct Answer: B

Case Study continued: The above patient has a prostate health index that is elevated with a score of 59. He undergoes mpMRI of the prostate, which shows a PIRADS 4 lesion in the left mid-gland peripheral zone. Prostate biopsy is recommended.

4) What are his options?
   A) TRUS-biopsy.
   B) MRI fusion TRUS-biopsy.
   C) Transperineal biopsy.
   D) All of the above.

Expert Perspective: The definitive diagnosis of prostate cancer requires pathologic specimen. This is traditionally done via transrectal ultrasound (TRUS)-guided biopsy of the prostate, which is usually performed in office under regional anesthesia and samples the prostate transrectally. To adequately sample a prostate, systematic biopsy of the gland (particularly the peripheral zone) is performed. In the current MRI era, the diagnostic yield of biopsy is further enhanced by fusing MRI with transrectal US, allowing for specific targeting of MRI-visible lesions.

Risks associated with transrectal biopsy include hematuria, hematospermia, pain, infection, and sepsis. The risk of infection is of significant concern, particularly sepsis for which antimicrobial prophylaxis with a 24-hour dose of either a fluoroquinolone or first-, second-, or third-generation cephalosporin has been recommended. There is now a growing concern about fluoroquinolone and extended beta-lactamase resistant E. coli among men undergoing a prostate biopsy, which can be mitigated by employing a rectal swab culture to identify fluoroquinolone resistant bacteria in the rectum and directing antibiotic therapy.

More recently, the transperineal approach to prostate biopsy has been developed. This approach guides needles through the perineal skin and does not require antibiotic prophylaxis as it has no reported infectious complications. Additionally, it is thought to provide better sampling of the gland, especially of the anterior horn of the prostate, which tends to be under-sampled in TRUS-biopsy. Like TRUS-biopsy, this can also be done under regional anesthesia in office.

Correct Answer: D

Case Study 2

A 53-year-old male was referred to your clinic for continued rising PSA over the past three years in the setting of two prior negative biopsies. His most recent PSA is 9.8 ng/mL.

5) **What is the management for a patient with multiple prior negative biopsies and continued clinical concern for prostate cancer?**

Expert Perspective: Given the patient's rising PSA, he is at high risk for harboring prostate cancer. His workup should include mpMRI, which has been shown to have a high negative predictive value of 80–96% for a clinically significant cancer in patients with prior negative biopsies. If a suspicious lesion is detected, the MRI should be followed with targeted biopsy, which has been shown to have cancer detection rates of 34–56% in men with prior negative biopsies. Per NCCN guidelines, consideration can also be given to several biomarker tests such as %free PSA, prostate health index, 4Kscore, PCA3, and ConfirmDx before repeating a biopsy in assessing the patient's risk of having a clinically significant prostate cancer.

Case Study 3

Low- and Very Low-risk Disease

A 65-year-old Caucasian male with an elevated PSA of 5.7 ng/mL underwent a prostate biopsy revealing one core of Grade Group 1 (3 + 3 = 6) disease in the right mid-prostate and one core of Grade Group 1 in the left base-prostate; both cores are < 50% involved. His prostate cancer was not palpable on physical exam, and his prostate was 50 cc in size.

6) **How do you determine the best treatment plan for a patient with clinically localized prostate cancer when choosing between active surveillance, radical prostatectomy, and radiation therapy?**

Expert Perspective: It can be difficult to define a standardized treatment plan for patients with localized prostate cancer. The decision must take into consideration several factors, including age, life expectancy, comorbidities, logistics, and patient preferences.

Active surveillance should be considered the gold standard for men with very low-risk clinically localized prostate cancer and a preferred option among men with low-risk disease (Table 33.3). This is defined as the observation of disease with intent to treat definitively when necessary. Active surveillance is the preferred standard in very low-risk patients (such as the above example) with Grade Group 1 [Grade 6 (3 + 3)] prostate cancer that involves no more than three cores and no more than 50% of any one core, clinical stage T1c, and PSA density < 0.15 mg/mL/g. Active surveillance involves serial PSA, clinical exams, imaging, and serial biopsies. While the active surveillance protocol varies by institution, the AUA recommends serial PSA testing and digital rectal exam along with confirmatory biopsy within two years of diagnosis and surveillance biopsies thereafter with consideration given to MRI as well.

The rationale for active surveillance in the low-risk population is that it can avoid any intervention for the men who will never symptomatically or objectively progress. Its safety is demonstrated in large active surveillance cohorts from Johns Hopkins and Memorial Sloan Kettering Cancer Center, reporting 0.4–1.5% risk of metastasis at 15 years and 0.1% risk of prostate cancer mortality at 15 years.

Definitive treatment of low-risk disease with either radical prostatectomy or radiation therapy can be considered in some men who may be at higher risk of clinical progression on active surveillance. This includes men with PSA density > 0.15; African American race; extensive Grade Group 1 cancer on systematic biopsy; known pathogenic or likely pathogenic mutations in *BRCA2, 1* or, *ATM*; and/or with a family history of aggressive prostate cancer. The recommendation for early treatment is mainly to reduce the risk of clinical progression. These observations come from two large, randomized trials: the Prostate Cancer Intervention Versus Observation trial (PIVOT) and the more modern Prostate Testing for Cancer Treatment trial (ProtecT). Both trials demonstrated improvement in rates of disease progression with the PIVOT trial showing progression in only 5% of the treatment arm versus 10% of the active surveillance arm, while the ProtecT trial observed progression in 3% of the treatment arm vs 6% of the active surveillance arm.

The benefits in oncological outcomes must be weighed against the side effects and quality of life implications for radical treatment (discussed in greater detail later in the chapter). Patients undergoing treatment often develop erectile dysfunction and can have urinary or bowel (in the case of radiotherapy) morbidity. Hence, the decision to pursue treatment versus active surveillance should be based on informed decision-making.

Table 33.3 NCCN risk stratification for localized prostate cancer.

Risk group	Description	
Very low	PSA < 10 ng/mL and	
	Grade Group 1 (score 6 [3 + 3]) and	
	T1c (tumor identified by needle biopsy found in one or both sides, but not palpable) and	
	fewer than 3 prostate biopsy fragments/cores positive, ≤ 50% cancer in each fragment/core and	
	PSA density < 0.15 ng/mL/g	
Low	Does not qualify for very low risk and	
	PSA < 10 ng/mL and	
	T1 (clinically inapparent tumor that is not palpable) to T2a (tumor involves one-half of one side or less) and	
	Grade Group 1(score 6 [3 + 3])	
Intermediate	Has all of the following	*Favorable Intermediate*
	- No high- or very high-risk features	One intermediate factor and
	- One or more intermediate risk factor: T2b (tumor involves more than one-half of one side but not both sides) to T2c (tumor involves both sides) or Grade Group 2 (score 7 [3 + 4]) or 3 (score 7 [4 + 3]), or PSA 10–20 ng/mL	Grade Group 1 (score 6 [3 + 3]), or 2 (score 7 [3 + 4]) and % of positive biopsy cores < 50%
		Unfavorable Intermediate
		2 or more intermediate factors and/or Grade Group 3 (score 7 [4 + 3]) and/or ≥ 50% of positive biopsy cores
High	No very high-risk features and	
	T3a (extraprostatic extension) or Grade Group 4 (score 8 [4 + 4, 3 + 5] or [5 + 3]) or 5 (score 9 or 10 [4 + 5, 5 + 4, or 5 + 5]) or PSA > 20 ng/mL	
Very high	T3b (tumor invades seminal vesicle[s]) to T4 (tumor is fixed or invades adjacent structures other than seminal vesicles such as external sphincter, rectum, bladder, levator muscles, and/or pelvic wall) or primary Gleason pattern 5 or two or three high-risk features or > 4 cores with Grade Group 4 (score 8 [4 + 4, 3 + 5, or 5 + 3]) or 5 (score 9 or 10 [4 + 5, 5 + 4, or 5 + 5])	

Adapted from: NCCN Clinical Practice Guidelines in Oncology (NCCN Guidelines®): Prostate Cancer.

Case Study 4

Intermediate-risk Disease

A 68-year-old came in for routine history and physical examination and was found to have a concerning digital rectal exam consistent with clinical T2a disease (tumor involving less than one half of one side of the gland). His PSA was 8.9 ng/mL, and subsequent biopsy demonstrated Gleason Grade Group 2 (3 + 4 = 7) prostatic adenocarcinoma on his transrectal biopsy. He is asymptomatic and in relatively good health with an estimated survival of over 10 years.

7) What are his management options?
A) Radical prostatectomy.
B) Radiation therapy.
C) Focal therapy.

Expert Perspective: This patient has clinically localized, favorable intermediate-risk prostate cancer. Treatment of intermediate-risk prostate cancer with radical prostatectomy has shown to be effective in improving overall survival (OS) and cancer-specific survival (CSS). The SPCG-4 trial randomized men to radical prostatectomy versus observation and showed improvement in both OS and CSS for men undergoing radical prostatectomy. The absolute OS favoring radical prostatectomy was 12%, which translated into 2.9 years of life gained at the median follow-up of 23 years.

For men with intermediate-risk disease considering radiotherapy, the addition of short-term androgen deprivation therapy (ADT) improves oncological outcomes. The duration of ADT in these cases is typically four to six months. ADT is often omitted in favorable intermediate-risk cases such as the above example. Since ADT can have morbidity and has not shown absolute risk reduction in hard clinical endpoints in a subset of men with unfavorable intermediate-risk disease, biomarker trials are ongoing, which may facilitate omission of ADT in select group of patients (discussed later in this chapter).

Are there tools to predict oncologic outcomes based on prostate biopsy tissue?

The efforts are ongoing to improve upon risk stratification through biomarkers. Some of these tests include Polaris, OncotypeDx Prostate, and Decipher. These tests are based on RNA expression derived from routinely collected pathologic tissue. Polaris provides a cell cycle progression score, which has been retrospectively validated in predicting oncological outcomes including prostate cancer–specific mortality. OncotypeDx is a 17-gene expression assay covering several oncological pathways that has been validated to predict adverse pathology at prostatectomy. The Decipher test is a genome-wide array that outputs multiple signatures in different stages of validation. The most heavily studied signature is the Decipher genomic classifier, a 22-feature-based score that was initially developed to predict metastasis following prostatectomy but has also been validated for prediction of adverse pathological features, biochemical progression, prostate cancer–specific survival, and overall survival. Due to the breadth of its platform, the Decipher test has been used in retrospective exploratory analyses of randomized controlled trials and more recently in preplanned risk stratification for therapeutic clinical trials. All three tests may aid in clinical decision-making. The decipher genomic classifier can aid in postoperative decision-making regarding use of radiation therapy and intensification with adjuvant ADT, as well.

Case Study 5

A 58-year-old male is diagnosed with cT1c, Gleason Grade Group 2 (3 + 4 = 7), PSA 7 ng/mL prostate adenocarcinoma. The patient is considering treatment but is concerned about his treatment options.

8) When helping this patient decide, he asks about the side effects of each intervention. How does the side effect profile vary between prostatectomy, external beam radiotherapy (EBRT), and brachytherapy?

Expert Perspective: The PROST-QA prospective questionnaire-based study following definitive therapy showed that radical prostatectomy was generally associated with worse sexual function and urinary incontinence, with some recovery observed in nerve-sparing surgeries over time. Those who underwent EBRT showed more irritative and obstructive urinary symptoms as well as increased bowel toxicity. The size of prostate was critical in brachytherapy, as those with larger prostates experienced greater urinary irritation. These findings were largely echoed by the quality-of-life studies under the ProtecT trial and the CEASAR study. Radical prostatectomy and radiation-based therapy were both associated with negative effects on sexual function, while radical prostatectomy also demonstrated effects on urinary continence, and radiation therapy also showed worse bowel function.

9) What minimally invasive treatment options exist for this patient besides the more standard options of radiation or surgery?

Expert Perspective: Focal or subtotal glandular therapy is increasingly being explored as a treatment option for a select group of patients. The premise of therapy is to treat localized prostate cancer while sparing men from sexual and urinary morbidity. Modalities used in subtotal therapy include cryoablation, high-intensity focused ultrasound (HIFU), focal laser ablation, irreversible electroporation, photodynamic therapy, and focal radiation. Though functional outcomes after treatment appear favorable, subtotal or focal therapy is still considered investigational with only short- to intermediate-term follow-up currently available.

10) What are the potential EBRT options for a patient with favorable intermediate-risk prostate cancer?

Expert Perspective: Three main EBRT techniques fall under the umbrella of image-guided radiotherapy (IGRT). The first is three-dimensional conformal RT (3DCRT), which was developed in the 1990s by utilizing computed tomography (CT)-based treatment planning. By incorporating newly acquired three-dimensional anatomic and spatial information, it allowed treatment planning that could more focally concentrate dose on the target while staying off adjacent areas—this served to decrease the risk of toxicity compared to conventional 2D techniques and allowed for dose escalation and improved biochemical control. The second, more advanced, next-generation iteration of three-dimensional planned therapy is intensity-modulated radiotherapy (IMRT). IMRT uses CT-based inverse treatment planning to modulate the intensity of the radiation beam over small surface areas. This allows for steep dose gradients, further reducing dose exposure to adjacent organs at risk. IMRT in some iteration (such as volumetric modulated arc therapy, or VMAT) is currently considered the standard of care. EBRT has historically been delivered in small daily doses in up to 8+ weeks of daily treatment. With technological advancements such as IMRT, it is possible to deliver more dose per day, abbreviating treatment into a shorter hypofractionated course. Several large, randomized studies have shown that it is both safe and effective to abbreviate treatment into a course of 20–28 fractions, with total duration of 4–5.5 weeks. The third technique is stereotactic body radiotherapy (SBRT). SBRT uses very large doses per fraction (also known as "extreme hypofractionation") with the advantage of a higher biologic effective dose and a lower total number of treatments, typically a total of five or less.

All the above technologies are employed with IGRT techniques to verify patient and prostate positioning, such as cone beam CT, live MRI or ultrasound, or fiducials implanted in the prostate prior to treatment initiation. IGRT is considered standard of care. Additionally, other aids for treatment can include a transperineal-placed rectal spacing hydrogel ("SpaceOAR") to allow more distance between the prostate and rectum. The use of this intervention was demonstrated in a company-sponsored study utilizing conventional fractionated radiotherapy; many clinicians prefer to reserve its use for hypofractionated or SBRT treatments. Some centers and patient series have demonstrated excellent outcomes without its utilization. In practice, its use varies quite a bit by center and provider.

Most commonly, photons (produced by a linear accelerator) are used for radiation therapy. However, charged-particle therapy can also be utilized as an alternative to photon-based treatment. Charged-particle therapy refers to mass- and charge-carrying particles (i.e. ions) that give off their energy while traversing tissue—allowing for theoretical preferential lower-dose sparing of certain tissues. While the choice of the particle can include options such as carbon ions, in the United States most commonly protons (i.e. hydrogen atoms stripped of their electrons) are utilized. Recent implementation of more facilities has allowed for their widespread utilization. Some data showing limited benefit matched with their higher cost of implementation has yielded some controversy and limited more routine use. Direct comparison of the two sources is currently under investigation by the COMPPARE trial.

11) Which patients are eligible for definitive brachytherapy?

Expert Perspective: Definitive brachytherapy as monotherapy is considered an acceptable option for patients in low-risk and favorable intermediate-risk disease. The RTOG 0232 trial randomized patients with intermediate risk (not routinely planned to undergo ADT) to either brachytherapy monotherapy or brachytherapy with an external beam boost to the prostate; the trial demonstrated no improvement in freedom from progression from the dual modality approach. The ASCENDE trial showed significant improvement in freedom from progression at five years with the use of a brachytherapy boost (vs EBRT alone), albeit in a study population where the majority of patients had high-risk disease. One major critique of this study is the incorporation of only 12 months of ADT, which for high-risk prostate cancer represents a significantly lower duration than what is considered the standard of care (approximately two years). This limits the conclusion of the study significantly.

The American Brachytherapy Society recommended relative contraindications to brachytherapy including prostate size > 60 mm in width and 50 mm in height, severe urinary irritative or obstructive symptoms, extensive transurethral resection of the prostate defect, substantial median lobe hyperplasia, severe pubic arch interference, gross seminal vesicle involvement, prior pelvic radiation therapy, inflammatory bowel disease, and pathologic involvement of pelvic lymph nodes. Absolute contraindications include distant metastases and life expectancy less than five years.

Case Study 6

A patient with known cT2b, PSA 9.3 ng/mL, and Gleason score 4 + 3 = 7 in 7 out of 12 total biopsy cores wants to undergo external-beam radiation therapy. He presents to your department for further discussion regarding treatment options.

12) Should this unfavorable intermediate-risk patient also undergo ADT?

Expert Perspective: Yes, this should be considered standard of care. D'Amico et al. (2008), demonstrated in a randomized trial from Dana-Farber Cancer Institute that short-term (six months) ADT yielded an overall survival benefit. Similarly, RTOG 9408 demonstrated an overall survival benefit with ADT in patients with intermediate-risk disease but no benefit in low-risk disease. A now validated subdivision of patients further classifying those with intermediate-risk disease into either with or without only favorable features reveals that the former approximates outcomes of low-risk prostate cancer—allowing omission of ADT. Taken together, it is reasonable to omit ADT with favorable intermediate-risk disease and recommend concurrent and adjuvant ADT with radiation therapy of duration four to six months in the setting of unfavorable intermediate-risk disease.

Case Study 7

A 62-year-old was diagnosed with T1c disease, a Gleason score of 3 + 4 = 7, PSA 8.9 ng/mL prostate adenocarcinoma. He underwent radical prostatectomy, and his final pathology was Gleason 4 + 3 = 7 in less than 50% of cores. The patient had focal extracapsular extension on the left side (pT3a) with negative surgical margins and lymph node–negative disease (0 of 16). His PSA at three months postop was undetectable.

13) Which pathologic or clinical features are indications for adjuvant radiotherapy?

Expert Perspective: Postoperative radiation therapy may broadly occur in one of two manners: in the adjuvant (i.e. based on pathologic features) or salvage (clinical or biochemical evidence of disease observed following radical prostatectomy) setting. Pathologic risk factors for which adjuvant radiation therapy might be considered include extracapsular extension, seminal vesicle invasion, and/or positive margins. As discussed later, contemporary clinical trial data seem to suggest that initial biochemical monitoring even in the setting of adverse features may be an acceptable strategy.

14) In the setting of the above risk factors, should he undergo adjuvant radiation therapy or wait for biochemical progression and proceed with early salvage radiation therapy?

Expert Perspective: While both are options to the patient (and should be discussed), contemporary data seem to suggest that close monitoring may be a viable option in the setting of an undetectable PSA. If men with high-risk features may not experience recurrent disease, they may be spared the side effects and risks of adjuvant radiotherapy that they may have never needed.

Three trials form the backbone of discussion regarding adjuvant radiation: SWOG 8794, EORTC 22911, and ARO 9602. These compared adjuvant radiotherapy versus observation in patients with high-risk pathologic features. A recent update of the EORTC 22911 trial (the largest of the three) with a median of 10 years follow-up continued to show improved biochemical progression-free survival for adjuvant radiotherapy; however, there was no difference in clinical progression-free survival, metastasis-free survival, or OS compared with observation. The long-term update of the SWOG 8794 (the second largest) trial showed an improvement in biochemical progression-free survival with adjuvant radiation over observation. However, while it also showed an improved metastasis-free survival and OS, this trial is often criticized for having a liberal approach to study enrollment and treatment, e.g. an undetectable PSA was not required before being randomized to adjuvant treatment or observation. ARO 9602, the smallest trial of the three, mandated an undetectable PSA before randomization—this trial found an improvement in biochemical progression-free survival but no benefit in more important clinical endpoints.

More recently, data from the RADICALS and RAVES trials comparing adjuvant radiation therapy versus early salvage radiation therapy have been published. These trials compared adjuvant radiation to close biochemical monitoring serving as a trigger for radiation therapy. In the RADICALS trial, after a median follow-up of 4.9 years, there was no significant difference in biochemical progression-free survival or freedom from hormonal therapy between the two arms. However, adjuvant radiation therapy increased the risk of urinary morbidity. The RAVES trial was closed prematurely due to low event rate. While not meeting statistical significance for non-inferiority, early salvage radiation therapy was shown to have a similar biochemical control to adjuvant radiation therapy. Like the RADICALS trial, the RAVES trial showed that salvage radiation therapy could avoid the increased (and potentially unnecessary) morbidity associated with adjuvant radiation therapy.

The above patient is lost to follow-up and returns two years later with a PSA of 1.2 ng/mL. Bone scan shows no evidence of distant metastatic disease, but MRI pelvis shows some concern for locally recurrent disease.

15) How is treatment failure defined after radiation therapy versus radical prostatectomy?

Expert Perspective: Following prostatectomy, biochemical failure has historically been defined as PSA ⩾ 0.2 ng/mL on a confirmatory check; trials such as RADICALS and RAVES emphasized a trend (e.g. three consecutive rising values) as opposed to an absolute value. Many clinicians have adopted a similar approach. In the setting of radiation therapy, because noncancerous prostatic tissue is retained, the PSA does not generally become undetectable after radiation therapy. Instead, a failure is defined as a PSA rise ⩾ 2 ng/mL above the nadir. This is often termed the "Phoenix" definition of failure, named after the consensus, reached in the city bearing its name.

16) When is the correct time to start androgen deprivation therapy (ADT)?

Expert Perspective: Use and timing of ADT should be determined after establishing a purpose of the treatment. In the case of a loco-regional recurrence (clinical or biochemical) after prostatectomy, ADT is often combined with radiation therapy for a finite duration of up to 6 to 24 months. For metastatic disease, ADT use is likely to be prolonged and could be combined with other agents such as abiraterone and enzalutamide (among other possibilities) or chemotherapy. For concern of local disease recurrence after definitive radiation therapy, first a biopsy is typically undertaken to confirm recurrent disease, and then salvage local therapy options should be considered. If ADT is being considered for a local recurrence that will not be treated with local therapy, ADT use is often determined by the patient's comorbidities, preferences, and other important metrics such as PSA kinetics and doubling time.

17) What newer imaging technology can be used to identify recurrence in the prostatic bed and systemically?

Expert Perspective: Routine imaging such as CT of the abdomen and pelvis, mpMRI of the prostatic fossa, or technetium bone scan may reveal sites of locally recurrent disease. However, these studies often are negative when PSAs are low after therapy and can yield equivocal results.

Determining if a recurrence is localized or systemic is critical, as local salvage options can often be curative but may have marginal to no effect in metastatic disease. Moreover, in low volume metastatic disease, metastasis-directed therapy (i.e. with stereotactic radiation) may improve oncological outcomes. Newer functional imaging modalities have been developed that allow for more accurate localization of disease. These include PET imaging utilizing 18F-fluciclovine or small molecules recognizing prostate-specific membrane antigen (PSMA). 18F-fluciclovine, commonly termed "PET Axumin" when used in PET, is a leucine amino acid analog radiolabeled with fluorine that can be used for positron-emission tomography and is preferentially taken up by prostate cancer cells. 18F-DCFPyL and other small molecules, commonly termed "PET PSMA" when used in PET, bind to PSMA, which is over-expressed in prostate cancer cell membranes. PET imaging in prostate cancer allows for detection of disease even when PSA levels are low. For example, in the postsurgical biochemically recurrent population with PSAs < 0.5 ng/mL, PET imaging with Axumin or PSMA detects disease in roughly 30% and 40%, respectively, of men imaged (Chapter 34).

Case Study 8

High-risk Disease

A 63-year-old male presents with an initial PSA screening showing an elevated PSA of 8.0 ng/mL. He was, therefore, referred to a urologist for a prostate biopsy. His PSA three months later was 13.0 ng/mL. The patient had a normal rectal exam. A biopsy at the time showed Gleason score 4 + 5 = 9 disease in 4 of 12 cores. He had an mpMRI of the prostate that showed a high-suspicion lesion with extracapsular extension.

18) How would you stage this patient?

Expert Perspective: Formal staging of prostate cancer is typically based on the American Joint Committee on Cancer (AJCC) staging manual, currently in its 8th edition. Primary tumor ("T") staging is based on extension of the disease; organ-confined disease is considered T2 or less in both clinical and pathologic staging. Based on palpability alone, this patient's stage would be consistent with clinical T1 disease; however, the MRI is concerning for T3a disease. His AJCC Group Stage would be IIIC.

A practical risk stratification system is typically utilized in the setting of non-metastatic cases. These are defined by the NCCN with patients falling in one of five categories: very low-, low-, intermediate-, high-, and very high-risk disease. The intermediate category is further divided into either favorable or unfavorable disease (Table 33.3). Patients are stratified based on anatomic extent of tumor, Gleason score, and PSA levels. Therapeutic recommendations are then largely guided by the risk strata. In the case of the above patient, he would fall into the very high-risk stratification due to T3a disease in combination with Gleason Grade Group 5 (Gleason score 9) disease.

19) What preoperative imaging studies would be needed for accurate staging of this high-risk patient?

Expert Perspective: The patient has already received mpMRI of the prostate. However, given his very high-risk disease, the patient should also undergo abdominal and pelvic imaging. Additionally, this very high-risk patient should undergo bone imaging typically in the form of a technetium-99 bone scan or sodium fluoride scan. Imaging of prostate cancer is a rapidly evolving arena; the use of novel PET radiotracer-based imaging for staging (as opposed to more conventional imaging) is actively under investigation, with some preliminary data showing promise for the approach.

20) Now that this patient is considered to have clinical T3a (extraprostatic extension) disease, what are his treatment options?

Expert Perspective: Observation is not a recommended option for high-risk prostate cancer unless the patient has a limited life expectancy of less than 5 years. The two treatment options for this patient include radical prostatectomy and radiation with prolonged ADT.

Radical prostatectomy may be an option for some patients with high- or very high-risk prostate cancer. Most notably, radical prostatectomy allows for more accurate pathologic staging, local cancer control, and relief of local symptoms if present. From an oncologic outcomes standpoint, patients with high- or very high-risk disease undergoing radical prostatectomy alone are more likely to have worse biochemical recurrence–free survival, metastasis-free survival, and cancer-specific survival. These outcomes are even worse in men with very high-risk disease. Hence, high-risk patients, particularly very high-risk patients, often require multimodal therapy with the use of adjuvant radiation.

Patients receiving radiation for high-risk disease are also typically recommended to be treated with long-term androgen deprivation therapy. One option is definitive EBRT to the prostate and lymph nodes with long-term ADT of two years duration. Validating conclusions from earlier trials (when lower radiation therapy doses were typically used), long-term ADT was confirmed to play a vital role alongside radiation therapy per the more modern DART 01/05 GICOR trial, which randomized mostly high-risk patients to either short-term ADT of goserelin for four months or long-term ADT of goserelin for 28 months, with both arms receiving modern dose-escalated EBRT of 76–82 Gy. Long-term ADT yielded significantly increased OS at five years of follow-up of 95% compared to short-term ADT of 86% ($P = 0.009$). An additional option includes the use of a brachytherapy boost following definitive EBRT with concurrent and adjuvant long-term ADT. This allows for additional delivery of radiation to the prostate in a conformal manner and was shown to prolong biochemical progression-free survival in the ASCENDE-RT trial when compared to full-course EBRT. However, the use of low-dose-rate brachytherapy was associated with higher rates of genitourinary toxicity, and the conclusions of the trial are limited by incorporating a less than standard duration of ADT (only 12 months) for a majority high-risk study population. Finally, if the patient were to undergo radical prostatectomy for high-risk pathologic features or nodal involvement, this could necessitate postoperative radiation therapy. Some argue that this may be a reason to consider radiation therapy up front (i.e. to avoid the morbidity of two local treatments), but this is controversial.

21) **The patient elects for surgery to treat his prostate cancer. Should he undergo bilateral pelvic lymphadenectomy?**

Expert Perspective: The American Urology Association (AUA) recommends bilateral pelvic lymphadenectomy for patients with unfavorable intermediate- or high-risk disease. On the other hand, the NCCN recommends bilateral pelvic lymphadenectomy for MSKCC nomogram predicted risk of ≥ 2% of pelvic lymph node involvement. This is a validated nomogram that uses pretreatment PSA, clinical stage, and Gleason sum to predict the risk of pelvic lymph node metastases.

The bilateral pelvic lymphadenectomy can be performed in a limited (external iliac nodes) or extended fashion. The NCCN argues for extended bilateral pelvic lymphadenectomy, which involves dissection of nodal tissues from an area bounded by the external iliac vein anteriorly, the pelvic side wall laterally, the bladder wall medially, the floor of the pelvis posteriorly, Cooper's ligaments distally, and the internal iliac artery proximally. The staging benefits of extended bilateral pelvic lymphadenectomy are well documented, but its therapeutic benefits remain controversial. Unlike in other malignancies, randomized controlled trials suggest that extended bilateral pelvic lymphadenectomy may not provide oncological benefit over more limited dissections. At this stage, larger studies with longer follow-up are needed to firmly establish any therapeutic benefits of extended bilateral pelvic lymphadenectomy.

Case Study 9

A 60-year-old male comes to your clinic after being diagnosed with cT3aN0M0 prostatic adenocarcinoma on MRI, Gleason 4 + 5 = 9 adenocarcinoma on biopsy involving 5 of 12 cores, with PSA 21 ng/mL on initial measurement. He expresses desire to forego surgical intervention and wants to discuss treatment with radiotherapy. During discussion, he asks about the role of hormonal therapy.

22) **Is there any advantage to undergoing radiation therapy in addition to ADT?**

Expert Perspective: The standard of care for patients with locally advanced, high-risk prostate cancer with no evidence of distant metastases is radiation therapy with long-term (28–36 months) ADT based on multiple randomized trials showing an overall survival advantage to radiation therapy with ADT over radiation therapy alone. The overall survival benefit of radiation therapy with ADT over ADT alone was demonstrated in the SPCG-7 trial, where after a median follow-up of 7.6 years, 79 men in the ADT alone group versus 37 men in the ADT plus radiation therapy group had died of prostate cancer. Cumulative 10-year prostate cancer–specific mortality was 23.9% for ADT alone versus 11.9% for ADT plus radiation therapy (95% CI 4.9–19.1%), for a relative risk of 0.44 (0.30–0.66).

23) What is the appropriate duration of ADT with radiotherapy in patients with locally advanced, high-risk prostate cancer?

Expert Perspective: The cumulative data from many trials overwhelmingly support the use of prolonged ADT in this setting. The largest trial to date, RTOG 9202, randomized 1,554 patients with T2c–T4 prostate cancer with no extrapelvic lymph node involvement and PSA less than 150 ng/mL to receive four months of goserelin and flutamide and EBRT to the prostate/nodes with either no additional ADT or 24 months of additional goserelin. The long-term ADT arm showed significant improvement in disease-free survival, cancer-specific survival, time to biochemical failure, time to distant metastases, and time to local progression, but it failed to show a difference in OS. However, in a subset of patients with Gleason 8–10 prostate cancer, long-term ADT had significantly better OS. EORTC 22961 randomized patients who had received EBRT and six months of ADT to no further treatment or 2.5 years of further ADT. Unlike the RTOG 9202 trial, EORTC 22961 showed an OS benefit with a five-year overall mortality of 15.2% in the long-term group versus 19.0% in the short-term group. These findings were corroborated in the DART 01/05 trial utilizing modern, dose-escalated EBRT. This trial included intermediate- and high-risk patients but showed improved disease-free survival, metastasis-free survival, and OS in the entire cohort with use of long-term ADT (goserelin for 28 months) over short-term ADT (goserelin for four months). Again, a more pronounced OS benefit was observed in the high-risk patients with long-term ADT yielding a hazard ratio 3.43 (95% CI 1.26–9.32; $P = 0.015$). For a patient with locally advanced prostate cancer (Gleason score 8 to 10) who are opting for EBRT, long-term concomitant, continuous ADT is recommended.

Case Study 10

A 65-year-old male comes to your clinic after screening PSA of 8.5 ng/mL with subsequent transrectal biopsy showing Gleason 4 + 4 = 8 prostatic adenocarcinoma in 5/12 cores. After being diagnosed with high-risk disease, he underwent a CT of the abdomen and pelvis as well as a bone scan. While the bone scan showed no observable lesions, the CT revealed multiple enlarged internal iliac nodes up to 1.3 cm in diameter that are clinically suspicious for metastatic disease.

24) What treatments should be offered with clinically node-positive prostate cancer?

Expert Perspective: ADT and pelvic radiation therapy should be considered. A subset of the RTOG 85–31 trial (examining locally advanced prostate cancer patients) of clinically positive lymph nodes randomized to radiation therapy + ADT or radiation therapy alone demonstrated a 10-year absolute survival rate improvement in the radiation therapy + ADT arm: 49% versus 39% ($P = 0.002$). Local failure, distant metastasis, and disease-specific mortality were all improved. Conversely, several large patient series looking at outcomes of patients treated with ADT for prostate cancer with node involvement demonstrate benefit from the addition of radiation therapy to ADT.

Case Study 11

Low Volume Metastatic Prostate Cancer

A 75-year-old male presents with new onset lower back pain. He has a significant history of prostatic adenocarcinoma diagnosed at T1c after presenting PSA of 7.8 ng/mL, Gleason 4 + 3 = 7 in 4/12 cores. He underwent radical prostatectomy seven years ago that revealed no adverse features at the time, with postoperative PSA initially undetectable. He was lost to follow-up until recently, at which point his PSA was elevated at 2.5 ng/mL. Bone scan reveals a single lesion in the lumbar spine that is consistent in location with a sclerotic lesion observed at L4 vertebral body on dedicated MRI of the lumbar spine.

25) What is the standard definition of oligometastatic disease?

Expert Perspective: Oligometastatic disease refers to a theoretical state between localized and widespread metastatic disease, a limited volume of metastasis that could be amenable to aggressive local therapy typically not utilized for metastatic disease. Several trials such as ORIOLE and STOMP have examined the role of local therapy for treatment of oligometastatic prostate cancer (as below) finding benefits in outcomes such as clinical progression and freedom from initiation of ADT. More recently, the SABR COMET phase II randomized trial included 99 patients who were distributed in 2:1 fashion to either standard of care or ablative SBRT to sites of oligometastatic disease. In this trial, oligometastatic disease was defined as a maximum of three metastases in any single organ or no more than five sites of metastases in total. This trial showed an overall survival benefit for those receiving SBRT over standard of care, with five-year rates of OS measuring 42.3% versus 17.7%, respectively ($P = 0.006$). However, this trial contained not only prostate cancer patients but also those with metastatic disease from other primary cancers.

26) What is the role of SBRT in management of oligometastatic prostate cancer, specifically?

Expert Perspective: Definitive treatment of oligometastatic disease can be performed by surgical excision or by ablation using high doses of radiotherapy via SBRT. This was investigated in the STOMP trial, a phase II randomized trial of either surveillance or metastasis-directed therapy in a total of 62 patients. Patients in the intervention arm underwent either metastectomy or SBRT, with the large majority receiving SBRT. The primary endpoint was time from enrollment to initiation of ADT with symptomatic progression or objective progression of disease. Median ADT-free survival was improved in the intervention arm when compared to surveillance, with 13 months in the surveillance group and 21 months in the intervention group (HR 0.60; $P = 0.11$).

Similar results were found in the ORIOLE study, a phase II randomized trial of 54 men with recurrent hormone-sensitive prostate cancer and one to three metastatic lesions. These patients were randomized to observation or SBRT directed to sites of recurrent or oligometastatic disease. Their primary endpoint was progression-free survival at six months, with progression defined as increased PSA, objective progression of disease on imaging, initiation of ADT, or death. Overall, they found reduced rates of progression of

19% and 61% (*P* = 0.005) at six months in the intervention arm when compared to observation, respectively.

Taken together, results of these phase II trials show signal of benefit in treatment of prostate cancer when in the oligometastatic state. This benefit may be in the form of freedom from ADT or freedom from objective progression. Higher-level data and further validation with phase III trials are planned and awaited. When relating these data to our patient, it is certainly an option for the patient to undergo metastasis-directed therapy to his site of disease in the lumbar spine with SBRT. However, the risks and benefits of this must be thoroughly discussed with the patient before moving forward.

Case Study 12

High-volume Metastatic Prostate Cancer

A 68-year-old male has a significant history of prostatic adenocarcinoma diagnosed at T1c after presenting with a PSA of 11ng/mL. His TRUS biopsy showed Gleason Grade Group of 4 in 7 of 12 cores. His metastatic workup with CT abdomen and pelvis and bone scan were negative for metastatic cancer. He subsequently underwent a successful radical prostatectomy with the final pathology of pT3a without positive nodes but had a small positive apical margin. At six months postoperative follow-up, the PSA was undetectable. Patient was subsequently lost to follow-up but returns four years later with a new onset back pain. A repeat PSA is obtained which is 15 ng/mL. A CT of abdomen and pelvis is also obtained, which shows multiple metastatic lesions in the pelvic bone, right 8th rib, and in thoracic and lumbar spines. These were then confirmed on the bone scan as well. Patient is subsequently started on ADT with two weeks of bicalutamide.

27) What is his least appropriate treatment option?
   A) ADT.
   B) ADT+docetaxel.
   C) ADT+androgen recetpor signaling inhibitor (ARSI) (i.e. apalutamide, enzalutamide, abiraterone).
   D) ADT+decetaxel+ARSI (i.e. abiraterone, darolutamide).

Expert Perspective: The backbone of treatment of metastatic hormone-sensitive prostate cancer remains ADT. This can be achieved with surgical castration (bilateral simple orchiectomy), LHRH agonists (leuprolide, goserelin), or LHRH antagonists (degarelix, relugolix), with chemical castration being the most common. These agents are generally given intramuscularly except for relugolix, which is administered orally. Additionally, both AUA and NCCN guidelines recommend intensification of therapy by combining ADT with either androgen pathway-directed therapy (abiraterone acetate plus prednisone, apalutamide, enzalutamide) or chemotherapy (docetaxel) for optimal oncologic outcome.

Although there is no universally accepted definition of high-volume disease, the current standard is adopted from the CHAARTED trial. This includes presence of visceral metastases and/or four or more bony metastasis with at least one metastatic lesion outside of the vertebral column and pelvis. This distinction was deemed important by the CHAARTED trial as it showed that chemo-hormonal therapy with docetaxel and ADT significantly improved OS to 51.2 months versus 34.4 months for ADT only for men with high-volume disease, with no survival benefit noted in low volume–disease patients. The survival benefits of up-front chemo-hormonal therapy were further confirmed by the STAMPEDE trial, but it did not detect any differences in treatment effect based on the metastatic burden. Of note, patient populations of CHAARTED and STAMPEDE differed in composition. The STAMPEDE trial primarily consisted of patients having metastatic disease at their initial presentation rather than progressing to this state following local therapy.

Additionally, multiple, large, randomized controlled trials have shown significant improvement in OS and progression-free survival with antiandrogen intensification by combining ADT with androgen pathway-directed therapy. The combination of abiraterone and prednisone with ADT has been evaluated in two clinical trials—LATITUDE and STAMPEDE (arm G). The LATITUDE showed OS benefit of 53.3 months in the combination arm versus 36.5 months in the ADT arm. The STAMPEDE similarly noted a 37% relative improvement in survival at the median follow-up of 40 months. Apalutamide, which is a nonsteroidal antiandrogen, was evaluated in the TITAN trial, which showed that the combination of apalutamide and ADT reduced the risk of death by 35% at the median follow-up of 44 months. It additionally showed a delay in progression-free survival and progression to castration resistance. The ENZAMENT trial evaluating the combination of ADT with enzalutamide, another nonsteroidal antiandrogen, also showed similar survival benefits at the median follow-up of 34 months.

More recently, combining androgen deprivation, chemotherapy and androgen-receptor signaling inhibitors has shown significant improvement in overall survival and delay in progression to castrate-resistant disease. These effects are most substantial in men with high volume metastatic disease. The ARASENS trial combined Darolutamide with androgen deprivation with docetaxel. It randomized men to Darolutamide with androgen deprivation with docetaxel vs. placebo with androgen deprivation and docetaxel. At a median follow-up of 43.7 months in Darolutamide vs. 42.4 months in placebo group, it showed a significant improvement in overall survival (HR 0.68) and a significant delay in progression to castrate-resistant prostate cancer (HR 0.36). Similarly, PEACE-1 is a multi-arm trial involving men with denovo mHSPC that compared men receiving Abiraterone with ADT and docetaxel vs. ADT and docetaxel alone. The combination of Abiraterone with ADT/docetaxel improved the progression free survival from 2.03 years to 4.46 years (HR 0.50) and overall survival from 4.43 years to 'not reached' at the time of data cut-off. When these patients were further stratified by disease volume as defined in CHAARTED trial, the combination treatment improved the overall survival in men with high-volume disease from 3.47 years to 5.14 years.

Our Patient: The patient is initiated on ADT and docetaxel and experiences a decrease in PSA to 9.8 ng/mL with relief of back pain at his next follow-up. He remained stable with decreasing PSA until approximately one year following initiation of ADT with docetaxel, at which time he began experiencing worsening right-sided chest wall pain consistent with known metastasis. Imaging shows objective enlargement of the above lesions without evidence of visceral disease, and PSA has risen to 12.5 ng/mL. He initiates a novel hormonal therapy of abiraterone with prednisone but experiences no improvement in symptoms or objective findings.

Correct Answer: A

28) What radiotherapeutic options can be considered in this patient with high-volume castrate-resistant metastatic prostate cancer?

Expert Perspective: The most widely used radiopharmaceutical is Radium-223, trade named Xofigo. It is administered once a month for up to six months via intravenous injection. It is ideal in patients without visceral metastases. The radium isotope is preferentially taken up in bone due to its chemical similarity to calcium and acts on skeletal metastases via emission of alpha particles. This radiation has a low radius of activity and produces a very localized effect. Its efficacy was demonstrated by the phase III randomized, controlled ALSYMPCA trial in which 921 men with castrate-resistant prostate cancer who had failed or refused docetaxel were randomized to radium-223 or placebo. The trial was terminated early due to its benefits, as it showed significantly improved overall survival at interim analysis in the intervention arm, with median value of 14.0 months versus 11.2 months (HR 0.70; 95% CI 0.055–0.88; $P = 0.002$). These benefits were confirmed on long-term analysis, leading to FDA approval.

With the use of PSMA PET imaging (discussed in earlier sections), there exists the possibility of utilizing the ligand for therapeutic intervention. Lutetium-177 PSMA-617 utilizes a similar molecule to bind the PSMA on prostate cancer cells while employing beta particles for treatment. Use of this radioligand requires prior imaging with PSMA PET to ensure appropriate binding of the ligand. However, the therapeutic molecule can also be used for imaging due to release of gamma rays during the decay. This can allow for tracking of response with treatment. The efficacy of Lu-177 PSMA was investigated in the phase III randomized, controlled VISION trial. Patients with metastatic, castrate-resistant prostate cancer who had failed ADT and one taxane-based chemotherapy were randomly assigned to Lu-177 PSMA or standard care alone. After a median follow-up of 20.9 months, an OS benefit was observed in the intervention arm versus the standard of care with 15.3 months versus 11.3 months, respectively (HR 0.62; $P < 0.001$). There was also benefit favoring Lu-177 PSMA regarding imaging-based progression-free survival. This came at the cost of increased grade 3 or higher adverse events in the intervention arm, at 52.7% versus 38.0%, respectively.

Recommended Readings

Calais, J., Ceci, F., Eiber, M., Hope, T.A., Hofman, M.S., Rischpler, C. et al. (2019). 18F-fluciclovine PET-CT and 68Ga-PSMA-11 PET-CT in patients with early biochemical recurrence after prostatectomy: a prospective, single-centre, single-arm, comparative imaging trial. *Lancet Oncol* 20 (9): 1286–1294. https://doi.org/10.1016/S1470-2045(19)30415-2.

Chi, K.N., Agarwal, N., Bjartell, A., Chung, B.H., Pereira de Santana Gomes, A.J., Given, R. et al. (2019). Apalutamide for metastatic, castration-sensitive prostate cancer. *N Engl J Med* 381 (1): 13–24. https://doi.org/10.1056/NEJMoa1903307.

Davis, I.D., Martin, A.J., Stockler, M.R., Begbie, S., Chi, K.N., Chowdhury, S. et al. (2019). Enzalutamide with standard first-line therapy in metastatic prostate cancer. *N Engl J Med* 381 (2): 121–131. https://doi.org/10.1056/NEJMoa1903835.

Hofman, M.S., Lawrentschuk, N., Francis, R.J., Tang, C., Vela, I., Thomas, P. et al. (2020). Prostate-specific membrane antigen PET-CT in patients with high-risk prostate cancer before curative-intent surgery or radiotherapy (proPSMA): a prospective, randomised, multicentre study. *Lancet (London, England)* 395 (10231): 1208–1216. https://doi.org/10.1016/S0140-6736(20)30314-7.

Hamdy, F.C., Donovan, J.L., Lane, J.A. et al. (2023 April 27). ProtecT study group. Fifteen-year outcomes after monitoring, surgery, or radiotherapy for prostate cancer. *N Engl J Med* 388 (17): 1547–1558. https://doi.org/10.1056/NEJMoa2214122. Epub 2023 Mar 11. PMID: 36912538.

James, N.D., de Bono, J.S., Spears, M.R., Clarke, N.W., Mason, M.D., Dearnaley, D.P., et al. (2017). Abiraterone for prostate cancer not previously treated with hormone therapy. *N Engl J Med* 377 (4): 338–351. https://doi.org/10.1056/NEJMoa1702900.

Kasivisvanathan, V., Rannikko, A.S., Borghi, M., Panebianco, V., Mynderse, L.A., Vaarala, M.H. et al. (2018). MRI-targeted or standard biopsy for prostate-cancer diagnosis. *N Engl J Med* 378 (19): 1767–1777. https://doi.org/10.1056/NEJMoa1801993.

Ma, T.M., Sun, Y., Malone, S., Roach, M. 3rd et al. (2023 February 1). Meta-analysis of randomized trials in cancer of the prostate (MARCAP) consortium investigators. Sequencing of Androgen-deprivation therapy of short duration with radiotherapy for nonmetastatic prostate cancer (SANDSTORM): a pooled analysis of 12 randomized trials. *J Clin Oncol* 41 (4): 881–892. https://doi.org/10.1200/JCO.22.00970. Epub 2022 Oct 21. PMID: 36269935; PMCID: PMC9902004.

Phillips, R., Shi, W.Y., Deek, M., Radwan, N., Lim, S.J., Antonarakis, E.S. et al. (2020). Outcomes of observation vs stereotactic ablative radiation for oligometastatic prostate cancer: the ORIOLE phase 2 randomized clinical trial. *JAMA Oncol* 6 (5): 650–659. https://doi.org/10.1001/jamaoncol.2020.0147.

Sachdev, S., Carroll, P., Sandler, H., Nguyen, P.L., Wafford, E., Auffenberg, G. et al. (2020). Assessment of postprostatectomy radiotherapy as adjuvant or salvage therapy in patients with prostate cancer: a systematic review. *JAMA Oncol* 6 (11): 1793–1800. https://doi.org/10.1001/jamaoncol.2020.2832.

34

Metastatic Prostate Cancer

Priyanka Chablani, Natalie Reizine, and Walter Stadler

University of Chicago, Chicago, IL

Introduction

According to the SEER database, in 2022, there will be an estimated 268,490 new cases of prostate cancer (14% of all new cancer cases) and an estimated 34,500 deaths. Seventy-four percent of patients present with localized, 13% with regional, and 7% with distant disease (6% unknown/unstaged). The five-year relative cancer-specific survival is 100% for localized or regional disease but only 30.6% for distant disease. Death rates are higher in African American men with advanced prostate cancer, men with advanced-stage cancer compared to early stage of the disease, and older men, i.e. 75–84 years of age. Extent of disease can be categorized as biochemically recurrent following definitive local therapy, locally advanced, oligometastatic (generally fewer than four or five metastatic sites), or metastatic (low volume versus high volume). Given the availability of more sensitive PET-based imaging, there is an increasing need to define the optimal imaging modalities to use to assess the extent of metastatic disease. Therapy is also driven by whether the patient has normal testosterone levels, referred to as castrate-sensitive, or eugonadal, disease, or whether cancer progression is occurring in the castrate state (testosterone < 50 ng/dL), referred to as castrate-resistant disease. In the past decade, many new therapies have been added to the armamentarium for recurrent or metastatic prostate cancer. There is also an emerging role for metastasis-directed therapy in oligometastatic disease. Additionally, adjunct therapies such as calcium/vitamin D and bone-strengthening agents play an important role in reducing morbidity. Please refer to Figure 34.1 for an overview of the treatment options discussed in this chapter. Localized prostate cancer is discussed in Chapter 33, and hereditary cancer syndromes in Chapters 45–47.

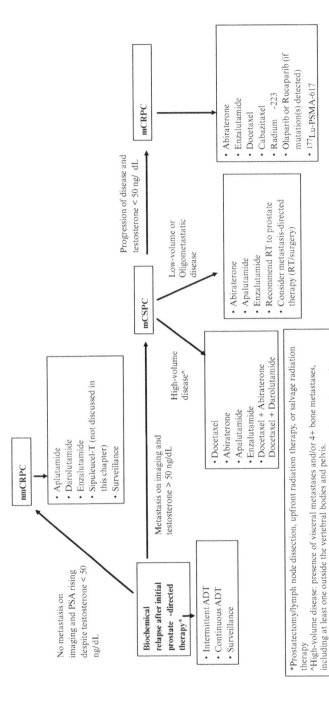

Figure 34.1 Overview of treatment options for biochemically recurrent and metastatic prostate cancer.

Case Study 1

A 72-year-old man with clinical T1c (tumor is found during a needle biopsy that was performed because of an elevated PSA level) Gleason score 3 + 4 adenocarcinoma was treated with definitive external beam radiation three years ago, with PSA nadir of 0.3 ng/mL. Over the last few years, his PSA has slowly risen and is currently at a level of 4 ng/mL. Conventional imaging with computed tomography (CT) and nuclear medicine bone scan is negative for recurrent or metastatic disease.

1) What is the role of PET-based imaging in this case?

Expert Perspective: Following definitive prostate-directed therapy, the first sign of recurrent disease is typically an asymptomatic rising PSA. Biochemical recurrence after radical prostatectomy is defined as PSA ⩾0.2 ng/mL confirmed on serial measurements, and after definitive radiation treatment (brachytherapy or external beam radiation) as a rise of 2 ng/mL or more above the nadir PSA. Conventional imaging in biochemical recurrence has historically included CT and NM bone scans; however, these imaging modalities have limited sensitivity at PSA levels <10–20 ng/mL.

- F-18 fluciclovine positron-emission tomography (PET)-CT, also known as Axumin PET-CT, is an FDA approved imaging modality utilized to evaluate men with biochemical recurrence. It has a sensitivity and specificity of 91% and 40%, respectively, although this is dependent on PSA levels (rarely positive if PSA <1 ng/mL).

- Prostate-specific membrane antigen (PSMA) PET-CT has demonstrated even greater sensitivity and can detect disease at PSA levels as low as 0.5 ng/mL using one of two FDA approved radiotracers (^{68}Ga-PSMA-11 or ^{18}F-DCFPyl). These radiotracers are approved for men with suspected prostate cancer recurrence, but insurance and supply chain issues may limit access.

In this case, detection of oligometastatic disease by PET imaging could support the use of focal radiotherapy to the metastatic sites in an effort to delay further systemic therapy. In biochemical recurrence after prostatectomy, the lack of distant PET-positive lesions would help support salvage radiotherapy to the prostate bed in addition to short or long-course androgen deprivation therapy (6 or 24 months) depending on risk factors present at prostatectomy.

Case Study 2

A 65-year-old male underwent radical prostatectomy for clinical T2b (confined to more than one half of one lobe of gland but not both), Gleason score 4 + 4 prostate adenocarcinoma two years ago. PSA postoperatively was detectable; thus, he received salvage radiation therapy to the prostate bed. Unfortunately, his PSA has risen to 5 ng/mL on the most recent follow-up, with a doubling time of about six months. Testosterone level is normal. PSMA-PET ordered for evaluation of biochemical recurrence does not detect recurrent or metastatic disease.

2) What is the best management strategy?

Expert Perspective: The definition of biochemical recurrence after radical prostatectomy is serum PSA ⩾0.2 ng/mL, which is confirmed by a second determination with a

PSA ≥0.2 ng/mL. This person has biochemical recurrence with a PSA of 5 ng/mL, with a rapid doubling time of less than one year and no radiologically detectable disease. The history of prior salvage radiation therapy to prostate bed generally precludes additional local therapy. Importantly, the the definition of biochemical recurrence is different after definitive external beam radiation therapy—a PSA rise of ≥2 ng/mL from the nadir PSA. The ideal timing for initiating systemic therapy for biochemical recurrence is debated, as many men will not develop overt metastatic disease for years. In the presence of advanced age, decreased life expectancy, or significant comorbidities, active surveillance may be a reasonable option. Clinical features suggestive of more aggressive pathology or disseminated disease include Gleason score of 8–10 or rapid PSA doubling time (defined as <10–12 months). Systemic therapy would be recommended given this patient's young age, high-risk disease, and rapid PSA doubling time.

Androgen deprivation therapy (ADT) monotherapy is the mainstay of treatment for castrate-sensitive biochemical recurrence. However, ADT can result in significant side effects affecting quality of life, including fatigue, cognitive changes, osteoporosis, decreased muscle mass, hot flashes, erectile dysfunction, and increased cardiovascular risk. To minimize these long-term treatment-related effects, intermittent ADT has been proposed. Intermittent androgen deprivation program consists of cyclic administration of ADT (induction treatment followed by temporary withdrawal) with close monitoring of PSA and testosterone levels, with ADT reinitiation once PSA begins to rise. A landmark non-inferiority trial evaluated intermittent ADT with resumption of treatment at PSA > 10ng/mL vs continuous ADT trial in patients who had received definitive radiotherapy (primary or salvage) with biochemical recurrence and no distant metastasis on conventional imaging (Crook et al. 2012). Median OS was 8.8 years in the intermittent ADT arm vs 9.1 years in the continuous ADT arm (no difference, HR 1.02), demonstrating that intermittent ADT was non-inferior to continuous ADT in patients with biochemical recurrence. Intermittent ADT provided benefits with respect to decreased hot flashes, sexual function, and urinary symptoms. As such, intermittent ADT is a reasonable treatment option for biochemically recurrent disease. Of note, in a similar study investigating intermittent ADT vs continuous ADT in patients with metastatic castrate-sensitive prostate cancer, using intermittent ADT did not meet the non-inferiority threshold (Hussain et al. 2013) and thus should not be utilized in men with overt metastatic disease on imaging. The increasing utilization and demonstrated value of combination hormonal therapy in patients with high risk and metastatic castration-sensitive disease further limits the applicability of intermittent androgen ablation (see below).

Case Study 3

A 65-year-old male underwent radical prostatectomy for clinical T2b (tumor has spread to more than one-half of one side of the prostate but not to both sides), Gleason score 4 + 4 prostate adenocarcinoma eight years ago. PSA postoperatively was detectable; thus, he received salvage radiation therapy to prostate bed with six months of concurrent ADT. Unfortunately, his PSA has now risen to 2 ng/mL with a doubling time of about 18 months on the most recent check. Testosterone level is normal. PSMA-PET demonstrates an isolated osseous lesion in the lateral right 9th rib consistent with metastatic disease.

3) What is the best management strategy?

Expert Perspective: In contrast to Case 2, which presented a patient with rapid recurrence, short PSA doubling time, and PSMA–PET-negative disease, this patient presents with a delayed recurrence of prostate cancer, a long PSA doubling time, and a single metastatic focus seen on PET-CT. With the advent of next-generation molecular imaging techniques, an increasing number of patients with biochemical recurrence will likely be diagnosed with oligometastatic (or isolated) disease, such as in this case. Options for these patients include (i) androgen ablation alone, (ii) androgen ablation plus potent androgen receptor signaling inhibitor, (iii) metastases-directed therapy only, or (iv) metastasis-directed therapy plus either hormonal therapy approach. We recommend engaging in a multidisciplinary discussion for such cases. Numerous ongoing studies will help define optimal therapy, but in this case, focal high-intensity radiotherapy alone to delay toxicity from hormonal therapy is reasonable.

4) What are the options for treating a patient presenting with high-volume metastatic prostate cancer with no prior therapy (eugonadal or castration sensitive)?

Expert Perspective: High-volume metastatic disease in prostate cancer is defined as the presence of visceral metastases and/or at least four bone lesions with at least one lesion outside of the vertebral column and/or pelvis. Treatment options for these men include (i) ADT (medical or surgical orchiectomy) combined with second-generation androgen receptor signaling inhibitor alone—abiraterone, enzalutamide, or apalutamide, or (ii) ADT combined with a second-generation androgen receptor signaling inhibitor and docetaxel (Table 34.1).

Two large randomized trials demonstrated the benefit of abiraterone in patients with metastatic castrate-sensitive prostate cancer—STAMPEDE (James et al. 2017) and LATITUDE (Fizazi et al. 2019). In both of these trials, patients were randomized to ADT plus abiraterone/steroid (prednisolone or prednisone) vs ADT alone. Both of these trials showed significantly improved OS in the abiraterone plus ADT arms vs ADT alone. Given that early studies of abiraterone showed increased absorption with food, a phase II study investigated abiraterone at standard dosing (1,000 mg daily) vs 250 mg with a low-fat meal in patients with castrate-resistant prostate cancer (Szmulewitz et al. 2018). The study demonstrated non-inferiority of the lower dose with regard to PSA response and rmacodynamic biomarkers, and as such, abiraterone 250 mg with a low-fat meal is now included as an option in NCCN Guidelines.

The androgen receptor signaling inhibitors enzalutamide, apalutamide, and darolutamide were approved to treat metastatic castrate-sensitive prostate cancer after they were shown to have superior clinical outcomes compared to control arms in the ENZAMET and ARCHES trials (enzalutamide), TITAN trial (apalutamide), the ARASENS trial (Table 34.1). Given the results the recent ARASENS trial (Smith et al, 2022) showing improved OS in patients who received ADT + docetaxel + darolutamide vs. ADT + docetaxel alone, ADT + docetaxel alone is no longer considered an appropriate standard in patients with high volume metastatic castration-sensitive disease despite the findings of the earlier CHAARTED, STAMPEDE, and GETUG AFU 15 trials of ADT alone with or without docetaxel. The PEACE-1 trial (Fizazi et al, 2022) also showed an OS benefit in patients who received ADT + docetaxel + abiraterone). Of note, the value of triplet therapy with androgen ablation, an androgen receptor signaling inhibitor and docetaxel compared to ADT + androgen receptor signaling inhibitor alone in high risk/

Table 34.1 Key phase III trials in metastatic castrate-sensitive prostate cancer.

Trial	N	Experimental Arm	Control	Primary Endpoint
CHAARTED Kyriakopoulos et al. (2018)	790	Docetaxel + ADT	ADT	OS: 57.6 vs 47.2, HR 0.72 (long-term OS results)
STAMPEDE James et al. (2017)	1,917	Abiraterone/ prednisolone + ADT	ADT	OS at 40 months: 184 vs 262 deaths, HR 0.63. Failure-free survival at 40 months: 248 vs 535 events, HR 0.29
LATITUDE Fizazi et al. (2017)	1,199	Abiraterone/ prednisone + ADT	ADT	Radiologic PFS: 33 vs 14.8 months, HR 0.47. OS: not reached vs 34.7 months, HR 0.62
ENZAMET Davis et al. (2019)	1,125	Enzalutamide + ADT	Bicalutamide, nilutamide, or flutamide	OS at 34 months: 102 vs 143 deaths, HR 0.67
ARCHES Armstrong et al. (2019)	1,150	Enzaluatmide + ADT	ADT	Radiologic PFS: not reached vs 19 months, HR 0.39
TITAN Chi et al. (2019)	1,052	Apalutamide + ADT	ADT	Radiologic PFS at 24 months: 68.2% vs 47.5%, HR 0.48. OS at 24 months: 82.4% vs 73.5%, HR 0.67
ARASENS Smith et al. (2022)	1306	Darolutamide + Docetaxel + ADT	Docetaxel + ADT	OS: not estimable vs. 48.9 months (HR 0.68)

high volume patients is still being debated due to the lack of phase III data comparing these two approaches. When selecting between abiraterone, enzalutamide, darolutamide, and apalutamide, clinicians should consider the agent's side effect profile.

- Abiraterone/prednisone can cause hypertension, hyperglycemia, hypokalemia, and edema, and may not be the best choice in patients with poorly controlled hypertension or diabetes. Enzalutamide, darolutamide and apalutamide are more commonly associated with fatigue, cognitive changes, and joint/muscle aches. Darolutamide has less brain penetration, and may have fewer cognitive effects, but comparative trials are pending. In addition, enzalutamide and apalutamide are contraindicated in those with a history of seizures.

5) **What are the treatment options for a patient presenting with low-volume metastatic prostate cancer who has not received prior therapy (eugonadal or castration-sensitive setting)?**

Expert Perspective: For patients with low-volume metastatic castrate-sensitive prostate cancer, we recommend ADT combined with abiraterone, enzalutamide, or apalutamide based on the results of the studies described in the previous explanation (Table 34.1). We do not recommend ADT plus docetaxel or triplet therapy due to decreased benefit and worse toxicity observed in patients with low-volume metastatic disease in the CHAARTED trial. Radiation therapy to the prostate is generally recommended in patients with newly diagnosed prostate cancer and low-volume metastatic disease. This is based on results of an arm on the STAMPEDE trial that randomized patients with newly diagnosed metastatic prostate cancer to standard of care vs standard of care plus radiation therapy to the prostate. While the results did not show an OS benefit for the overall group that received radiation therapy, there was a three-year OS benefit in the subgroup of men with low metastatic burden (81% vs 73%; HR 0.68) (Parker et al. 2018). Additionally, radiation therapy to the prostate improved three-year failure-free survival for the overall group recieving radiation therapy (32% vs 23%; HR 0.76). Several phase II randomized clinical trials have evaluated the benefit of metastases-directed therapy in men with oligometastatic prostate cancer (STOMP Trial, Ost et al. 2018; ORIOLE Trial, Phillips et al. 2020). These trials did not specifically investigate OS; however, they demonstrated significantly improved ADT-free survival and progression-free survival with metastasis-directed therapy, which may have a positive impact on the quality of life of patients and supports consideration of metastasis-directed therapy (see also Case 1 above).

6) **What are the treatment options for a patient presenting with non-metastatic castrate-resistant prostate cancer who has received prior ADT?**

Expert Perspective: Non-metastatic castrate-resistant prostate cancer is the state referred to when a patient has a rising PSA despite castrate levels of testosterone (<50 ng/mL) and there is no evidence of metastasis on imaging. Treatment options for patients in this situation include enzalutamide, apalutamide, and darolutamide, all of which resulted in significant improvement in metastasis-free survival compared to placebo in randomized phase III trials of patients with nonmetastatic castrate-resistant prostate cancer. In each of these studies, patients were enrolled if they had no lesions detectable on conventional imaging (CT/MRI and bone scan), and a PSA doubling time of ≤10 months. In the enzalutamide trial, patients also needed to have a PSA ≥2 ng/mL. Later analyses demonstrated an OS benefit of all three agents. When discussing these options with patients, the benefit of improving metastasis-free survival and OS should be weighed against the side effects of these therapies and drug-drug interactions.

Abiraterone is not formally approved for patients with nonmetastatic castrate-resistant prostate cancer, although it can be offered if patients are unable to tolerate or have a contraindication to the other androgen receptor signaling inhibitor.

7) **If a patient with metastatic castrate-resistant prostate cancer has progressed on ADT plus first-line androgen receptor signaling inhibitor (abiraterone, enzalutamide, or apalutamide), is there any benefit to using a different androgen-receptor signaling inhibitor as subsequent sequential therapy?**

Expert Perspective: There is limited data regarding the benefit of sequencing androgen-receptor signaling inhibitors. In one study, patients with newly diagnosed metastatic castrate-resistant prostate cancer were randomized to abiraterone until progression followed by crossover to enzalutamide (group A) vs enzalutamide followed by abiraterone (group B) (Khalaf et al. 2019). The time to second PSA progression was a median of 19.3 months in group A vs 15.2 months in group B (HR 0.66; $P = 0.036$). PSA responses after second-line therapy were seen in 36% of patients given enzalutamide and 4% given abiraterone ($P < 0.0001$). Although this data suggests that abiraterone should be given first and then enzalutamide, in clinical practice, responses to second-line androgen receptor signaling inhibitor after progression on first-line androgen receptor signaling inhibitor are short-lived and of unknown long-term benefit. However, second-line androgen receptor signaling inhibitor may be favored over docetaxel or cabazitaxel in elderly or frail patients who cannot tolerate chemotherapy.

In the CARD trial, 255 men who had received docetaxel and abiraterone or enzalutamide were randomized to cabazitaxel vs the other androgen receptor signaling inhibitor (Wit et al. 2019). All men must have had progression on an androgen receptor signaling inhibitor within 12 months. Third-line cabazitaxel was found to be superior to androgen receptor signaling inhibitor with regard to the outcomes of imaging-based progression or death (74% vs 80%; HR 0.54), median OS (13.6 months vs 11 months; HR 0.64), and other endpoints. Thus, if eligible for chemotherapy, this regimen should be prioritized in appropriate patients (Table 34.2).

One biomarker proposed to assist with selecting anti-androgen therapies is AR-V7, a splice variant resulting in a truncated androgen receptor, leading to constitutive activation. In the PROPHECY study, the presence of AR-V7 was examined with circulating tumor cell assays in 118 patients with metastatic castrate-resistant prostate cancer initiating abiraterone or enzalutamide (Armstrong et al. 2019). AR-V7 was associated with fewer confirmed PSA responses (0–11%) or soft tissue responses (0–6%) and shorter progression-free survival and OS. As reproducible testing methods for AR-V7 are not yet commercially available, we do not routinely test for AR-V7 to help guide therapeutic decisions in clinical practice.

Case Study 4

A 75-year-old male with Gleason 4 + 5 prostate cancer and PSA of 70 ng/mL presents with newly diagnosed metastatic disease in his bilateral pelvis, sacrum, sternum, bilateral ribs, and skull base. He is started on ADT + abiraterone. A baseline DEXA scan shows no evidence of osteopenia or osteoporosis. His teeth are intact, with no evidence of dental issues.

8) **What is the best treatment for bone health in this patient?**
   A) Denosumab 60 mg SQ every six months.
   B) Denosumab 120 mg SQ every month.
   C) Zoledronic acid 5 mg IV every year.
   D) Zoledronic acid 4 mg IV every month.
   E) Calcium and vitamin D supplement and weight-bearing exercise.

Expert Perspective: According to the National Osteoporosis Foundation guidelines, men on ADT should receive calcium 1000–1200 mg daily from food and supplements and vitamin D_3 400–1000 IU daily. We generally obtain DEXA scans at the start of ADT to obtain a baseline and identify osteopenia or osteoporosis, followed by every two years thereafter. There are currently no guidelines on how often to monitor vitamin D levels, but they can be assessed simultaneously when obtaining a DEXA scan, and vitamin D levels should be repleted to normal levels as appropriate.

Table 34.2 Key phase III trials in metastatic castrate-resistant prostate cancer.

Trial	N	Experimental Arm	Control	Primary Endpoint
COU-AA-301 de Bono et al. (2011)	1,195	Abiraterone/ Prednisone	Placebo/ Prednisone	OS: 14.8 vs 10.9 months, HR 0.65
AFFIRM Scher et al. (2012)	1,199	Enzalutamide	Placebo	OS: 18.4 vs 13.6 months, HR 0.63
TROPIC de Bono et al. (2010)	755	Cabazitaxel	Mitoxantrone	OS: 15.1 vs 12.7 months, HR 0.70
ALSYMPCA Parker et al. (2013)	921	Radium-223	Best standard of care	OS: 14.9 vs 11.3 months, HR 0.70
PROfound de Bono et al. (2020)	Cohort A: 245 (*BRCA1/2* or *ATM*) Cohort B: 142	Olaparib	Abiraterone or enzalutamide	Radiologic PFS in Cohort A: 7.4 vs 3.6 months, HR 0.34
VISION Sartor et al. (2021)	831	^{177}Lu-PSMA-617	Standard of care	Radiologic PFS: 8.7 vs 3.4 months, HR 0.40 OS: 15.3 vs 11.3 months, HR 0.62

There are two classes of osteoclast inhibitors used in prostate cancer: bisphosphonates and denosumab. Denosumab is a fully human monoclonal antibody that binds to the RANK ligand, disrupting the interaction between the RANK ligand and the RANK receptor on osteoclast precursors and osteoclasts. These medications result in decreased bone resorption and increased bone density. There are two indications for using bone-strengthening agents, i.e. denosumab and bisphosphonates in patients with prostate cancer: (i) for the treatment of osteopenia or osteoporosis and (ii) for the prevention of skeletal-related events in patients with bone metastasis and castrate-resistant prostate cancer. The term "skeletal-related event" refers to the complications secondary to bone metastases—pain, fracture, spinal cord compression, or need for radiation therapy or surgery. There is no indication for bone strengthening agents to decrease skeletal-related event in patients with bone metastasis and castrate-sensitive prostate cancer. In fact, a trial demonstrated that zoledronic acid did not affect the time to first skeletal-related event or OS in patients with castrate-sensitive prostate cancer and bone metastasis (Smith et al. 2014).

9) When are bone strengthening agents indicated in advanced prostate cancer?

Expert Perspective: Treatment options for patients with prostate cancer and osteopenia/ osteoporosis include denosumab (60 mg subcutenous every six months), zoledronic acid (5 mg intravenous annually), or alendronate (70 mg oral/week). All of these agents carry a risk for osteonecrosis of the jaw, with the risk being increased for patients with tooth extractions, poor dental hygiene, or dental appliances. Patients should have a dental evaluation if there is any concern for dental issues before being started on osteoclast inhibitors. There is also a risk for kidney injury with zoledronic acid, so creatinine should be checked before each dose. Denosumab does not require monitoring of creatinine; however, the risk of severe hypocalcemia increases with CrCL <60 mL/min. Both zoledronic acid and denosumab are not recommended for patients with CrCl <30 mL/min. In men with castrate-resistant prostate cancer and bone metastases, the dose of zoledronic acid to prevent skeletal-related events is 4 mg intravenous every 3–4 weeks; however, there is data to support dosing every 12 weeks instead. When initiating zoledronic acid or when used in conjunction with radium-223, it is recommended to use the 4 mg intravenous every four weeks dose. The dose of denosumab to prevent skeletal-related events in men with castrate-resistant prostate cancer and bone metastases is 120 mg every four weeks. Denosumab has been shown to be more effective than zoledronic acid in preventing skeletal-related events in patients with bone metastasis and castrate-resistant prostate cancer. In a phase III trial, 1,904 men with castrate-resistant prostate cancer and at least one bone metastasis were randomized to denosumab (120 mg) or zoledronic acid (4 mg) every four weeks (Fizazi et al. 2011). The time to first on-study skeletal-related event was significantly prolonged with denosumab compared to zoledronic acid (median 20.7 months vs 17.1 months; HR 0.82; 95% CI 0.71–0.95). However, there was no significant difference between the two groups in OS (19.4 months vs 19.8 months; HR 10.3) or time to disease progression (8.4 months in both regimens; HR 1.06). Hypocalcemia was more frequent with denosumab (13% vs 6%). Given the much higher cost of denosumab, zoledronic acid is an appropriate alternative for patients/centers where cost is a concern. All patients on osteoclast inhibitors should take calcium and vitamin D to prevent secondary hyperparathyroidism and hypocalcemia. The optimal duration to continue monthly therapy with an osteoclast inhibitor to prevent skeletal-related events is unknown; however, patients in the major trials were treated for a maximum of 24 months.

Correct Answer: E

10) What are the recommendations for germline testing and molecular phenotyping of the tumor in advanced prostate cancer?

Expert Perspective: NCCN guidelines recommend germline genetic testing for men with (i) high-risk, very high-risk regional, or metastatic prostate cancer, (ii) Ashkenazi Jewish ancestry, (iii) family history of high-risk germline mutations (eg, *BRCA1/2*, Lynch mutations), or (iv) a strong positive family history of cancer. An estimated 12% of patients with metastatic prostate cancer will carry a germline pathogenic variant in a DNA repair gene. The most commonly mutated gene is *BRCA2* (5.3%), followed by *CHEK2* (1.9%), *ATM* (1.6%), *BRCA 1* (0.9%), *RAD51D* (0.4%), and *PALB2* (0.4%) (Pritchard et al. 2016). Current guidelines recommend testing for DNA homologous recombination genes (*BRCA1/2, ATM, PALB2,* and *CHEK2*), and mismatch repair genes to evaluate for Lynch syndrome (*MLH1, MSH2, MSH6, PMS2*). Testing for additional genes such as *HOXB13* can also be considered depending on the clinical context (refer to Chapters 46 and 47).

Somatic tumor testing to evaluate for alterations in DNA repair genes is recommended for all men with metastatic prostate cancer and can be considered in men with regional prostate cancer. We suggest somatic tumor testing mainly in men with progressive castrate-resistant disease, as it can inform the use of platinum chemotherapy, PARP inhibitors, or specific clinical trials (refer to Chapter 18).

Germline-only testing will unfortunately miss a significant proportion of *BRCA1/2* alterations that are somatic in origin. While somatic-only testing could theoretically detect both somatic and inherited variants present in the tumor sample, germline variants can be missed or misclassified due to limitations of testing and tissue sample availability. Presently, germline and somatic testing are complementary, and interpretation together increases the sensitivity of testing (refer to Chapters 32, 45, and 46).

11) What is the role of PARP inhibitors in metastatic castrate-resistant prostate cancer?

Expert Perspective: The PARP inhibitors olaparib, niraparib, talazoparib and rucaparib are approved for patients with metastastic castrate-resistant prostate cancer and DNA repair mutations. In the phase III PROfound trial, 387 men with metastatic castrate-resistant prostate cancer, progression on an androgen receptor signaling inhibitor, and alterations in 15 predefined genes hypothesized to be involved (directly or indirectly) with homologous recombination repair were randomized to either physician's choice of androgen receptor signaling inhibitor (abiraterone or enzalutamide) or olaparib 300 mg twice daily (de Bono et al. 2020). Study cohort A was composed of men with pathogenic variants in *BRCA1*, *BRCA2*, and *ATM*; cohort B was composed of men with alterations in 12 other prespecified genes (*CDK12*, *CHEK1/2*, etc.). Patients in the olaparib arm in cohort A had improved radiographic progression-free survival (median 7.4 months vs 3.6 months; HR 0.34), OS (median 19.1 months vs 14.7 months; HR 0.69) and objective response rate (33% vs 2%; $P < 0.0001$) compared to those receiving androgen receptor signaling inhibitor. The benefits from olaparib compared to the control arm in cohort B were lower; however, the FDA approved olaparib for all 15 genes, based on the combined radiographic progression-free survival benefit with olaparib in cohorts A and B vs control (median 5.8 months vs 3.5 months; HR 0.49). Notably, the gene-level data for many of the involved alterations was inconclusive, and the magnitude of benefit was primarily derived from men with *BRCA1/2* alterations in cohort A. Efficacy of olaparib for men with alterations in DNA repair genes other than *BRCA1/2* is likely limited.

In contrast to olaparib, the PARP inhibitor, rucaparib is FDA approved for patients with *BRCA1/2* alterations and only after disease progression on androgen receptor signaling inhibitor and taxane therapy. Rucaparib was approved based on TRITON2, which was a single-arm phase II study that demonstrated an objective response rate of 44% and radiographic progression-free survival of 9 months (95% CI 8.3–13.5). Objective response rates were similar for patients with germline or somatic *BRCA* alterations and *BRCA1* vs *BRCA2* alterations (Abida et al. 2020). Most recently, TRITON3 study reported that at 62 months, the duration of imaging-based PFS was significantly longer in the rucaparib (600 mg twice daily) group than in the control group (docetaxel or a second-generation ARPI [abiraterone acetate or enzalutamide]), both in the *BRCA* subgroup (median, 11.2 months and 6.4 months, respectively; hazard ratio, 0.50; 95% CI, 0.36 to 0.69) and in the intention-to-treat group (median, 10.2 months and 6.4 months, respectively; hazard ratio, 0.61; 95% CI, 0.47 to 0.80; $P<0.001$ for both comparisons). In an exploratory analysis in the *ATM* subgroup, the median duration of imaging-based PFS was 8.1 months in the rucaparib group and 6.8 months in the control group (hazard ratio, 0.95; 95% CI, 0.59 to 1.52). Common side effects of olaparib and rucaparib include anemia, fatigue, nausea, and anorexia. Most recently, the FDA approved the fixed dose combination of niraparib and abiraterone acetate with prednisone, for adult patients with deleterious or suspected deleterious BRCA-mutated castration-resistant prostate cancer (MAGNITUDE study) and talazoparib with enzalutamide for homologous recombination repair (HRR) gene-mutated metastatic castration-resistant prostate cancer (TALAPRO-2 study). Please see Table 34.2 for a summary of the key trials in metastatic castrate-resistant prostate cancer.

Case Study 5

A 75-year-old male with Gleason 4 + 4 prostate cancer initially presented with a PSA of 70 ng/mL and osseous metastasis that were considered high-volume disease. He was treated with ADT + docetaxel with a good response and upon repeat PSA rise with abiraterone, once again with a good response and a PSA nadir of 4 ng/mL. After three years of therapy, PSA has started to rise and is now 30 ng/mL. CT scans of abdomen and pelvis and NM bone scan demonstrate new osseous lesions in the lumbar and sacral spine and bilateral ribs with no visceral or lymph node disease. The patient is complaining of significant pain in his lower back limiting his ability to be active. MRI of the lower spine is unremarkable for cord compression.

12) What is the best treatment strategy?
   A) Enzalutamide.
   B) Radium-223.
   C) Radium-223 + abiraterone.
   D) Radium-223 + an osteoclast inhibitor.

Expert Perspective: Radium-223 is a bone-seeking, alpha-particle-emitting radioisotope that deposits high-energy radiation over a short distance, allowing for treatment of the tumor with decreased toxicity to the normal bone marrow. Radium-223 is a treatment option for patients with symptomatic metastatic castrate-resistant prostate cancer with predominantly bone metastasis without visceral disease and in the absence of large nodal metastasis (> 3–4 cm). Radium-223 was approved based on results of the phase III ALSYMPCA trial, in which 921 patients were randomized to best supportive care plus radium-223 or best supportive care plus placebo. All patients had castrate-resistant prostate cancer and had either progressed on docetaxel chemotherapy or were not candidates for docetaxel. Overall survival was significantly increased in the radium-223 group (median 14.9 months vs 11.3 months; HR 0.70; 95% CI 0.58–0.83). The time to first symptomatic skeletal event was also significantly delayed with radium-223 compared to placebo (median 15.6 months vs 9.8 months; HR 0.66; 95% CI 0.52–0.83). The approved schedule of radium-223 is six doses given every four weeks. Common side effects include anemia, thrombocytopenia, neutropenia, nausea, vomiting, and diarrhea.

The optimal sequencing of radium-223 in metastatic castrate-resistant prostate cancer is unclear, as newer agents such as abiraterone, enzalutamide, and the chemotherapy agent cabazitaxel were not utilized by patients in the ALSYMPCA trial. Notably, the ERA 223 trial showed an increased rate of fractures when radium-223 was combined with abiraterone—29% of patients receiving combined therapy vs 11% in the control group (Smith et al. 2019). However, after further analysis, this was thought to be due to low utilization of osteoclast inhibitors (only approximately 40% of patients in either group). A trial is evaluating enzalutamide plus radium-223 vs enzalutamide alone in asymptomatic or mildly symptomatic men with metastatic castrate-resistant prostate cancer (PEACE III, EORTC 1333). Due to the results of the ERA 223 trial, PEACE III was amended to mandate that all patients be treated with osteoclast inhibitors. In a preliminary report of a subset of 253 patients, the risk of fracture at 1.5 years was 46% with enzalutamide plus radium-223 vs 22% with enzalutamide alone. However, after mandating use of an osteoclast inhibitor, the risk of fracture at 1.5 years dropped to 4.3% in the enzalutamide plus radium-223 group and 2.6% in the enzalutamide alone group (Gillessen et al. presentation at ASCO 2021).

Given the currrent data, NCCN guidelines recommend against combining radium-223 with any other systemic therapy including abiraterone and docetaxel. Radium-223 can be combined safely with ADT. All patients receiving radium-223 should be treated with an osteoclast inhibitor.

Correct Answer: D

Case Study 6

A 75-year-old male with Gleason 4 + 4 prostate cancer initially presented with a PSA of 70 ng/mL and osseous metastasis that were considered high-volume disease. He was treated with ADT + docetaxel with a good response and upon repeat PSA rise, with abiraterone, once again with a good response and a PSA nadir of 4 ng/mL. After three years of therapy, PSA has started to rise and is now 30 ng/mL. CT scans of abdomen and pelvis and NM bone scan demonstrate new liver and osseous lesions in the lumbar and sacral spine and bilateral ribs. The biopsy of liver lesion shows prostate adenocarcinoma. The patient is complaining of significant pain in his lower back limiting his ability to be active. MRI of the lower spine is unremarkable for cord compression.

13) What is the next best management strategy?
   A) Cabazitazel 20 mg/m^2.
   B) Cabazitaxel 25 mg/m^2.
   C) Radium-223 + an osteoclast inhibitor.
   D) Olaparib.

Expert Perspective: Cabazitaxel can be used as a second-line chemotherapy agent for those who have progressed on docetaxel or as first-line therapy in chemo-naive patients with metastatic castrate-resistant prostate cancer. Cabazitaxel was approved based on results of the phase III TROPIC trial in patients with metastatic castrate-resistant prostate cancer who had disease progression on prior docetaxel (deBono et al. 2010). In all, 755 patients were randomized to cabazitaxel 25 mg/m^2 vs mitoxantrone 12 mg/m^2, and there was a significant difference in OS in men treated with cabazitaxel vs mitoxantrone (median OS 15.1 vs 12.7 months; HR 0.70; 95% CI 0.59–0.83). The most common grade 3 or higher adverse events were neutropenia, leukopenia, anemia, and diarrhea; importantly, grade 3 peripheral neuropathy was uncommon. Cabazitaxel may be used as a first-line chemotherapy agent in patients who are elderly (such as our patient in the case study) and/or frail or at high risk for peripheral neuropathy. Cabazitaxel 20 mg/m^2 is the preferred dose of cabazitaxel based on comparison to cabazitaxel 25 mg/m^2 and docetaxel 75 mg/m^2 in the first-line setting in patients with metastatic castrate-resistant prostate cancer (Oudard et al. 2017). The median OS was similar between the three groups (24–25 months), but the toxicity profile of cabazitaxel 20 mg/m^2 was better than that of cabazitaxel 25 mg/m^2 (Figure 34.1).

Correct Answer: A

14) What is the data supporting the use of PSMA-based therapies in metastatic castrate-resistant prostate cancer?

Expert Perspective: Prostate-specific membrane antigen (PSMA) is a transmembrane protein (glutamate carboxypeptidase) that has high expression on prostate cancer cells, including metastatic prostate cancer lesions in patients with castrate-resistant prostate cancer. Several PSMA-targeting radioligand therapies are currently in development.

Lutetium-177 (^{177}Lu)-PSMA-617 is a PSMA-targeting radioligand that was approved by the FDA based on results of the phase III VISION trial (Sartor et al. 2021). The VISION trial enrolled patients with metastatic castrate-resistant prostate cancer who had previously been treated with at least one androgen receptor signaling inhibitor and one or two taxane chemotherapies and had PSMA-positive gallium-68 (^{68}Ga)-labeled PSMA-11 PET-CT scans. PSMA-positive PET was defined as having at least one tumor lesion with gallium Ga 68 gozetotide uptake greater than normal liver. A total of 831 patients were randomized to either ^{177}Lu-PSMA-617 plus protocol-permitted standard of care (n = 551) or standard of care alone (n = 280). ^{177}Lu-PSMA-617 was administered at a dose of 7.4 GBq (200 mCi) every six weeks for four cycles, intravenously; up to two additional cycles could be given. Patients who received ^{177}Lu-PSMA-617 plus standard of care had a significantly longer radiographic progression-free survival (median 8.7 months vs 3.4 months; HR 0.40) and OS (median 15.3 months vs 11.3 months; HR 0.62) compared to standard of care alone. The median time to first symptomatic skeletal event was also significantly improved in patients who received ^{177}Lu-PSMA-617 (11.5 months vs 6.8 months; HR 0.50). Common adverse events with ^{177}Lu-PSMA-617 were anemia, thrombocytopenia, lymphopenia, fatigue, dry mouth, nausea, and constipation.

It is unclear what the optimal sequencing will be of ^{177}Lu-PSMA-617 in relation other treatment options for metastatic castrate resistant prostate cancer. (There is data suggesting that Lu-PMSA is superior to cabazitaxel, so would just keep this statement general)., in patients with metastatic castrate-resistant prostate cancer. A PSMA-positive PET is required for ^{177}Lu-PSMA-617 therapy. Many trials are underway evaluating PSMA radioligand therapies earlier in the disease course and in combination with other therapies.

Recommended Readings

Crook, J.M., O'Callaghan, C.J., Duncan, G. et al. (2012 September 6). Intermittent androgen suppression for rising PSA level after radiotherapy. *N Engl J Med* 367 (10): 895–903.

Davis, I.D., Martin, A.J., Stockler, M.R. et al. (2019 July 11). Enzalutamide with standard first-line therapy in metastatic prostate cancer. *N Engl J Med* 381 (2): 121–131.

de Bono, J., Mateo, J., Fizazi, K. et al. (2020 May 28). Olaparib for metastatic castration-resistant prostate cancer. *N Engl J Med* 382 (22): 2091–2102.

Fizazi, K., Carducci, M., Smith, M. et al. (2011 March 5). Denosumab versus zoledronic acid for treatment of bone metastases in men with castration-resistant prostate cancer: a randomised, double-blind study. *Lancet* 377 (9768): 813–822.

Fizazi, K., Foulon, S., Carles, J. et al., PEACE-1 investigators. (2022 Apr 30). Abiraterone plus prednisone added to androgen deprivation therapy and docetaxel in de novo metastatic castration-sensitive prostate cancer (PEACE-1): a multicentre, open-label, randomised, phase 3 study with a 2×2 factorial design. *Lancet* 399 (10336): 1695–1707. doi:10.1016/S0140-6736(22)00367-1. Epub 2022 Apr 8. PMID: 35405085.

Fizazi, K., Piulats, J.M., Reaume, M.N., et al. (2023 Feb 23). TRITON3 Investigators. rucaparib or physician's choice in metastatic prostate cancer. *N Engl J Med* 388 (8): 719–732. doi: 10.1056/NEJMoa2214676. Epub 2023 Feb 16. PMID: 36795891; PMCID: PMC10064172.

James, N.D., de Bono, J.S., Spears, M.R. et al. (2017 July 27). STAMPEDE investigators. Abiraterone for prostate cancer not previously treated with hormone therapy. *N Engl J Med* 377 (4): 338–351.

Kyriakopoulos, C.E., Chen, Y.H., Carducci, M.A. et al. (2018 April 10). Chemohormonal therapy in metastatic hormone-sensitive prostate cancer: long-term survival analysis of the randomized phase III E3805 CHAARTED Trial. *J Clin Oncol* 36 (11): 1080–1087.

Parker, C., Nilsson, S., Heinrich, D. et al. (2013 July 18). ALSYMPCA investigators. Alpha emitter radium-223 and survival in metastatic prostate cancer. *N Engl J Med* 369 (3): 213–223.

Parker, C.C., James, N.D., Brawley, C.D. et al. (2018 December 1). Radiotherapy to the primary tumour for newly diagnosed, metastatic prostate cancer (STAMPEDE): a randomised controlled phase 3 trial. *Lancet* 392 (10162): 2353–2366.

Sartor, O., de Bono, J., Chi, K.N. et al. (2021 June 23). Lutetium-177-PSMA-617 for metastatic castration-resistant prostate cancer. *N Engl J Med* doi: 10.1056/NEJMoa2107322. Epub ahead of print.

Smith, M.R., Hussain, M., Saad, F. et al., ARASENS Trial Investigators. (2022 Mar 24). Darolutamide and survival in metastatic, hormone-sensitive prostate cancer. *N Engl J Med* 386 (12): 1132–1142. doi:10.1056/NEJMoa2119115. Epub 2022 Feb 17. PMID: 35179323; PMCID: PMC9844551.

Trabulsi, E.J., Rumble, R.B., and Vargas, H.A. (2020 April). Optimum imaging strategies for advanced prostate cancer: ASCO guideline summary. *JCO Oncol Pract* 16 (4): 170–176.

35

Germ Cell Tumors

Hamid Emamekhoo[1], Syed A. Abutalib[2], and Timothy Gilligan[3]

[1] *University of Wisconsin Carbone Cancer Center, Madison, WI*
[2] *Aurora St. Luke's Medical Center, Milwaukee, WI*
[3] *Taussig Cancer Institute, Cleveland Clinic, Cleveland, OH*

Introduction

Germ cell tumors are the most common malignancies among men between ages 15 and 35. It is estimated that 9,910 cases and 460 deaths occurred in the United States in 2022. Germ cell tumors most frequently originate in the gonads (testis or ovary) and less commonly in the retroperitoneum and mediastinum. Germ cell tumors are derived from the malignant transformation of premeiotic germ cells. For a discussion of germ cell tumors in women, see Chapter 42, "Uncommon Gynecologic Cancers." Retroperitoneal germ cell tumors are often associated with an invasive tumor or carcinoma *in situ* within the testis, even in the absence of a palpable testicular mass. Primary mediastinal germ cell tumors are not associated with testicular involvement. Primary extragonadal germ cell neoplasms also arise rarely in the sacrum, pineal gland, paranasal sinuses, and liver. Regardless of the stage or extent of disease, the therapeutic objective is cure, which requires an integrated multidisciplinary approach.

1) **Which of the following statements about germ cell tumors is correct?**
   A) Testicular nonseminomas compared to seminomas occur more frequently in men with AIDS.
   B) Klinefelter syndrome is a risk factor for the development of mediastinal germ cell tumors.
   C) A metachronous or synchronous testicular primary germ cell tumor occurs in the contralateral testis in 10% of patients.
   D) Men in whom *in situ* disease is identified during a testicular biopsy as part of an infertility evaluation have a 10% risk of an invasive tumor within a five-year period.
   E) Treatment of an undescended testis does not decrease the risk of testicular cancer.
   F) An isochromosome of the short arm of chromosome 12—i(12p)—is present in 30% of all germ cell tumors.

Expert Perspective: Abdominal and inguinal cryptorchidism, spermatic or testicular dysgenesis, and a positive family history are known risk factors for germ cell tumors. Treatment of an undescended testis before puberty decreases the risk of testicular cancer as compared to correction after puberty; however, orchiopexy or surgical correction of abdominal cryptorchidism after puberty allows improved ability to monitor the testis for cancer. Factors associated with increased testicular cancer mortality include age older than 40, nonwhite race, and lower socioeconomic status. Testicular seminoma occurs more frequently in men with AIDS, and the treatment by stage is the same as for the non-infected population—of note, the incidence of this has been decreasing with advent of successful therapy. Klinefelter syndrome is a risk factor for the development of mediastinal germ cell tumors. Carcinoma *in situ* (intratubular germ cell neoplasia) is found in all cases of testicular germ cell tumors. Men in whom *in situ* disease is identified during a testicular biopsy as part of an infertility evaluation have a 50% risk of an invasive tumor within a five-year period. A metachronous or synchronous testicular primary germ cell tumor occurs in 2% of patients, with seminoma as the most common histology. An isochromosome of the short arm of chromosome 12—i(12p)—is present in 80% of all histologic subtypes, including carcinoma *in situ* and extragonadal tumors. The remaining 20% of cases have excess 12p genetic material as an increase in copy number, tandem duplication, or transposition, which indicates that one or more genes on 12p participate in malignant transformation.

Correct Answer: B

2) At what time point should serum tumor markers be drawn to determine the prognosis and stage of testicular germ cell tumors?
   A) Prior to orchiectomy.
   B) Post orchiectomy.
   C) On day 1 of cycle 1 of chemotherapy.
   D) Use the highest tumor marker numbers.

Expert Perspective: For men with disseminated germ cell tumors, prognosis should be based on the burden of disease at the time that systemic therapy is started. Therefore, the optimal time to measure serum β-hCG (beta-human chorionic gonadotropin), α-fetoprotein (AFP), and lactate dehydrogenase (LDH) is immediately before initiating chemotherapy, which is almost always after orchiectomy. Postorchiectomy serum tumor marker staging used for risk classification is displayed in Table 35.1. Nonetheless, the serum tumor markers β-hCG and AFP should be drawn before orchiectomy but not for prognostic purposes. The serum tumor marker levels before orchiectomy reflect the primary tumor as well as any metastatic disease and thus are an unreliable indicator of the extent of any disseminated disease. The value of pre-orchiectomy β-hCG and AFP is twofold: an elevated AFP excludes a diagnosis of pure seminoma regardless of the histopathological findings (unless an alternative, non-germ cell tumor explanation for the AFP elevation is established) and having pre-orchiectomy markers facilitates interpretation of post-orchiectomy markers. The serum half-lives of β-hCG and AFP are 30 hours and five to seven days, respectively. If β-hCG or AFP is persistently elevated or rising following orchiectomy, this is indicative of disseminated disease even in the absence of any radiographic evidence of metastases, and the standard treatment is chemotherapy. In contrast to β-hCG and AFP, the only role for measurement of serum LDH is to establish prognosis at the start of chemotherapy. An

Table 35.1 On day 1 of cycle 1 of chemotherapy serum tumor marker staging used for risk classification.

S category	S criteria
Sx	Marker studies not available or not performed
S0	Marker study levels within normal limits
S1	β-hCG (mIU/mL) < 5,000 and AFP (ng/mL) < 1,000 and LDH < 1.5 × ULN*
S2	β-hCG (mIU/mL) 5,000 to 50,000 or AFP (ng/mL) 1,000 to 10,000 or LDH 1.5–10 × ULN
S3	β-hCG (mIU/mL) > 50,000 or AFP (ng/mL) > 10,000 or LDH > 10 × ULN

* ULN: upper limit of normal.

elevated LDH may result from myriad different conditions and is often unrelated to the patient's cancer. There is no clear reason to measure LDH levels before or after orchiectomy unless the patient is going to start treatment with chemotherapy for metastatic disease. A low-level elevation of β-hCG can occur in certain benign conditions such as hypothyroidism (cross-reactivity with the thyroid-stimulating hormone), hypogonadism (cross-reactivity with luteinizing hormone and/or β-hCG production by the pituitary), and marijuana use in men. AFP can be elevated in patients with liver disease. β-hCG may be elevated in both seminoma and nonseminoma, and AFP may be elevated in nonseminoma but not in pure seminomas. Elevations in any one marker or combination are found in approximately 20% of patients with stage I disease, 40% of patients with stage II disease, and ≥ 60% of patients with stage III disease. Of note, neither serum β-hCG nor AFP, alone or in combination, is sufficiently sensitive or specific to establish the diagnosis of testicular cancer in the absence of histologic confirmation.

Correct Answer: C

Stage I disease

3) **Which of the following is/are reasonable option(s) for patients with clinical stage I testicular seminoma?**
   A) Surveillance.
   B) Radiation therapy.
   C) Carboplatin for one cycle.
   D) Carboplatin for two cycles.
   E) Any of the above.

Expert Perspective: Approximately 70% of patients with seminoma have stage I disease. Surveillance is the best option for most but not all men with stage I testicular seminoma. Following orchiectomy, the risk of relapse for clinical stage I seminoma of the testis is about 15–18% mostly in the retroperitoneum: surveillance spares more than four out of five men unnecessary additional therapy. Moreover, surveillance results in long-term disease-specific survival of over 99%. However, to capture any potential late relapses, prolonged follow-up is needed, which can result in associated anxiety and noncompliance. So, as the long-term disease specific survival is over 99% with surveillance, adjuvant treatment with carboplatin chemotherapy or radiation therapy after orchiectomy does not increase either disease-specific or overall survival. The rationale for treating clinical stage I seminoma is not based on preventing deaths from testis cancer but rather on wanting to lower the risk of relapse because relapse and the subsequent need for treatment can be highly disruptive.

Treatment options for clinical stage I seminoma include surveillance, one or two cycles of single-agent carboplatin chemotherapy (AUC = 7 dose), or radiation therapy to either a paraaortic strip field (preferred) or a dogleg (aka hockey-stick) field that includes the paraaortic strip plus the proximal ipsilateral hemipelvis. Relapse rates are 15–18% with surveillance, 5% with a single cycle of carboplatin, 4% with radiation therapy, and 2% with two cycles of carboplatin. However, case series have reported higher relapse rates for high-risk stage I seminomas after a single cycle of carboplatin, and single-arm studies have reported lower relapse rates when two cycles of carboplatin are given (2% overall, 3% in high-risk patients). Therefore, some experts prefer two cycles of carboplatin for patients who chose chemotherapy for stage I seminoma. Radiation therapy has been less popular over the past decade because of extensive data showing an increased risk of variety of cancers; it is also avoided in patients with inflammatory bowel disease and patients with underlying anatomical issues. A minimum of five years surveillance is recommended for all stage I patients. Patients on surveillance have the highest risk of late relapse according to population-based data from the SWENOTECA group, and their practice is 10 years of surveillance. In a retrospective report by Fischer and colleagues on patients who experienced a relapse after adjuvant carboplatin (one or two cycles of carboplatin), 15% of the relapses occurred more than three years after adjuvant treatment. Whether carboplatin at the doses used in this setting is associated with significant late toxicity is not yet clear, but both cisplatin and carboplatin have been associated with a higher risk of second cancers when used at higher doses. The bottom line is that surveillance is the preferred option for most men, but two doses of carboplatin produce the lowest relapse rate for men who prefer active treatment.

Correct Answer: E

4) **Which of the following are management option(s) for patients with stage I nonseminoma testicular germ cell tumors?**
   A) Surveillance.
   B) Bleomycin, etoposide, and cisplatin (BEP) for one cycle.
   C) Bleomycin, etoposide, and cisplatin (BEP) for two cycles.
   D) Retroperitoneal lymph node dissection.
   E) All of the above.

Expert Perspective: About 30–40% of patients with nonseminomatous germ cell tumors present with stage I disease. It is important to note that most patients with stage I disease have stage T1 (tumor limited to testis [including rete testis invasion] without lymphovascular invasion) or T2 (tumor limited to testis [including rete testis invasion] with lymphovascular invasion or tumor invading hilar soft tissue or epididymis or penetrating visceral mesothelial layer covering the external surface of tunica albuginea with or without lymphovascular invasion) tumors, and this discussion applies to them. The optimal management of T3 (tumor directly invades spermatic cord soft tissue with or without lymphovascular invasion) and T4 (tumor invades scrotum with or without lymphovascular invasion) tumors is not well defined and such cases should be referred to centers of excellence whenever feasible. Surveillance is an excellent option for most men with clinical stage I nonseminomatous germ cell tumors but is not the best option for everyone. It does not make logical sense to choose surveillance if the patient will not be able to comply with the surveillance schedule. There may be psychological, economical, geographical, or other obstacles to compliance. Assessing the feasibility of frequent visits for blood tests and physical examination and less frequent visits for imaging studies is essential before deciding on surveillance as a management strategy. Primary chemotherapy using one or two cycles of BEP (bleomycin 30 units on days 1, 8, and 15; etoposide 100 mg/m^2 on days 1–5; cisplatin 20 mg/m^2 on days 1–5) lowers the risk of relapse from about 30% to about 2%, and thus the benefit of surveillance and the risk associated with noncompliance with surveillance are much smaller in a patient who has been treated with primary chemotherapy. It is not clear that a second cycle of BEP significantly lowers the relapse rate compared to one cycle, so most guidelines recommend one rather than two cycles of BEP for patients receiving chemotherapy in this setting. Nerve-sparing retroperitoneal lymph node dissection also lowers the risk of relapse in nonseminomatous germ cell tumors but by a lesser degree compared to primary chemotherapy. A second reason that surveillance may not be the best option for some men with clinical stage I nonseminomatous germ cell tumors has to do with patient preference. Being diagnosed with cancer is often psychologically traumatic and disruptive, resulting in time away from work or school and lost income, as well as anxiety and distress. Relapse of the cancer repeats this trauma and disruption, typically with greater severity. Moreover, relapse comes at an unpredictable time and cannot be planned or incorporated into the patient's schedule regarding education, career, or family. For some patients, the ability to choose to have chemotherapy now (rather than to possibly receive it at an unpredictable future time) and to have greater peace of mind because of a near-zero risk of relapse outweighs the downsides of receiving chemotherapy that they probably do not need. Shared decision-making is thus appropriate regarding management of stage I nonseminomatous germ cell tumors so that the patient's values and priorities can be incorporated into the decision-making process.

In choosing a management strategy, assessing risk of relapse is important. The most used risk factor for relapse is the presence of lymphovascular invasion in the primary tumor. Another often-used risk factor is predominance of embryonal carcinoma in the tumor. Roughly half of men with lymphovascular invasion will relapse, and in some studies a predominance of embryonal carcinoma further increases that risk. While it is well documented that men with a high risk of relapse can be safely managed with surveillance, surveillance is often less attractive to men with such characteristics. Some experts prefer a risk-adapted approach, while others prefer surveillance for all patients. A risk-adapted approach typically means treating men with lymphovascular invasion while using surveillance in men without lymphovascular invasion.

In summary, surveillance is a good option for all men with clinical stage I nonseminomatous germ cell tumors who are willing to comply with the surveillance schedule, but some men may prefer treatment with chemotherapy. In patients with stage I nonseminomatous germ cell tumor without risk factors (lymphovascular invasion or invasion of spermatic cord or scrotum or predominance of embryonal carcinoma) surveillance is the preferred approach. For patients with stage I disease with risk factors, all options including surveillance, chemotherapy (with one cycle of BEP), or nerve-sparing retroperitoneal lymph node dissection should be carefully considered. If retroperitoneal lymph node dissection is considered, it should only be performed by an experienced surgeon in testicular cancer (high-volume center). Retroperitoneal lymph node dissection performed by surgeons who perform the operation infrequently yield inferior results. The decision to recommend adjuvant chemotherapy after a retroperitoneal lymph node dissection is made on the basis of pathologic findings, as described for patients with pathologic stage II disease. Patients without evidence of clinical disease and persistently elevated tumor markers, including, β-hCG and/or AFP, after orchiectomy (stage IS), should receive standard chemotherapy for advanced disease rather than surgery.

Correct Answer: E

5) What are the preferred surveillance schedules for clinical stage I seminomas and nonseminomas tumors?

Expert Perspective: For patients with clinical stage I germ cell tumors, surveillance schedules must balance the benefit of detecting a relapse as early as possible against the potential harm of CT radiation exposure and the need not to waste medical resources on unnecessarily intensive testing. Recent data support MRI as an alternative to CT for imaging the abdomen and pelvis but, while this eliminates exposure to ionizing radiation, it adds cost and requires greater technology and expertise.

- **Stage I seminoma** typically relapses in the retroperitoneum with normal serum tumor marker (β-hCG and/or LDH) levels. The median time to relapse is 14 months, which is twice as long as for clinical stage I nonseminomatous tumors, and late relapses at greater than five years may occur. As a result, cross-sectional imaging is the only reliable way to detect relapse. Fortunately, seminomas tend to grow more slowly than nonseminomas. There are a variety of different scanning schedules that have been published with a trend over time toward fewer imaging studies. NCCN currently recommends scans every six months for the first two to three years and every 12 to 24 months in years 4–5. Chest X-ray is optional because data suggests that chest surveillance very rarely contributes to detecting relapse. It now appears that magnetic resonance imaging can replace abdominopelvic CT scans and thus eliminate ionizing radiation, but this adds cost and is less widely available.
- **Stage I nonseminomatous germ cell tumors:** Most recurrences of nonseminomatous germ cell tumors will occur within two years of orchiectomy although late recurrences are also observed. A more intensive serum tumor marker surveillance schedule is used because many relapses first present with elevated BHCG or AFP. An international study compared a surveillance schedule that obtained CT scans at months 3 and 12 to a schedule that included scans at months 3, 6, 9, 12, and 24. No difference in outcome was reported. Nonetheless, many experts are uncomfortable with stopping CT scans at 12 months since a significant number of relapses occur in the second and third year. The surveillance schedule shown in Table 35.2 is thus recommended.

Table 35.2 Surveillance schedule of clinical stage I nonseminomatous germ cell tumors.

	Serum tumor markers AFP and beta-hCG and physical exam	Chest X-ray	CT abdomen and pelvis
Year 1	Every 2 months	Every 4 months	At 3 and 9 months
Year 2	Every 3 months	Every 4–6 months	At 18 months (1.5 yrs)
Year 3	Every 4 months	Every 6 months	At 30 months (2.5 yrs)
Year 4	Every 6 months	Every 12 months	At 42 months (3.5 yrs)
Year 5	Every 12 months	Optional	At 60 months (5 yrs)
Years 6–10	Every 12 months	Only as clinically indicated	

AFP: alpha-fetoprotein; CT: computed tomography; hCG: human chorionic gonadotropin.

Case Study 1

A 32-year-old man presents with a newly diagnosed mixed germ cell tumor of the right testis that shows lymphovascular invasion (pT2) and consists of 80% embryonal carcinoma and 20% seminoma. A chest X-ray and CT of the abdomen and pelvis show no evidence of metastases, and his serum tumor markers are normal following orchiectomy. He elects to undergo chemotherapy.

6) Which of the following would be the most appropriate regimen for this man?
   A) Bleomycin, etoposide, and cisplatin (BEP) for one cycle.
   B) One cycle of carboplatin chemotherapy.
   C) Bleomycin, etoposide, and cisplatin (BEP) for two cycles.
   D) Two cycles of carboplatin chemotherapy.

Expert Perspective: There is no data to support the use of carboplatin in patients with nonseminomatous germ cell tumors, and the substitution of carboplatin for cisplatin in multi-agent regimens has been shown to result in inferior outcomes in patients with metastatic disease.

- One versus two cycles of BEP (bleomycin, etoposide, and cisplatin): In the past, if adjuvant chemotherapy was considered the preferred approach, treatment with one or two cycles of BEP was recommended for patients with stage I nonseminoma. Patients were considered at high risk for disease relapse if the orchiectomy surgical specimen indicated lymphovascular invasion, invasion of spermatic cord or scrotum, or predominance of embryonal carcinoma. More intensive treatment with two cycles of BEP chemotherapy was recommended for patients with stage I nonseminoma with these risk factors. However, this recommendation was changed based on the results of a prospective clinical trial by the Swedish and Norwegian Testicular Cancer Group (SWENOTECA). In this study, patients with stage I nonseminoma with or without lymphovascular invasion received one course of adjuvant BEP. The five-year overall survival was 100% in both groups, and the five-year relapse rates were 3.2% for patients with lymphovascular invasion and 1.6% for patients without lymphovascular invasion, and these rates remained stable at a longer median follow-up of 7.9 years. In addition, this high relapse-free survival rate with only one cycle of BEP for patients with lymphovascular invasion was similar to survival rates in other studies that used two cycles of BEP. Considering the late and chronic consequences of cisplatin-based chemotherapy (which include neuropathy, cardiovascular conditions, hearing nerve damage, and secondary malignancies as well as an increased risk of death from causes other than testis cancer) later in life in younger patients that are likely cured of their cancer, minimizing unwanted treatment-related sequela is very important. Therefore, only one cycle of adjuvant BEP is recommended for patients with stage I nonseminoma with or without risk factors due to a lower risk of treatment-related toxicity. For patients without risk factors, surveillance is the preferred approach, but for those with risk factors, all three options (surveillance, BEP chemotherapy, and retroperitoneal lymph node dissection) should be carefully considered and discussed with the patient.

- **Clinical stage I pure seminomas:** In general, surveillance is the preferred approach in patients with stage I pure seminoma. If adjuvant chemotherapy is considered for a patient, then one or two cycles of carboplatin (AUC 7) is recommended. Multiple groups have studied the use of one or two cycles of carboplatin in the adjuvant setting for stage I seminoma. A non-randomized retrospective study of 897 patients with stage I seminoma who were treated with one cycle of carboplatin noted higher rates of relapse in patients with tumor size greater than 4 cm, rete testis invasion, or both. A recent prospective trial by the German Testicular Cancer Study Group compared the relapse rate with surveillance, radiotherapy, and one or two cycles of carboplatin in 725 patients with stage I seminoma. At a median follow-up of 30 months, they reported that disease-specific survival was 100% and relapse rates were 8.2%, 2.4%, 5.0%, and 1.5% for surveillance, radiotherapy, one cycle of carboplatin, and two cycles of carboplatin, respectively. Therefore, two cycles of carboplatin could be considered for high-risk patients with stage I seminoma.

Correct Answer: A

Stage II disease

7) Should all stage II testicular cancer patients be treated with chemotherapy?

Expert Perspective: No. Chemotherapy is an option but not the preferred treatment for all men with stage IIA (pT/TX, N1, M0, S0-1) seminoma or nonseminomas who have normal serum tumor markers levels (S0) (Table 35.3).

Seminoma

- The false-positive rate on CT scan for clinical stage IIA seminomas is unknown because these patients rarely undergo retroperitoneal lymph node dissection to confirm their stage. Men with borderline normal scans can be closely observed for progression, but the standard treatment for stage IIA seminoma (i.e. the diameter of involved nodes ≤ 2 cm in greatest dimension) is either radiation therapy or chemotherapy. There are no randomized controlled trials comparing outcomes after these two approaches, so the practice is based on individual patient characteristics (such as the location of the enlarged nodes) as well as physician habit and experience.

Table 35.3 Stage II and its therapy in seminoma and nonseminoma testicular germ cell tumors.

	IIA	IIB	IIC
	Any T		
	N1S0	N2S0	N3S0
	N1S1	N2S1	N3S1
Seminoma	RT is preferred	BEP × 3 or EP × 4 or RT	BEP × 3 or EP × 4
Nonseminoma*	• Normal tumor markers: RPLND or chemo (BEP × 3 or EP × 4) • Persistently elevated tumor markers: chemo (BEP × 3 or EP × 4)	BEP × 3 or EP × 4	

* Mediastinal primary nonseminoma is considered poor risk and should be treated with BEP × 4.
RT: radiation therapy; chemo: chemotherapy; RPLND: retroperitoneal lymph node dissection; N1: metastasis with a lymph node mass 2 cm or smaller in greatest dimension or multiple lymph nodes, none larger than 2 cm in greatest dimension; N2: metastasis with a lymph node mass larger than 2 cm but not larger than 5 cm in greatest dimension or multiple lymph nodes, any one mass larger than 2 cm but not larger than 5 cm in greatest dimension; N3: metastasis with a lymph node mass larger than 5 cm in greatest dimension; S0 and S1: see Table 35.1.

- Men with stage IIB seminomas are also managed with either radiation therapy or chemotherapy with BEP × 3 (or etoposide and cisplatin [EP] × 4), but some guidelines prefer chemotherapy for men with nodes larger than 3.0 cm in greatest dimension. Chemotherapy is also preferred for men with IIA or IIB disease with enlarged nodes in multiple regions of the retroperitoneum. In general, the acute side effects of radiation are milder than those of three cycles of BEP chemotherapy, but there are insufficient data to compare chronic and late toxicity. Both radiation therapy and germ cell tumor chemotherapy have been associated with an increased risk of secondary cancers.
- Patients with stage IIC seminoma should be treated with BEP × 3 (or EP × 4).

Nonseminoma

- Not all stage IIA nonseminomas are the same. Depending on individual patient characteristic, chemotherapy (BEP × 3 or EP × 4), retroperitoneal lymph node dissection or even close surveillance may be preferred. A finding of a single 11 × 15 mm lymph node is different from a 19 × 19 mm node or four enlarged nodes. Mildly enlarged nodes in the primary landing zone are more concerning than mildly enlarged nodes elsewhere. Careful review of imaging studies is essential for clinical stage IIA nonseminomatous germ cell tumors because the false-positive rate on CT scans has been reported to be

10–40%. Three cycles of BEP chemotherapy are an appropriate option for men with convincing evidence of nodal metastases but represents substantial overtreatment for a considerable number of men with very early clinical stage IIA disease. Therefore, in men with borderline or ambiguous findings on imaging, close surveillance, or retroperitoneal lymph node dissection to confirm stage of disease is preferred to chemotherapy. It is also important to note that RPLND is strongly preferred for men with teratoma with somatic malignant transformation.
- For clinical stage IIB/C nonseminomatous germ cell tumors cisplatin-based chemotherapy is preferred.

Of note, men with persistently elevated serum tumor markers following orchiectomy (seminoma or nonseminoma) should undergo chemotherapy for disseminated disease (discussed in next section) regardless of the presence or absence of retroperitoneal adenopathy.

8) What are the preferred workup and management if a patient with stage II nonseminomatous tumor was found to have residual masses (≥ 1 cm in size) with negative serum tumor markers after completion of adjuvant chemotherapy?
   A) Obtain a PET scan
   B) Obtain a CT-guided biopsy of the residual mass
   C) Bilateral retroperitoneal lymph node dissection
   D) Treat with two additional cycles of etoposide and cisplatin (EP) or paclitaxel, ifosfamide and cisplatin (TIP) chemotherapy

Expert Perspective: Nonseminoma post chemotherapy: Referral to a high-volume center for bilateral retroperitoneal lymph node dissection is the recommended management if the residual masses are larger than 1 cm in the CT scan. PET scan has no role in assessing treatment response and residual masses following chemotherapy in patients with nonseminomatous germ cell tumors. If the pathology from retroperitoneal lymph node dissection reveals teratoma or no viable tumor, surveillance is appropriate. If there is viable tumor in the retroperitoneal lymph node dissection specimen, an additional two cycles of chemotherapy should be recommended.

Seminoma post chemotherapy: In patients with pure seminoma, residual masses less than 3 cm in greatest transverse dimension should be closely observed. Larger masses can also be closely observed, or a PET scan can be used to assess them. A positive PET scan should be followed by a biopsy or complete resection of the residual mass. If the resected mass contains viable tumor, additional two cycles of chemotherapy could be considered. Recent studies have reported an alarmingly high false-positive rate for PET scans in this setting, and enthusiasm for such scans is thus in decline. If a PET scan is obtained and the results are ambiguous, surveillance is preferred over invasive procedures.

Correct Answer: C

9) **If the decision is made to perform a retroperitoneal lymph node dissection, should the patient be referred to a surgeon who performs a high volume of these operations?**

Expert Perspective: Yes. The favorable outcomes that have been reported for retroperitoneal lymph node dissections come almost exclusively from centers and surgeons who have extensive experience with performing the operation. In contrast, data from urologists without extensive experience are disappointing. For instance, a randomized control trial comparing a single cycle of BEP chemotherapy to retroperitoneal lymph node dissection in clinical stage I nonseminomatous germ cell tumors testis cancer patients that was conducted at community hospitals rather than specialized centers reported that more than half the relapses after retroperitoneal lymph node dissection (over 4% of patients) occurred in the retroperitoneum. In contrast, the expected rate of retroperitoneal relapse at centers of excellence for this procedure is fewer than 2% in their clinical stage I and clinical stage II patients treated with retroperitoneal lymph node dissection. In addition, a skilled surgeon can preserve antegrade ejaculation in almost all men with clinical stage I nonseminomatous germ cell tumors without compromising the oncologic effectiveness of the operation by applying nerve-sparing techniques.

Advanced stage disease

10) **For men with good-risk disseminated germ cell tumors, which of the following is the preferred option?**
    A) BEP for three cycles
    B) EP for four cycles

Expert Perspective: Although both regimens are entirely acceptable, the data supporting BEP for three cycles are stronger for good-risk disseminated germ cell tumors. Numerous trials have been conducted comparing regimens that include bleomycin to regimens that do not include bleomycin, and in each trial, the trend has favored the bleomycin arm. The one randomized controlled trial comparing three cycles of standard-dose BEP to four cycles of standard-dose EP reported that the risk of death for men in the EP × 4 arm was more than twice as high as in the BEP × 3 arm (HR 0.42; 95% CI 0.15–1.20), but the difference was not statistically significant. Most centers prefer BEP × 3 over EP × 4, but both are highly effective. EP × 4 is the preferred regimen for men with a contraindication to bleomycin (patients > 50 years of age, heavy smokers, those with underlying lung disease and at risk for pulmonary complications) and for men started on BEP who develop signs or symptoms of bleomycin pulmonary toxicity. In addition, because bleomycin is cleared by the kidneys, patients with compromised renal function due to comorbidity or advanced age may be better off receiving EP × 4. For patients with a GFR less than 50 cc/min, bleomycin either should not be used or dose should be reduced as recommended in the package insert. Bleomycin is renally cleared, and patients with renal insufficiency are at high risk of bleomycin pulmonary toxicity.

Correct Answer: A

11) **In which of the following scenarios should etoposide, ifosfamide, and cisplatin (VIP) × 4 most definitively be used instead of bleomycin, etoposide, and cisplatin (BEP) × 4 to treat disseminated germ cell tumors?**
   A) When the patient has brain metastases
   B) When the patient has liver or bone metastases
   C) When the patient has a mediastinal primary nonseminomatous germ cell tumor
   D) When the patient has lung metastases
   E) When patient has moderately severe emphysema

Expert Perspective: BEP × 4 is preferred because it is less toxic, with a lower rate of high-grade hematologic toxicity and a lower incidence of renal failure. However, in two randomized controlled trials, there was no significant difference to treatment-related deaths, overall survival, or other cancer outcomes. For men with a contraindication to bleomycin and for men who develop evidence of bleomycin pulmonary toxicity during treatment, VIP is an alternative therapy that is equally effective. Significant lung disease is a contraindication to bleomycin. In addition, VIP for four cycles is preferred by some but not all centers for men with a primary mediastinal nonseminomatous germ cell tumors because they will require major chest surgery following chemotherapy and exposure to bleomycin would place them at high risk for perioperative pulmonary complications. For the same reason, VIP may be preferred for men with intermediate- or poor-risk nonseminomatous germ cell tumors and bulky lung metastases who are likely to require post-chemotherapy resection of residual masses.

Correct Answer: E

12) **How does the risk stratification according to the International Germ Cell Consensus (IGCC) Classification affect the treatment selection in germ cell tumors?**

Expert Perspective:

Seminoma: Based on the IGCC classification, all seminomas are considered good risk except for those with visceral (nonpulmonary) metastases, which are considered intermediate risk. There is no poor-risk seminoma (Table 35.4). However, recent data indicates that men with good-risk seminomas with a serum LDH greater than 2.5 times the upper limit of normal have a similar prognosis as those with intermediate-risk disease. Whether an LDH greater than 2.5 times the upper limit of normal at the start of chemotherapy should be an indication to give more than three cycles of BEP (i.e. BEP × 4 or BEP × 3 plus EP × 1) remains controversial in the absence of a trial investigating this question.

   Seminoma Treatment: According to current guidelines, only patients with stage III seminoma who have metastases to organs other than the lungs are considered intermediate risk and should be treated with BEP × 4 or VIP × 4. Patients with good-risk seminoma are treated with BEP × 3 (or EP × 4). Some centers treat good-risk patients with an LDH > 2.5 × ULN with BEP × 3 plus a fourth cycle using EP, but this is controversial.

   Nonseminoma: Having intermediate-risk serum tumor markers (S2) in the absence of nonpulmonary visceral metastases is classified as intermediate-risk nonseminoma. Patients with mediastinal primary site or those with poor-risk serum tumor markers (S3) or those with nonpulmonary visceral metastases are considered poor risk.

Table 35.4 IGCC risk stratification.

Seminoma	**Good risk**
	Metastases limited to lymph nodes and/or lungs
	Intermediate risk
	Presence of metastases to organs other than the lungs (e.g. liver or bone)
Nonseminoma	**Good risk**
	Testis/retroperitoneal primary and good-risk tumor markers (S1) and no metastases to organs other than the lungs
	Intermediate risk
	Testis/retroperitoneal primary and intermediate serum tumor markers (S2) and no metastases to organs other than the lungs
	Poor risk
	Mediastinal primary site or metastases to organs other than the lungs or poor-risk serum tumor markers (S3)

Nonseminoma Treatment: Patients with good-risk nonseminoma should receive BEP × 3 (or EP × 4). Patients with intermediate or poor-risk nonseminoma should receive BEP × 4 or VIP × 4.

13) Should men with brain metastases be treated with whole-brain radiation therapy?

Expert Perspective: Brain metastases from gonadal and extragonadal germ cell tumors in men are rare, and there are no trials that inform us about optimal management. Brain MRI for evaluation should be considered in patients with β-hCG > 5,000 IU/L, non-pulmonary visceral metastases, extensive lung metastasis, AFP > 10,000 ng/mL, and those with neurological symptoms. In practice, systemic chemotherapy is the primary treatment of brain metastases in germ cell tumors in men. Most brain tumors occur in the setting of widespread metastatic disease, and in the absence of a neurological emergency necessitating local therapy first, the initial treatment is typically four cycles of BEP chemotherapy. If there is a residual mass, then resection is preferred when feasible to resect chemo-resistant and potentially radiation-resistant tumor. When surgery is not feasible, stereotactic radiosurgery should be considered. Whole-brain radiation should be reserved for patients with multiple residual tumors or an extensive solitary residual mass not amenable to stereotactic radiosurgery.

14) If a man has reduced renal function, should carboplatin be substituted for cisplatin?

Expert Perspective: With rare exceptions, carboplatin should not be substituted for cisplatin, because randomized controlled trials have demonstrated that cisplatin results in superior outcomes. When carboplatin was substituted for cisplatin in BEP chemotherapy, the number of deaths doubled in one trial and quadrupled in another. When etoposide plus carboplatin was compared to etoposide plus cisplatin, there were four times as many relapses in the carboplatin arm. In general, the thinking is that it is better to be alive with renal failure (after cisplatin) than dead with normal kidneys (after carboplatin). However, even though carboplatin is not as effective as cisplatin, it is still highly effective. For instance, among good-risk patients with normal renal function who are treated with four cycles of etoposide and carboplatin for metastatic disease, fewer than 20% relapse.

Men with disseminated germ cell tumor and renal insufficiency should be referred to centers with extensive experience with treating testis cancer, and they should be treated with cisplatin and etoposide. There are case reports of administration of full-dose cisplatin and etoposide to patients on hemodialysis. For patients with intermediate- or poor-risk disease, VIP is the preferred regimen in the setting of renal failure, but there is little data to guide the management of these patients.

15) **If a patient is receiving chemotherapy for a germ cell tumor, under which circumstances should you delay chemotherapy and/or reduce the dose?**
   A) When the neutrophil count is less than $1,000/mm^3$
   B) When the platelet count is less than $50,000/mm^3$
   C) When the creatinine is above 1.7 mg/dL
   D) When the patient has febrile neutropenia

Expert Perspective: Febrile neutropenia represents a clear reason to delay chemotherapy and to consider a dose reduction for subsequent cycles (etoposide, ifosfamide, and paclitaxel doses should be reduced by 20% if dose reducing, but the cisplatin dose should not be reduced). An alternative to dose reduction in this setting is to add a granulocyte colony-stimulating factor to subsequent cycles if it was not used in the cycle complicated by febrile neutropenia. Thrombocytopenic bleeding is also an indication to reduce doses for subsequent cycles. Chemotherapy doses should not be delayed due to myelosuppression alone. Generally, no dose adjustments are indicated for a serum creatine less than 2.0 mg/dL, but switching to a non-bleomycin regimen should be considered for patients with compromised renal function. See Question 8 for additional information on chemotherapy in the setting of renal failure.

Second-line therapy

16) **What is the preferred second-line chemotherapy regimen?**
   A) Vinblastine, ifosfamide, and cisplatin (VeIP)
   B) Paclitaxel, ifosfamide, and cisplatin (TIP)
   C) Two cycles of high-dose carboplatin and etoposide
   D) Any of the above

Expert Perspective: Data support all three of these regimens, and there is no persuasive evidence that one is better than the others. However, for most centers, four cycles of either vinblastine, ifosfamide, and cisplatin or paclitaxel, ifosfamide, and cisplatin represent the best option. Although promising results have been reported for tandem cycles of high-dose carboplatin and etoposide, these data come from a center where hematopoietic stem cell collection and subsequent high-dose chemotherapy could begin almost immediately without the need to give cycles of standard-dose chemotherapy while waiting for insurance approval for stem cell transplantation. At most centers, there is a substantial delay involved in waiting for insurance approval and scheduling pheresis, and patients typically receive several cycles of paclitaxel, ifosfamide, and cisplatin or vinblastine, ifosfamide, and cisplatin while waiting, which can make them less fit for high-dose chemotherapy. It is not clear that the exciting single-center results of high-dose carboplatin and etoposide can be replicated elsewhere at this time. The role of high-dose chemotherapy as salvage therapy is currently being investigated in an international randomized controlled trial.

Correct Answer: D

Recommended Readings

Beyer, J. et al. (2013). Maintaining success, reducing treatment burden, focusing on survivorship: highlights from the third European consensus conference on diagnosis and treatment of germ-cell cancer. *Ann Oncol* 24 (4): 878–888. PMID: 23152360.

Culine, S. et al. (2007). Refining the optimal chemotherapy regimen for good-risk metastatic nonseminomatous germ-cell tumors: a randomized trial of the Genito-urinary group of the french federation of cancer centers (GETUG T93BP). *Ann Oncol* 18 (5): 917–924. PMID: 17351252.

Einhorn, L.H. et al. (2007). High-dose chemotherapy and stem-cell rescue for metastatic germ-cell tumors. *N Engl J Med* 357 (4): 340–348. PMID: 17652649.

Gilligan, T. et al. (2019). Testicular cancer, Version 2.2020, NCCN clinical practice guidelines in oncology. *J Natl Compr Canc Netw* 17 (12): 1529–1554. PMID: 31805523.

Gilligan, T.D. et al. (2010). American society of clinical oncology clinical practice guideline on uses of serum tumor markers in adult males with germ cell tumors. *J Clin Oncol* 28 (20): 3388–3404. PMID: 20530278.

Honecker, F. et al. (2018). ESMO consensus conference on testicular germ cell cancer: diagnosis, treatment and follow-up. *Ann Oncol* 29 (8): 1658–1686. PMID: 30113631.

Oldenburg, J. et al. (2013). Testicular seminoma and non-seminoma: ESMO clinical practice guidelines for diagnosis, treatment and follow-up. *Ann Oncol* 24 (Suppl 6): vi125–32. PMID: 24078656.

Sanchez, V.A., Shuey, M.M., Dinh, P.C. Jr, et al. (2023 April 20). Patient-reported functional impairment due to hearing loss and tinnitus after cisplatin-based chemotherapy. *J Clin Oncol* 41 (12): 2211–2226. https://doi.org/10.1200/JCO.22.01456. Epub 2023 Jan 10. PMID: 36626694.

Schmoll, H.J. et al. (2010a). Testicular seminoma: ESMO clinical practice guidelines for diagnosis, treatment and follow-up. *Ann Oncol* 21 (Suppl 5): v140–v146. PMID: 20555065.

Schmoll, H.J. et al. (2010b). Testicular non-seminoma: ESMO clinical practice guidelines for diagnosis, treatment and follow-up. *Ann Oncol* 21 (Suppl 5): v147–v154. PMID: 20555066.

Stephenson, A. et al. (2019). Diagnosis and treatment of early stage testicular cancer: AUA guideline. *J Urol* 202 (2): 272–281. PMID: 31059667.

Part 6

Skin Malignancies

36

Melanoma

Ana M. Ciurea[1] and Kim Margolin[2]

[1] The University of Texas MD Anderson Cancer Center, Houston, TX
[2] St. John's Cancer Institute, Santa Monica, CA

Introduction

Melanoma is currently the fifth most common cancer in the United States, resulting in more than 7,000 deaths each year. The incidence of melanoma continues to rise and is the leading cause of death from cutaneous malignancies, accounting for 1–2% of all cancer deaths in the United States. Melanoma affects all age groups, with a median age at diagnosis of 63; however, melanoma is the most common cancer in young adults aged 25–29. Risk factors for melanoma include sun exposure, dysplastic (atypical) nevi, increased number of benign nevi, family history of melanoma, and skin type with tendency to burn. Germline mutation in the *CDKN2A* gene is the most common cause of familial or inherited melanoma. However, sporadic melanomas represent the majority of melanomas (Chapter 45). The melanoma field has seen an unprecedented set of clinical advances over the past decade, which transformed management of the disease. However, despite numerous advances in the management of advanced melanoma, the cornerstone to ensuring a cure remains early detection. The outcome is highly dependent on the stage of the disease; primary cutaneous early melanoma, when excised appropriately, is highly curable, whereas metastatic melanoma comes with an extremely poor prognosis despite contemporary treatment. Studies have led to the development of immunotherapy using checkpoint inhibitors and LAG-3 inhibitors (e.g. relatlimab) and targeted therapy (*BRAF* plus *MEK* inhibitors). Both checkpoint inhibitor immunotherapy and targeted therapy prolong progression-free and overall survival (OS) compared with chemotherapy.

Case Study 1

1) A 31-year-old man with multiple freckles, history of two invasive melanoma, and a family history of melanoma in parents and sister is concerned about hereditary melanoma. In discussing with the patient, which genetic mutation is highly likely to be detected upon testing?
   A) TERT.
   B) CDK4.
   C) CNKN2A.
   D) BAP-1.

Expert Perspective: Melanoma pathogenesis is complex and heterogeneous, with genetic, phenotypic, and environmental factors contributing to its development. The main risk factors involved in the pathogenesis of cutaneous melanoma are phenotypic factors (light skin, eyes and hair, inability to tan, burns easily), a large number of common acquired melanocytic nevi (>50), atypical melanocytic nevi (>5), exposure to ultraviolet radiation, and personal and family history of melanoma. Familial melanoma is defined as a family in which either two first-degree relatives or three or more melanoma patients on the same side of the family (irrespective of degree of relationship) are diagnosed with melanoma (Chapter 45). Familial melanoma accounts for approximately 5–14% of all melanoma cases. Melanoma is not linked to a single gene, but several high- and intermediate-penetrance melanoma susceptibility genes have been identified to date. Germline susceptibility has been associated with mutations in high-penetrance melanoma predisposition genes, *CDKN2A* (cyclin-dependent kinase 2A), and less frequently in *CDK4* (cyclin-dependent kinase 4), *BRCA-1* associated protein-1 (*BAP1*, breast cancer associated protein-1), *TERT* (telomerase reverse transcriptase), and *POT1* (protection of telomeres 1), or with variants in intermediate-risk genes, MC1R (melanocortin 1 receptor) and *MITF* (microphthalmia-associated transcription factor) (Chapter 46). The most commonly known melanoma genetic mutation is *CDKN2A* (p16INK4a), which accounts for approximately 20–50% of familial melanoma cases. Mutated gene shows impaired capacity to inhibit the cyclin D1-*CDK4* complex, allowing for unchecked cell cycle progression. Mutations in *CDK4* are extremely rare and manifest by impairing the inhibitory interaction with p16INK4a. *BAP1* mutations predisposes to uveal/cutaneous melanoma, atypical melanocytic tumors, meningioma, and other internal malignancies (renal cell carcinoma, cholangiocarcinoma, basal cell carcinoma). It enhances the metastatic potential of uveal melanoma, a distinct variant in which mutations in *BRAF, NRAS,* and *KIT* are rarely, if ever, seen. This variant of melanoma more often has *BAP1* (increased risk of metastasis and worsened prognosis), *GNAQ, GNA11, SF3B1*, and *EIF1AX. ERT* and *POT1* mutations are associated with melanoma via uncertain mechanisms. Genes involved in the melanoma biosynthetic pathway (*MITF* [microphthalmia-associated transcription factor] and MC1R [MelanoCortin-1 receptor]) have been implicated in melanoma development likely due to accumulation of pheomelanin, which appears to have a carcinogenic effect regardless of ultraviolet exposure.

Correct Answer: C

2) Should this patient see a genetic counselor?

Expert Perspective: Yes. Identification of patients with a germline mutation predisposing to cancer enables genetic testing and counseling of patients, family members, and appropriate surveillance, reducing morbidity and mortality in this patient population. However, no widely accepted guidelines for management of families with hereditary melanoma risk have been developed. Genetic testing for high-penetrance melanoma susceptibility genes should be considered when a patient has a personal or family history of cancer. Prior to testing, adequate pre- and post-test counseling including risk assessment, the potential impact of which involves complex factors related to having increased risk without risk-reducing intervention, with possible effects on family members, insurance coverage, and concerns regarding confidentiality should be addressed.

3) How can one best manage subjects with *CDKN2A* mutation?

Expert Perspective: Carriers of a *CDKN2A* mutation are at high risk of developing multiple melanomas and, in some families, pancreatic cancer. The identification of a deleterious *CDKN2A* mutation suggests that carriers should be included in intensive skin surveillance programs with complete skin examination performed every 3–12 months, planned on the basis of the patient's risk factors; digital dermoscopy and clinical photography are highly recommended for monitoring these patients. With regard to pancreatic cancer, patients should be aware of the current lack of effective screening guidelines. Overall, *CDKN2A* carriers are candidates for annual pancreatic cancer screening via endoscopic ultrasonography or magnetic resonance cholangiopancreatography (Chapter 47). The recommendation of avoiding tobacco has been suggested for germline *CDKN2A* mutation carriers. It is also prudent for children from familial melanoma kindreds to undergo routine skin examinations beginning at puberty.

Case Study 2

A 45-year-old woman was referred to dermatology clinic for surveillance due to history of melanoma, multiple atypical nevi, and tanning bed use.

4) Which of the following diagnostic techniques is the most useful in the diagnosis of melanoma?
   A) Dermoscopy.
   B) *In vivo* reflectance confocal microscopy.
   C) Electrical impedance spectroscopy.
   D) Total body photography.

Expert Perspective: Dermoscopy (dermatoscopy, epiluminescence microscopy) is an established *in vivo*, noninvasive tool that has been shown to significantly improve the diagnosis of several skin disorders including tumors. The procedure allows for the visualization of skin structures in the epidermis, at the dermoepidermal junction and the upper dermis; these structures are not usually visible to the naked eye. The images can be photographed and stored digitally for sequential analysis. The visualization of colors and structures in the epidermis and papillary dermis has generated a new terminology for the morphologic description of skin lesions. A histologic correlation has been established for most of the structures seen with dermoscopy. Melanoma detection remains the most important indication of dermoscopy. The discipline of dermoscopy has improved the detection of melanoma and other skin cancers, which has resulted in the detection of thinner melanomas. Moreover, it has helped improve the ability to differentiate benign nevi from melanomas, which has resulted in fewer biopsies and excisions of benign cutaneous lesions. In the last few years, three meta-analyses and two randomized studies have definitely proven that dermoscopy allows improving sensitivity for melanoma compared with the naked eye examination alone. Reflectance confocal microscopy (RCM) is one of the most studied diagnostic methods that are emerging in the field of melanoma imaging. It allows dynamic imaging of the skin at cellular resolution in real time, akin to an optical biopsy. Most probably in the future, RCM will be more frequently available in tertiary referral centers. In electrical impedance spectroscopy, the varying electrical properties of human tissue are used to categorize cellular structures and thereby detect malignancies. The system is designed to be used when a clinician chooses to obtain additional information when considering excisions. Total body photography (TBP) can facilitate the detection of melanoma in high-risk individuals. However, the accuracy of TBP in diagnosing melanoma remains unclear. None of these imaging tools is meant to be used to confirm a clinical diagnosis of melanoma which can only be achieved with histologic analysis.

Correct Answer: A

Case Study 3

A 62-year-old woman with a history of stage IV melanoma, *BRAF V600E* tumor mutation positive, is undergoing treatment with vemurafenib and cobimetinib treatment for three weeks. She presents with rapidly progressing diffuse erythema involving the oral mucosa, lips, scalp, face, trunk, and lower legs and 2 cm flaccid nontender bullae on the back. Patient denies fever, malaise, or loss of appetite.

5) What is the most likely diagnosis?
 A) Disseminated zoster.
 B) Bullous drug hypersensitivity eruption.
 C) Toxic epidermal necrolysis.
 D) Staphylococcal scalded skin syndrome.
 E) Drug rash with eosinophilia and systemic symptoms.

Expert Perspective: *BRAF* and *MEK* inhibitors (*BRAF/MEK*i) are a standard of care in patients with *BRAF*-mutated metastatic melanomas. Combination *BRAF* and *MEK* inhibition results in improved outcomes compared to single-agent *BRAF* inhibition. These agents are usually administered until disease progression or unacceptable toxicity occurs. *BRAF* and *MEK* inhibitors have been associated with life-threatening adverse cutaneous reactions, including toxic epidermal necrolysis (TEN), Steven-Johnson syndrome (SJS), drug rash with eosinophilia and systemic symptoms (DRESS), acute generalized exanthematous pustulosis (AGEP), and generalized bullous fixed eruption (GBFE). These drug reactions often require hospitalization and could be fatal. The onset of the skin adverse reaction is 9.3 days, and full resolution of symptoms occurs usually in 10–14 days. The immune checkpoint inhibitors (ipilimumab, pembrolizumab) may predispose patients to drug hypersensitivity reactions implicated in SJS/TEN in patients treated with *BRAF-MEK* inhibitors (Chapter 50). Although the discontinuation of the offending drug is the mainstay treatment of these life-threatening complications, continuing treatment of metastatic melanoma is also critical. It is suggested that switching the *BRAF* inhibitor to a different drug of the same class may not lead to cross-reactivity. A prompt dermatologic evaluation is necessary in order to achieve proper diagnosis and management of these severe cutaneous toxicities in patients undergoing targeted therapy with *BRAF-MEK* inhibitors.

Correct Answer: C

6) Which cutaneous immune-related, adverse event occurs most commonly in patients treated with immune checkpoint inhibitors?
   A) Lichenoid drug eruption.
   B) Psoriasis.
   C) Hypersensitivity drug eruption (maculopapular rash).
   D) Pruritus (correct answer).
   E) Vitiligo.

Expert Perspective: Checkpoint inhibitors can cause a wide-spectrum immune-related adverse event due to their triggering cytotoxic CD4+/CD8+ cytotoxic T-cell activation. More than 60% of patients develop these adverse events, which theoretically can involve any organ. Dermatological toxicities are the most common immune related adverse effects in modern cancer immunotherapy.

Nonspecific immune activation may lead to immune-related adverse events, wherein the skin and its appendages are the most frequent targets. Cutaneous immune-related adverse events include a diverse group of inflammatory reactions, with maculopapular rash, pruritus, psoriasiform and lichenoid eruptions being the most prevalent subtypes. These reactions occur early, with maculopapular rash presenting within the first six weeks after the initial immune checkpoint inhibitor dose. Management involves the use of topical corticosteroids for mild to moderate (grades 1–2) rash, addition of systemic corticosteroids for severe (grade 3) rash, and discontinuation of immunotherapy with grade 4 rash. Of interest, cutaneous immune-related adverse event may occur with a median time of 13.3 months.

The treatment of bullous pemphigoid eruptions is similar to the treatment of maculopapular rash and lichenoid eruptions, with the addition of rituximab in grade 3 and 4 rashes. Skin hypopigmentation/depigmentation does not require specific dermatologic treatment aside from photoprotective measures. In addition to topical corticosteroids, psoriasiform dermatitis may be managed with vitamin D3 analogues, narrowband ultraviolet B-light phototherapy, retinoids, or immunomodulatory biologic agents. Stevens-Johnson syndrome and toxic epidermal necrolysis require inpatient care as well as urgent dermatology consultation. (Also refer to Chapter 50.)

Correct Answer: C

Staging in Melanoma

7) Which statement about the AJCC 8th edition for melanoma is correct?
   A) The tumor mitotic rate is not incorporated into melanoma staging system for the primary tumor.
   B) Ulceration is not used to define patient subsets for tumor thickness.
   C) Regional lymph node involvement is classified as either "microscopic" or "macroscopic."
   D) Serum LDH level is not part of the staging system.

Expert Perspective: Although little has changed over the past decade in the surgical practice of melanoma management, there is a new staging system, AJCC 8, that improves on AJCC 7 by recognizing and fine-tuning the relationship between prognosis and assigned stage. AJCC 8 was widely adopted for use in clinical practice and trials, but it remains suboptimal in lacking the power to distinguish prognostic substages that account for substantial differences in the outcome of patients in each stage. Although the tumor mitotic rate is not incorporated into melanoma staging system for the primary tumor, it remains a significant prognostic factor within all tumor thickness categories, and it should be assessed and recorded in all primary melanomas. Ulceration is defined as the absence of an intact epithelium over the melanoma. It is used to define patient subsets for each tumor thickness group. Regional lymph node involvement is classified as either "clinically occult" (found microscopically, usually based upon a sentinel lymph node biopsy) or "clinically detected" (on physical examination or by imaging). Serum LDH is an important independent prognostic factor in patients with disseminated melanoma and is part of staging system (Table 36.1).

Correct Answer: A

8) Which of the following statements about stages of melanoma is/are correct?
    A) Stage I disease does not present with an ulcerated tumor.
    B) Stage II disease may have presence of in-transit or satellite metastases in regional lymph nodes.
    C) Stage III disease includes pathologically documented involvement of regional lymph nodes.
    D) All of the above.

Expert Perspective: Stage I melanoma is limited to patients with low-risk primary melanomas (T1a, T1b, and T2a) without evidence of regional or distant metastases. Stage II disease includes primary tumors that are at higher risk of recurrence (T2b, T3a, T3b, T4a, and T4b) but do not have any evidence of lymphatic disease or distant metastases. Stage III disease includes pathologically documented involvement of regional lymph nodes and/or the presence of in-transit or satellite metastases (incorporated using N subcategory). Patients with stage III disease are substaged as having stage IIIA, IIIB, IIIC, or IIID disease (Table 36.1).

Correct Answer: C

Adjuvant and Neoadjuvant Therapy

9) What is the role of completion lymph node dissection in patients with positive sentinel lymph node biopsy?

Expert Perspective: Surgical practice and some of the statistical assumptions now forming the basis of surgical adjuvant trials have been most heavily impacted by the results of the MSLT-I and MSLT-II trials, which were essentially designed to test the impact – predominantly on overall survival, but secondarily on locoregional control – of reducing the amount of surgery that is routinely used to both stage and treat microscopic nodal disease in patients with early stage disease.

- The MSLT-I trial demonstrated that sentinel lymph node biopsy itself did not enhance the survival for the entire population of early stage melanoma patients when studied in a proper "intent-to-treat" fashion. However, when only those patients with node-positivity

Table 36.1 AJCC 8th edition melanoma TNM* definitions.

TNM	Description	
T category	Thickness	Ulceration
T1a	<0.8 mm	—
T1b	<0.8 mm	+
	0.8 to 1 mm	+/−
T2a	>1 to 2 mm	—
T2b	>1 to 2 mm	+
T3a	>2 to 4 mm	—
T3b	>2 to 4 mm	+
T4a	>4 mm	—
T4b	>4 mm	+
N category	Number of tumor-involved regional lymph nodes	Presence of in-transit, satellite, and/or microsatellite metastases
N1a	One clinically occult (i.e. detected by sentinel lymph node biopsy)	No
N1b	One clinically detected	No
N1c	No regional lymph node disease	Yes
N2a	Two or three clinically occult (i.e. detected by sentinel lymph node biopsy)	No
N2b	Two or three, at least one of which was clinically detected	No
N2c	One clinically occult or clinically detected	Yes
N3a	Four or more clinically occult (i.e. detected by sentinel lymph node biopsy)	No
N3b	Four or more, at least one of which was clinically detected, or presence of any number of matted nodes	No
N3c	Two or more clinically occult or clinically detected and/or presence of any number of matted nodes	Yes
M category	Location	LDH
M1a	Distant metastasis to skin, soft tissue including muscle, and/or nonregional lymph node	Not recorded
-M1a(0)		Not elevated
-M1a(1)		Elevated
M1b	Distant metastasis to lung with or without M1a sites of disease	Not recorded
-M1b(0)		Not elevated
-M1b(1)		Elevated

(Continued)

Table 36.1 (Continued)

M category	Location	LDH
M1c	Distant metastasis to non-CNS visceral sites with or without M1a or M1b sites of disease	Not recorded
-M1c(0)		Not elevated
-M1c(1)		Elevated
M1d	Distant metastasis to CNS with or without M1a, M1b, or M1c sites of disease	Not recorded
-M1d(0)		Not elevated
-M1d(1)		Elevated

* Tumor, node, metastasis.

were considered – either at the time of sentinel lymph node biopsy or later, at the time of clinical/macroscopic nodal relapse – the survival was superior for those whose nodal involvement had been diagnosed by sentinel lymph node biopsy. Delayed therapeutic lymph node dissection did not control melanoma as well as removal of microscopically positive disease. Thus, a procedure that did not improve overall population survival and certainly carried some morbidity remained the standard for all (except those with the shallowest and ulceration-negative melanomas) patients while benefiting only a small subset of patients.

- In the MSLT-II trial, the benefit of completion lymph node dissection was studied. Patients with one or more positive sentinel lymph node biopsies were randomized between completion lymph node dissection and observation with close surveillance consisting of frequent (every four months) ultrasound examinations of the pertinent nodal bed. This trial too was negative for a survival benefit from completion lymph node dissection – and it was reported nearly simultaneously with the results of an almost identical multicenter German Dermatologic Cooperative Oncology Group trial (DeCOG; n = 483) – but in this case, the trial results set a new standard for sentinel lymph node biopsy-positive melanoma, which was to forgo the completion lymph node dissection in favor of close ultrasonograpic surveillance and to perform therapeutic lymph node dissection for only those patients who relapse.

Patients benefit by fewer days of recovery from surgical procedures and avoidance of the morbidities of completion lymph node dissection, particularly the frequent bacterial infections complicating lymph node dissection and the high rate of often-irreversible lymphedema following the procedure. The adjuvant therapy decision is thus based on the initial sentinel lymph node biopsy findings. Replacing the nodal US (ultrasound) with other forms of surveillance such as PET-CT, often performed more frequently than once a year in patients at particularly high risk of distant relapse, is not recommended because the nodal US in the hands of experienced radiologists is believed to be both more sensitive and more specific.

10) Which agents are FDA approved for adjuvant therapy in melanoma?

Expert Perspective: Currently used adjuvant systemic therapies were based on the drugs with the highest activity in advanced melanoma and a favorable therapeutic index. Patient characteristics such as age, comorbidities, *BRAF V600E/K*, and treatment preferences influence the choice of therapy. Dabrafenib plus trametinib in patients with *BRAF V600E/K* mutation (COMBI-AD study), nivolumab (CheckMate 238), and pembrolizumab (KEYNOTE 054/EORTC1325) are acceptable adjuvant therapies for stage III B/C/D disease. Adjuvant therapy for stage IIIA melanoma is not recommended if the nodal involvement is a single-focus and < 1 mm in diameter, while intervention remains controversial for stage IIIA with greater involvement of the node. Ipilimumab (EGOG 1609 and EORTC 18071) is approved by the FDA but is not used due to superior alternate options. Pembrolizumab is also approved as adjuvant therapy for up to approximately one-year for stage IIB or IIC melanoma (KEYNOTE 716). Also, nivolimab is approved for adjuvant treatment of completely resected stage IIB or IIC melanoma (CheckMate -76K study). For patients with stage IV disease, regardless of *BRAF V600E/K* mutation status, who have undergone definitive treatment of all sites of disease with either surgery or radiation therapy, adjuvant therapy of nivolumab. The data from a small randomized study (IMUNED) of adjuvant nivolimab plus ipilimumab at standard doses showed twice as great a relpase-free survival benefit for combination (HR 0.56) as for nivolimab (HR 0.23) when compared to placebo, at a cost of higher toxicity a subsequent trial (CheckMate 915) nivolumab showed efficacy consistent with previous adjuvant studies reaffirming nivolumab as a standard of care for melanoma adjuvant treatment.

11) What is the overarching theme of adjuvant therapy in melanoma?

Expert Perspective: By the time interferon-alpha (IFNα) was discarded as inactive (without survival benefit) and excessively toxic in both in the adjuvant setting (as single agent) and for advanced disease (in complex combinations termed "bio chemotherapy"), the immune checkpoint blocking antibodies had established their activity and tolerability in advanced melanoma as well as some other malignancies. At the present time, PD-1–blocking antibodies such as nivolumab and pembrolizumab have firmly established roles in the adjuvant treatment of high-risk melanoma (indications discussed in Question 10). These agents are generally given at the same dose and schedule that are used for metastatic melanoma, and their activity, expressed by the hazard ratio for relapse-free survival in treated patient versus those randomized to placebo or observation, is associated with a reduction in relapse rates ranging from 25 to 50%.

In addition to the evidence that can be used effectively as adjuvant therapy in high-risk stage III disease, similar benefits have been shown in combination with small-molecule agents targeting the mitogen-activated protein (MAP) kinase pathway which are activated by *BRAF V600E/K* mutations and further enhanced by downstream *Mitogen-activated protein kinase kinase (MEK)*. The adjuvant therapy data with targeted agents appear almost identical to those of the immune checkpoint blocking antibodies (including the lack of benefit for stage IIIA patients with nodal involvement Breslow depth < 1 mm in diameter), and the decision about how to select the optimal adjuvant therapy for patients with targetable *BRAF* mutant melanoma remains to be further investigated in studies that are carefully designed to stratify for important clinical factors and to test for the presence of biomarkers that will reveal tumor and host parameters with predictive impact on the relapse-free survival and OS outcomes. Patterns of toxicity, particularly regarding irreversible effects of immunotherapy, and responsiveness to treatment of relapse for those not benefiting from adjuvant therapy will also be important endpoints for comparative studies.

12) What are the principles and uncertainties for the treatment of high-risk stage IIB/C (without nodal disease) melanoma?

Expert Perspective: Recent trial randomizing patients with resected stage IIB and IIC melanoma demonstrated the relapse-free survival benefit of adjuvant pembrolizumab (see Question 10), given in the same dose and schedule as for advanced disease. Most recently, nivolumab demonstrated a statistically significant improvement in recurrence-free survival compared to placebo (CheckMate -76K). It remains to be seen, as for all of the adjuvant trials of current-day therapies, whether there is an overall survival benefit. It has been difficult to show a survival benefit for adjuvant interventions to date because patients who relapse are currently treated with essentially the same classes of drugs for metastatic disease as those used for adjuvant therapy, so the advantage of early therapy is not yet proven. Adjuvant therapy is not indicated in patient with stage I and stage IIA.

13) What is the role of neoadjuvant therapy in melanoma?

Expert Perspective: Neoadjuvant systemic therapy has been used for many other malignancies with favorable outcomes and is considered standard in rectal cancer, selected sarcomas, subsets of breast cancer, and a growing number of less common tumors, such as Merkel cell carcinoma (Chapter 37). More recent studies in melanoma, primarily resectable but bulky nodal disease, have shown very high response rates, including pathologic complete, near complete, and partial responses. A recent randomized trial of pembrolizumab given either as neodjuvant therapy for 3 cycles followed by surgery and then followed by 15 more cycles versus all 18 cycles given as adjuvant therapy demonstrated a significant relapse-free survival in favor of sandwich approach (HR 0.58).

14) What is the surveillance protocol during and after curative therapy?

Expert Perspective: Surveillance of patients during and after adjuvant therapy is generally recommended at intervals that reflect the risk of relapse over time, which follows an inverted S-shaped curve with plateaus that look different for different stages (paradoxically, the plateaus are reached more quickly in higher-stage disease, whereas the shape of the relapse versus time curve for early stage melanoma falls slowly and steadily with a later plateau). Higher-risk patients are generally examined and imaged more often than lower-risk patients, and the extent of such surveillance is also based on the disease stage prior to adjuvant therapy.

Although guidelines for the type and precise frequency of surveillance are based on retrospective data and educated guess, it is customary to restage patients approximately once or twice during the year of adjuvant therapy and then use any one of a number of published guidelines to select the surveillance plan going forward, usually consisting of physician examinations every few months and scanning (contrast CT or ^{18}FDG-PET-CT without iodinated contrast) yearly for about five years. Imaging of the brain (MRI with gadolinium contrast) should be considered at the time of yearly surveillance scans, particularly for patients who were originally high-risk, because brain metastases are common in patients with melanoma, even occurring in a small percentage of patients as the first and/or only site of metastatic disease.

Advanced Melanoma

The last decade has seen a major paradigm shift, with melanoma leading the way, in the treatment of immunoresponsive tumors. Melanoma patients have also benefited from the identification of driver oncogenes and targetable mutations, although to a degree far less than some other malignancies, notably lung cancers. The result has been a dramatic improvement of relapse-free and OS and has also pushed the field forward in the development of new immunotherapy strategies and treatments for a wider range of molecular targets.

In patients without a targetable oncogenic driver mutation, *BRAF* (specifically *V600E/K* mutants) is the only targetable mutation in melanoma so far, with three approved *BRAF V600E/K* plus *MEK* inhibitor combinations. The major therapy decision for patients who cannot enroll in a clinical trial of frontline therapy is whether to use (a) single-agent PD-1 blockade, nivolumab (CheckMate 066) or pembrolizumab (KEYNOTE 006) or (b) combination CTLA-4 plus PD-1 blockade as first-line therapy (CheckMate 069). In favor of the former is its low toxicity (low incidence of immune-related adverse events, occasionally requiring steroid, other immunosuppressants, or, rarely, discontinuation of therapy), whereas the latter regimen has a higher response rate (approximately 55%) with higher toxicity therefore appears most applicable to patients with unfavorable tumor features including low expression of PD-L1 or presence of a *BRAF* mutation.

15) Is there a relationship between the development of one or more immune-related toxicities and the likelihood of response in melanoma?

Expert Perspective: There is a strong but not guaranteed relationship between the development of one or more immune-related toxicities and the likelihood of response to therapy. Regimens designed to reduce toxicity and retain therapeutic activity are clearly needed, and so far, the only regimen that appears to meet these needs is the so-called flipped dose ipilimumab plus nivolumab, in which the doses of ipilimumab and nivolumab during the initial four-cycle induction period are reversed (ipilimumab 1 mg/kg and nivolumab 3 mg/kg), and the subsequent maintenance nivolumab is given at the original dose of 3 mg/kg.

16) Which statement about the combination therapy of *BRAF V600E/K* plus *MEK−* inhibitors is/are correct?
   A) Dabrafenib plus trametinib is superior to encorafenib plus binimetinib.
   B) Vemurafenib plus cobimetinib is superior to dabrafenib plus trametinib.
   C) Cardiomyopathy has been identified in patients treated with *MEK* inhibitors.
   D) Dabrafenib can cause hemolytic anemia.
   E) C and D.

Expert Perspective: Treatment of advanced melanoma with mitogen-activated protein kinase *MAPK* inhibitors evolved from inhibition of a single protein, the mutated *BRAF*, to inhibition of mutant *BRAF V600E/K* and hyperactivated downstream *MEK-* double inhibition. Three pairs of *BRAF V600E/K* plus *MEK* inhibitors are available (dabrafenib plus trametinib, encorafenib plus binimetinib, and vemurafenib plus cobimetinib [coBRIM study]) with similar antitumor activity (overall response rates of about 70%) and minimally varying toxicity spectra. There are, however, a few dose-limiting toxicities that dictate the selection and potential changes in *MAPK*-directed therapy. Cardiomyopathy has been identified in patients treated with *MEK* inhibitors. Patients receiving *MEK* inhibitors should undergo assessment of left ventricular ejection fraction prior to initiation of and during therapy. Also, risk of reversible central serous retinopathy from *MEK* inhibitors should be monitored by pretreatment and periodic eye exams while on therapy. Prolongation of the QTc interval can occur with administration of the *BRAF* inhibitors, vemurafenib and encorafenib. Dabrafenib should be avoided in patients with glucose-6-phosphate dehydrogenase deficiency due to hemolytic anemia.

Correct Answer: E

17) What are the advances and limitations in treatment of noncutaneous (uveal, acral and mucosal) melanomas? Is there role of imatinib in these patients?

Expert Perspective: On the horizon are new treatments for unique subsets of melanoma such as uveal, which is generally divided into two or more subsets for relapse risk based on patterns of gene expression in the primary. Uveal melanoma has a strong propensity to metastasize to the liver and is traditionally resistant to all forms of antineoplastic therapy. Remarkably, the investigational bispecific fusion molecule, tebentafusp, which consists of a T-cell receptor specific to gp-100 and restricted by HLA-A-0201 that is fused to an agonistic anti-CD3 antibody, has recently been shown to prolong survival over physician's choice of either dacarbazine or single-agent immune checkpoint blockade for patients with metastatic uveal melanoma (IMCgp100-202) and is FDA approved for metastatic uveal melanoma in patient carrying HLA-A-0201. In addition, HEPZATO KIT (melphalan for Injection/Hepatic Delivery System) containing melphalan is FDA approved as a liver-directed treatment for adult patients with uveal melanoma with unresectable hepatic metastases affecting less than 50% of the liver and no extrahepatic disease, or extrahepatic disease limited to the bone, lymph nodes, subcutaneous tissues, or lung that is amenable to resection or radiation. Although the numbers for subsets of melanoma are small and the studies are not powered to report them separately, it is generally accepted that acral melanoma has a somewhat lower response rate and that mucosal melanoma is substantially less responsive to the therapies used for cutaneous melanoma, so combination immune checkpoint blockade is generally recommended, with the attendant immune-related toxicities (Chapter 50). Of interest, metastatic acral or mucosal melanoma with an activating *c-KIT* mutation in exon 11 and 13 who progress on or are ineligible for immunotherapy are candidates for imatinib.

Case Study 4

A 35-year-old woman undergoes dermatologic and then surgical management of a pathologic stage IIIB (T2b, 1.6 mm with ulceration; N2a, two microscopically involved lymph nodes) cutaneous melanoma on her posterior neck.

18) When considering the selection of adjuvant therapy, which of the following characteristics is recommended in decision-making for this patient?
    A) *BRAF* V600E/K mutation status of the primary.
    B) Number of mitoses per mm^2 on light microscopy.
    C) Tumor mutation burden.
    D) Expression of PD-L1 on tumor.

E) Expression of PD-1 on infiltrating T cells.
F) Size of the nodal micro metastases (< 1 mm or > 1 mm) on light microscopy.

Expert Perspective: This patient is expected to benefit equally by receiving MAPK inhibitors or PD-1 blockade for one year. It is important in discussing and deciding that the BRAF V600E/K status of the tumor be available to the patient and oncologist. The number of mitoses is not clearly associated with predictivity for adjuvant therapy and is no longer used in staging. Tumor mutation burden is not considered in adjuvant therapy recommendations and, in melanoma, does not vary widely across the spectrum of cutaneous primaries. Expression of PD-L1 on tumor and PD-1 on lymphocytes is not predictive of the outcome of adjuvant therapy and is not used to select the type of therapy recommended.

The size of nodal micrometastasis in Na (occult nodal) disease does not contribute to the decision to offer adjuvant therapy when the overall pathologic stage is IIIB or higher (in this case, the ulcerated primary upstaged the lesion to B) and thus the risk of relapse is elevated. To date, all of the features used to select therapy except for the BRAF V600E/K mutation are considered prognostic and not predictive.

Correct Answer: A

Case Study 5

A 40-year-old woman developed lupus following her last pregnancy at age 33 and eventually went on to develop renal failure, requiring dialysis and then a living related donor renal transplant. She remains on tacrolimus and has to be treated once with steroid for an episode of acute rejection. She developed an ulcerated T3 melanoma on her back, underwent sentinel lymph node biopsy, and had two nodes with 3 mm and 4 mm implants of melanoma. The primary tumor has BRAF V600K mutation.

19) What advice should you give her?
 A) Avoid adjuvant therapy, because immunotherapy may cause rejection and MAPK inhibitors will cause nephrotoxicity.
 B) Take MAPK inhibitors, which have the highest activity in the adjuvant setting.
 C) Immunotherapy with a PD-1 antibody has the highest activity in the adjuvant setting, so it is worth taking the risk of losing the kidney.
 D) Immunotherapy and MAPK inhibitor therapy have similar activity in the adjuvant setting, but immunotherapy has a higher likelihood of causing loss of the kidney.
 E) She should undergo a completion lymphadenectomy to improve her survival.

Expert Perspective: This unfortunate patient has a high-risk melanoma that does not appear to have been caused by immunosuppression, because despite all of the recent advances in treating melanoma with immunotherapy, the role of immunodeficiency in enhancing the risk of melanoma is minimal; rather, the nonmelanoma skin cancers, particularly squamous cancer, which is very common, and Merkel cell cancer, which is very rare, are markedly increased in incidence in immunosuppressed individuals (Chapter 37).

In immunocompetent subjects, the hazard ratio of improved relapse-free survival (over no further therapy) attributable to immunotherapy with a PD-1 antibody or MAPK inhibition for BRAF V600E/K mutant melanomas is essentially identical, although the treatments have not been compared head-to-head. It is therefore important to consider toxicities and quality of life issues as well as comorbidities and other medical issues, such as potentially interacting medications, when selecting adjuvant therapy.

In the case of this patient, who requires immunosuppression, there is substantial risk of immunostimulation leading to a rejection episode and possibly even irreversible loss of the transplanted organ and her life. However, there is no absolute or even relative contraindication to the use of *MAPK* inhibitor, which is not nephrotoxic and should not interact with her transplant rejection prophylaxis. Further, any toxicities emerging from the agents used in *MAPK* inhibitor are reversible by holding the dose(s) and adjusting them upon reintroduction.

If the patient relapses, a similar decision between immunotherapy and molecularly targeted therapy will have to be made, but at that point the risk versus benefit ratio of the therapy choices may be different than at the present time, and new agents may also be available.

Correct Answer: D

Case Study 6

A 65-year-old man with a history of shallow T1a, N0, M0 melanoma six years ago presents with palpable adenopathy in the lymph node bed closest to the primary site in the left upper leg. Core needle biopsy shows metastatic melanoma, and genomic analysis reveals mutations of *NRAS* and *hTERT*, while *BRAF* and *KIT* are wild-type. The PET-CT scan shows an equivocal focus of uptake in a node close to the large nodal mass, which has a diameter of 6 cm with an SUV (standardized update value) of 18. The surgical oncologist has determined that based on the proximity to vessels, this mass is borderline resectable.

18) **Which of the following would be consider optimal therapy?**
    A) Proceed with surgical excision of both sites followed by radiotherapy.
    B) Empiric trial of *MAPK* inhibitors followed by surgery if the mass does not regress.
    C) Ipilimumab at decremented dose plus nivolumab plus augmented dose for two cycles, then surgery.
    D) Radiation plus pembrolizumab followed by surgery.
    E) Binimetinib to best response, followed by radiation.

Correct Answer: C

Expert Perspective: Surgery followed by radiotherapy for a large, borderline resectable mass is reasonable in the absence of effective systemic therapies but has decreased its appeal with the advent of highly-active immunotherapy. *MAPK* inhibitors do not have sufficient activity in patients without a *BRAF V600E/K* activating mutation and in patients without *V600E/K* mutant *BRAF* and should not be used. Moreover, in the presence of an *NRAS* mutation and given the possibility that paradoxical activation of the *NRAS* pathway could stimulate the growth of *NRAS*-mutant melanomas as well as precipitating a new cancer, particularly squamous cancer of the skin, is another reason not to use the *MAPK* inhibitors (particularly *BRAF* inhibitors unaccompanied by *MEK* inhibitors. The use of so-called flipped-dose ipilimumab plus nivolumab, using lower ipilimumab in the induction cycles and higher nivolumab in the induction cycles, has demonstrated activity comparable with standard doses of therapy with those agents and greater safety. Patients treated with that regimen in a randomized phase II trial of neoadjuvant immunotherapy given in one of three sequences, showed about 70% overall objective response rate and nearly 50% pathologic complete response rate, and relapse-free status was maintained even without postoperative adjuvant therapy. Radiation plus PD-1 blockade is unlikely to provide durable control of bulky nodal disease and has also rarely been associated with an abscopal effect on any distant disease. This patient needs to have a relatively rapid and substantial cytoreduction to achieve disease control, and only surgery or the above-detailed immunotherapy is likely to provide that degree of control. The *MEK* inhibitor, binimetinib has minimal activity against *NRAS*-mutant melanoma and should not be used in this setting, where substantial reduction of tumor bulk from systemic therapy with or without additional surgery is needed.

Correct Answer: C

Case Study 7

A 53-year-old woman with a history of melanoma on the left abdominal wall treated with surgery and one year of adjuvant pembrolizumab almost four years ago is found to have new lung, liver, and skin metastases. A brain MRI is negative. A biopsy of a lung lesion was tested for melanoma mutations and found to carry an activating *BRAF V600E/K* mutation. Her laboratory tests are within normal except for an LDH level. Her performance status is 1 (fatigue), and she continues to work part-time.

20) **Which of the following should be considered optimal therapy at this point?**
   A) Combination of cobimetinib, vemurafenib, and atezolizumab.
   B) Two cycles of ipilimumab plus nivolumab at full dose, followed by maintenance therapy with encorafenib and binimetinib for one year.
   C) Dabrafenib plus trametinib for three years.
   D) Four cycles of ipilimumab plus nivolumab at full dose, followed by nivolumab maintenance therapy for 22 months.
   E) Dabrafenib plus trametinib given intermittently, two months on and two weeks off, until relapse.
   F) Talimogene laherparepvec (T-VEC) injected into all of the accessible skin lesions, plus pembrolizumab.

Expert Perspective: Although the combination of targeted and PD-L1-directed therapy (using cobimetinib, vemurafenib and atezolizumab) has been shown superior to targeted therapy alone in largest Phase III study, leading to FDA approval of this regimen, its benefit is modest and may not outweigh its toxicities. Therefore, this regimen is not recommended for routine use in patients with advanced melanoma with a *BRAF* mutation. Similarly, the regimens that involve switch strategies either from immunotherapy to targeted therapy or from targeted therapy to immunotherapy prior to progression, are promising but have not yet proven superior to single-modality or switch-upon-failure approaches. The use of double *MAPK* (*BRAF* plus *MEK*) inhibition is valid in this setting and is being tested head-to-head against the other combination therapy. However, it is rare that patients with unfavorable risk factors, including liver metastases and elevated LDH, would maintain disease control for as long as three years. The only standard regimen for this patient's characteristics among the available answers is combination ipilimumab and nivolumab, with treatment extended to two years in patients benefiting (objective response and acceptable tolerance) from therapy (CheckMate 069). It was recently shown that intermittent dosing of *MAPK* inhibitors did not provide superior activity over continuous dosing, and it is not recommended. T-VEC has a high regression rate for individual injected lesions, but its ability to provide an abscopal effect and induce regression of visceral and distant lesions is minimal.

Correct Answer: D

Case Study 8

A 76-year-old man with acral melanoma that arose in the left 4th fingertip was managed with amputation and sentinel lymph node biopsy. There was no evidence of nodal or metastatic disease, but in order to be complete in case of a future metastasis, the whole genome sequencing was performed and showed a *KIT* mutation and a loss of part of the *NF1* gene. The patient did well until three years later, when a CT scan during workup for a minor injury showed several pulmonary nodules. Follow-up PET-CT confirmed the high likelihood of metastatic disease (SUV ranging from 10 to 17 for the pulmonary nodules), and he underwent a brain MRI to complete his staging, which showed three masses measuring 1.0 cm, 1.2 cm, and 1.8 cm in diameter without edema. He was neurologically asymptomatic with normal laboratory values.

22) **Which of the following treatments should be offered now?**
    A) Imatinib 800 mg/day.
    B) Whole brain radiotherapy followed by ipilimumab and nivolumab at standard doses, standard regimen.
    C) Pembrolizumab.
    D) Stereotactic radiotherapy followed by nivolumab.
    E) Ipilimumab plus nivolumab at standard doses, standard schedule and duration of therapy.

Expert Perspective: Melanoma has a strong predilection to metastasize to the brain and, much less often, the meninges. Although imatinib is a commonly used targeted therapy for *KIT*-mutated solid tumors and related hematologic malignancies, it is not very active against *KIT*-mutated melanoma (with few exceptions in metastatic acral or mucosal melanoma-discussed earlier) and has not been tested in patients with brain metastases. Whole brain radiotherapy has minimal activity against brain metastases of melanoma. Stereotactic radiosurgery has long been the mainstay of definitive management for small, single to oligometastatic disease in the brain but leaves nontargeted areas of the brain untreated and does not address systemic metastatic disease. Although CTLA-4 blockade alone had only modest activity, similar to its low activity in extracranial disease, the combination of

CTLA-4 blockades with PD-1 blockade was highly active. The activity of ipilimumab and nivolumab is substantial (see Question 5), and whole brain radiation is unlikely to provide additional benefit. Single-agent PD-1 blockade appears to be about half as active as double checkpoint blockage against brain metastases and is similarly less active against extracranial metastatic melanoma. Furthermore, these responses with double blockade have been shown to be quite durable, with the median progression-free survival not reached at 36+ months and the overall survival 72% at 39+ months. The addition of stereotactic brain radiotherapy to single PD-1 blockade is reasonable therapy for advanced melanoma, but double immune checkpoint therapy has superior activity, which appears to be sufficiently high to allow omission of the radiotherapy unless the patient fails to respond or develops an "escape" metastasis that requires radiotherapy for control. Full-dose and full-duration ipilimumab and nivolumab have shown activity against brain metastases that is similar to their activity against extracranial metastatic disease in patients with or without brain metastases. Therefore, this is the recommended combination until better and less toxic drugs are shown to possess high activity against not only extracranial but also brain metastases. Regimens that combine SRT and immunotherapy have been reported to slightly increase the risk of radionecrosis, whihc may be difficult to distinguish from lesion progression and may require surgery and/or agents such as bevacizumab with its attendant risk and cost.

Within this group of patients with melanoma metastatic to the brain are also those with a *BRAF V600E/K*-mutated tumor, and in general they have a moderately high response to targeted agents. These drugs, however, are not as effective in patients with brain metastases, and responses in both the brain and extracranial sites are of more limited duration. Thus, first-line systemic therapy for these individuals should also be immunotherapy according to the same principles detailed earlier. If the patient had contraindication to immunotherapy, then the preferred *BRAF/MEK* combo in brain disease would be dabrafenib plus trametinib (COMBI-MB study).

Correct Answer: E

23) **Would you have treated this patient differently if he had neurologic symptoms related to brain metastatic disease?**

Expert Perspective: Yes. In contrast with remarkable results for immunotherapy in patients without neurologic symptoms or requirement for steroid therapy, patients with neurologic symptoms or a requirement for steroid have much less favorable results and are likely to require stereotactic radiosurgery and possibly surgery, and they should expect improved outcomes from immune checkpoint blockade only if they are able to wean off steroids prior to starting immunotherapy.

24) **Where do we stand with immune checkpoint blocking antibody in combination with other inhibitor(s)?**

Expert Perspective: Several additional scenarios exist for advanced melanoma therapy where available treatments are suboptimal, but new regimens are very close to being approved or, in the case of available agents, assuming greater use. The general approach to optimizing immunotherapy for advanced melanoma is to identify one or more agents that can be safely combined with PD-1 or PD-L1 blockade, with the goal of matching or exceeding the response rate reported for ipilimumab plus nivolumab and reducing the rate of immune-related toxicities. Many drugs are undergoing testing with these goals, and so far, the most promising appear to be combinations of PD-1 blockade with either LAG-3 antibodies (LA3 is another important immune checkpoint) or in combination with the broad-spectrum kinase inhibitor, lenvatinib.

To date, most of these agents remain investigational, but the addition of LAG3 antibody to nivolumab has shown marked improvement in the progression-free interval, likely to predict a prolongation of survival once the data are mature and a fixed-dose formulation of the combination of LAG-3 antibody plus nivolumab is now approved by FDA and undergoing trials in neoadjuvant and adjuvant settings.

25) Which of the following statements about T-VEC is correct?
A) T-VEC is an adenovirus-derived oncolytic immunotherapy.
B) T-VEC was compared with GM-CSF in patients with unresected stage IIIB–IV melanoma.
C) Durable response rate was significantly higher with T-VEC than GM-CSF in the OPTiM study.
D) B and C.

Expert Perspective: T-VEC is a herpes simplex virus type 1–derived oncolytic immunotherapy designed to selectively replicate within tumors and produce granulocyte macrophage colony-stimulating factor (GM-CSF) to enhance systemic antitumor immune responses. T-VEC was compared with GM-CSF in patients with unresected stage IIIB–IV melanoma in a randomized, open-label phase III trial. Patients with injectable melanoma that was not surgically resectable were randomly assigned at a 2:1 ratio to intralesional T-VEC or subcutaneous GM-CSF. The primary end point was durable response rate (objective response lasting continuously ⩾ 6 months) per independent assessment. Among 436 patients randomly assigned, durable response rate was significantly higher with T-VEC (16.3%; 95% CI 12.1–20.5%) than GM-CSF (2.1%; 95% CI 0–4.5%; odds ratio, 8.9; $P <0.001$). Overall response rate was also higher in the T-VEC arm (26.4%; 95% CI 21.4–31.5% vs 5.7%; 95% CI 1.9–9.5%). Median OS was 23.3 months (95% CI 19.5–29.6 months) with T-VEC and 18.9 months (95% CI 16.0–23.7 months) with GM-CSF (HR 0.79; 95% CI 0.62–1.00; $P =0.051$). T-VEC efficacy was most pronounced in patients with stage IIIB, IIIC, or IV-M1a disease and in patients with treatment-naive disease. The most common adverse events with T-VEC were fatigue, chills, and pyrexia. The only grade 3 or 4 adverse events occurring in ⩾ 2% of T-VEC-treated patients was cellulitis (2.1%). No fatal treatment-related adverse events occurred. When T-VEC is injected directly into tumor, its mechanism of action is due to a combination of a direct oncolytic effect from the viral infection and lytic replication, as well as the induction of a systemic immune response. Based on the results of this study, the FDA approved T-VEC to treat unresectable, injectable cutaneous, subcutaneous, and nodal melanoma with limited visceral disease. However, the addition of T-VEC did not provide statistical benefit of progression-free or overall survival when added to pembrolizumab in patients with injectable and non-injected metastatic melanoma (KEYNOTE-265).

Correct Answer: D

26) Which of the following statements about desmoplastic melanoma is correct?
   A) There is a high frequency of *NF1* mutations.
   B) This variant does not respond to immunotherapy.
   C) Adjuvant radiation therapy for local control has no role in this variant.
   D) All of the above.

Expert Perspective: Desmoplastic melanoma is a rare melanoma variant that has unique biology and pathology compared with conventional melanoma. Whole-exome sequencing in these patients has revealed a high mutational frequency of *NF1* mutations. Surgery followed by adjuvant radiation appears to provide superior local control compared with surgery alone for patients with desmoplastic melanoma. These subtypes of melanoma are highly responsive to immunotherapy.

Correct Answer: A

Future Directions

Make sure the font is same style as the remaining chapter/book. There is growing enthusiasm and data favoring the use of neoadjuvant therapy, either immunotherapy agents or *MAPK* inhibitors, as initial treatment of bulky, unifocal or oligometastatic melanoma that is amenable to curative resection. While awaiting the data from ongoing large, randomized trials, many patients are already suitable candidates for such an approach and should be considered for neoadjuvant therapy and managed by expert multidisciplinary teams. The use of assays for circulating tumor cell DNA based either on common mutations or on patient-specific mutations detected at the time of tumor DNA sequencing has begun to permeate the practice of oncology across many tumor types. Although the data for these assays are very promising, their validation and regulatory approval in clinical practice remains to be determined. Like other blood tumor markers, it is likely that these assays will play a greater role in the assessment of patients with active disease on therapy or in the selection of patients for adjuvant therapy following initial surgery than in the identification and treatment of relapse. Also, novel vaccines as the mRNA vaccines based on the patient-specific mutations has shown promising adjuvant activity when added to pambrolizumab and similar approaches in the advanced disease settings have been observed. Noncutaneous subsets of melanoma are less responsive to available immunotherapy, rarely carry a targetable *BRAF V600E/K* mutation, and include acral and mucosal melanomas. Although acral melanoma responds somewhat less well to immunotherapy than cutaneous melanoma arising in non-acral sites to, mucosal melanoma is far less responsive and requires better regimens than we now have to achieve and maintain response.

Recommended Readings

Andtbacka, R.H., Kaufman, H.L., Collichio, F. et al. (2015). Talimogene laherparepvec improves durable response rate in patients with advanced melanoma. *J Clin Oncol* 33 (25): 2780–2788. doi: 10.1200/JCO.2014.58.3377. Epub 2015 May 26. PMID: 26014293.

Ascierto, P.A., McArthur, G.A., Dréno, B. et al. (2016). Cobimetinib combined with vemurafenib in advanced BRAF(V600)-mutant melanoma (coBRIM): Updated efficacy results from a randomised, double-blind, phase 3 trial. *Lancet Oncol* 17 (9): 1248–1260. doi:10.1016/S1470-2045(16)30122-X. Epub 2016 Jul 30. PMID: 27480103.

Davies, M.A., Saiag, P., Robert, C. et al. (2017). Dabrafenib plus trametinib in patients with BRAF^{V600}-mutant melanoma brain metastases (COMBI-MB): A multicentre, multicohort, open-label, phase 2 trial. *Lancet Oncol* 18 (7): 863–873. doi: 10.1016/S1470-2045(17)30429-1. Epub 2017 Jun 4. PMID: 28592387; PMCID: PMC5991615.

Dummer, R., Ascierto, P.A., Gogas, H.J. et al. (2018). Encorafenib plus binimetinib versus vemurafenib or encorafenib in patients with BRAF-mutant melanoma (COLUMBUS): A multicentre, open-label, randomised phase 3 trial. *Lancet Oncol* 19 (5): 603–615. doi:10.1016/S1470-2045(18)30142-6. Epub 2018 Mar 21. PMID: 29573941.

Eggermont, A.M., Chiarion-Sileni, V., Grob, J.J. et al. (2015). Adjuvant ipilimumab versus placebo after complete resection of high-risk stage III melanoma (EORTC 18071): A randomised, double-blind, phase 3 trial. *Lancet Oncol* 16 (5): 522–530. doi: 10.1016/S1470-2045(15)70122-1. Epub 2015 Mar 31. Erratum in: (2015 June) Lancet Oncol 16 (6): e262.Erratum in: (2016 June). Lancet Oncol 17 (6): e223.PMID: 25840693.

Eggermont, A.M.M., Blank, C.U. et al. (2018 May 10). Adjuvant pembrolizumab versus placebo in resected stage III melanoma. *N Engl J Med* 378 (19): 1789–1801. doi: 10.1056/NEJMoa1802357. Epub 2018 Apr 15. PMID: 29658430.

Faries, M.B., Thompson, J.F., Cochran, A.J. et al. (2017). Completion dissection or observation for sentinel-node metastasis in melanoma. *N Engl J Med* 376 (23): 2211–2222. doi: 10.1056/NEJMoa1613210. PMID: 28591523.

Gutzmer, R., Stroyakovskiy, D., Gogas, H. et al. (2020). Atezolizumab, vemurafenib, and cobimetinib as first-line treatment for unresectable advanced BRAF^{V600} mutation-positive melanoma (IMspire150): Primary analysis of the randomised, double-blind, placebo-controlled, phase 3 trial. *Lancet* 395 (10240): 1835–1844. doi:10.1016/S0140-6736(20)30934-X. Erratum in: (2020 August 15). Lancet 396 (10249): 466.PMID: 32534646.

Larkin, J. et al. (2019). Five-year survival with combined nivolumab and ipilimumab in advanced melanoma. *N Engl J Med* 381 (16): 1535–1546.

Long, G.V., Atkinson, V., Lo, S. et al. (2018). Combination nivolumab and ipilimumab or nivolumab alone in melanoma brain metastases: A multicentre randomised phase 2 study. *Lancet Oncol* 19 (5): 672–681. doi:10.1016/S1470-2045(18)30139-6. Epub 2018 Mar 27. PMID: 29602646.

Long, G.V., Hauschild, A., Santinami, M. et al. (2017). Adjuvant dabrafenib plus trametinib in stage III BRAF-mutated melanoma. *N Engl J Med* 377 (19): 1813–1823. doi: 10.1056/NEJMoa1708539. Epub 2017 Sep 10. PMID: 28891408.

Postow, M.A., Chesney, J., Pavlick, A.C. et al. (2015). Nivolumab and ipilimumab versus ipilimumab in untreated melanoma. *N Engl J Med* 372 (21): 2006–2017. doi: 10.1056/NEJMoa1414428. Epub 2015 Apr 20. Erratum in: (2018 November 29). N Engl J Med 379 (22): 2185. PMID: 25891304; PMCID: PMC5744258.

Robert, C. et al. (2019). Five year survival outcomes with dabrafenib plus trametinib for metastatic melanoma. *N Engl J Med* 381 (7): 626–636.

Robert, C., Long, G.V., Brady, B. et al. (2015). Nivolumab in previously untreated melanoma without BRAF mutation. *N Engl J Med* 372 (4): 320–330. doi: 10.1056/NEJMoa1412082. Epub 2014 Nov 16. PMID: 25399552.

Weber, J., Mandala, M., Del Vecchio, M. et al. (2017). CheckMate 238 collaborators. Adjuvant nivolumab versus ipilimumab in resected stage III or IV melanoma. *N Engl J Med* 377 (19): 1824–1835. doi: 10.1056/NEJMoa1709030. Epub 2017 Sep 10. PMID: 28891423.

Weber, J.S., Schadendorf, D., Del Vecchio, M. et al. (2023 Jan 20). Adjuvant therapy of nivolumab combined with ipilimumab versus nivolumab alone in patients with resected stage IIIB-D or stage IV melanoma (CheckMate 915). *J Clin Oncol* 41 (3): 517–527. doi:10.1200/JCO.22.00533. Epub 2022 Sep 26. PMID: 36162037; PMCID: PMC9870220.

37

Nonmelanoma Skin Cancers

Chrysalyne D. Schmults and Danielle A. Parker

Brigham and Women's Department of Dermatology, Jamaica Plain, MA

Introduction

Although most cases of cutaneous squamous cell carcinoma are easily cured with surgical excision, advanced disease occurs. Approximately 10,000 metastatic events are expected in the United States in 2022 at cost as high $50,000 per patient per month, with a cost approaching $6 billion for newly diagnosed patients. Because cutaneous squamous cell carcinoma is excluded from US cancer registries and detailed information is lacking in most European registries, basic questions remain regarding to nodal staging, adjuvant therapy, and surveillance for recurrence. For patients failing surgery and radiation, the only approved treatment is PD-1 inhibition. It is effective in less than 50% of patients. Consequently, deaths from cutaneous squamous cell carcinoma are expected to continue to approximate those from melanoma (7,000 annually in the United States). Basal cell carcinoma is the most common cancer in white-skinned individuals with increasing incidence rates worldwide. Similar to cutaneous squamous cell carcinoma, the incidence of basal cell carcinoma is also increasing, and this cancer places a large burden on healthcare systems because of the high incidence and the increased risk of synchronous and metachronous presentation and other ultraviolet radiation related skin cancers (i.e. field cancerization). The cases herein highlight areas of incomplete and emerging knowledge in these two nonmelanoma skin cancers plus two other malignancies in the skin, dermatofibrosarcoma protuberans (sarcoma) and Merkel cell carcinoma (neuroendocrine tumor).

Cutaneous Squamous Cell Carcinoma

Case Study 1

A 90-year-old woman who suffered from hypertension and hyperlipidemia developed a 6.5 cm lesion on her left cheek. There were no evidence of clinically palpable lymph nodes, and bone invasion was ruled out. The tumor was surgically removed, and the skin biopsy revealed a moderately differentiated cutaneous squamous cell carcinoma, with perineural invasion of deep nerves that were ≥0.1 mm in diameter, which involved beyond the

Cancer Consult: Expertise in Clinical Practice, Volume 1: Solid Tumors & Supportive Care,
Second Edition. Edited by Syed A. Abutalib, Maurie Markman, Al B. Benson III, and Hope S. Rugo.
© 2024 John Wiley & Sons Ltd. Published 2024 by John Wiley & Sons Ltd.

subcutaneous fat and areas of acantholisis (Figure 37.1a–c). Other high-risk features such as desmoplasia were also observed.

1) **Which of the following are high-risk factors for recurrence in this patient?**
   A) Size ⩾4 cm
   B) Perineural invasion ⩾0.1 mm
   C) Involvement of the tumor beyond the subcutaneous fat
   D) Desmoplasia
   E) All the above

Expert Perspective: When treating a patient diagnosed with a cutaneous squamous cell carcinoma, the first question we should try to answer is whether or not we are confronting a high-risk cutaneous squamous cell carcinoma. There is not a clear consensus on the definition of high-risk cutaneous squamous cell carcinoma and advanced cutaneous squamous cell carcinoma. In practical terms, the presence of one of the factors of poor prognosis is what defines a cutaneous squamous cell carcinoma as being high risk. In Table 37.1, we show the prognostic factors that increase the risk for recurrence and metastasis in cutaneous squamous cell carcinoma that the National Comprehensive Cancer Network (NCCN) clinical guidelines consider.

The NCCN guidelines raise the term "very high-risk," which is used to describe cutaneous squamous cell carcinoma ⩾4 cm in greatest clinical dimension, with poor degree of differentiation, desmoplastic type, with deep invasion (>6 mm in thickness or invasion beyond the subcutaneous fat), perineural invasion (deep or large nerves), or lymphovascular invasion (Table 37.1). A cutaneous squamous cell carcinoma is considered high-risk when it is ⩾2 cm in its greatest clinical dimension, it involves some high-risk areas (irrespective of its size),

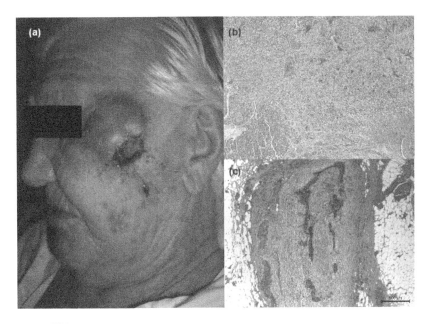

Figure 37.1

it shows poorly defined borders, it is recurrent, it happens in immunosuppressed patient, it occurs in a site of prior radiation therapy or chronic inflammatory process, it is rapidly growing, or it shows neurologic symptoms. Also, some histopathologic subtypes are considered high-risk as well, and perineural invasion when it is not found in large or deep nerves. There is some controversy concerning the prognostic significance of some risk factors. The acantholytic subtype has long been considered high-risk, but recent works have pointed toward its not partic-

Table 37.1 Cutaneous squamous cell carcinoma and risk groups.

Risk group	Low risk	High risk	Very high risk
Location/size	Trunk, extremities <2 cm	Trunk, extremities 2 to <4 cm	≥4 cm (any location)
		Head, neck, hands, feet, pretibial, and anogenital (any size)	
Borders	Well-defined	Poorly defined	
Primary vs recurrent	Primary	Recurrent	
Immunosuppression	(−)	(+)	
Site of prior RT or chronic inflammatory process	(−)	(+)	
Rapidly growing tumor	(−)	(+)	
Neurologic symptoms	(−)	(+)	
Pathology			
Degree of differentiation	Well or moderately differentiated		Poor differentiation
Histologic features: Acantholytic (adenoid), Adenosquamous (showing mucin production), or metaplastic (carcinosarcomatous) subtypes	(−)	(+)	Desmoplastic SCC
Depth: Thickness or level of invasion	≤6 mm and no invasion Beyond subcutaneous fat		>6 mm or invasion beyond subcutaneous fat
Perineural involvement	(−)	(+)	Tumor cells within the nerve sheath of a nerve lying deeper than the dermis or measuring ≥0.1 mm
Lymphatic or vascular involvement	(−)	(−)	(+)

Adopted from NCCN.

ularly aggressive behavior. Considering the features of the tumor described in our patient, we can deem it as high or even very high risk.

Correct Answer: E

2) **What would be the next step once you identify your patient display a high or very-high-risk cutaneous squamous cell carcinoma?**
   A) Schedule surgical treatment as soon as possible.
   B) Rule out locoregional involvement (nodal staging).
   C) Rule out invasion into deep structures.
   D) Calm the patient and tell the patient this is a not aggressive tumor and has a very good prognosis.
   E) B and C.

Expert Perspective: Imaging may be useful in the management of high-risk cutaneous squamous cell carcinoma for evaluating both the local invasion and the nodal and/or distant progression of the tumor. Using imaging tests at diagnosis may modify the management in one-third of high-risk cutaneous squamous cell carcinomas, which impacts prognosis by increasing disease-free survival over those patients in which no imaging is performed (Konidaris et al. 2021). Concerning the evaluation of local/deep invasion, depending on the tissue to be evaluated, we should select the imaging technique. Thus, a CT with contrast is especially useful for exploring the bone, and an MRI is recommended for perineural invasion and involvement of soft tissue. Imaging may be implemented for nodal staging (Canueto et al. 2020). Cutaneous squamous cell carcinoma may evolve metastasis, mainly to the lymph nodes, and for this reason, nodal staging at diagnosis may be useful in selective cases. A CT with contrast is the preferred imaging test for nodal staging (Canueto et al. 2018). Sentinel lymph node biopsy is another way of performing nodal staging. However, in the head and neck area, the lymphatic drainage may be less predictive, and thus the technique may be less reliable. Nodal staging has been suggested in high-risk cutaneous squamous cell carcinoma (T2b/T3– per Brigham and Women's Hospital's [BWH]) (Canueto et al. 2020) and it might be useful in certain T3/T4 (per American Joint Committee on Cancer 8th edition [AJCC8] cases as well.

Correct Answer: E

3) **What would be the T stage in this patient using both, the AJCC8 and BWH systems?**
   A) T2-AJCC8 and T2a-BWH.
   B) T3-AJCC8 and T2b-BWH.
   C) T4-AJCC8 and T3-BWH.
   D) T3-AJCC8 and T3-BWH.
   E) The tumor cannot be staged based on the information here presented.

Expert Perspective: Cancer-staging systems stratify tumors according to their risk of recurrence. There are currently two widely used staging systems in CSCC, the AJCC8 (Tschetter et al. 2020) staging system and the BWH alternative staging system (Hanna et al. 2020; Maubec et al. 2018). Both these systems are shown in Table 37.2. Several groups have compared AJCC8 staging system with AJCC7, and it was found to be better than the former but with clear limitations (Canueto et al. 2019; Fox et al. 2019).

Table 37.2 AJCC8 staging system and BWH alternative staging system.

	AJCC8 staging system		BWH staging system (***)	
Low risk	T1	Diameter <2 cm	T1	No high-risk factors
	T2	Diameter ≥2–4 cm	T2a	1 high-risk factor
High risk	T3	Diameter ≥4 cm Deep invasion (Thickness >6 mm or invasion beyond the subcutaneous fat) Perineural invasion (according to AJCC8)*	T2b	2–3 high-risk factors
	T4	T4a tumor with gross cortical bone/marrow involvement T4b tumor with skull base invasion or skull base foramen involvement	T3	≥4 high-risk factors

(*) Perineural invasion according to the AJCC8 consists of the involvement of nerves with a diameter of ≥0.1 mm, with the involvement of nerves located deeper than the dermis, or by clinical or radiologically evident perineural invasion.
(***) High-risk factors: Tumor diameter ≥2 cm, invasion beyond subcutaneous fat, poorly differentiated, and perineural invasion ≥0.1 mm. Adapted from Amin M, et al. 2017 and Morgan FC, et al 2015.

The BWH system considers four risk factors and, depending on their combination, classifies cutaneous squamous cell carcinoma into four T stages. (Hanna et al. 2020; Maubec et al. 2018) Using the BWH staging system in clinical practice is straightforward, allowing the stratification of tumors beyond the head and neck, and it is the most popular staging system after the AJCC. Most clinical guidelines consider BWH as the staging system to guide clinical management of cutaneous squamous cell carcinoma. Based on the BWH is the considering of the accumulation of risk factors, which is clearly relevant in prognosis. The BWH system is more distinctive than the official AJCC8. A group from the University Hospital of Tübingen provided a risk stratification system based on the accumulation of risk factors that proved useful for predicting disease-specific death from cutaneous squamous cell carcinoma (Oncology NCCN 2022). They consider the tumor thickness to shape the T stage and immunosuppression and desmoplasia as additional risk factors. To date, it is less widely used than the AJCC and BWH staging systems.

Considering the tumor in our patient, it should be staged T3-AJCC8 and T2b-BWH (with three risk factors, size ≥2 cm, perineural invasion ≥0.1 mm, and invasion beyond subcutaneous fat). According to the current staging systems, high-risk cutaneous squamous cell carcinoma would be considered as T3/T4-AJCC8 or T2b/T3-BWH (Table 37.2). However, many tumors within these T stages will display a nonaggressive behavior. Thus, the positive predictive value and sensitivity is low within these stages, and an improvement in the risk stratification of high-risk cutaneous squamous cell carcinoma would be desirable. Indeed, only 24–38% of patients with T2b/T3-BWH tumors and 14–17% of T3/T4-AJCC8 patients develop metastasis (Pickering et al. 2014).

Concerning the AJCC8 staging system, several limitations have been highlighted. First, some high-risk features are not considered in the AJCC8 (such as the poor degree of differentiation, which was excluded despite its prognostic impact). Those T3-AJCC8 that show poor degree of differentiation are much more aggressive (Conde-Ferreiros et al. 2020; van Lee et al. 2019), and up to one-third may evolve nodal metastasis (van Lee et al. 2019). Second, AJCC8 gives the same prognostic relevance to all the risk factors, although all risk factors are not equally relevant in terms of prognostic effect (van Lee et al. 2019). Finally, it does not consider the influence of the combination of risk factors, which show greater prognostic impact than an isolated risk factor (Fox et al. 2019). It has been demonstrated that two or more risk factors combined are more predictive of poor prognosis than an isolated risk factor (Morgan et al. 2021; Paulson et al. 2017), which is the basis of BWH.

By combining the AJCC8 risk factors, different prognostic subgroups have been identified within T3-AJCC8. (Bichakjian et al. 2021) In that proposal, those T3-AJCC8 cutaneous squamous cell carcinoma that show 3 or more risk factors at the same time displayed the poorest prognosis (T3c). Both BWH and T3-AJCC8 subclassification, and the Tübingen's system are better for high-risk cutaneous squamous cell carcinoma classification than the official AJCC8 [16]. These alternative staging systems allow a more reliable risk stratification of high-risk cutaneous squamous cell carcinoma, but their prognostic accuracy is still low, and thus staging still needs improvement [16], which might come from the incorporation of additional risk factors or by the inclusion of genomic data (Pickering et al. 2014).

Correct Answer: B

4) What is the best therapy for this patient?
   A) Surgery and adjuvant radiation therapy
   B) Salvage radiation therapy
   C) Cemiplimab
   D) Cetuximab
   E) Any of the above

Expert Perspective: Surgery, with the histopathological evaluation of margins, is the cornerstone in the management of cutaneous squamous cell carcinoma, including high-risk cases. The main objective is the complete clearance of the tumor, with acceptable functional and cosmetic results. Conventional surgery may be considered, but guidelines recommend at least 10 mm margins for high-risk cutaneous squamous cell carcinoma. However, the recommendations on surgical margins for high-risk cutaneous squamous cell carcinoma is difficult to establish. It is important not to cover the surgical defect until there is evidence of complete tumor clearance. Thus, linear or delay repair should be considered if conventional surgery is chosen.

Mohs micrographic surgery or other forms of complete circumferential peripheral and deep margin assessment (CCPDMA) can be considered as standard of care in high-risk cutaneous squamous cell carcinoma and especially for very high-risk cases. Several retrospective [17, 18] and prospective studies have also shown such a benefit of Mohs over standard excision [19, 20]. Cutaneous squamous cell carcinoma treated with Mohs shows five-year local recurrence, nodal metastasis-free survival, and disease-free survival were 99.3%, 99.2%, and 99.4%, respectively [19]. Five-year cure rates were higher for Mohs micrographic surgery over any other technique in all tumor subgroups in that study [21]. Also, Mohs micrographic surgery can reduce the size of the surgical defect and thus facilitate reconstruction.

The outcome benefit of adjuvant radiation therapy following a cutaneous squamous cell carcinoma resection with clear surgical margins is controversial. However, even when free margins are obtained, guidelines recommend multidisciplinary consultation and considering adjuvant radiation therapy when extensive perineural, large, or named nerve involvement exist. For high-risk cutaneous squamous cell carcinoma with clear margins after surgery, a study demonstrated no usefulness for radiotherapy even when they stratified by perineural invasion [22], which has been demonstrated in other studies too [23], although it is generally recommended in cutaneous squamous cell carcinoma with perineural invasion of gross nerves (irrespective of the margin status after surgery) [23, 24], and guidelines recommend it as well. The patient's context should be considered.

Our patient: Surgery and adjuvant radiation therapy was chosen after discussion by the multidisciplinary tumor board. High-risk cutaneous squamous cell carcinoma should be discussed in specialized tumor boards to define therapeutic and follow-up recommendations.

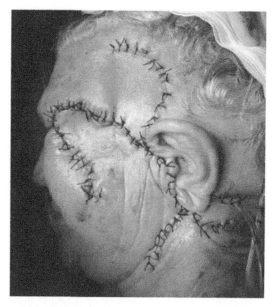

Figure 37.2 Case Study 1 patient following Mohs micrographic surgery while waiting for adjuvant radiation therapy.

Correct Answer: A

Case Study 2

An 82-year-old male is diagnosed with a recurrent cutaneous squamous cell carcinoma of 4.5 cm × 3.0 cm on the left temporal area. His medical history also states two kidney transplantations, of which the last transplantation resulted in a stable kidney function.

Three mapping biopsies of the lesion show poorly differentiated cutaneous squamous cell carcinoma with a maximum invasion depth of 5.2 mm (Figure 37.3). One of the biopsies also shows perineural invasion of a small (defined as <0.1mm) superficial nerve without signs of lymphatic or vascular involvement. There were no palpable regional lymph nodes, and ultrasound guided evaluation of the regional lymph nodes was negative.

5) What would be the preferred management option for a patient with a local very-high-risk cutaneous squamous cell carcinoma?
   A) Standard excision
   B) Mohs surgery or another form of complete circumferential peripheral and deep margin assessment (CCPDMA)
   C) Primary radiotherapy
   D) Immune checkpoint inhibitor

37 Nonmelanoma Skin Cancers

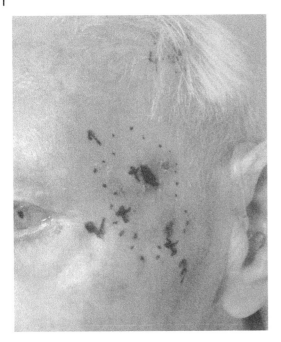

Figure 37.3

Expert Perspective: According to the NCCN, cutaneous squamous cell carcinoma patients with a local cutaneous squamous cell carcinoma can be stratified into low, high, or very high risk for local recurrence, metastases, or death from disease to determine treatment options and follow-up. Patients with a cutaneous squamous cell carcinoma equal or larger than 4 cm are considered very high-risk patients (Table 37.1). Cutaneous squamous cell carcinoma patients with a very high risk should preferably be treated with Mohs micrographic surgery or other forms of complete circumferential peripheral and deep margin assessment. Another option would be standard excision, but only with wider surgical margins and postoperative margin assessment and delayed or otherwise linear repair. Standard excision with wide surgical margins is usually not preferred for cutaneous squamous cell carcinoma on the face, as previously discussed in Question 1. Primary radiotherapy is also an option for a cutaneous squamous cell carcinoma but is generally reserved for patients that are nonsurgical candidates. Finally, in solid organ transplant recipients, therapy with an immune checkpoint inhibitor has a significant risk of organ rejection and is therefore avoided in cutaneous squamous cell carcinoma.

Correct Answer: B

6) This patient is treated with Mohs micrographic surgery. After two stages of excision, the margins are negative, but there i6s extensive perineural involvement of nerves deep to the dermis. Now what would be the preferred management option?
    A) Additional wide local excision
    B) An additional stage of Mohs surgery

C) Adjuvant radiotherapy
D) Adjuvant systemic therapy

Expert Perspective: Patients with extensive perineural invasion of large (defined as ⩾0.1mm), deep to the dermis, or named nerves have an indication for an adjuvant radiotherapy, and it is therefore recommended to discuss those patients in a multidisciplinary setting. Only in complicated cases where radiotherapy is not feasible can adjuvant systemic therapy be considered. Additional surgery, including further Mohs micrographic surgery, has no evidence of benefit as an adjuvant therapy beyond initial complete surgical margins.

Correct Answer: C

Case Study 3

An 88-year-old otherwise healthy man developed a 2.2 cm cutaneous lesion on the right temple, which was surgically excised (Figure 37.4A). The histopathological evaluation was consistent with a poorly differentiated cutaneous squamous cell carcinoma, 7 mm in thickness, with an infiltrative pattern of invasion. The lesion was excised with free margins. The patient underwent clinical surveillance, and 14 months later, he developed parotid involvement, confirmed through fine needle aspiration. He was managed by salvage radiotherapy, and despite initial clinical response, five months after treatment, the lesion recurred (Figure 37.4B) and an ulcerated lesion later began to appear immediately under his right ear, which gradually enlarged. When we saw him in the clinic, the patient showed a tumoral lesion on the lateral right part of his neck, 7 cm in diameter, which consisted with an ulcerated tumor that invaded into deep structures. The patient complaint about intense pain, and he said the tumor sometimes profusely bled (Figure 37.4C).

7) Which would be your initial approach in this patient?
   A) Immediate surgery
   B) Further imaging
   C) Analgesia only and hospice
   D) Elective radiotherapy
   E) Other

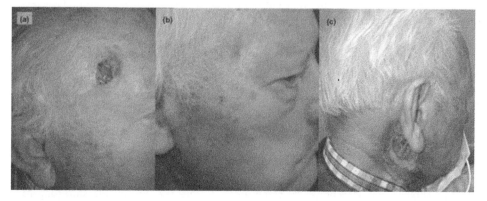

Figure 37.4

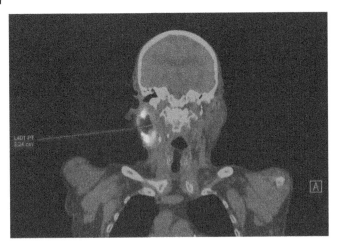

Figure 37.5

Expert Perspective: A PET-CT was indicated, and it demonstrated morphometabolic progression of the lesion in the right parotid cell, which showed approximate dimensions of 7.2 × 3.2 cm (coronal plane) and SUVmax 48 (Figure 37.5). The lesion extended up to the skin surface and down close to vascular structures.

Imaging may be useful in the management of cutaneous squamous cell carcinoma for evaluating both the local invasion and the nodal/distant progression of the tumor. Using imaging tests at diagnosis can change management in up to one-third of high-risk cutaneous squamous cell carcinoma and imaging impacts prognosis by increasing disease-free survival over those patients in which no imaging was performed. Concerning the evaluation of local/deep invasion, depending on the tissue to be evaluated, we should select the imaging technique. Thus, CT with contrast is especially useful for exploring the bone, and MRI is recommended for perineural invasion and involvement of soft tissue. Imaging may be implemented for nodal staging as well and for evaluating distant involvement. CT with contrast is the preferred test for nodal staging. PET has demonstrated usefulness and even greater accuracy for restaging. In this case, we chose PET-CT to provide both functional and structural imaging and because it was a restaging context. The information helped us decide the treatment because the tumor was deemed irresectable with curative intention.

Correct Answer: B

8) **What is the next best step for this patient?**
   A) Immediate surgery
   B) Cetuximab
   C) Hostage therapy
   D) Elective radiotherapy
   E) Immunotherapy with cemiplimab or another anti-PD1.

Expert Perspective: This patient was managed with cemiplimab 350 mg every 21 days. The tumor showed rapid response to cemiplimab. Before the second infusion (day 21), the patient already reported significant improvement on his pain and bleeding. Also, a

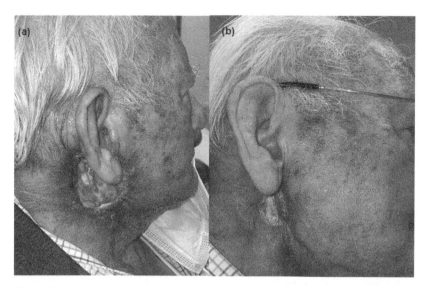

Figure 37.6

decrease in the margin thickness of the lesion could be observed, which corresponded with clinical improvement (Figure 37.6a). After four cycles, there was almost complete remission both clinically (Figure 37.6b) and on the PET-CT.

Tumors with high mutational burden show a higher likelihood of response to immune checkpoint inhibitors, and cutaneous squamous cell carcinoma shows the greatest mutational burden of solid tumors. The immune system is important in fighting against cancer, and cutaneous squamous cell carcinoma is much more common in immunosuppressed patients. Both these factors supposed the rationale for developing clinical trials with immune checkpoint inhibitors for cutaneous squamous cell carcinoma. Several case reports initially showed efficacy of immunotherapy in cutaneous squamous cell carcinoma immunocompetent patients, and clinical trials came later.

Cemiplimab was the first FDA- and European Medicines Agency (EMA)-approved drug for locally advanced and metastatic cutaneous squamous cell carcinoma. Cemiplimab boosts the immune system by avoiding the PD-1 connection to its ligand, thus preventing T cell exhaustion. Cemiplimab is a human IgG4 monoclonal antibody against PD-1, and it has showed safety and efficacy in locally advanced and metastatic cutaneous squamous cell carcinoma, with response rates of 50% and 47%, respectively. Real-world data show comparatively lower response, 31.5% of responses compared with 48% in clinical trials. Other anti-PD1 molecules have been used to treat advanced cutaneous squamous cell carcinoma. Pembrolizumab has been FDA approved for advanced cutaneous squamous cell carcinoma.

Correct Answer: E

Table 37.3 AJCC 8 and BWH T-staging systems for basal cell carcinoma.

Tumor-staging system	Definition
AJCC8 T-staging cutaneous carcinoma of the head and neck	
T1	<2 cm in greatest diameter
T2	≥2 cm but <4 cm in greatest diameter
T3	≥4 cm in greatest diameter or minor bone invasion or perineural invasion or deep invasion
T4a	Tumor with gross cortical bone and/or marrow invasion
T4b	Tumor with skull bone invasion and/or skull base foramen involvement
BWH T-staging for BCC	
T1	Tumor diameter of <2 cm or tumor diameter of ≥2 cm with 0 or 1 risk factors
T2	Tumor diameter of ≥2 cm with 2 or 3 risk factors

Sources: M. Amin et al., eds., AJCC Cancer Staging Manual, 8th ed. (Springer, 2017); F. C. Morgan et al., Brigham and Women's Hospital tumor classification system for basal cell carcinoma identifies patients with risk of metastasis and death, *J Am Acad Dermatol* 85, no. 3 (2021): 582–587.

Basal Cell Carcinoma

Case Study 4

An 80-year-old women is diagnosed with a large primary basal cell carcinoma on her right upper leg. An MRI of the leg showed a large tumor with significant invasion of the subcutaneous tissue and the quadriceps femoris muscle (Figure 37.7) without satellite lesions or inguinal lymphadenopathy.

9) **Which of the following risk factors of patients with locally advanced basal cell carcinomas is associated with a high risk of metastasis and/or death?**
   A) Female gender
   B) Location on the extremities
   C) Invasion beyond fat
   D) Micronodular or infiltrative histopathological subtype

Expert Perspective: Most basal cell carcinomas are easily cured with surgical excision. Depending on the treatment provided, five-year recurrence rates vary from 1–3% when treated with Mohs micrographic surgery to 2–10% when treated with standard surgical excision. The risk of developing metastasis in the overall group of basal cell carcinoma patients is extremely low (0.0028–0.55%). This is expected to be higher among patients with locally advanced basal cell carcinomas, demonstrating the need of improved prognostic information to also improve outcomes in this subgroup.

The NCCN has established low- and high-risk criteria for basal cell carcinoma. However, these criteria are intended to identify tumors that may recur locally, but not those who metastasis or can even lead to death. Until recently, only the AJCC8 T-staging system for

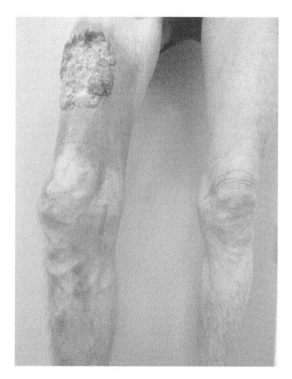

Figure 37.7

cutaneous carcinoma of the head and neck was available to determine the risk of metastasis/death (M/D) in basal cell carcinoma, but this has now been expanded with the BWH T-staging system specifically developed for basal cell carcinoma (Table 37.2). Although both systems can capture all tumor metastasis and deaths in the higher stages, the BWH staging system has a high specificity and positive predictive value. Risk factors associated with metastasis and death in the BWH system include tumor diameter of 4 cm or greater, head or neck location, and tumor depth beyond fat.

Correct Answer: C

10) **Surgery is expected to be very debilitating considering the tumor invasion in the quadriceps femoris muscle. What systemic treatment can be considered if this patient is deemed inoperable?**
    A) Vismodegib or sonidegib
    B) Cemiplimab-rwlc
    C) Ustekinumab
    D) Cetuximab

Expert Perspective: Vismodegib and sonidegib are oral hedgehog pathway inhibitors that are approved by the FDA for the treatment of locally advanced basal cell carcinomas in patients who are not candidates for surgery or radiation, whereas only vismodegib is also approved for metastatic cases. They are small-molecule inhibitors of Smoothened that acts on the Sonic Hedgehog pathway, which is mutated in most basal cell carcinomas.

Hedgehog inhibitors have shown good overall response rates, which can lead to a decrease in size of some basal cell carcinomas and result in complete clearance of others. A limiting factor for these medications are their effect on quality of life, such as ageusia, alopecia, and debilitating cramps. Management of these side effects is often difficult, requiring drug holidays, reduced dosages, or even treatment discontinuation.

Since February 2021 the FDA also approved cemiplimab-rwlc, a PD-1 antibody, for patients with locally advanced basal cell carcinoma previously treated with hedgehog pathway inhibitors or for whom hedgehog pathway inhibitors is not appropriate and granted accelerated approval to cemiplimab-rwlc for patients with metastatic basal cell carcinoma previously treated with a hedgehog pathway inhibitors or for whom a hedgehog pathway inhibitors is not appropriate. In this patient, this would be an option in case of tumor progression or if the patient becomes intolerant to hedgehog pathway inhibitors therapy.

Correct Answer: A

Dermatofibrosarcoma Protuberans

Case Study 5

A 51-year-old healthy male patient with a medical history of a dermatofibrosarcoma protuberans for which he underwent two prior excisions on his scalp almost thirty years ago presents again with an indurated, ulcerated plaque within the old scar (Figure 37.8). The plaque is fixated to the underlying tissue. There is no clinical evidence of enlarged lymph nodes. Three mapping biopsies all show CD34+ spindled cells arranged in a storiform pattern and fibrosis, matching a recurrent dermatofibrosarcoma protuberans.

11) What is the preferred initial radiological workup for this patient with dermatofibrosarcoma protuberans?
    A) MRI of the scalp with contrast
    B) CT of the chest, abdomen, and pelvis

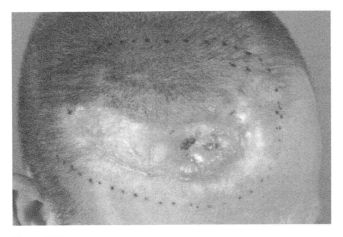

Figure 37.8

C) Ultrasound of the lymph nodes in the head and neck area
   D) CT of the lungs
   E) Total body PET CT

Expert Perspective: Dermatofibrosarcoma protuberans is a rare, slowly growing, soft-tissue tumor that, unlike most skin cancers, is a non-UV-related skin cancer. Dermatofibrosarcoma protuberans is commonly located on the trunk and proximal extremities and, in 10–15% of cases, on the head and neck area.

Dermatofibrosarcoma protuberans rarely metastasize, and an extensive workup aimed at detecting metastasis is therefore not routinely indicated unless there are suggestive aspects in the history and physical examination. It has been suggested that signs of a histopathological fibrosarcomatous transformation or a high mitotic rate within a dermatofibrosarcoma protuberans may have a prognostic value, and it is thus recommended that these features are mentioned in the pathology report.

Dermatofibrosarcoma protuberans are usually difficult to delineate, so a preoperative MRI with contrast is advised for treatment planning, especially in case of a recurrent tumor and if extensive extracutaneous extension is expected. In case involvement of the underlying bone is expected, a CT should be performed. (Also refer to Chapter 44.)

Correct Answer: A

12) **The MRI of this patient was suggestive of extensive subcutaneous extension, and the CT showed no invasion of the underlying bone. What would be the preferred treatment for a recurrent dermatofibrosarcoma protuberans?**
   A) Wide local excision with standard bread loaf pathology assessment
   B) Mohs micrographic surgery or another form of complete circumferential peripheral and deep margin assessment
   C) Radiotherapy
   D) Imatinib

Expert Perspective: Dermatofibrosarcoma protuberans should preferably be resected whenever possible. The irregular shape and tentacle-like extension often lead to incomplete removal with conventional excision and recurrences often occur. Wide local excision margins of typically 2–4 cm result in a large defect but still do not allow complete assessment of the deep margins. Therefore, a form of histologic assessment of the entire peripheral and deep surgical margins before reconstruction is the preferred treatment for primary and recurrent dermatofibrosarcoma protuberans. Radiation is usually not used as a primary therapeutic modality for dermatofibrosarcoma protuberans but can be considered for positive margins if further resection is not feasible. Imatinib is generally reserved for patients where the disease is unresectable or if a resection will lead to unacceptable functional or cosmetic outcomes. It works well especially in patients with t(17;22). The use of imatinib in the neoadjuvant and/or adjuvant setting is not a standard practice.

Correct Answer: B

Merkel Cell Carcinoma

Case Study 6

An 83-year-old woman with a history of atrial fibrillation and chronic lymphocytic leukemia (CLL) develops a 1.5 cm nodule on the right temple (Figure 37.9). There is no evidence of clinically palpable lymph node involvement. A small biopsy from the edge of the tumor is performed and reveals a

13) What is the recommended initial treatment approach for this patient and tumor?
   A) Wide local excision with 1–2 cm margins alone
   B) Wide local excision with 1–2 cm margins and sentinel lymph node biopsy
   C) Narrow margin excision and sentinel lymph node biopsy
   D) Narrow margin excision, sentinel lymph node biopsy, and adjuvant post-operative radiation therapy
   E) Primary radiation therapy alone

Expert Perspective: Merkel cell carcinomas are rare cutaneous neoplasms of neuroendocrine cells most frequently seen in elderly male patients in their 70s or 80s with a history of extensive sun exposure. Merkel cell carcinoma is one of the most aggressive skin cancers with a mortality rate exceeding melanoma. The five-year relative or Merkel cell carcinoma–specific survival rates range from 41 to 77%. Often the disease metastasizes early, with 26–36% of tumors presenting with lymph node involvement and 6–16% presenting with distant metastatic disease.

The most common sites affected are sun-exposed areas, especially the head and neck. Risk factors include increasing age, Caucasian ethnicity, geographic locations with higher UV indices, and a history of immunosuppression (especially organ transplantation, lymphoproliferative disorders such as CLL, and HIV infection). Merkel cell carcinoma–specific survival is worse in patients who are immunosuppressed.

Merkel cells, so-called touch cells, reside predominantly in the basal layer of the epidermis and follicular epithelium and play a role in light touch sensory responses, nerve guidance, somatostatin synthesis, and other endocrine and paracrine effects. Recent advances in

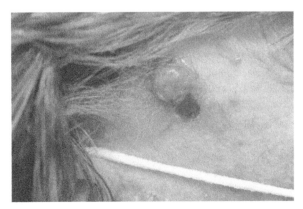

Figure 37.9

immunohistochemistry have helped identify that Merkel cell carcinoma has a characteristic perinuclear dot pattern staining of CK-20. Other stains positive in Merkel cell carcinoma include CK7, neuron-specific enolase, chromogranin, and synaptophysin. Notably, thyroid transcription factor 1 is negative and helps rule out a potential cutaneous metastases from other small-cell carcinomas, such as lung carcinoma.

Surgery is the primary treatment modality for Merkel cell carcinoma along with sentinel lymph node biopsy. Sentinel lymph node biopsy positivity has been reported between 30 and 38% and is thus recommended. Every effort to coordinate sentinel lymph node biopsy at the time of definitive primary resection of the tumor is advised. Postoperative radiation is frequently used and recommended depending on the clinical scenario, tumor stage, and risk factors. Merkel cell carcinoma is widely regarded as a radiosensitive tumor, and a meta-analysis demonstrated a survival advantage for patients with stage I and II disease treated with combination surgery and adjuvant radiation. If adjuvant radiation is planned, narrow margin excision may be sufficient and preferred to allow for less complicated closure of the wound (primary closure, avoiding extensive tissue movement) and expeditious initiation of radiation therapy. In patients with one or more risk factor (tumor >2 cm, immunosuppression, head/neck primary site, lymphovascular invasion), narrow margin excision with concurrent sentinel lymph node biopsy followed by postoperative adjuvant radiation therapy is the recommended initial treatment approach. Lastly, based on the results of PODIUM-201 study, the FDA granted accelerated approval to the PD-1 inhibitor retifanlimab-dlwr for adult patients with metastatic or recurrent locally advanced Merkel cell carcinoma. The objective response rate was 52% (95% confidence interval [CI] = 40%–65%), with a complete response rate of 18%. Twenty-six patients (76%) had a duration of response lasting at least 6 months, and 21 (62%) had a duration of response of 12 months or more.

14) Which of the following statements about the workup and tumor surveillance in this patient is correct?
   A) Serology testing of Merkel cell polyomavirus (MCPyV) is unnecessary in routine workup of Merkel cell carcinoma.
   B) The absence of MCPyV oncoprotein (T-antigen) antibodies is associated with favorable recurrence and survival outcomes.
   C) The absence of MCPyV viral capsid (VP1) antibodies is associated with favorable recurrence and survival outcomes.
   D) VP1 antibodies may be monitored during tumor surveillance for early signs of recurrence.
   E) MCPyV oncoprotein (T-antigen) antibodies may be monitored during tumor surveillance for early signs of recurrence.

Expert Perspective: Merkel cell polyomavirus was first discovered in 2008 after analysis of four Merkel cell carcinoma tumors, utilizing digital transcriptome subtraction, revealed previously unknown viral transcripts. The Merkel cell polyomavirus is a double-stranded DNA virus that is now known to be ubiquitous in the human population. Serum antibodies to MCPyV appear during the first decade of life, after an asymptomatic infection, and are subsequently found in 80% of all adults. Causality is still unproven, but 75–80% of tumors contain the viral genome. It has been shown to integrate within the cellular genome of Merkel cell carcinoma, and even metastatic Merkel cell carcinomas demonstrate the viral DNA. The remaining 20–25% of Merkel cell carcinoma that are MCPyV-negative have been recently noted to have a significantly higher mutational burden and UV signature of cytosine to thymine (C to T) mutations. These patients also have a worse prognosis compared with MCPyV-positive patients.

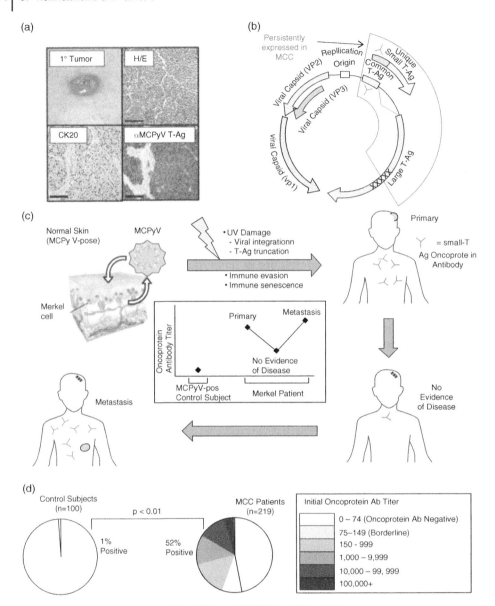

Figure 37.10 (a-d). *Source:* Paulson KG et al. 2017/John Wiley & Sons.

Recently, the significance of antibodies to Merkel cell polyomavirus has been elucidated and can now be utilized for prognostication as well as tumor surveillance. There are two major classes of Merkel cell polyomavirus serologies that are now commercially available and should be utilized during the workup and management of Merkel cell carcinoma patients. Antibodies to MCPyV viral capsid (VP) as well as oncoproteins (T-antigens) may be present in patients. Low baseline antibodies to the major MCPyV capsid protein (VP1) correspond with a higher risk of recurrence and increased mortality, but do not vary with disease burden.

MCPyV oncoprotein antibodies are found in approximately half of Merkel cell carcinoma patients at diagnosis. The absence of MCPyV oncoprotein antibodies at baseline is associated with a 42% higher risk of recurrence, and these patients may benefit from more aggressive surveillance as well. But more importantly, in patients who were seropositive for MCPyV oncoprotein antibodies, monitoring of the antibody levels correlate with tumor burden and recurrence and thus may be utilized in ongoing surveillance because rising titers can be an early marker for tumor recurrence.

Correct Answer: E

Recommended Readings

Bichakjian, C.K. et al. (2021). Merkel cell carcinoma. *J Natl Compr Canc Netw* 16 (6): 742–774.

Canueto, J., Burguillo, J., Moyano-Bueno et al. (2018). Comparing the eighth and the seventh editions of the American Joint Committee on Cancer staging system and the Brigham and Women's Hospital alternative staging system for cutaneous squamous cell carcinoma: Implications for clinical practice. *J Am Acad Dermatol* 80: 106–113.e2. PMID: 30003984. DOI: 10.1016/j.jaad.2018.06.060.

Canueto, J., Jaka, A., Corchete et al. (2019). Postoperative radiotherapy provides better local control and long-term outcome in selective cases of cutaneous squamous cell carcinoma with perineural invasion. *J Eur Acad Dermatol Venereal* 34: 1080–1091. PMID: 31587379. DOI: 10.1111/jdv.16001.

Canueto, J., Tejera-Vaquerizo, A., Redondo, P. et al. (2020). A review of terms used to define cutaneous squamous cell carcinoma with a poor prognosis. *Actas Dermosifiliogr* 111: 281–290.

Conde-Ferreiros, A., Corchete, L.A., Puebla-Tornero, L. et al. (2020). Definition of prognostic subgroups in the T3-AJCC8 stage for cutaneous squamous cell carcinoma: Tentative T3 stage subclassification. *J Am Acad Dermatol* 85: 1168–1177. PMID: 32278798. DOI: 10.1016/j.jaad.2020.03.088.

Fox, M., Brown, M., Golda, N. et al. (2019). Nodal staging of high-risk cutaneous squamous cell carcinoma. *J Am Acad Dermatol* 81: 548–557.

Hanna, G.J., Ruiz, E.S., LeBoeuf, N.R. et al. (2020). Real-world outcomes treating patients with advanced cutaneous squamous cell carcinoma with immune checkpoint inhibitors (CPI). *Br J Cancer* 123: 1535–1542.

Konidaris, G., Paul, E., Kuznik, A. et al. (2021). Assessing the value of cemiplimab for adults with advanced cutaneous squamous cell carcinoma: A cost-effectiveness analysis. *Value Health* 24 (3): 377–387. doi: 10.1016/j.jval.2020.09.014 Epub 2021/03/02. PubMed PMID: 33641772.

Maubec E.B.M., Petrow, P. et al. (2018). Pembrolizumab as first line therapy in patients with unresectable squamous cell carcinoma of the skin: Interim results of the phase 2 CARSKIN trial. *J Clin Oncol* 36.

Morgan, F.C. et al. (2021). Brigham and Women's Hospital tumor classification system for basal cell carcinoma identifies patients with risk of metastasis and death. *J Am Acad Dermatol* 85 (3): 582–587.

Oncology NCCN. (2022). Squamous cell skin cancer. NCCN Guidelines.

Paulson, K.G. et al. (2017). Viral oncoprotein antibodies as a marker for recurrence of Merkel cell carcinoma: A prospective validation study. *Cancer* 123 (8): 1464–1474.

Pickering, C.R., Zhou, J.H., Lee, J.J. et al. (2014). Mutational landscape of aggressive cutaneous squamous cell carcinoma. *Clin Cancer Res* 20: 6582–6592.

Tschetter, A.J., Campoli, M.R., Zitelli, J.A., and Brodland, D.G.. (2020). Long-term clinical outcomes of patients with invasive cutaneous squamous cell carcinoma treated with Mohs micrographic surgery: A 5-year, multicenter, prospective cohort study. *J Am Acad Dermatol* 82: 139–148.

van Lee, C.B., Roorda, B.M., Wakkee, M. et al. (2019). Recurrence rates of cutaneous squamous cell carcinoma of the head and neck after Mohs micrographic surgery vs. standard excision: A retrospective cohort study. *Br J Dermatol* 181: 338–343.

Part 7

Gynecological Cancers

38

Ovarian Cancer: Primary Treatment and Approach to Recurrent Disease

Rani Bansal[1], Don Dizon[2], and Martina Murphy[3]

[1] Duke University, Durham, NC, USA
[2] Alpert Medical School of Brown University, Division of Hematology-Oncology, RhodeIsland Hospital, Providence, RI, USA
[3] University of Florida, Division of Hematology-Oncology, Gainesville, FL, USA

Introduction

Ovarian cancer is the seventh most common cancer among women in the world and is the second most common gynecologic malignancy in the United States with an average age at diagnosis of 63 years old. Risk factors for ovarian cancer include increasing age, endometriosis, polycystic ovarian syndrome, cigarette smoking, and infertility. Several susceptibility genes for ovarian cancer have been identified such as *BRCA1*, *BRCA2*, and mismatch repair genes associated with hereditary nonpolyposis colorectal cancer (Lynch syndrome; Chapters 45–47). Most patients typically present with late stage of disease, when the five-year relative survival rate is only 29%, compared with those few cases that are diagnosed at stage I, where five-year relative survival is 92%. Thus, it is important to understand treatment options for patients with ovarian cancer and how genetics and mutation pathways play a role.

Case Study 1

Ms. A is a 69-year-old woman who presents with progressive abdominal distention over several months. A CT scan of the chest, abdomen, and pelvis reveals a 4.7 cm left-sided adnexal mass, diffuse carcinomatosis involving the large bowel, and large-volume ascites. Biopsy of an omental implant reveals high-grade serous carcinoma of the ovary. The cancer antigen 125 (CA125) level is 1,357.

1) What is the optimal sequence of initial treatment for this patient?

Expert Perspective: The initial step in assessing treatment options for this patient is to first determine the clinical stage. The International Federation of Gynecology and Obstetrics (FIGO) classification system is a single-staging system for ovarian, fallopian tube, and peritoneal carcinomas based on the tumor, node, and metastasis (TNM) classification (Table 38.1). At this point, we can only assign a clinical stage. However, complete surgical staging is important for prognostication and treatment planning.

After clinical staging, patients suspected of having ovarian malignancy should be evaluated for primary surgical cytoreduction followed by systemic chemotherapy, which is the

Table 38.1 FIGO staging criteria for ovarian cancer.

TNM	FIGO	Description
Tx		Primary tumor cannot be assessed
T0		No evidence of primary tumor
T1	I	Tumor limited to ovaries (one or both) or fallopian tube(s)
T1a	IA	Tumor limited to one ovary (capsule intact) or fallopian tube
T1b	IB	Tumor limited to both ovaries; (capsules intact) or fallopian tubes
T1c	IC	Tumor limited to one or both ovaries or fallopian tubes with any of the following:
	IC1	Surgical spill
	IC2	Capsule ruptured before surgery/tumor on ovarian or fallopian tube surface
	IC3	Malignant cells in ascites or peritoneal washings
T2	II	Tumor involves one or both ovaries or fallopian tubes with pelvic extension below pelvic brim or PPC
T2a	IIA	Extension and/or implants on the uterus and/or fallopian tube(s) and/or ovaries
T2b	IIB	Extension to and/or implants on other pelvic tissues
T3	III	Tumor involves one or both ovaries or fallopian tubes, or PPC, with microscopically confirmed peritoneal metastasis outside the pelvis and/or metastasis to the RP LNs
T3a	IIIA2	Microscopic extrapelvic (above the pelvic brim) peritoneal involvement ± metastasis to the RP LNs
T3b	IIIB	Macroscopic peritoneal metastasis beyond pelvis 2 cm or less in greatest dimension with or without metastasis to the RP LNs
T3c	IIIC	Macroscopic peritoneal metastasis beyond the pelvis more than 2 cm in greatest dimension with our without metastasis to the RP LNs (includes extension of tumor to capsule of liver and spleen without parenchymal involvement of either organ)
NX		Reginal LN cannot be assessed
N0		No regional LN metastasis
N1	IIIAI	Positive RP LN only
N1a	IIIAIi	Metastasis ≤10mm
N1b	IIIAIii	Metastasis > 10mm
M0		No distant metastasis
M1	IV	Distant metastasis including pleural effusion with positive cytology; liver or splenic parenchymal metastasis; metastasis to extra-abdominal organs and transmural involvement of intestine
M1a	IVA	Pleural effusion with positive cytology
M1b	IVB	Liver or splenic parenchymal metastases; metastases to extra-abdominal organs (including inguinal LNs and LNs outside the abdominal cavity) and transmural involvement of intestine

PPC, primary peritoneal cancer; RP, retroperitoneal; LN, lymph node.

preferred initial management for most patients. These patients should have an upfront gynecologic surgical assessment to review whether their cancer can be optimally debulked. Optimal cytoreduction is defined by residual disease <1 cm, although every effort should be made to remove all gross disease because this is associated with better patient outcomes. After primary surgery, patients with advanced-stage epithelial ovarian cancer should begin adjuvant chemotherapy, ideally within two to four weeks (Bristow 2002).

For patients who are not candidates for primary surgery due to poor performance status or medical comorbidities, or because their disease is unlikely to be optimally cytoreduced, neoadjuvant chemotherapy is commonly administered. The goal of this approach is a clinical response that would allow for or increase the likelihood of optimal cytoreduction at surgery.

Our patient has clinical stage III disease. Given the extent of her disease with diffuse carcinomatosis and large-volume ascites, which is not amenable to definitive resection, she would meet criteria for neoadjuvant therapy.

Another important assessment for patients with newly diagnosed ovarian, fallopian tube, or primary peritoneal cancer is for genetic risk evaluation and germline and somatic testing. This is a National Comprehensive Cancer Network (NCCN) recommendation at diagnosis because this will play a potential role regarding maintenance therapies (Chapter 46).

Studies have shown comparable results for neoadjuvant chemotherapy versus upfront surgery for patients with stage IIIC or IV disease. In a review of five randomized controlled trials of 1,713 patients with stage IIIC/IV ovarian cancer randomized to neoadjuvant chemotherapy followed by interval debulking surgery or primary debulking surgery followed by chemotherapy, there was little or no different regarding overall survival (OS). This data also showed that neoadjuvant chemotherapy may reduce need for stoma formation, bowel resection, and postoperative mortality. Thus, the sequence of therapy can be tailored to each individual patient and can consider surgical resectability, age, histology, stage, and performance status (Coleridge 2021).

2) What is the first line chemotherapy for patients with ovarian cancer?

Expert Perspective: The international standard adjuvant chemotherapy consists of a platinum agent with a taxane. The platinum-taxane combination has shown improved survival when compared with platinum monotherapy or a platinum plus non-taxane combination (Kyrgiou 2006). Carboplatin/paclitaxel regimen is the standard regimen used for patients and can achieve a clinical complete remission in most patients.

As we establish a greater understanding of the molecular pathways involved in carcinogenesis and tumor growth, many potential therapeutic targets have been identified. Perhaps the most mature concept is abrogation of blood vessels that tumors require to grow and metastasize. Among the antiangiogenic agents is bevacizumab, a monoclonal antibody against vascular endothelial growth factor (VEGF) and that is approved for use in the first-line setting in many countries, including the United States, based on two seminal adjuvant treatment trials showing that compared with chemotherapy alone, bevacizumab given with chemotherapy and then as single-agent maintenance treatment improves progression-free survival, though it does not improve OS (Burger

2011). A recent study to determine the length of bevacizumab maintenance treatment has shown no difference in progression free survival or OS for patients who received 15 months versus 30 months of bevacizumab maintenance. This trial of the AGO Study group randomized FIGO stage IIB–IV epithelial ovarian, fallopian tube, or primary peritoneal carcinoma patients who received 6 cycles of carboplatin/paclitaxel to 15 months of bevacizumab maintenance versus 30 months of bevacizumab maintenance. For patients who received 15 months of bevacizumab, median progression-free survival was 24.2, and median OS was 54.3 months compared to median progression-free survival of 26.0 and median OS of 60.0 for patients who received 30 months of bevacizumab, with no significant difference between the groups (Pfisterer 2021).

3) What is the role for intraperitoneal (IP) chemotherapy?

Expert Perspective: Given that the majority of ovarian cancer recurrences are confined to the peritoneal cavity, there is a strong rationale for administering cytotoxic drugs directly into the abdominal cavity, thereby increasing the dose intensity delivered to residual tumor implants while simultaneously avoiding additional systemic toxicity associated with increased systemic dose intensity. While three large phase III randomized trials comparing IP-containing chemotherapy with intravenous chemotherapy regimen consistently showed improved outcomes (including disease-free and OS) with IP treatment, the most recent trial conducted in the United States showed no benefit to IP treatment when bevacizumab was utilized as well. This was seen in the GOG 252 study, which included 1,560 patients with newly diagnosed ovarian cancer randomly assigned to received six cycles of intravenous paclitaxel (80 mg/m^2, weekly) with intravenous carboplatin (AUC 6) versus intravenous paclitaxel (weekly) with IP carboplatin (AUC 6) versus intravenous paclitaxel (135 mg/m^2 on day 1 every 3 weeks), IP cisplatin (75 mg/m^2 on day 2), and IP paclitaxel (60 mg/^{2} on day 8). All study participants also received bevacizumab every 3 weeks in cycles 2–22. There was no significant difference in median progression-free survival duration between each group. Patient reported toxicity scores were statistically worse in the IP cisplatin arm (Walker 2019).

Given these challenges and considering advances in the treatment of ovarian cancer (including the role of maintenance treatment), IP therapy has been utilized far less frequently. However, for the patient who undergoes an optimal cytoreduction at the time of diagnosis, IP-containing treatment is reasonable, especially if bevacizumab is not planned.

4) What is the role of hyperthermic intraperitoneal chemotherapy?

Expert Perspective: For patients who undergo neoadjuvant chemotherapy, there has also been interest in the utilization of hyperthermic intraperitoneal chemotherapy (HIPEC) at the time of surgical cytoreduction. This is based on one randomized phase III trial conducted in Amsterdam that randomly assigned 245 patients with stage III epithelial ovarian cancer who had at least stable disease after three cycles of intravenous carboplatin and intravenous paclitaxel to interval cytoreductive surgery with or without administration of HIPEC with cisplatin (100 mg/m^2). Three additional cycles of intravenous carboplatin and intravenous paclitaxel were given after surgery. The results showed that the addition of HIPEC to interval cytoreductive surgery resulted in longer recurrence free survival (14.2 months in HIPEC group vs 10.7 months in non-HIPEC group) and longer OS (45.7 months in

HIPEC group vs 33.9 months in non-HIPEC group). Also of note, the percentage of patients who had adverse events of grade 3 or 4 was similar in the two groups (27% in HIPEC group vs 25% in non-HIPEC group; $P = 0.76$) (Van Driel 2018). However, ongoing studies are needed to determine whether there is truly a significant benefit of HIPEC because some studies have suggested clinical benefit but with significant toxicity.

5) What is the role for PARP inhibitor maintenance therapy?

Expert Perspective: As previously discussed, germline and somatic testing is a recommendation for all patients with newly diagnosed ovarian, fallopian tube, or primary peritoneal carcinoma because it may influence decisions regarding maintenance therapy with poly (adenosine diphosphate-ribose) polymerase (PARP) inhibitor.

Multiple trials have evaluated the benefit of the addition of PARP inhibitors as maintenance therapy after chemotherapy.

- The SOLO-1 trial evaluated the benefit of olaparib maintenance therapy in 388 patients with stage II or IV ovarian, fallopian tube or primary peritoneal cancer with a mutation in *BRCA1*, *BRCA2*, or both (*BRCA1/2*) who had a partial or complete response to platinum-based chemotherapy. Participants were randomized in a 2:1 fashion to maintenance therapy with olaparib 300 mg twice daily versus placebo. The results showed that there was a significant improvement in progression-free survival among those on olaparib maintenance therapy compared with placebo and 70% lower risk of disease progression of death with olaparib compared with placebo. This study showed the significance that PARP inhibitors can have in the setting of advanced ovarian cancer for patients with a *BRCA* mutation (Moore 2018).
- The PRIMA trial then evaluated the benefit of niraparib, a different PARP inhibitor, in patients regardless of *BRCA* mutation status. This phase III trial randomized patients in a 2:1 ratio to receive niraparib 200 mg daily versus placebo daily after response to platinum-based chemotherapy. The primary end point was to evaluate efficacy in patients with homologous-recombination deficiency and those in the overall population. For patients with homologous-recombination deficiency, the median progression-free survival was significantly longer in the niraparib group compared with placebo (21.9 months vs 10.4 months) and in the overall population (13.8 months vs 8.2 months). Of note, in patients with homologous-recombination proficiency, progression-free survival was only 8.1 months in the niraparib group compared with 5.4 months in the placebo group (González-Martín 2019).
- In the PAOLA-1 trial, the addition of olaparib to bevacizumab maintenance therapy was evaluated in patients with ovarian cancer regardless of *BRCA* mutation status. The study randomized 806 patients who had a response after first-line platinum-taxane therapy plus bevacizumab in a 2:1 ratio to olaparib 300 mg twice daily versus placebo for 24 months. All patients received bevacizumab for 15 months. Significant benefit was seen in patients who received bevacizumab with olaparib compared with those who received bevacizumab alone for those who had *BRCA* mutations (median progression-free survival 22.1 months vs 16.6 months) and homologous-recombination deficiency (median progression-free survival 37.2 vs 17.7 months). Interestingly, patients who did not have a *BRCA* mutation and were homologous-recombination

deficiency proficient had no benefit with the addition of olaparib. One limitation of the study was that there was no monotherapy arm of olaparib without bevacizumab, and thus it is not clear if the benefit in patients with *BRCA* mutation or homologous-recombination deficiency was due to olaparib alone (Ray-Coquard 2019).

For our patient, Ms. A, germline and somatic testing would aid in the decision regarding the addition of PARP inhibitor maintenance therapy. As discussed earlier, if she was to have a *BRCA* mutation or homologous-recombination deficiency, there would be significant progression-free survival benefit in the addition of PARP inhibitor maintenance therapy. However, for patients who are *BRCA*-wild-type and homologous recombination proficient, there is a modest benefit to the use of niraparib maintenance therapy regarding progression-free survival and observation only or bevacizumab maintenance therapy are other reasonable options.

Case Study 2

Ms. A undergoes three cycles of neoadjuvant chemotherapy with carboplatin/paclitaxel, optimal debulking surgery, followed by three additional cycles of chemotherapy. Genetic testing reveals no clinically significant germline or somatic mutations. She declines first-line maintenance with PARP inhibitor. She was followed with surveillance imaging, and one year after completion of her systemic therapy, she was noted to have recurrence on imaging with increased pelvic lymphadenopathy and a peritoneal implant. Her CA125 was also elevated.

6) **What is the role of secondary cytoreduction in a patient with platinum-sensitive recurrent ovarian cancer?**

Expert Perspective: The question of secondary cytoreduction was addressed in three phase III trials, and the bulk of the data support surgery in selected patients.

The GOG-0213 trial reported that for women with platinum-sensitive recurrent disease, secondary cytoreductive surgery did not result in longer OS when compared with chemotherapy alone. The hazard ratio for death (surgery vs no surgery) was 1.29 (95% CI 0.97–1.72; $P = 0.08$), which corresponded to a median OS of 50.6 months and 64.7 months, respectively. The hazard ratio for disease progression or death (surgery vs no surgery) was 0.82 (95% CI 0.66–1.01; median progression-free survival, 18.9 months, and 16.2 months, respectively) (Coleman 2019).

However, both the DESKTOP III trial and SOC-1 trials did report a benefit of secondary cytoreductive surgery for carefully selected patients. In the DESKTOP III trial, volunteers were selected if they had no evidence of ascites at recurrence, had no residual disease after their first surgery, and had an excellent performance status (KPS 0). Among these volunteers, secondary cytoreductive surgery resulted in significant improvement in OS compared to chemotherapy alone (median 53.7 vs 46.2 months, respectively; HR 0.76; 95% CI 0.59–0.97; $P = 0.03$) and progression-free survival (18.4 vs 14 months; HR 0.66; 95% CI 0.54–0.82; $P < 0.001$). Of importance in this study is that this benefit was only seen in patients who had a complete resection, and thus it highlights that patient selection and surgical expertise are important factors (Du Bois 2020).

The SOC-1 trial allowed patients who met criteria based on a clinical model (the iModel). The criteria included FIGO stage, presence of residual disease after primary surgery, platinum-free interval, performance status, CA125 level, and presence of ascites. Compared with chemotherapy treatment only, secondary cytoreduction significantly improved progression-free survival (median 17.4 vs 11.9 months HR 0.58; 95% CI 0.45–0.74; $P < 0.0001$). OS data is not yet mature (Shi 2021).

In total, the data support surgery in women with a platinum-sensitive recurrence, but careful selection is required to identify those most likely to benefit from it.

7) What is the standard treatment of platinum-sensitive recurrent ovarian cancer?

Expert Perspective: Relapsed disease is managed based on the time to relapse since platinum-based therapy. Patients are considered platinum-sensitive if their progression-free interval is six months or longer. Patients with a progression-free interval of less than six months are considered to have platinum-resistant disease. Those patients within this group who progress while receiving platinum therapy are considered platinum-refractory.

Ms. A would be considered platinum sensitive, and as discussed earlier, options would be for secondary cytoreduction versus second-line chemotherapy of platinum/taxane with or without bevacizumab.

Data has suggested that patients with platinum-sensitive disease achieve better response and progression-free survival using maintenance treatment, which can consist of bevacizumab, olaparib, or niraparib. If bevacizumab was used in the platinum-based regimen, it is recommended to continue with bevacizumab maintenance therapy. The GOG 213 trial evaluated patients with platinum-sensitive recurrent ovarian cancer and randomly assigned them to secondary cytoreduction versus no secondary cytoreduction and separately to chemotherapy of carboplatin and paclitaxel with or without bevacizumab. For those patients who received bevacizumab, it was continued as maintenance therapy until progression. When compared with chemotherapy alone, the addition of bevacizumab improved progression-free survival from 10 months to 14 months and improved in OS from 37 months to 43 months. Of note, there were increased rates of serious grade 3/4 gastrointestinal complications and infections in the bevacizumab arm (Coleman 2017). However, if patients had previously received bevacizumab in the first-line setting, a rechallenge with bevacizumab prolonged progression-free survival but did not improve OS as seen in the MITO-16B trial (Pignata 2021).

The use of PARP inhibitor for maintenance therapy for patients with recurrent platinum-sensitive ovarian cancer has shown an improvement in progression-free survival, but OS outcomes are still pending. In the NOVA study, 553 patients with platinum-sensitive recurrent ovarian cancer were randomly assigned to chemotherapy then niraparib maintenance versus placebo. Niraparib was shown to increase progression-free survival in all cohorts, even in patients who were non-germline *BRCA* mutated (9.3 vs 3.9 months) (Mirza 2016). Olaparib has also been studied in patients regardless of *BRCA* status in Study 19, and maintenance therapy for platinum-sensitive relapsed disease and has shown a similar progression-free survival benefit (Friedlander 2018). Rucaparib also showed similar progression-free survival benefit in the ARIEL3 trial, which allowed patients to enroll even if they had residual bulky disease (Coleman 2017).

Case Study 3

Suppose Ms. A had recurrence of her disease within six months of receiving platinum-based therapy.

8) What treatment options are available for her?

Expert Perspective: For patients with platinum-resistant disease, options for first-line therapy depend on prior therapies they have received. One Cochrane systemic review of trials that included 1,323 patients with platinum-resistant ovarian cancer showed that single-agent topotecan, paclitaxel, and pegylated liposomal doxorubicin have similar efficacy but differ in patterns of side effects, such as increased hematologic toxicity with topotecan compared with paclitaxel and liposomal doxorubicin (Lihua 2008).

Certain patients who have received less than two prior regimens, have not received bevacizumab previously, and have no recent history of bowel obstruction may be candidates for single-agent chemotherapy with bevacizumab based on the AURELIA trial. This phase III randomized trial included patients with platinum-resistant ovarian cancer and randomly assigned them to single-agent chemotherapy alone or with bevacizumab until progression of toxicity. Options for single-agent chemotherapy included pegylated liposomal doxorubicin, weekly paclitaxel, or topotecan. Adding bevacizumab to single-agent chemotherapy significantly improved progression-free survival from 3.4 months to 6.7 months and improved overall response rate from 11.8% to 27.3% (Pujade-Lauraine 2014).

Some studies have also suggested some benefit of PARP inhibitors for recurrent platinum resistant disease. In the phase II CLIO trial, 85 *BRCA*-wild-type patients with platinum-resistant disease were treated with olaparib and demonstrate an overall response rate of 13% compared with 6% with chemotherapy alone. Progression-free survival was similar between the groups (Vanderstichele 2019). A single-arm trial of niraparib for women with a median of four previous lines of therapy with resistant or refractory disease showed response rate of 8% with a median duration of response of 9.4 months (Moore 2019).

Patients with recurrent ovarian cancer should have genomic testing for DNA mismatch repair (MMR)-deficient (dMMR) or microsatellite-instable (MSI) disease. The immune checkpoint inhibitor pembrolizumab is FDA approved for treatment of ovarian cancer that is dMMR or MSI. This was based on KEYNOTE-158, which looked at 233 patients with 27 tumor types with confirmed dMMR/MSI tumors refractory to prior therapy. Among the participants were 15 patients with ovarian cancer with an overall response rate of 33% and 3 complete responses (Marabelle 2020).

Palliative care is also an important part of oncologic care, especially for patients with recurrent disease that is platinum refractory. Malignant bowel obstruction is a common problem faced by women with recurrent ovarian cancer, and for the majority, it can be a terminal event. Options for treatment are to improve symptoms and provide palliation such as with placement of percutaneous endoscopic gastrotomy tube to improve vomiting. Chemotherapy and surgery may be options. Recurrent ascites is also seen in a large proportion of women with platinum-resistant disease, and therapeutic paracentesis provides relief but is temporary, and thus consideration for a more permanent catheter such as a Pleurx catheter can be placed to offer relief of symptoms and drainage at home. There is some evidence to suggest that an angiogenesis inhibitor such as bevacizumab can be used to manage refractory ascites and provide symptom relief (Numnum 2006).

Case Study 4

Ms. B is a 30-year-old female who presents to the emergency department because of a few days of nausea, vomiting, and diarrhea due to norovirus, but she is incidentally found to have a concerning mass on her right ovary from a CT of the abdomen and pelvis imaging. She undergoes a CT chest with contrast without signs of other areas of disease. Her CA125 is elevated. She is not planning on having more children. She undergoes surgery with finding of complete replacement of right ovary with a cystic mass. Post-op pathology shows grade 1 endometrioid adenocarcinoma.

9) What is the role of chemotherapy in early stage ovarian cancer?

Expert Perspective: Women with stage I epithelial ovarian cancer typically have an excellent prognosis. Complete surgical staging is important to ensure that there is no microscopic spread that would "upgrade" the patient.

Whether adjuvant chemotherapy is required for people with early stage disease was addressed in two European phase III randomized studies. The Adjuvant Clinical Trial in Ovarian Neoplasms (ACTION) enrolled women with surgically respected early stage ovarian cancer and randomly assigned them to observation or to adjuvant platinum-based chemotherapy. The International Collaborative Neoplasm Studies (ICON1) trial randomly assigned volunteers to similar treatment but did not require surgical staging (ICON1 2004; Trimbos 2003).

A total of 924 patients were randomized to both trials. In a combined analysis with over four years of median follow-up, adjuvant chemotherapy resulted in an absolute 11% improvement in relapse-free survival (HR 0.64; 95% CI 0.50–0.82; $P = 0.001$) and an absolute 8% improvement in OS (HR 0.67; 95% CI 0.50–0.90; $P = 0.008$). Subgroup analysis demonstrated in the ACTION trial that completeness of surgical staging was an independent factor for prognosis, both for progression-free survival and for OS (along with histological type and tumor grade). In suboptimally staged patients, adjuvant chemotherapy did improve the outcome. A report of a 10-year follow-up of the ICON1 trial has revealed that the improvement in 5-year OS persists even one decade following the completion of adjuvant chemotherapy (Swart 2007).

Given the added clarity to the question of surgical staging provided by the ACTION and ICON1 trials and subsequent analyses, the question remains whether individuals with high-risk early stage epithelial ovarian cancer are overtreated systemically. The Gynecologic Oncology Group conducted a phase III trial regarding the management of early stage disease. This study compared three versus six cycles of carboplatin and paclitaxel combination chemotherapy as the treatment regimen for women with high-risk, surgically staged disease. The results showed that there was an approximately 25% increased risk of relapse associated with the truncated course of chemotherapy, although this difference did not reach statistical significance, mainly due to the inadequate sample size. The risk of recurrence in this patient population seems to have remained relatively unchanged over the years, leaving opportunities for innovative research.

Overall, it is felt that the subset of patients with early stage disease with greatest increased risk of relapse are those with high-risk features. This includes stage IC disease, which indicates the tumor is confined to the ovary with positive peritoneal washing, or stage II disease, in which the tumor involves the pelvis, clear cell histology at any stage, or a high-grade tumor (at least grade 3). Five-year disease-free survival rates for women with early stage disease with high-risk features range from 40 to 80% (Chan 2008).

The overall recommendation from NCCN guidelines is for women with resected and fully staged grade 1, stage IA, or stage IB disease is to consider observation alone rather than the use of adjuvant therapy. For women with high-risk disease (defined as stage IC or II, high grade, or clear cell cancers of any stage), the recommendation would be for adjuvant chemotherapy. The role of adjuvant therapy for patients with grade 2 tumors is controversial but may be beneficial in a subgroup of patients.

Case Study 5

10) If Ms. B were interested in fertility preservation, what options would she have?

Expert Perspective: A small proportion of women with invasive epithelial ovarian cancer are diagnosed in the reproductive age group. Approximately 25% are stage I, and bilaterality is dependent on cell type. Most mucinous and clear cell tumors are unilateral, but approximately 50% of serous tumors are bilateral. Thus, fertility-sparing surgery may be performed in selected young patients with apparent disease confined to one ovary (stage 1A). There is generally a greater risk of relapse in this patient cohort. When relapse occurs in the residual ovary alone, salvage treatment may result in cure. However, if disseminated recurrence with peritoneal carcinomatosis occurs, cure is uncommon. In a study that examined the natural history of stage I ovarian cancer managed without chemotherapy, the five-year survival rate was 94% for stage IA lesions, 92% for stage IB tumors, and 84% for stage IC neoplasm.

Comprehensive surgical staging is the overarching surgical principal for those women with clinically apparent stage I ovarian cancer. Comprehensive surgical staging generally consists of peritoneal cytologic washings, systematic inspection and palpation of all peritoneal contents, multiple biopsies of upper abdominal and pelvic peritoneal surfaces, omentectomy, and pelvic and para-aortic lymphadenectomy. In general, if extraovarian disease is apparent at the time of surgical intervention, maximal surgical resection to achieve no gross residual disease is the goal. Postoperatively, if the tumor was a low-grade serous carcinoma, mucinous carcinoma, or well-differentiated endometrioid subtype, most would recommend surveillance without postoperative therapy. Cure rates for women with low-risk stage I tumors are in the 80–90% range. However, for those women with high-grade serous carcinoma, undifferentiated carcinoma, transitional carcinoma, and high-grade endometrioid carcinoma, or for women with stage IC disease, standard chemotherapy with carboplatin and paclitaxel is recommended. Cure rates for these high-risk women range from 50 to 60%.

A major concern after conservative therapy for early stage ovarian cancer centers around the ability to achieve pregnancy after treatment, particularly because many patients with stage I disease will receive adjuvant chemotherapy. Studies of young women with germ cell tumors of the ovary, breast cancer, and Hodgkin's lymphoma have indicated that many women will resume menstrual function after cytotoxic chemotherapy. Among women with early stage ovarian cancer who underwent fertility conserving surgery, menstrual function was preserved in 94% of patients in one series. Reports of pregnancy outcomes after fertility-sparing surgery for invasive epithelial ovarian cancer are limited to retrospective case series because no prospective randomized study on this specific issue has been published. Park et al. (2008) reviewed records of 62 patients with invasive epithelial ovarian cancer who underwent fertility-sparing surgery, defined as the preservation of ovarian tissue in one or both adnexa and the uterus, between May 1990 and October 2006. Most patients had stage IA disease and mucinous histology with a median follow-up of 56 months. Eleven patients had a tumor recurrence, 6 died of disease, 2 were alive with disease, and 54 were alive without disease. Patients with greater than stage IC or grade 3 tumors had significantly worse survival. Nineteen women attempted to conceive; there were 22 term pregnancies and no congenital anomalies in any of the offspring. Interestingly, none of the patients with serous histology recurred (Bristow 2002).

Finally, the question of whether completion oophorectomy and/or hysterectomy should be undertaken in women after the conclusion of childbearing frequently arises. Completion surgery is appealing because many of the recurrences in patients who initially underwent conservative surgery occur in the contralateral adnexa. Whether completion surgery alters long-term outcome is unknown; thus, the decision to undergo completion surgery should be individualized.

Recommended Readings

Burger, R.A., Brady, M.F., Bookman, M.A. et al. (2011). Incorporation of bevacizumab in the primary treatment of ovarian cancer. *N Engl J Med* 365: 2473–2783.

Coleman, R.L., Oza, A.M., Lorusso, D. et al. (2017b). ARIEL3 investigators. Rucaparib maintenance treatment for recurrent ovarian carcinoma after response to platinum therapy (ARIEL3): A randomised, double-blind, placebo-controlled, phase 3 trial. *Lancet* 390 (10106): 1949–1961. doi:10.1016/S0140-6736(17)32440-6. Epub 2017 Sep 12. Erratum in: Lancet. 2017 Oct 28;390(10106):1948. PMID: 28916367; PMCID: PMC5901715.

Coleman, R.L. et al. (2019). Secondary surgical cytoreduction for recurrent ovarian cancer." *N Engl J Med* 381 (20): 1929–1939.

Du Bois, A., Sehouli, J., Vergote, I. et al. (2020). Randomized phase III study to evaluate the impact of secondary cytoreductive surgery in recurrent ovarian cancer: Final analysis of AGO DESKTOP III/ENGOT-ov20. 6000.

Kyrgiou, M., Salanti, G., Pavlidis, N. et al. (2006). Survival benefits with diverse chemotherapy regimens for ovarian cancer: Meta-analysis of multiple treatments. *J Natl Cancer Inst* 98 (22): 1655–1663. doi:10.1093/jnci/djj443. PMID: 17105988.

Moore, K., Colombo, N., Scambia, G. et al. (2018). Maintenance olaparib in patients with newly diagnosed advanced ovarian cancer. *N Engl J Med* 379 (26): 2495–2505.

Pignata, S., Lorusso, D., Joly, F. et al. (2021). MITO16b/MANGO–OV2/ENGOT–ov17 Investigators. Carboplatin-based doublet plus bevacizumab beyond progression versus carboplatin-based doublet alone in patients with platinum-sensitive ovarian cancer: A randomised, phase 3 trial. *Lancet Oncol* 22 (2): 267–276. doi:10.1016/S1470-2045(20)30637-9. PMID: 33539744.

Van Driel, W.J., Koole, S.N., Sikorska, K. et al. (2018). Hyperthermic intraperitoneal chemotherapy in ovarian cancer. *N Engl J Med* 378 (3): 230–240.

Walker, J.L., Brady, M.F., Wenzel, L. et al. (2019). Randomized trial of intravenous versus intraperitoneal chemotherapy plus bevacizumab in advanced ovarian carcinoma: An NRG oncology/gynecologic oncology group study. *J Clin Oncol* 37 (16): 1380.

39

Ovarian Cancer: Second-line Treatment Strategies
Maurie Markman

City of Hope, Phoenix, AZ

Introduction

Although more than 80% of patients with epithelial ovarian cancer respond to primary platinum-based therapy, most individuals will unfortunately ultimately experience recurrence of their illness and be candidates for second-line (or later) therapeutic options. Patients who experience disease recurrence after a relatively long treatment (platinum)-free interval (>6–12 months) are generally considered for possible reintroduction of a platinum-based regimen. The addition of bevacizumab to either a platinum or a non-platinum-based chemotherapy program in the second-line setting has been shown in several randomized trials to improve progression-free survival, although documenting superior overall survival in this setting has been difficult due to the availability of multiple therapeutic options following disease progression of participants in a randomized trial. There is evidence that a patient who has received bevacizumab as a component of treatment in the first-line setting may also benefit from use of the drug in later lines of treatment. More recently, several poly adenosine diphosphate-ribose polymerase (PARP) inhibitors have been revealed to be of clinical utility in the second-line (or later) setting when used either as a single-agent "maintenance strategy" (after a response to a platinum-based regimen) or as a single-agent treatment approach in the presence of known disease. Existing data indicate that patients with *BRCA* mutations (germline or somatic) or with molecular evidence of "homologous recombination deficiency" (in the absence of a documented *BRCA* mutation) are more likely to benefit from PARP inhibitor therapy compared with individuals with evidence of a proficient DNA repair process. Large-panel somatic molecular testing is increasingly utilized to discover the objectively small number of ovarian cancer patients who may benefit from other individual targeted therapeutic strategies (e.g. checkpoint inhibitor therapy in the presence of a high microsatellite instability phenotype).

Case Study 1

A 66-year-old ovarian cancer patient develops abdominal pain and bloating nine months after the completion of carboplatin–paclitaxel chemotherapy. The serum CA25 level is now 395 U/mL (repeat value 436 U/mL), having declined to 27 U/mL at the end of the first-line treatment program. A computed tomography (CT) scan of the abdomen and pelvis reveals a small amount of ascites and possible peritoneal wall nodules. Germline testing performed at the time of ovarian cancer diagnosis does not reveal *BRCA* mutation.

1) **All of the following would be reasonable subsequent management strategies except which one?**
    A) Initiate chemotherapy with a non-platinum-containing regimen.
    B) Initiate chemotherapy with a platinum-containing regimen.
    C) Obtain a biopsy of the peritoneal wall nodule to confirm the presence of ovarian cancer.
    D) Initiate cytotoxic chemotherapy plus bevacizumab.

Expert Perspective: With a treatment-free interval of nine months (greater than six months), the cancer in this patient would be considered to have a modest opportunity to again respond to a platinum agent, and either employing or not employing platinum (cisplatin or carboplatin) in the second-line setting would be an appropriate option. Knowledge of the severity of toxicity experienced by the patient during primary chemotherapy can be helpful in deciding the wisdom of resuming platinum-based treatment versus employing a non-platinum-based strategy. Several randomized trials have shown the addition of bevacizumab to platinum or non-platinum chemotherapy improves progression-free survival compared with cytotoxic chemotherapy alone. There is no need to rebiopsy a patient with known ovarian cancer who has recurrent symptoms and a definite increase in the serum CA125 level if this procedure is being performed solely for the purpose of confirming the presence of recurrent disease.

Correct Answer: C

2) **Which of the following statements regarding the second-line treatment of epithelial ovarian cancer is correct?**
    A) There is no rationale for delivering more than three different chemotherapy regimens in ovarian cancer because the chances of producing serious side effects beyond this number of regimens far outweighs the opportunity for clinical benefit.
    B) The overall "duration of survival" following initial disease progression in ovarian cancer now frequently exceeds the time from diagnosis to the date of initial progression.
    C) There are no oral agents with known activity in ovarian cancer currently available for routine clinical use.
    D) None of the above.

Expert Perspective: Increasingly, patients with ovarian cancer are able to experience extended survival (including prolonged survival after initial progression following front-line platinum-taxane chemotherapy) due to the activity of multiple active antineoplastic agents in this malignancy. There are no reasonable arbitrary limits on the number of chemotherapy regimens that may be employed, assuming care is taken to minimize the risk of excessive and sustained toxicity. Several oral antineoplastic agents (e.g. tamoxifen, etoposide, and altretamine) are utilized in routine clinical practice in the management of ovarian cancer. Oral PARP inhibitors are also approved for treatment of recurrent ovarian cancer in the setting of a documented *BRCA* mutation, either germline or somatic.

Correct Answer: B

3) **Which of the following molecular markers have been shown to be clinically relevant in the selection of second-line therapy of ovarian cancer?**
   A) Activating mutations in epidermal growth factor receptor.
   B) *BRCA* mutations.
   C) *BRAF* mutations.
   D) None of the above.

Expert Perspective: Several PARP inhibitors (olaparib, niraparib, rucaparib) are currently approved for both maintenance treatment of recurrent ovarian cancer following a response to platinum-based therapy or as single-agent treatment of the malignancy. This is a rapidly evolving area, as PARP inhibitors are also being employed as a maintenance strategy in the front-line setting. It remains unknown whether a patient who has received one PARP inhibitor as treatment of recurrent disease may respond to a different PARP inhibiting agent at the time of disease progression.

Correct Answer: B

Case Study 2

A 52-year-old female with epithelial ovarian cancer develops recurrent disease with a treatment-free interval of 19 months following the completion of her primary chemotherapy regimen (carboplatin-paclitaxel).

4) **Which of the following statements regarding the opportunity for this individual to respond to another platinum-based chemotherapy regimen is incorrect?**
   A) There is at least a 50% chance for an objective response to be observed.
   B) Compared with single-agent platinum, platinum-based combination chemotherapy has been shown to improve both progression-free and overall survival in this setting.
   C) Cure is a realistic goal in this clinical setting.
   D) None of the above.

Expert Perspective: There is a high probability (greater than 50%) that a patient with this prolonged treatment-free interval will achieve a second response following reintroduction of a platinum strategy. Several phase III trials have documented the superiority of combination platinum-based compared with single-agent platinum in recurrent ovarian cancer. Although second-line therapy in ovarian cancer has been shown to improve both progression-free and overall survival, there is currently no evidence that such therapy can cure the malignancy.

Correct Answer: C

Case Study 3

A 65-year-old asymptomatic female with epithelial ovarian cancer is found to have a rising serum CA125 antigen level approximately 16 months following the completion of her primary chemotherapy regimen. A CT scan of the abdomen reveals a small amount of ascites as well as several small (less than 3 cm in maximum diameter) pelvic and peritoneal nodules.

5) Which of the following statements regarding the clinical utility of secondary surgical cytoreduction in this clinical setting is correct?
   A) A phase III trial has revealed the superiority of an attempt at secondary cytoreduction in epithelial ovarian cancer compared with initiating treatment with chemotherapy (and no surgery).
   B) A phase III trial has failed to document the benefits associated with secondary cytoreduction in epithelial ovarian cancer.
   C) Phase III trial data suggest that secondary cytoreduction surgery is of value only if it is possible to resect all visible macroscopic disease
   D) Existing data support all of the above conclusions.

Expert Perspective: Several phase III randomized clinical trials examining the issue of the benefits, or harm, associated with secondary cytoreductive surgery in epithelial ovarian cancer have been reported with quite conflicting results. However, existing data support careful consideration of this approach in a setting where it is believed to be reasonably possible to safely resect all visible macroscopic disease prior to the initiation of second-line chemotherapy.

Correct Answer: D

6) For several reasons, randomized phase III trials have been required to answer the question of the utility of secondary cytoreduction in ovarian cancer, versus simply accepting the results of retrospective analyses comparing patients undergoing or not undergoing such procedures. Which of the following is correct?
   A) Any benefit of surgery may result from selection bias associated with the patient population chosen to undergo such surgery (e.g. superior performance status and fewer comorbidities).
   B) Any benefit of surgery may result from similar biological factors that influence the ability to successfully surgically cytoreduce the cancer and that determine the growth, spread, and development of drug resistance.
   C) Both A and B.
   D) Neither A nor B.

Expert Perspective: Both issues of selection bias and similar biological factors are critical factors in any discussion of the relevance of retrospective analyses in defining the utility of secondary cytoreduction in ovarian cancer. As a result of the compounding influence of these factors, only the conduct of a well-designed randomized phase III trial can resolve the issue. Unfortunately, existing phase III trial data have revealed conflicting results as to the actual benefits of this therapeutic strategy in ovarian cancer.

Correct Answer: C

Case Study 4

A 47-year-old woman with a 2-year history of ovarian cancer undergoes secondary cytoreduction and is left with only microscopic residual disease. She inquires about the potential role of intraperitoneal chemotherapy in her management.

7) **Which of the following statements regarding this strategy in the second-line management of ovarian cancer is correct?**
    A) Phase III trial data have revealed a survival advantage for this approach compared with systemic administration in this clinical setting.
    B) This strategy should not be employed in the second-line setting due to the potential for severe intraperitoneal side effects in multiple clinical trials.
    C) Phase II trial data have revealed the opportunity to achieve surgically documented complete responses following second-line intraperitoneal cisplatin-based chemotherapy.
    D) None of the above.

Expert Perspective: Multiple phase II trials have revealed the biological and clinical activity (including surgically confirmed complete responses) associated with the second-line delivery of platinum-based chemotherapy in epithelial ovarian cancer. However, there remains no phase III trial data to demonstrate the therapeutic superiority of this approach compared with systemic drug administration in this clinical setting.

Correct Answer: C

Case Study 5

A 53-year-old female will be initiating second-line carboplatin-based chemotherapy for ovarian cancer.

8) **Which of the following platinum-associated toxicities are somewhat unique to this clinical setting?**
    A) Hypersensitivity reactions.
    B) Peripheral neuropathy.
    C) Severe emesis.
    D) Cardiac dysfunction.

Expert Perspective: Considerable retrospective data have revealed that the incidence of platinum-associated (most frequently, carboplatin) hypersensitivity increases dramatically after a total of at least five to six cumulative doses of the agent, which in most circumstances will occur in the second-line setting. This is presumably due to a requirement for multiple exposures of the susceptible immune system to very low concentrations of free platinum that may be present within the antineoplastic drug preparation.

Correct Answer: A

Case Study 6

A 62-year-old ovarian cancer patient experiences recurrent abdominal pain following completion of her second-line carboplatin treatment regimen.

9) **Which of the following statements regarding the ability to retreat this patient with another platinum program is correct?**
   A) Platinum-based regimens should be used a maximum of two times due to the development of excessive side effects with additional treatment.
   B) The probably of another response (third-line) to a platinum program will be dependent on the duration of time the patient has been off treatment from the second-line regimen.
   C) Phase III trial data have revealed that non-platinum therapy is superior to a platinum regimen for third-line treatment of ovarian cancer.
   D) Because of the low probably of a response to any cytotoxic therapy in ovarian cancer, there is essentially no role to readminister a platinum regimen in this setting.

Expert Perspective: As with second-line therapy of ovarian cancer, the probability of a third response to a platinum agent appears to be related to the duration of time a patient has been off treatment from a second-line platinum program. Of course, this assumes that the patient exhibited a response to that regimen. If not, alternative non-platinum-based options will need to be considered. It should also be noted that in the presence of a *BRCA* mutation (germline or somatic), an alternative approach in platinum-sensitive recurrent ovarian cancer is the delivery of one of several commercially available noninvestigative PARP inhibitors.

Correct Answer: B

Case Study 7

A 49-year-old female with ovarian cancer experiences abdominal pain and is found to have a new pelvic mass on imaging studies four months after the completion of her primary chemotherapy program.

10) **Which of the following statements concerning her future management is correct?**
    A) The cancer is considered to be platinum resistant.
    B) High-dose chemotherapy with stem cell rescue has not been shown to be of value in this clinical setting.
    C) The administration of a two-drug cytotoxic chemotherapy program has been shown to result in improved survival compared with single-agent cytotoxic delivery.
    D) Both A and C.

Expert Perspective: This cancer is considered to be platinum resistant (recurrence within six months of the completion of primary chemotherapy). High-dose chemotherapy plays no role in patients with platinum-resistant disease, and there is no evidence that combination cytotoxic therapy is superior to single-cytotoxic-agent treatment in this setting. However, phase III trial data have revealed the superiority of cytotoxic chemotherapy plus bevacizumab compared with chemotherapy alone in this clinical setting.

Correct Answer: A

Case Study 8

A 52-year-old ovarian cancer patient experiences recurrence of her disease 22 months following the completion of primary chemotherapy.

11) **Which of the following statements regarding management of recurrent potentially platinum-sensitive ovarian cancer is correct?**
    A) Compared with single-agent platinum, combination platinum-based chemotherapy has been shown in randomized trials to improve both the time to subsequent disease progression and overall survival in this clinical setting.
    B) Cisplatin has been documented to be more active than carboplatin in recurrent ovarian cancer.
    C) On the basis of existing phase III trial data, there is currently no evidence for the superiority of any one platinum-based combination chemotherapy regimen compared with another in the setting of recurrent ovarian cancer.
    D) None of the above.

Expert Perspective: Two phase III randomized trials have revealed the superiority of a platinum-based combination regimen compared with single-agent platinum in improving progression-free survival. One such study has demonstrated an improvement in overall survival. There is no evidence for the superiority of cisplatin compared with carboplatin in recurrent disease. In a phase III trial, the combination of carboplatin plus pegylated liposomal doxorubicin improved progression-free survival compared with carboplatin plus paclitaxel in recurrent ovarian cancer.

Correct Answer: A

12) **In the phase III randomized trial of carboplatin plus paclitaxel versus carboplatin plus pegylated liposomal doxorubicin (PLD) in recurrent ovarian cancer, patients treated with the PLD-containing regimen experienced an unexpectedly low incidence of which carboplatin-associated toxicity (compared with that observed in the paclitaxel-containing program)?**
    A) Emesis.
    B) Bone marrow suppression.
    C) Peripheral neuropathy.
    D) Hypersensitivity reactions.

Expert Perspective: In this trial, 5.6% of patients treated on the pegylated liposomal doxorubicin arm experienced a carboplatin-associated hypersensitivity reaction (at least grade 2) compared with an incidence of 18.8% with paclitaxel. A biological explanation for this highly provocative finding remains elusive, although a second smaller, randomized trial has reached a similar conclusion. The lower risk of carboplatin hypersensitivity may explain (at least in part) the statistically significant improvement in time to disease progression noted in this trial in favor of the pegylated liposomal doxorubicin-containing regimen because a lower percentage of patients on this study arm had treatment with carboplatin discontinued because of this potentially highly relevant side effect.

Correct Answer: D

13) An overall survival advantage was revealed in favor of single-agent pegylated liposomal doxorubicin in a phase III trial that compared this agent to topotecan as a second-line therapy of epithelial ovarian cancer. This survival advantage was confined to what subset of patients?
    A) Platinum-resistant disease.
    B) Platinum-sensitive disease.
    C) An overall survival advantage was observed in both subgroups.
    D) There was no overall survival advantage observed in this trial, only an improvement in progression-free survival.

Expert Perspective: In this important phase III trial, patients with potentially platinum-sensitive (treatment-free interval of >6 months) recurrent ovarian cancer treated with pegylated liposomal doxorubicin experienced superior overall survival compared with second-line therapy with topotecan. There was no difference in survival for patients with platinum-resistant disease.

Correct Answer: B

14) Which statement is correct regarding the activity of weekly paclitaxel in patients previously treated with every-three-week paclitaxel delivery in the front-line setting?
    A) Weekly paclitaxel administration is inactive in this clinical setting.
    B) An objective response rate of 20% can be anticipated with weekly paclitaxel delivery.
    C) Weekly paclitaxel is associated with an unacceptably high risk of peripheral neuropathy in patients previously treated with every-three-week paclitaxel.
    D) None of the above.

Expert Perspective: Several phase II studies have revealed an objective response rate of approximately 20% when weekly paclitaxel is administered to patients who have previously received and progressed on a regimen where the agent was delivered on an every-three-week schedule. In addition, in most patients with which this approach is associated had a favorable side effect profile.

Correct Answer: B

15) Single-agent pegylated liposomal doxorubicin is commonly administered in the management of platinum-resistant ovarian cancer at a dose of 40 mg/m^2 (delivered on an every-28-day schedule). This has been done to reduce the risk of patients experiencing highly clinically relevant toxicity (e.g. hand-foot-syndrome, mucositis, and stomatitis) commonly observed at the dose level, which received US Food and Drug Administration approval for delivery as second-line therapy of ovarian cancer. What is this dose level?
    A) 50 mg/m^2 every 28 days.
    B) 60 mg/m^2 every 28 days.
    C) 70 mg/m^2 every 28 days.
    D) None of the above.

Expert Perspective: Although there have been no direct comparison studies of pegylated liposomal doxorubicin administered at a dose of 40 versus 50 mg/m^2 in ovarian cancer, retrospective data from several centers have suggested equivalent activity of the two dose levels. Further, randomized trials have compared the same control arm (gemcitabine) with pegylated liposomal doxorubicin at either the 40 or 50 mg/m^2 levels with equivalent survival outcomes. Of greatest relevance, however, is the observation that the lower dose level is associated with a substantially more favorable toxicity profile for the agent in this palliative clinical setting.

Correct Answer: A

Case Study 9

A 67-year-old female with epithelial ovarian cancer has received several prior chemotherapy regimens and is considering possible options for her again-progressing malignancy.

16) Which of the following clinical factors in this individual's medical history would suggest the possible inadvisability of employing bevacizumab?
    A) Several recent episodes of medically managed partial small-bowel obstruction.
    B) Medication-controlled hypertension.
    C) Platinum-resistant ovarian cancer.
    D) History of carboplatin-associated hypersensitivity reaction.

Expert Perspective: Existing clinical trial data have suggested a considerable risk of bowel perforation (10%) associated with bevacizumab administration in heavily pretreated patients with ovarian cancer, with the greatest risk noted in individuals with evidence of bowel involvement with tumor. The presence of small-bowel obstruction likely suggests such involvement and would be a relative contraindication for the use of this antineoplastic medication.

Correct Answer: A

17) Despite the documented benefits of bevacizumab when combined with cytotoxic chemotherapy in several tumor types, the single-agent activity of this antiangiogenic agent in these cancers has been quite modest. What is the reported single-agent response rate in the second-line (or later) setting for bevacizumab in epithelial ovarian cancer?
    A) <2%.
    B) 5%.
    C) 15%.
    D) 35%.

Expert Perspective: In one well-designed and well-conducted single-agent phase II trial involving heavily pretreated patients with epithelial ovarian cancer, an objective response rate of 15% was observed. Of note, this level of activity is comparable with several cytotoxic agents routinely employed in this clinical setting (e.g. pegylated liposomal doxorubicin, topotecan, paclitaxel, and docetaxel).

Correct Answer: C

18) In two reported phase III trials comparing chemotherapy with or without bevacizumab in recurrent platinum-sensitive ovarian cancer, what was the cytotoxic regimen examined?
   A) Cisplatin plus paclitaxel.
   B) Carboplatin plus paclitaxel.
   C) Carboplatin plus gemcitabine.
   D) Both B and C.

Expert Perspective: Carboplatin plus gemcitabine and carboplatin plus paclitaxel were the control arms in two reported randomized phase III trials with the experimental regimen in each study adding bevacizumab.

Correct Answer: D

19) In the several phase III trials examining PARP inhibitors as "maintenance therapy" following a response to platinum-based chemotherapy in recurrent ovarian cancer, what was the patient population most likely to achieve clinical benefit?
   A) *BRCA* mutation positive (germline or somatic).
   B) *BRCA* wild-type.
   C) Homologous recombination proficient.
   D) Somatic *BRCA* mutation positive only (not germline positive).

Expert Perspective: The phase III trials examining several PARP inhibitors as a maintenance strategy in recurrent ovarian cancer have shown that patients with *BRCA* mutations (germline or somatic) exhibit the greatest clinical benefit (improvement in progression-free survival compared to nontreated control populations). Patients with *BRCA* wild-type or with evidence of homologous recombination proficient cancers (no defect in DNA repair) exhibit less statistically defined clinical benefit.

Correct Answer: A

20) In a phase III trial that compared the administration of cytotoxic chemotherapy with or without bevacizumab in platinum-resistant ovarian cancer, there was a choice of three different cytotoxic regimens. These included all of the following except which one?
   A) Topotecan.
   B) Pegylated liposomal doxorubicin.
   C) Weekly paclitaxel.
   D) Pemetrexed.

Expert Perspective: The times to disease progression on each of the three chemotherapy regimens (topotecan, pegylated liposomal doxorubicin, and weekly paclitaxel) included in this study were shown to be prolonged with the addition of bevacizumab. Refer to Chapter 38 for neoadjuvant, adjuvant, and further discussion on surgical issues in ovarian cancer.

Correct Answer: D

Recommended Readings

Baert, T., Ferrero, A., Sehouli, J. et al. (2021). The systemic treatment of recurrent ovarian cancer revisited. *Ann Oncol* 32 (6): 710–725.

Harrison, R., Zighelboim, I., Clobern, N.G. et al. (2021). Secondary cytoreductive surgery for recurrent ovarian cancer: An SGO clinical practice statement. *Gynecol Oncol* 163: 448–452.

Haunschild, C.E. and Tewari, K.S. (2021). The current landscape of molecular profiling in the treatment of epithelial ovarian cancer. *Gynecol Oncol* 160: 333–345.

Kristeleit, R., Lisyanskaya, A., Fedenko, A. et al. (2022). Rucaparib versus standard-of-care chemotherapy in patients with relapsed ovarian cancer and a deleterious *BRCA1* or *BRCA2* mutation (ARIEL4). *Lancet Oncol* 23: 465–478.

Laine, A., Sims, T.T., Le Saux, O. et al. (2021). Treatment perspectives for ovarian cancer in Europe and the United States: Initial therapy and platinum-sensitive recurrence after PARP inhibitors or bevacizumab therapy. *Curr Oncol Rep* 23: 148.

Markman, M. (2019a). Genomic-based therapy of gynecologic malignancies. *Acta Med Acad* 48 (1): 84–89.

Markman, M. (2019b). Pharmaceutical management of ovarian cancer: Current status. *Drugs* 79 (11): 1231–1239.

Monk, B.J., Parkinson, C., Lim, M.C. et al. (2022). A randomized, phase III trial to evaluate rucaparib monotherapy as maintenance treatment in patients with newly diagnosed ovarian cancer (ATHENA-MONO/GOG-3020/ENGOT-ov45). *J Clin Oncol* JCO2201003. doi: 10.1200/JCO.22.01003. Epub ahead of print. PMID: 35658487.

Tew, W.P., Lacchetti, C., Ellis, A. et al. (2020). PARP inhibitors in the management of ovarian cancer: ASCO guidelines. *J Clin Oncol* 38: 3468–3493.

40

Endometrial Cancer

Maurie Markman

City of Hope, Phoenix, AZ

Introduction

There are approximately 60,000 new cases of endometrial cancer diagnosed in the United States each year, making this the most common gynecologic cancer. It should be noted that in contrast with other malignancies, the incidence of endometrial cancer is increasing in the United States, presumably due to the epidemic of obesity, which is increasingly recognized as a serious risk factor for development of the malignancy. Another important risk factor is increased estrogen exposure. The most common symptom of endometrial cancer is abnormal uterine bleeding. The major treatment modality is surgery (total hysterectomy, bilateral salpingo-oophorectomy, and examination of local/regional lymph nodes), with most cases being diagnosed at an early and curable stage. However, recurrences are not rare, especially in the presence of high-grade morphology, serous, clear cell, or carcinosarcoma subtypes. With disease recurrence or in the presence of metastatic disease, the combination of carboplatin-paclitaxel is the generally preferred regimen in high-grade disease or carcinosarcoma, whereas hormonal therapy (single agent or a combination drug regimen) may be attempted initially in low-grade cancer in the absence of extensive organ involvement. Alternatively, hormonal therapy may be employed in this situation following progression on a platinum-based regimen. Recent data has revealed a relatively high percentage of metastatic endometrial cancers have microsatellite instability (MSI-H). Such patients with MSI-H have shown greater than 40–50% response rate to one of several commercially available checkpoint inhibitors. Further, the combination of pembrolizumab plus lenvatinib has been revealed to improve overall survival compared with cytotoxic chemotherapy (doxorubicin or weekly paclitaxel) in advanced endometrial cancer patients whose disease had progressed on a platinum regimen. Recently, two paradigm changing randomized trials have been reported which reveal the combination of checkpoint inhibitor therapy plus chemotherapy is superior to chemotherapy alone as initial systemic therapy of advanced or recurrent endometrial cancer. It should be noted that bevacizumab has been shown to have clinical activity in endometrial cancer, but unfortunately the trials conducted to date have not been sufficient to permit its approval by the FDA in endometrial cancer. Uterine leiomyosarcoma, carcinosarcomas, endometrial stromal sarcomas, and adenosarcomas comprise approximately 4% of uterine cancers and will be discussed in this chapter as well as in Chapter 42.

Cancer Consult: Expertise in Clinical Practice, Volume 1: Solid Tumors & Supportive Care,
Second Edition. Edited by Syed A. Abutalib, Maurie Markman, Al B. Benson III, and Hope S. Rugo.
© 2024 John Wiley & Sons Ltd. Published 2024 by John Wiley & Sons Ltd.

40 Endometrial Cancer

Case Study 1

A 73-year-old female is diagnosed as having adenocarcinoma of the endometrium. Computed tomography scan of the chest reveals multiple 0.5–1.0 cm lung nodules.

1) Because of her age, hormonal therapy is being considered as a possible therapeutic option. Hormonal therapy has been shown to be a useful strategy in metastatic endometrial adenocarcinoma in each of the following situations except which one?
   A) Low-grade cancers.
   B) High-grade cancers.
   C) Cancers expressing the progesterone receptor.

Expert Perspective: Patients with high-grade cancers rarely (if ever) respond to hormonal therapy (e.g. systemic progesterone delivery). As a result, in this setting systemic, chemotherapy or immunotherapy (in carefully selected patients) is the preferred initial treatment option even in patients who present with low-volume metastatic disease.

Correct Answer: B

2) Which of the following statements regarding the combination of chemotherapy and hormonal therapy in endometrial adenocarcinoma is correct?
   A) Randomized phase III trial data reveal the favorable impact of this strategy on progression-free survival in metastatic low-grade endometrial adenocarcinoma.
   B) Randomized phase III trial data reveal the favorable impact on overall survival when employed as an adjuvant strategy in low-grade endometrial adenocarcinoma.
   C) Randomized phase III trial data reveal an increase in treatment-related mortality when hormonal therapy is combined with chemotherapy in metastatic endometrial adenocarcinoma.
   D) None of the above.

Expert Perspective: There is no solid, evidence-based data supporting the combination of chemotherapy and hormonal therapy (medroxyprogesterone or alternating medroxyprogesterone and tamoxifen) in endometrial adenocarcinoma. In addition, any toxicity benefits associated with the use of hormonal therapy will be lost only if combined with cytotoxic chemotherapy. To date, randomized trial data have not revealed a positive impact on overall survival when hormonal therapy is employed as an adjuvant strategy in low-grade endometrial adenocarcinoma

Correct Answer: D

3) Which of the following non-cytotoxic drug combinations demonstrated improvement in clinical outcomes in advanced endometrial cancer when compared with cytotoxic chemotherapy?
   A) Lenvatinib plus bevacizumab.
   B) Lenvatinib plus olaparib.
   C) Lenvatinib plus pembrolizumab.
   D) Lenvatinib plus erlotinib.

Expert Perspective: The combination of lenvatinib plus pembrolizumab (vs non-platinum cytotoxic chemotherapy; KEYNOTE-775 study) significantly improved both median progression-free (6.6 vs 3.8 months) and median overall survival (18.3 vs 11.4 months), respectively. Adverse events of grade 3 or greater occurred in 88.9% of the patients who received lenvatinib plus pembrolizumab and in 72.7% of those who received chemotherapy (doxorubicin or weekly paclitaxel). The most common grade 3 or higher adverse events were hypertension, hypothyroidism, diarrhea, and nausea in the experimental arm. Fatal adverse reactions occurred in four patients, including gastrointestinal perforation, reversible posterior leukoencephalopathy syndrome with intraventricular hemorrhage, and intracranial hemorrhage

Correct Answer: C

4) **The earlier noted randomized phase III study (KEYNOTE-775) was conducted in what clinical setting?**
    A) Second-line treatment after failure of at least one platinum-based chemotherapy.
    B) Primary treatment for metastatic or stage III disease (grade 3 only).
    C) Second-line therapy in patients who have not previously received a platinum agent.
    D) First- or second-line therapy in patients with serous histology only.

Expert Perspective: This paradigm-changing study was conducted in patients with advanced endometrial cancer who had failed at least one platinum-based chemotherapy regimen.

Correct Answer: A

5) **Which of the following statements about use of pembrolizumab as a single agent for patients with advanced endometrial carcinoma that is MSI-H or mismatch repair deficient (dMMR) is correct?**
    A) Patients without disease progression could be treated for up to 24 months.
    B) Objective response rate was close to 50%.
    C) The median duration of response was 2 months.
    D) Both A and B.

Expert Perspective: Approximately 25–31% of patients with endometrial cancer have tumors with high levels of microsatellite instability (MSI-H) and mismatch repair deficiency (dMMR). Note that dMMR occurs as an inherited mutation (known as Lynch syndrome) in one of the mismatch repair (MMR) genes *MLH1, MSH2, PMS2* and *MSH6* or as sporadic methylation of the MLH1 promoter. MSI-H/dMMR endometrial cancer is associated with a higher neoantigen load and increased CD3-positive, CD8-positive, and programmed death-1 (PD-1)–expressing tumor-infiltrating lymphocytes and programmed death ligand-1 (PD-L1)–expressing intraepithelial and peritumoral immune cells compared with microsatellite stable endometrial cancers. Most recently, the FDA approved pembrolizumab as a single agent for patients with advanced endometrial carcinoma that is MSI-H or dMMR who have disease progression following prior systemic therapy in any setting and who are not candidates for curative surgery or radiation.

Efficacy was evaluated in KEYNOTE-158 a multicenter, nonrandomized, open-label, multicohort trial in 90 patients with unresectable or metastatic MSI-H or dMMR endometrial carcinoma in Cohorts D and K. Patients received pembrolizumab 200 mg intravenously every three weeks until unacceptable toxicity or 400 mg every six weeks or documented disease progression. Patients treated with pembrolizumab without disease progression could be treated for up to 24 months.

The major efficacy outcome measures were objective response rate and duration of response as assessed by blinded independent central review according to RECIST v1.1, modified to follow a maximum of 10 target lesions and a maximum of 5 target lesions per organ. The objective response rate was 48% (95% CI 37–60), and median duration of response was not reached (2.9–49.7+ months). Median progression-free survival was 13.1 (95% CI 4.3–34.4) months, and median overall survival was not reached (95% CI 27.2 months to not reached). Among all treated patients, 76% had ≥ 1 treatment-related adverse event (grades 3–4, 12%). There were no fatal treatment-related events. Immune-mediated adverse events or infusion reactions occurred in 28% of patients (grades 3–4, 7%; no fatal events).

Correct Answer: D

6) **What is the lifetime risk for developing endometrial cancer in women with Lynch syndrome (hereditary nonpolyposis colorectal cancer)?**
   A) 0–5%.
   B) 10–15%.
   C) 20–30%.
   D) 40–60%.

Expert Perspective: Women with germline mismatch repair genes mutations have a 40–60% lifetime risk of developing endometrial cancer at a median age of 48 years. Similar risk of colorectal cancer is observed with these germline mismatch repair gene mutations (also refer to Chapter 47). Patients with germline *BRCA1* and *PTEN* mutations have increased risk for endometrial cancer as well.

Correct Answer: D

Case Study 2

A 52-year-old female is diagnosed with stage IV endometrial cancer with evidence of metastatic spread to the peritoneal cavity, lung, and liver.

7) **Which combination chemotherapy regimen has been found in a phase III randomized trial to improve overall survival compared with doxorubicin plus cisplatin in metastatic endometrial adenocarcinoma?**
   A) Carboplatin-paclitaxel.
   B) Cisplatin-doxorubicin-paclitaxel.
   C) Cisplatin-docetaxel.
   D) Carboplatin-paclitaxel-doxorubicin.

Expert Perspective: In a phase III trial conducted by the Gynecologic Oncology Group, the combination of cisplatin-doxorubicin-paclitaxel improved overall survival (median: 15.3 months vs 12.3 months; $P = 0.037$) compared with doxorubicin plus cisplatin.

Correct Answer: B

8) **Despite the favorable survival outcome associated with cisplatin-doxorubicin-paclitaxel regimen in stage IV disease, there was a statistically significant increase in all of the following toxicities for this program compared to cisplatin–doxorubicin except which one?**
   A) Secondary acute leukemia.
   B) Peripheral neuropathy.
   C) Metabolic abnormalities.

Expert Perspective: The phase III trial revealed an increased risk of clinically relevant peripheral neuropathy and metabolic dysfunction associated with the three-drug regimen, without an increase in secondary acute myeloid leukemia, possibly because patients received a limited number of total doses of platinum.

Correct Answer: A

Case Study 3

A 62-year-old female is diagnosed with metastatic endometrial cancer. Because of clinically relevant comorbidities, it is decided to treat her with sequential single-agent therapy.

9) **Based on phase III trial results, which is the most active individual cytotoxic agent in endometrial adenocarcinoma?**
   A) Cisplatin.
   B) Doxorubicin.
   C) Paclitaxel.
   D) All of the above.

Expert Perspective: Phase III trial data are not available to document the single most biologically and clinically active cytotoxic agent in endometrial adenocarcinoma. Unfortunately, only single-arm phase II trial data exist to draw any indirect comparisons. As a result, it is only appropriate to state that the platinum agents (cisplatin and carboplatin), doxorubicin, and paclitaxel are active drugs in this clinical setting.

Correct Answer: D

Case Study 4

A 51-year-old female is diagnosed with stage III (tumor involving serosa, adnexa, vagina, or parametrium) endometrial cancer with only microscopic residual disease remaining in the peritoneal cavity at the completion of exploratory surgery.

10) **Compared with the delivery of whole abdominal radiation in stage III endometrial adenocarcinoma, which cytotoxic chemotherapy program has been shown in a phase III randomized trial to improve overall survival?**
    A) Single-agent doxorubicin.
    B) Cisplatin-doxorubicin.
    C) Carboplatin-paclitaxel.
    D) Cisplatin-doxorubicin-paclitaxel.

Expert Perspective: In a landmark phase III trial, the combination of cisplatin and doxorubicin as primary therapy was shown to improve overall survival compared to whole abdominal radiation (without chemotherapy) (Table 40.1).

Correct Answer: B

Table 40.1 Role of adjuvant therapy in endometrial cancer based on risk category, grade, and stage.

Risk category	Definition	Clinical features	Adjuvant therapy
Low[†]	-Grade 1 or 2 -Cancer limited to the endometrium; or invading < 50% of the myometrium, with no lymphovascular space invasion -Cancer that is not a high-risk histologic type*	Endometroid carcinoma, stage IA, grade 1 or 2	None
Intermediate	-Absence of high-risk histologies* and Lymphovascular invasion- Invading > 50% of the myometrium-Grade 3 and invading < 50% of the myometrium-Occult cervical stromal invasion	Endometroid carcinoma, stage IA, and grade 1 or 2	Vaginal brachytherapy
		Endometroid carcinoma, stage IA, and grade 3	
		Endometroid carcinoma, stage IB, grade 1 or 2	
		Endometroid carcinoma, stage IB, grade 3	Vaginal brachytherapy +/– EBRT +/– chemotherapy
		Stage II (any grade)	EBRT +/– vaginal brachytherapy +/– chemotherapy
High	High-risk histologies (clear cell, serous, carcinosarcoma or dedifferentiated or undifferentiated)	Stage III (any grade) Stage IV (A and selected B with omental disease)	Chemotherapy +/– EBRT +/– vaginal brachytherapy

[†] Patients who did not undergo nodal evaluation are considered unstaged, but given that their risk of nodal involvement was < 5%, they may not get surgical staging.
* High-risk histologies (clear cell, serous, carcinosarcoma or dedifferentiated or undifferentiated)

Case Study 5

A 47-year-old female is diagnosed as having a stage I (tumor confined to the corpus uteri, including endocervical glandular involvement) papillary serous carcinoma of the endometrium.

11) Which of the following statements is correct regarding adjuvant chemotherapy for high-risk, early stage endometrial adenocarcinoma?
   A) A phase III trial has revealed the favorable impact of this strategy (employing carboplatin-paclitaxel) on overall survival.
   B) A phase III trial has documented inferior overall survival and quality of life associated with the administration of adjuvant chemotherapy (cisplatin-doxorubicin-paclitaxel) compared with an "observation" control arm.
   C) A phase III trial has documented the favorable impact on survival for this strategy in patients with specific subtypes of endometrial cancer, and no benefit was observed in other subtypes.
   D) None of the above.

Expert Perspective: High-risk histologic subtypes of endometrial carcinoma such as papillary serous and clear cell carcinomas have a poorer prognosis than endometrioid carcinomas. There is currently no evidence based on the results of phase III trials that the adjuvant delivery of cytotoxic therapy will improve overall survival in high-risk, early stage endometrial adenocarcinoma. However, retrospective data from several centers have suggested a possible benefit when comparing historical experiences for patients who received, or did not receive, some form of adjuvant therapy. Serous and clear cell histology endometrial cancers (except if surgical stage IA with no myometrial invasion) should be considered for treatment with chemotherapy with consideration of brachytherapy or external beam radiation therapy.

Correct Answer: D

Case Study 6

A 67-year-old female in otherwise excellent health is diagnosed as having metastatic endometrial adenocarcinoma. You are in the process of considering therapeutic options.

12) Compared with cisplatin-doxorubicin-paclitaxel, the combination of carboplatin-paclitaxel results in all of the following in patients with metastatic endometrial adenocarcinoma except which one?
    A) Equivalent progression-free survival.
    B) Equivalent overall survival.
    C) Increased toxicity.

Expert Perspective: A phase III randomized trial conducted by the Gynecologic Oncology Group revealed equivalent survival (progression-free and overall) for the combination of carboplatin-paclitaxel compared with cisplatin-doxorubicin-paclitaxel with a more favorable toxicity profile. As a result, the two-drug combination of carboplatin-paclitaxel should in most circumstances be considered the standard of care in the management of metastatic or recurrent endometrial adenocarcinoma. Most recently, based on the results of RUBY study, FDA approved dostarlimab with carboplatin and paclitaxel, followed by single-agent dostarlimab, for primary advanced or recurrent endometrial cancer that is mismatch repair deficient (dMMR).

Correct Answer: C

Case Study 7

A 65-year-old female is diagnosed with a stage I carcinosarcoma and is treated with adjuvant external-beam radiation. Unfortunately, nine months later, she experiences metastatic spread to the lung.

13) Compared with the combination of paclitaxel and ifosfamide, which combination chemotherapy regimen has been shown in a phase III randomized study to improve survival outcomes in this clinical setting?
    A) Ifosfamide-paclitaxel.
    B) Cisplatin-paclitaxel.
    C) Carboplatin-paclitaxel.
    D) Docetaxel-gemcitabine.

Expert Perspective: In a recently reported phase III trial, the combination of carboplatin and paclitaxel was shown to improve both progression free and overall survival compared with paclitaxel and ifosfamide (Chapter 42).

Correct Answer: C

Case Study 8

A 50-year-old female is diagnosed with a stage IV endometrial sarcoma.

14) **Which of the following statements regarding chemotherapy in this clinical setting is incorrect?**
    A) The combination of gemcitabine-docetaxel is an active strategy in metastatic endometrial leiomyosarcoma, but its superiority to other approaches has yet to be proven in a phase III randomized trial.
    B) In patients with endometrial carcinosarcoma, the metastatic sites has most commonly revealed adenocarcinoma component rather than sarcoma.
    C) The combination of a platinum agent and paclitaxel produces objective responses in endometrial carcinosarcomas.
    D) High-dose chemotherapy with stem cell rescue has been shown to have curative potential in a carefully defined subset of patients with metastatic endometrial sarcomas.

Expert Perspective: There is currently no evidence for the curative potential of high-dose chemotherapy in metastatic endometrial sarcomas. Metastatic components from carcinosarcoma have been shown to be principally composed of adenocarcinoma. Carcinosarcomas can be responsive to the combination of a platinum agent and paclitaxel, and the combination of docetaxel and gemcitabine or doxorubicin-based treatment is active in unresectable metastatic endometrial leiomyosarcomas. Endometrial stromal sarcomas are low-grade tumors and are therefore potentially sensitive to antihormonal therapy.

Correct Answer: D

Case Study 9

A 69-year-old female presents to your clinic after full surgical staging, including a total abdominal hysterectomy, bilateral salpingo-oophorectomy, and pelvic and para-aortic node dissection for grade 3 endometrial adenocarcinoma. The surgical pathology confirms the diagnosis. There is evidence of deep invasive of the myometrium and lymphovascular invasion without involving the lymph nodes.

15) **What is the next best step?**
    A) Adjuvant vaginal brachytherapy.
    B) Observation.
    C) Adjuvant chemotherapy.
    D) Adjuvant chemoradiation therapy.

Expert Perspective: This patient meets criteria for intermediate-risk endometrial cancer. The risk for recurrence in this group is about 27% with no additional treatment. One classification comes from the Gynecologic Oncology Group and is based on age and any of three pathologic factors: (i) outer-third invasion of the myometrium, (ii) grade 2 or 3 histology, or (iii) evidence for lymphovascular space invasion. Intermediate risk is characterized by the presence of any one factor in women older than 70 years of age, two risk factors in a woman aged 50–69 years (as in our patient), and all three factors in women aged 18–49 years. Patients with an intermediate-risk endometrial cancer should proceed with vaginal brachytherapy. The Post-Operative Radiation Therapy in Endometrial Cancer (PORTEC-2) trial provides evidence for the use of vaginal brachytherapy over whole pelvic radiation therapy, excluding papillary serous and clear cell carcinomas. In this trial, there were no differences in recurrence-free survival, rate of distant metastases, or five-year survival outcomes. Compared with pelvic radiation therapy, vaginal brachytherapy resulted in lower rates of treatment-related toxicity and superior quality of life.

Correct Answer: A

16) **All of the following features classify endometrial carcinoma as high-risk, except?**

   A) Stage III disease.
   B) Serous histology regardless of stage.
   C) Clear cell histology regardless of stage.
   D) Grade 3 deeply invasive endometrioid carcinoma.
   E) Positive peritoneal cytology.

Expert perspective: Endometrial cancers with high-risk characteristic should be considered to receive adjuvant chemotherapy (Table 40.1). Positive peritoneal cytology in otherwise low-risk disease does not imply by itself a high-risk feature. These patients have lower rate of recurrence compared with other patients with positive peritoneal cytology. Moreover, presence of POLE mutation is not a high-risk feature but appears to be a favorable characteristic in patients with aggressive histologic features. Two prospective studies assessing the possibility of de-escalation of therapy are ongoing: (i) PORTEC-4a is a multicenter randomized phase III trial in patients with high-intermediate risk endometrial cancer, and (ii) Tailored Adjuvant Therapy in POLE-mutated and p53-wildtype/no specific molecular profile (NSMP) Early Stage Endometrial Cancer (TAPER) is a prospective cohort study in early stage endometrial cancer. Patients with high-risk histology (serous, clear, undifferentiated/dedifferentiated, or carcinosarcoma) endometrial cancer should be considered to receive adjuvant chemotherapy with a carboplatin-paclitaxel regimen. Patients with IA should be considered to receive adjuvant vaginal brachytherapy, and patients with IB or later stage should be considered for vaginal brachytherapy with or without adjuvant external beam radiation therapy.

Correct Answer: E

17) **Which of the following statements about uterine sarcomas is true?**
   A) Carcinosarcomas have low rates of recurrence.
   B) Observation is the standard of care following resection of a uterus-limited leiomyosarcoma.
   C) Adenosarcomas with sarcomatous overgrowth are intermediate-risk tumors.
   D) Low-grade endometrial stromal sarcomas are hormone-insensitive tumors.

Expert perspective: Among the endometrial sarcomas, carcinosarcomas make up about 50%, leiomyosarcomas make up about 40%, and adenosarcomas and endometrial stromal sarcomas make up the remaining 10%. Careful histologic review is recommended for these rare and high-risk histologies, because the prognosis and management may vary depending on the specific type of uterine sarcoma. Carcinosarcomas have high rates of recurrence, even among patients with early stage disease. Except for stage IA disease (controversial), most patients receive adjuvant carboplatin-paclitaxel. In patients with unresectable or measurable carcinosarcoma, the combination of carboplatin-paclitaxel, ifosfamide-paclitaxel, or ifosfamide-cisplatin are reasonable options. Leiomyosarcoma is a high-risk cancer with a propensity for early hematogenous dissemination. The current standard of care after resection of uterus-limited leiomyosarcoma is observation. In patients with unresectable leiomyosarcoma, docetaxel plus gemcitabine is a reasonable regimen. Adenosarcomas with sarcomatous overgrowth are high-risk cancers, the prognosis and treatment of which is driven by the high-grade portion of the tumor. Low-grade endometrial stromal sarcomas are hormone-sensitive tumors.

Correct Answer: B

Recommended Readings

Amant, F., Coosemans, A., Debiec-Rychter, M. et al. (2009). Clinical management of uterine sarcomas. *Lancet Oncol* 10: 1188–1198.

Cosgrove, C.M., Bakes, F.J., O'Malley, D. et al. (2021). Endometrial cancer: Who lives, who dies, can we improve their story? *The Oncol* 26: 1044–1051.

Eskander, R.N., Sill M.W., Beffa L., et al. (2023) Pembrolizumab plus chemotherapy in advanced endometrial cancer. *N Engl J Med*. doi:10.1056/NEJMoa2302312

Fleming, G.F., Brunetto, V.L., Cella, D. et al. (2004). Phase III trial of doxorubicin plus cisplatin with or without paclitaxel plus filgrastim in advanced endometrial carcinoma: A Gynecologic Oncology Group study. *J Clin Oncol* 22 (11): 2159–2166.

Lu, K.H. and Broaddus, R.R. (2020). Endometrial cancer. *N Engl J Med* 383: 2053–2064.

Konstantinopoulos, P.A., Lee, E.K. et al. (2023 January 20). A phase II, two-stage study of Letrozole and Abemaciclib in estrogen receptor-positive recurrent endometrial cancer. *J Clin Oncol* 41 (3): 599–608. doi: 10.1200/JCO.22.00628. Epub 2022 Sep 29. PMID: 36174113.

Makker, V., Colombo, N., Herraez, A.C. et al. (2022). Lenvatinib plus pembrolizumab for advanced endometrial cancer. *N Engl J Med* 386: 437–448.

Mirza, M.R., Chase, B.M., Slomovitz, R., et al. (2023) Dostarlimab for primary advanced or recurrent endometrial cancer. *N Engl J Med*. doi:10.1056/NEJMoa2216334.

O'Malley, D.M., Bariani, G.M., Cassier, P.A. et al. (2022). Pembrolizumab in patients with microsatellite instability-high advanced endometrial cancer: Results from the KEYNOTE-158 study. *J Clin Oncol* 40 (7): 752–761. doi: 10.1200/JCO.21.01874. Epub 2022 Jan 6. PMID: 34990208; PMCID: PMC8887941.

Powell, M.A., Filiaci, V.L., Hensley, M.L. et al. (2022). Randomized phase III trial of paclitaxel and carboplatin versus paclitaxel and ifosfamide in patients with carcinosarcoma of the uterus or ovary: An NRG oncology trial. *J Clin Oncol* 40 (9): 968–977.

Randall, M.E., Filiaci, V.L., Muss, H. et al. (2006). Randomized phase III trial of whole-abdominal irradiation versus doxorubicin and cisplatin chemotherapy in advanced endometrial carcinoma: A Gynecologic Oncology Group study. *J Clin Oncol* 24 (1): 36–44.

Toboni, M.D. and Powell, M.A. (2021). New treatments for recurrent uterine cancer. *Curr Oncol Rep* 23: 139.

41

Cancer of the Cervix, Vulva, and Vagina

Sabrina M. Bedell and Peter G. Rose

Department of Obstetrics and Gynecology, Cleveland, OH

Introduction

Cancers of the cervix, vulva, and vagina are most commonly due to human papillomavirus (HPV) and are more commonly squamous cell histology. Risk factors for HPV-related cancers include multiple lifetime sexual partners, early age at first intercourse, and smoking. The HPV-related cancers generally have dysplastic precursor lesions named for their respective sites as cervical intraepithelial neoplasia (CIN), vaginal intraepithelial neoplasia (VAIN), and vulvar intraepithelial neoplasia (VIN).

Cervical cancer is the most common out of these entities and therefore the most well studied. For cervical cancer specifically, 99.7% are HPV-related; 70% are squamous cell carcinomas, 25% are adenocarcinoma, and the remaining 5% represent other rarer histologies. Vulvar and vaginal cancer are rarer cancer types. Approximately 83% of vaginal cancers are squamous cell carcinoma, 9% are adenocarcinoma, and 8% are other histologies including sarcomas and melanomas. Squamous cell carcinoma of the vulva can be HPV related or can arise in patients with lichen sclerosis. Approximately 75% of vulvar cancer are squamous cell carcinoma, 8% are melanoma, 10% are basal cell carcinoma, 1–2% are sarcoma, and <1% are extramammary Paget's disease.

Cervical Cancer

Case Study 1

A 59-year-old patient is diagnosed with FIGO 2018 stage IB1 (>5 mm depth of stromal invasion and ≤2 cm in greatest dimension) squamous cell carcinoma of the cervix and is a poor surgical candidate, so the decision is made to proceed with definitive chemoradiation.

1) **What data supports use of the addition of concurrent cisplatin-based chemotherapy in this patient?**
   A) Gynecologic Oncology Group 85 (GOG 85) and GOG 120 were prospective randomized trials that compared platinum-based chemotherapy with non-platinum-based chemotherapy and demonstrated superior outcomes with cisplatin-containing regimens for the treatment of cervical cancer.

B) A National Cancer Database (NCDB) study that compared outcomes following treatment with definitive external beam radiation therapy (EBRT)/brachytherapy alone or EBRT/brachytherapy with concurrent chemotherapy found that the addition of chemotherapy was superior.
C) RTOG 90–01 demonstrated an improvement in survival with the addition of concurrent chemotherapy to EBRT for patients with stage IB cervical cancer with pelvic nodal metastasis.
D) There is no data to support use of chemotherapy in this case, and use is based on expert opinion.

Expert Perspective: Prospective trials included patients with more advanced stage cervical cancer or patients with stage IB and poor prognostic factors (i.e. nodal metastasis). GOG 85 and GOG 120 did not include stage IB1 cervical cancer but included stages IIB (with parametrial involvement but not up to the pelvic wall), III, and IVA (spread to adjacent pelvic organs) and thus do not apply to this patient scenario. It is true that GOG 85 and GOG 120 found cisplatin-containing regimens to be superior with improvement in progression-free survival in both studies, and with overall survival (OS) in GOG 120 (Table 41.1).

In GOG 85, the relative risk of progression or death was 0.79 (90% CI 0.62–0.99) for the cisplatin and fluorouracil group compared with the hydroxyurea group. In GOG 120, the relative risk of progression or death was 0.57 (95% CI 0.42–0.78) for cisplatin alone and 0.55 (95% CI 0.40–0.75) for cisplatin, fluorouracil, and hydroxyurea compared with hydroxyurea alone. Again, in GOG 120, the relative risk of death was 0.61 (95% CI 0.44–0.85) for cisplatin alone and 0.58 (95% CI 0.41–0.81) for cisplatin, fluorouracil, and hydroxyurea compared with hydroxyurea alone.

RTOG 90–1 did demonstrate improvement in the five-year OS for patients treated with radiotherapy and chemotherapy compared with those treated with radiotherapy alone (73% vs 58%; $P = 0.004$). However, this paper was published in 1999 and thus uses FIGO

Table 41.1 FIGO staging of cancer of the cervix uteri.

Stage	Description
I	The carcinoma is strictly confined to the cervix (extension to the uterine corpus should be disregarded).
II	The carcinoma invades beyond the uterus, but has not extended onto the lower third of the vagina or to the pelvic wall.
III	The carcinoma involves the lower third of the vagina and/or extends to the pelvic wall and/or causes hydronephrosis or nonfunctioning kidney and/or involves pelvic and/or paraaortic lymph nodes.†
IV	The carcinoma has extended beyond the true pelvis or has involved (biopsy proven) the mucosa of the bladder or rectum. (Bullous edema, as such, does not permit a case to be allotted to stage IV.)

†Adding notation of r (imaging) and p (pathology) to indicate the findings that are used to allocate the case to stage IIIC. Example: If imaging indicates pelvic lymph node metastasis, the stage allocation would be stage IIIC1r, and if confirmed by pathologic findings, it would be stage IIIC1p. The type of imaging modality or pathology technique used should always be documented.

1995 staging for inclusion criteria. Lymph node status was not a part of staging until the 2018 FIGO staging for cervical cancer update, and by FIGO 2018 staging, if the patient had positive pelvic lymph nodes, she would be stage IIIC1 (pelvic lymph node metastasis only). A NCDB study published in 2017 by Haque et al. (2017) identified patients with stage IB1 or stage IIA1 (≤4 cm in greatest dimension) cervical cancer diagnosed 2004–2012 who received definitive radiation therapy and found a longer median OS for those who received concurrent chemotherapy, 121.1 months (radiation therapy alone) versus not reached (chemoradiation) with a hazard ratio (HR) of 0.719 (95% CI 0.549–0.945).

Correct Answer: B

Case Study 2

A 40-year-old patient is diagnosed with IIB (with parametrial involvement but not up to the pelvic wall) squamous cell carcinoma of the cervix based on an MRI. She has no enlarged lymph nodes on the MRI or PET-CT.

2) What is the highest level of data that provides guidance on whether we should surgically stage this patient via laparoscopic lymph node dissection?
   A) A retrospective review demonstrated no difference in survival for patients with locally advanced cervical cancer who undergo surgical staging versus radiographic staging prior to definitive chemoradiation.
   B) A randomized controlled trial comparing PET-CT to surgical staging demonstrated superior progression-free survival but no difference in overall survival in the surgically staged group.
   C) A randomized, controlled trial demonstrated improvement in disease-free survival for patients with stage II–IVA cervical cancer who underwent surgical staging prior to definitive chemoradiation.
   D) A randomized controlled trial demonstrated improvement in disease-free survival for patients with stage IIB cervical cancer who underwent surgical staging and subsequent chemoradiation.

Expert Perspective: Uterus-11 was an international multicenter study that randomized patients with locally advanced (stage IIB–IVA) cervical cancer to surgical staging or clinical staging followed by primary platinum-based chemoradiation. Results from Uterus-11 were published in 2018 by Marnitz et al. (2020), and although the overall cohort showed no difference in disease-free survival, in patients with stage IIB disease surgical, staging proved beneficial for disease-free survival with a hazard ratio of 0.51 (95% CI 0.30–0.86; $P = 0.011$). The GOG study that retrospectively analyzed survival outcomes for radiographic versus surgical staging prior to definitive chemoradiation as part of the GOG 85, 120, and 165 trials demonstrated both progression-free and OS benefit with surgical staging. We do not yet have randomized data comparing surgical staging with PET-CT in locally advanced cervical cancer, but there is an ongoing trial, PALDISC trial, that aims to address this question specifically.

Correct Answer: D

Case Study 3

A 32-year-old female is diagnosed with radiographic stage IIIC1 (pelvic lymph node metastasis only) cervical cancer. There are enlarged FDG-avid pelvic lymph nodes but not para-aortic lymph nodes on her staging PET-CT.

3) **Which of the following statements is supported by data regarding surgical staging via retroperitoneal lymph node dissection prior to definitive chemoradiation?**
   A) There is up to 25% risk of para-aortic lymph node positivity in the setting of positive pelvic node metastasis on PET-CT.
   B) There is less than 5% risk of para-aortic lymph node positivity in the setting of negative PET-CT.
   C) The combination of CT and MRI has the lowest rate of pathologically positive nodes in the setting of normal imaging.
   D) There is a 15% risk of para-aortic aortic lymph node positivity in the setting of negative PET-CT.

Expert Perspective: Gold et al. (2008) found that patients who have FDG-avid pelvic lymph nodes have a 2.4 times increased risk of recurrence over those that have negative nodes on imaging. Further, on pathologic evaluation there was a 25% false negative rate of para-aortic nodal metastasis when evaluated by PET-CT. Leblanc et al. (2007) found the rate of positive para-aortic lymph nodes increased from 9% with negative imaging to 24% if they had positive pelvic nodes on preoperative PET (with or without CT). A literature review on pretreatment surgical lymph node for locally advanced cervical cancer that included 15 prospective trials, 6 retrospective trials, and 1 randomized controlled trial compared reported detection rates for different imaging modalities including CT, MRI, and PET. Reported rates of surgically positive nodes that were deemed radiographically negative were 9–35% for CT ±MRI, 4–11% for PET, and 6–15% for combined PET-CT.

Correct Answer: A

4) **Which of the following statements regarding survival outcomes is correct?**
   A) A retrospective analysis of patients from GOG 85, 120, and 165 demonstrated no difference in progression-free survival or OS for patients with cervical cancer with radiographic or surgical lymph node staging treated with definitive chemoradiation.
   B) There is no survival difference for patients with surgically confirmed node-negative disease who received pelvic EBRT alone and patients with microscopic (≤5 mm) para-aortic nodal disease who received extended-field EBRT.
   C) Surgically identified para-aortic lymph node metastases of any size have significantly worse prognosis regardless of receipt of extended field EBRT.
   D) Retrospective analysis of GOG 85, 120, and 165 demonstrated superior progression-free but not OS for patients who had surgical staging over radiographically staged lymph nodes.

Expert Perspective: A prospective trial evaluating short- and long-term outcomes for patients with locally advanced cervical cancer who underwent laparoscopic staging prior to definitive radiation therapy demonstrated no survival difference for patients with surgically confirmed node-negative disease who received pelvic EBRT alone and patients with microscopic (≤5 mm) para-aortic nodal disease who received extended-field EBRT. On univariate analysis, survival was significantly worse when patients had any size para-aortic lymph node involvement ($P = 0.02$).

The GOG study that retrospectively analyzed survival outcomes for radiographic versus surgical staging prior to definitive chemoradiation as part of the GOG 85, 120, and 165 trials demonstrated a significant survival benefit with surgical staging despite the fact that the radiographically staged patients had significantly better performance status, less advanced stage of disease, and smaller tumor size. For those radiographically staged, the relative risk of disease progression was 1.35 (95% CI, 1.01–1.81; $P = 0.043$), and the relative risk of death was 1.46 (95% CI, 1.08–1.99; $P = 0.014$) on multivariate analysis.

Correct Answer: B

Case Study 4

A 70-year-old patient just completed six cycles of carboplatin, paclitaxel, and bevacizumab for treatment of recurrent squamous cell carcinoma of the cervix. She is then continued on maintenance bevacizumab.

5) What data supports the use of maintenance bevacizumab in this patient?
   A) A phase II trial found significant increase in median progression free survival with the use of maintenance bevacizumab over observation following carboplatin, paclitaxel, and bevacizumab chemotherapy in metastatic or recurrent cervical cancer patients.
   B) GOG 240 included an arm with maintenance bevacizumab that showed improvement in progression-free survival.
   C) An NCDB study found improvement in progression free survival for patients who received maintenance bevacizumab following chemotherapy for advanced cervical cancer.
   D) A small prospective study demonstrated a complete response rate of 40% for patients who received maintenance bevacizumab following platinum-based chemotherapy combined with bevacizumab.

Expert Perspective: A pilot study including 15 patients, published by Toyoshima et al. (2021), demonstrated an overall and complete response rate of 46.7% and 40%, respectively, for single agent bevacizumab following platinum-based combination chemotherapy plus bevacizumab in which the chemotherapy was discontinued due to adverse events. Although this is not the same scenario as the patient in the above scenario, the interesting results may indicate value to maintenance bevacizumab in the case of a complete response.

CECILIA was a phase II trial that primarily aimed to evaluate the safety and rate of adverse events with maintenance bevacizumab in persistent, recurrent, or newly diagnosed metastatic cervical cancer. CECILIA did not have a comparative arm of patients who did not receive maintenance therapy, and therefore conclusions on the benefit of maintenance bevacizumab compared to observation following carboplatin, paclitaxel, and bevacizumab cannot be made. CECILIA reports overall response rate of 61%, complete response in 14%, median progression-free survival of 10.9 months, and median OS of 25 months.

In GOG 240, 6.6% of patients who received a bevacizumab containing regimen had a complete response to treatment (compared with 2.7% of patients who received chemotherapy alone). There was no maintenance bevacizumab arm in GOG 240.

To the authors' knowledge, to date there is no NCDB study evaluating maintenance bevacizumab in cervical cancer.

Correct Answer: D

Case Study 5

A 39-year-old is diagnosed with a 5 cm cervical mass without vaginal or parametrial involvement on pretreatment MRI. Her biopsy confirms the diagnosis of cervical adenocarcinoma. She receives definitive cisplatin potentiated EBRT followed by brachytherapy and then a completion hysterectomy.

6) **What data supports completion hysterectomy in this patient?**
   A) On multivariate analysis, an NCDB study demonstrated significant improvement in OS for patients who received completion hysterectomy.
   B) An NCDB study indicates a decrease in local recurrence rate with adjuvant hysterectomy for stage IB2 (>2 cm and ≤ 4 cm in greatest dimension) to IIA2 (>4 cm in greatest dimension) disease.
   C) A randomized GOG study found improvement in OS with receipt of completion hysterectomy for cervical cancer tumors measuring 4–6 cm.
   D) A single institution retrospective review found that completion hysterectomy for patients with locally advanced cervical cancer had significant improvement in local and pelvic recurrence rates compared with definitive chemoradiation and brachytherapy alone.

Expert Perspective: GOG 71 was designed to determine whether completion hysterectomy improved survival in patients with bulky stage IB cervical cancer, that is, FIGO 2018 stage IB3 disease (Table 41.1), There was not a significant difference in progression-free survival with 46% of the radiation-only group progressing compared with 37% of the adjuvant hysterectomy group ($P = 0.09$ on log-rank test). The median progression-free survival for the radiation-only regimen was 7.4 years and was not reached in the adjuvant hysterectomy group. OS was also not different between the two groups. A test for interaction found that tumor size significantly affected OS rate (but not progression-free survival) with $P = 0.007$. For patients with tumor size 4–6 cm, the relative risk of death when adjuvant hysterectomy was done compared with radiation alone was 0.60. Patients with very bulky tumors (≥ 7 cm) actually had a higher risk of progression or death with adjuvant hysterectomy (relative risk 1.27 and 2.03, respectively).

It should be noted that the National Comprehensive Cancer Network (NCCN) Guidelines Version 1.2021 currently list completion hysterectomy for stage IB3 (>4 cm in greatest dimension) and IIA2 cervical cancer as category 3 for evidence to support this, specifically stating, "This approach can be considered in patients whose extent of disease, response to EBRT, or uterine anatomy precludes adequate coverage by brachytherapy" (Table 41.1).

There is an NCDB study that found a significantly improved four-year OS for patients who received adjuvant hysterectomy following chemoradiation (82.2% vs 74.9%; $P = 0.036$). However, this did not remain significant on multivariate Cox regression (HR 0.63; 95% CI 0.06–1.04; $P = 0.069$). This study did not evaluate local recurrence rates.

Cagetti et al. published a single-institution, retrospective review of completion hysterectomies performed at the Institut Paoli-Calmettes in Marseille, France. This study found no difference in three-year local or pelvic relapse survival rates between the group who received completion hysterectomy and those who did not, with HR 0.57 (95% CI 0.20–1.64; $P = 0.30$) and 0.37 (95% CI 0.10–1.31; $P = 0.12$), respectively. It should be noted that this population was relatively higher risk than those included in GOG 71 because it included stage II–IV disease, 51.7% had positive pelvic lymph nodes, and 16.5% had positive para-aortic lymph nodes on preoperative imaging.

Correct Answer: C

7) What is the rate of gastrointestinal fistula with bevacizumab use in cervical cancer?
   A) 6%.
   B) 1%.
   C) 3%.
   D) 0.3%.

Expert Perspective: GOG 240 evaluated the effectiveness of two chemotherapy regimens with and without the addition of bevacizumab. Reported rates of grade 3 or higher gastrointestinal fistula were 3% with bevacizumab-containing regimens, versus 0% with the non-bevacizumab regimens. In addition, a 3% rate of grade 3 or higher genitourinary fistula rate was reported for a total gastrointestinal and genitourinary fistula rate of 6%.

Correct Answer: C

Case Study 6

A 67-year-old Caucasian female is diagnosed with recurrent cervical squamous cell carcinoma nine months after definitive cis-EBRT (chemoradiation) for FIGO 2018 stage IIIC1 (pelvic lymph node metastasis only) cervical cancer. She has a new FDG-avid left iliac lymph node measuring 2 cm but no other evidence of disease. The decision is made to proceed with cisplatin, paclitaxel, and bevacizumab for her recurrent cervical cancer.

8) What factors indicate she would benefit from the addition of bevacizumab?
   A) Caucasian ancestry, lymph node involvement.
   B) Measurable pelvic disease, prior platinum therapy, disease-free interval <1 year.
   C) Disease-free interval <1year, age >65 years.
   D) Lymph node involvement, prior platinum therapy, age >50 years.

Expert Perspective: Tewari et al. published a prospective validation of the prognostic value of the Moore criteria in efforts to elucidate which advanced cervical cancer patients would benefit most from the addition of bevacizumab to a standard chemotherapy backbone. The Moore criteria is a set of five factors that were found to correlate with response to cisplatin-based chemotherapy for advanced/recurrent cervical cancer. The five factors associated with a poor response to treatment included (i) African-American ancestry, (ii) performance status >0, (iii) measurable pelvic disease, (iv) receipt of prior platinum radiosensitizer, and (v) disease-free interval <1 year. These factors were identified through multivariate analysis of patients included in three GOG studies (110, 169, and 179), and the study divided patients into three risk groups: low risk (0–1 factor), mid risk (2–3 factors), and high risk (4–5 factors). The initial application of the Moore criteria showed that patients in the high-risk group were estimated to have a poor response to cisplatin-based chemotherapy with response rate of 13%, median progression-free survival of 2.8 months, and median OS of 5.5 months.

In the present publication by Tewari et al. (2022), the Moore criteria were analyzed in the entire study population of GOG 240 to determine whether the risk categories had prognostic significance and whether these risk categories could be used to guide the choice of chemotherapy regimen. GOG 240 was a phase III randomized control trial evaluating two different chemotherapy backbones (cisplatin and paclitaxel vs topotecan and paclitaxel) with and without bevacizumab. When comparing the two chemotherapy backbones, there was no significant difference in response based on the Moore criteria risk stratification groups. When comparing the addition of bevacizumab to either chemotherapy backbone, the low-risk group (0–1 risk factor) did not appear to benefit from the addition of bevacizumab, with hazard ratios for death for treating with bevacizumab of 0.96 (95% CI 0.51–1.83; $P = 0.9087$) in the low-risk group, 0.673 (95% CI 0.5–0.91; $P = 0.0094$) in the mid-risk group, and 0.536 (95% CI 0.32–0.905; $P = 0.0196$) in the high-risk group.

Correct Answer: B

9) **Which of the following statements about adding pembrolizumab to chemotherapy with or without bevacizumab in the KEYNOTE-826 study with persistent, recurrent, or metastatic cervical cancer is correct?**
   A) Chemotherapy plus pembrolizumab with or without bevacizumab did not improve OS.
   B) Chemotherapy plus pembrolizumab with or without bevacizumab improved progression-free survival.
   C) Chemotherapy plus pembrolizumab with or without bevacizumab did not improve progression-free survival or OS.
   D) Chemotherapy plus pembrolizumab with or without bevacizumab improved OS and progression-free survival.

Expert Perspective: The KEYNOTE-826 trial showed that chemotherapy plus pembrolizumab with or without bevacizumab improved IS and progression-free survival in patients with metastatic cervical cancer based on subgroups including histology and prior treatment type. Investigators reported in the all-comer, squamous cell carcinoma population (n = 447), the median progression-free survival in the treatment arm was 10.4 months (95% CI, 8.4–12.1) versus 6.9 months in the control arm (95% CI, 6.2–8.3). Among the nonsquamous cell carcinoma population (n = 169), median progression-free survival was 11.6 months (95% CI, 9.1–23.3) in the treatment arm and 8.4 months (95% CI, 7.0–10.4) in the control arm. Similar to progression-free survival, the benefit conferred with the use of pembrolizumab also improved OS in all the key subgroups including histology, platinum use, bevacizumab use, and prior chemoradiation treatment

Correct Answer: D

10) **Which of the following statements about checkpoint inhibitor therapy in advance cervical cancer is correct?**
    A) Pembrolizumab has shown activity as second-line therapy in PD-L1-positive cancer if not used in first line with chemotherapy.
    B) Pembrolizumab has shown activity when used in first-line with chemotherapy.
    C) Cemiplimab has shown activity in patients with disease progression after platinum-based chemotherapy.
    D) All of the above.

Expert Perspective: Pembrolizumab has a role in the first-line setting for metastatic cervical cancers with chemotherapy (KEYNOTE-826 trial), but it may be used in the second-line setting (KEYNOTE-028 trial) as a single agent for those with PD-L1 CPS ⩾ 1%, per the FDA. In a randomized trial in patients with disease progression after platinum-based chemotherapy, the checkpoint inhibitor, cemiplimab (irrespective of PD-L1 expression), improved OS relative to single-agent chemotherapy (12.0 months vs 8.5 months) with fewer severe toxicities.

Correct Answer: D

11) **Which of the following statements about tisotumab vedotin-tftv in patients with previously treated recurrent or metastatic cervical cancer is correct?**
    A) It is a tissue factor-directed antibody and microtubule inhibitor drug conjugate.
    B) It has shown complete responses in the range of 24%.
    C) It does not cause alopecia.
    D) Ulcerative keratitis is a common adverse event.

Expert perspective: On 20 September 2021, the FDA granted accelerated approval to tisotumab vedotin-tftv, a tissue factor-directed antibody and microtubule inhibitor conjugate, for adult patients with recurrent or metastatic cervical cancer with disease progression on or after chemotherapy. The approval was based on the results of multicenter, open-label, single-arm, phase II GOG 3023 (innovaTV 204) study, which enrolled 102 patients. The confirmed objective response rate was 24% (95% CI 16–33), with 7% complete responses and 17% partial responses. The most common treatment-related adverse events included alopecia (38%), epistaxis (30%), nausea (27%), conjunctivitis (26%), fatigue (26%), and dry eye (23%). Grade 3 or worse treatment-related adverse events were reported in 28 (28%) patients and included neutropenia (3%), fatigue (2%), ulcerative keratitis (2%), and peripheral neuropathies (2% each with sensory, motor, sensorimotor, and neuropathy peripheral). Serious treatment-related adverse events occurred in 13% of patients, the most common of which included peripheral sensorimotor neuropathy (2%) and pyrexia (2%). One death due to septic shock was considered by the investigator to be related to therapy. Three deaths unrelated to treatment were reported, including one case of ileus and two unknown causes. The study included patients who had recurrent or metastatic squamous cell, adenocarcinoma, or adenosquamous cervical cancer; had disease progression during or after doublet chemotherapy with bevacizumab (if eligible by local standards); and had received two or fewer previous systemic regimens for recurrent or metastatic disease.

Correct Answer: A

Vulvar Cancer

Case Study 7

A 67-year-old is found to have vulvar squamous cell carcinoma with a 1 cm lesion on her left labia minora. She undergoes resection via modified radical left vulvectomy and left sentinel lymph node identification and sampling. Final pathology returns with positive left sentinel lymph node, with a tumor focus measuring 3 mm.

12) Which of the following statements is correct?
- A) Sentinel lymph node metastases >2 mm is associated with significantly lower disease-free survival; the role of concurrent chemoradiation is unclear.
- B) A single sentinel lymph node metastasis <5 mm has a less than 5% risk of nonsentinel lymph node involvement, and full lymphadenectomy is not indicated.
- C) Sentinel lymph node metastases >2 mm is associated with significantly lower disease-free survival; however, further treatment with EBRT is optional.
- D) A single sentinel lymph node metastasis >2 mm has a 40% risk of nonsentinel lymph node involvement and full lymphadenectomy as well as EBRT with concurrent chemotherapy is recommended.

Expert Perspective: GROINSS-V was a prospective multisite, randomized, controlled study evaluating outcomes following sentinel lymph node sampling for early stage vulvar cancer with lesions <4 cm. If a positive sentinel lymph node was identified (by frozen section or final pathology), a full inguinal lymphadenectomy was then performed. Measurements of the size of sentinel lymph nodes was not initially a part of the protocol. However, the risk of nonsentinel lymph node involvement based on size of sentinel node was performed in a blinded fashion on 307 patients from Dutch centers. The risk of nonsentinel node involvement increased with increasing sentinel node metastasis size, as seen in Table 41.2.

Table 41.2 Tumor size and likelihood of cases (per groin) with nonsentinel lymph node involvement.

Tumor focus size (mm)	Percentage of cases (per groin) with nonsentinel lymph node involvement
Isolated tumor cells	4.2%
≤1	10%
>1–2	11.1%
>2–5	13.3%
>5–10	38.5%
>10	62.5%

Five-year disease specific survival also correlated with the size of sentinel lymph node metastases: 97% for isolated tumor cells, 88% for 1–2 mm sentinel lymph node metastases, 70% for >2–5 mm sentinel lymph node metastases, and 69% for metastases >5 mm. This was a statistically significant difference for sentinel lymph node metastases ≤2 mm versus >2 mm with five-year disease specific survival of 94.4% and 69.5% ($P = 0.001$), respectively.

Current NCCN guidelines indicate that a full lymphadenectomy is preferred prior to proceeding with adjuvant EBRT for a sentinel lymph node metastasis >2 mm. However, any size positive sentinel lymph node (≤2 mm or >2 mm) should receive EBRT but is not recommended for full lymph node dissection. The role of concurrent chemotherapy use in this setting is not yet clarified. The GROINSS V authors suggest that concurrent chemotherapy be used for patients with sentinel lymph node metastases >2 mm based on the lower disease specific survival; however, to these authors' knowledge, to date there is not data to support that this strategy will provide benefit.

Correct Answer: A

Case Study 8

A 73-year-old female presents with a 6 cm left vulvar cancer with palpable left inguinal adenopathy. Given the size of resection that would be required, you elect not to resect the primary tumor. You recommend left inguinofemoral node dissection followed by at least pelvic and inguino-femoral radiation with concurrent cisplatin-based chemotherapy.

13) What data best supports this approach?
   A) A randomized controlled trial demonstrated superior progression-free survival for patients who received neoadjuvant chemoradiation prior to surgical resection of advanced stage vulvar cancer.
   B) A randomized controlled trial demonstrated no difference in survival but a decrease in surgical morbidity and improvement in quality of life for patients who received neoadjuvant chemoradiation prior to surgical resection for advanced-stage vulvar cancer.
   C) A phase II trial demonstrated superior progression-free survival for patients with advanced vulvar cancer who received neoadjuvant chemoradiation compared with a historical control group of patients who underwent up-front surgical resection.
   D) A phase II trial demonstrated a complete pathologic response rate of 50% for patients with advanced vulvar cancer who received neoadjuvant chemoradiation.

Expert Perspective: There is not a randomized controlled trial that directly compares up-front debulking of advanced vulvar cancer with neoadjuvant chemoradiation prior to surgical resection. The best data we have for neoadjuvant chemoradiation is from GOG 205. GOG 205 was a phase II trial that evaluated clinical and pathologic complete response rates for unresectable advanced vulvar cancer. Given GOG 88 had previously shown inferior outcomes for patients with stage I–III vulvar cancer that had radiation therapy to groin nodes without full lymph node dissection, the protocol for GOG 205 required inguinofemoral lymph node dissection for women with clinical negative or resectable groin nodes. GOG 205 found a complete clinical response rate of 64% and complete pathologic response rate of 50%.

Correct Answer: D

Case Study 9

A 61-year-old female is diagnosed with differentiated vulvar intraepithelial neoplasia on vulvar biopsy. She has a history of lichen sclerosis.

14) What is the best treatment?
  A) Imiquimod cream.
  B) Wide local excision.
  C) CO_2 laser ablation.
  D) Clobetasol cream.

Expert Perspective: Differentiated VIN is a precursor lesion to vulvar squamous cell carcinoma that often arises in the setting of chronic vulvar dermatoses, such as lichen sclerosis and lichen simplex chronicus. It is an HPV-independent entity. HPV-associated VIN (usual-type VIN) can be treated with excision, imiquimod cream, or laser ablation. Differentiated VIN should only be treated with excision due to a much higher risk of progression to vulvar cancer. Usual-type VIN has a 10% cumulative 10-year risk of progression to vulvar squamous cell carcinoma, whereas differentiated VIN has a 50% cumulative 10-year risk. Clobetasol cream is used for the treatment of lichen sclerosis, and treatment decreases the cancer risk in patients with lichen sclerosis. But clobetasol cream alone would not be appropriate treatment for a patient who already has differentiated VIN.

Correct Answer: B

Case Study 10

A 42-year-old patient with a history of liver transplant on tacrolimus is diagnosed with stage IIIA vulvar carcinoma with a 3 cm left labial primary tumor and an isolated tumor-metastasis (ITC) of the left sentinel lymph node.

15) What data best supports proceeding straight to radiation therapy for this patient?
  A) A prospective multicenter phase II trial found no increase in groin recurrence rate for patients who had a positive sentinel lymph node with tumor focus ≤ 2 mm and were treated with groin RT alone without full inguinofemoral lymphadenectomy.
  B) A prospective multicenter phase II trial found no increase in groin recurrence rate for patients with positive sentinel lymph nodes with tumor focus ≤ 5 mm in size and who were treated with groin RT alone without full inguinofemoral lymphadenectomy.
  C) A randomized controlled phase III trial found no difference in groin recurrence rates between patients who had sentinel lymph nodes ≤ 2 mm and underwent subsequent full inguinofemoral lymph node dissection then groin RT versus those who received groin RT alone.
  D) A randomized controlled phase III trial found no difference in groin recurrence rates between patients who had sentinel lymph nodes ≤ 5 mm and underwent subsequent full inguinofemoral lymph node dissection then groin versus those who received groin RT alone.

Expert Perspective: GROINSS-V II was a prospective multicenter phase II trial designed to evaluate whether radiotherapy could replace full inguinofemoral lymphadenectomy for patients with early stage vulvar cancer and positive sentinel lymph nodes. Results of this trial were presented at the Society for Gynecologic Oncology (SGO) Annual Meeting in 2020. Interim analysis at 54 months showed an increased risk for groin recurrence when the tumor focus of a sentinel node was 2 mm and/or there was extranodal extension. Isolated tumor cells are defined as a tumor focus measuring ≤ 2 mm. For nodal metastases ≤ 2 mm (isolated tumor cells), there was not an increased risk of groin recurrence when treated with radiation therapy alone without full lymph node dissection. Final publication of this data is yet to be released.

Correct Answer: A

16) **Which statement about vulvar melanoma is correct?**
    A) Vulvar melanomas have a very low rate of BRAF mutations.
    B) Staging of vulvar melanoma is different from staging for cutaneous melanomas.
    C) Pelvic exenteration is the preferred approach for localized disease.
    D) All of the above.

Expert Perspective: Vulvar melanomas are the second most common histological type of vulvar cancer, representing 7–10% of all malignant vulvar neoplasms. Compared with cutaneous (extragenital) melanoma, vulvar melanoma has a very low rate of mutations in BRAF and neuroblastoma RAS viral oncogene homolog (N-RAS). Staging of vulvar melanoma utilizes the same staging as for cutaneous melanomas. Wide local excision is the preferred approach in most localized cases (see Chapter 36).

Correct Answer: A

Vaginal Cancer

17) **Which one of the following is a risk factor for clear cell variant vaginal cancer?**
    A) Smoking.
    B) Prior history of cervical cancer.
    C) In utero diethylstilbestrol exposure.
    D) HPV infection.

Expert Perspective: Risk factors for squamous cell vaginal cancer are the same as cervical cancer and include HPV infection, smoking, early age at first intercourse, multiple lifetime sexual partners, and a history of prior cervix cancer. Other rare histologies of vaginal cancer include clear cell variant adenocarcinoma (in utero diethylstilbestrol exposure increases the risk for vaginal-cervical clear cell cancers), melanoma, and sarcoma and other adenocarcinomas. It is important to consider metastatic or recurrent disease from other sites (cervix, vulva, ovary, breast, endometrium, or uterus) in the evaluation of a new vaginal lesion because metastatic disease is more common than primary vaginal carcinoma.

Correct Answer: C

18) **A 50-year-old renal transplant patient is diagnosed with stage II vaginal cancer and undergoes concurrent chemoradiation based on which of the following supporting data?**
    A) An NCDB study found significant improvement in overall survival with the addition of concurrent chemotherapy to standard EBRT.
    B) A retrospective, single-institute study that demonstrated improvement in local control rate with the addition of concurrent chemotherapy to EBRT.
    C) A retrospective study found improvement in progression-free survival with the use of concurrent chemotherapy and EBRT.
    D) A Cochrane review found that use of concurrent chemotherapy improved OS in vaginal cancer patients undergoing definitive EBRT.

Expert Perspective: Rajagopalan et al. (2014) published an NCDB study including 8,222 patients who received radiation therapy for vaginal cancer, 3,932 of whom received concurrent chemotherapy. Median overall survival was significantly longer for the concurrent chemotherapy group compared with radiation alone, 56.2 months versus 41.2 months ($P < 0.0005$).

Correct Answer: A

Cervical Cancer Screening

19) **According to the United States Preventive Services Task Force, which of the following statements about cervical cancer screening is correct?**
    A) Screening should start at age 21, regardless of the age of initiation of sexual activity.
    B) Screening can be discontinued at age 65 in all patients.
    C) It is recommended to have annual Pap test from ages 21–29.
    D) Screening with annual HPV testing can be done in subjects older than age 30 years.
    E) Screening is not required for subjects who have had a hysterectomy with removal of the cervix even if they had a history of cervical intraepithelial neoplasia (CIN) 2.

Expert Perspective: Screening should start at age 21, regardless of the age of initiation of sexual activity, and it can be safely discontinued at age 65 only in subjects who have had adequate prior screening and are not otherwise at high risk for cervical cancer (no history of ≥ CIN 2 with evidence of prior adequate screening [≥3 negative cytology test results in a row, or two consecutive negative co-tests in the past 10 years, with the most recent within the past 5 years). It is recommended to have a Pap test every three years from ages 21–29. At age 30 and later, screening can continue with a Pap smear every three years, or subjects can elect to do primary HPV testing alone every five years (i.e. Cobas, BD Onclarity) or both tests every five years. Screening is not required for subjects who have had a benign hysterectomy with removal of the cervix who do not have a history of ≥ CIN 2. These guidelines are intended for the general population and are not intended for patients with a history of cervical cancer, high-grade cervical precancers, diethylstilbestrol in utero exposure, or who are immunocompromised (e.g. HIV infection).

Correct Answer: A

Prevention of HPV-related Cancers

20) **Which of the following statements about HPV-related cancers is correct?**
    A) HPV types 16 and 18 cause about 40% of all cervical cancers.
    B) HPV types 16 and 18 about 50% of anal cancers.
    C) HPV types other than types 16 and 18 do not cause cervical cancer.
    D) Gardasil 9 vaccination is specifically approved for prevention of cervical, vulvar, vaginal, anal, oropharyngeal, and other head and neck cancers.
    E) Both C and D.

Expert Perspective: HPV is a sexually transmitted pathogen that causes anogenital and oropharyngeal disease in males and females. HPV types 16 and 18 cause about 70% of all cervical cancers, nearly 90% of anal cancers, and a significant proportion of oropharyngeal cancer, vulvar and vaginal cancer, and penile cancer. Cervical cancers can also be caused by HPV types 31, 33, 45, 52, and 58. In the United States, the 9-valent vaccine (Gardasil 9; HPV types 6, 11, 16,18, 31, 33, 45, 52, and 58) is specifically approved for prevention of cervical, vulvar, vaginal, anal, oropharyngeal, and other head and neck cancers; anogenital precancerous and dysplastic lesions; and genital warts in females. It is used for the prevention of anal, oropharyngeal, and other head and neck cancers; anal precancerous and dysplastic lesions; and genital warts in males.

Correct Answer: D

Recommended Readings

Coleman, R.L., Lorusso, D., Gennigens, C. et al. innovaTV 204/GOG-3023/ENGOT-cx6 Collaborators. (2021). Efficacy and safety of tisotumab vedotin in previously treated recurrent or metastatic cervical cancer (innovaTV 204/GOG-3023/ENGOT-cx6): A multicentre, open-label, single-arm phase 2 study. *Lancet Oncol* 22 (5): 609–619. 10.1016/S1470-2045(21)00056-5. Epub 2021 Apr 9. PMID: 33845034.

Curry, S.J. (2018). Screening for cervical cancer: United States Preventive Services Task Force recommendation statement. *Jama* 320: 674.

Gold, M.A., Tian, C., Whitney, C.W. et al.(2008). Surgical versus radiographic determination of para-aortic lymph node metastases before chemoradiation for locally advanced cervical carcinoma: A Gynecologic Oncology Group study. *Cancer* 112: 1954–1963.

Haque, W., Verma, V., Fakhreddine, M. et al. (2017). Addition of chemotherapy to definitive radiotherapy for IB1 and IIA1cervical cancer: Analysis of the National Cancer Data Base. *Gynecologic Oncol* 144: 28–33.

Keys, H.M., Bundy, B.N., Stehman, F.B. et al. (2003). Radiation therapy with and without extrafascial hysterectomy for bulky stage IB cervical carcinoma: A randomized trial of the Gynecologic Oncology Group. *Gynecologic Oncol* 89: 343–353.

Leblanc, E., Narducci, F., Frumovitz, M. et al. (2007). Therapeutic value of pretherapeutic extraperitoneal laparoscopic staging of locally advanced cervical carcinoma. *Gynecologic Oncol* 105: 304–311.

Marnitz, S., Tsunoda, A.T., Martus, P. et al. (2020). Surgical versus clinical staging prior to primary chemoradiation in patients with cervical cancer FIGO stages IIB-IVA: Oncologic results of a prospective randomized international multicenter (Uterus-11) intergroup study. *Int J Gynecologic Cancer* 30: 1855–1861.

Rajagopalan, M.S., Xu, K.M., Lin, J.F. et al. (2014). Adoption and impact of concurrent chemoradiation therapy for vaginal cancer: A National Cancer Data Base (NCDB) study. *Gynecologic Oncol* 135: 495–502.

Tewari, K.S., Monk, B.J., Vergote, I. et al. Investigators for GOG Protocol 3016 and ENGOT Protocol En-Cx9 (2022). Survival with Cemiplimab in Recurrent Cervical Cancer. *N Engl J Med* 386 (6): 544–555. doi: 10.1056/NEJMoa2112187. PMID: 3513927.

Tewari, K.S., Sill, M.W., Long, H.J. et al. (2014). Improved survival with bevacizumab in advanced cervical cancer. *N Engl J Med* 370: 734–743.

Tewari, K.S., Sill, M.W., Monk, B.J. et al. (2015). Prospective validation of pooled prognostic factors in women with advanced cervical cancer treated with chemotherapy with/without bevacizumab: NRG oncology/GOG study. *Clin Cancer Res* 21 (24): 5480–5487.

Toyoshima, M., Shimada, M., Sasaki, S. et al. (2021). A single arm prospective pilot study examining the efficacy and safety of bevacizumab single maintenance therapy following platinum-based chemotherapy in patients with advanced or recurrent cervical cancer. *J Experimental Med* 254: 145–153.

42

Uncommon Gynecologic Cancers

Michael Frumovitz, Shannon Westin, and David M. Gershenson

Department of Gynecologic Oncology and Reproductive Medicine, The University of Texas MD Anderson Cancer Center, Houston, TX

Introduction

Our chapter presents clinical scenarios on nine different uncommon gynecologic cancers. Historically, these rare cancers were lumped with their more common counterparts and treated identically, both using standard of care therapies and in clinical trials. The following cases will provide the healthcare provider with valuable information regarding the specific clinical management of rare cervical, uterine, and ovarian cancers. We encourage readers to also refer to preceding chapters in this section on ovarian, endometrial, cervical, vulvar, and vaginal cancers.

Case Study 1

High-grade Neuroendocrine Carcinoma of the Cervix

A 27-year-old woman has a cervical biopsy that shows high-grade neuroendocrine carcinoma (small cell type) of the cervix.

1) **All of the following may be appropriate as initial therapy for newly diagnosed small-cell cervical cancer EXCEPT:**
   A) Surgical resection.
   B) Pelvic radiation.
   C) Systemic chemotherapy.
   D) Prophylactic brain irradiation.

Expert Perspective: Although prophylactic brain irradiation is commonly prescribed for patients with newly diagnosed small cell lung cancer, it is not employed in the treatment of women with neuroendocrine cervical cancers. The risk of occult brain metastases in the absence of disease spread to the liver or lung is exceedingly rare. Women with apparent early stage disease (stages IA1–IB2) may undergo surgical resection followed by chemotherapy with or without radiation. Women with locally advanced disease (stages IB3–IVA) will typically receive pelvic or extended field radiation with concurrent chemotherapy followed by systemic chemotherapy with cisplatin and etoposide. Finally, women

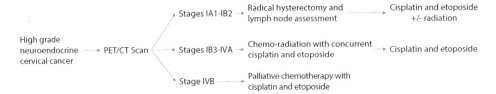

Figure 42.1 Management of newly diagnosed high-grade neuroendocrine carcinoma of the cervix.

with metastatic disease (stage IVB) will most frequently be given systemic chemotherapy with cisplatin and etoposide (Figure 42.1).

Correct Answer: D

Case continues: On pelvic exam, the tumor appears 2 cm in size with no vaginal or parametrial extension. Metastatic workup including a PET/CT scan is negative.

2) Which of the following is the most likely initial treatment for this patient?
    A) Radical hysterectomy, bilateral salpingo-oophorectomy, lymphatic mapping, and sentinel lymph node biopsy.
    B) Pelvic radiation with concurrent cisplatin.
    C) Extended-field radiation with concurrent cisplatin.
    D) Systemic chemotherapy with cisplatin and etoposide.

Expert Perspective: Because this patient has stage IB1 disease and a negative metastatic workup, initial treatment would consist of surgical resection including a radical hysterectomy and lymph node assessment. Although performing a bilateral salpingo-oophorectomy would be standard, one may consider bilateral salpingectomies with transposition of one or both ovaries if they appear grossly normal. Isolated microscopic disease to the ovaries is rare, so preventing surgical menopause in this 27-year-old patient with ovarian transposition is reasonable. In addition, pathologic assessment of pelvic lymph nodes should be undertaken. This may be in the form of lymphatic mapping and sentinel lymph node biopsies or via complete pelvic lymphadenectomy depending on surgeon preference.

Correct Answer: A

Case continues: Pathologic assessment of surgical specimens shows microscopic disease extension into the parametrial tissue with a positive parametrial margin. Lymph nodes are negative.

3) Which of the following adjuvant therapies is the best option?
    A) Pelvic radiation with cisplatin only.
    B) Pelvic radiation with cisplatin and etoposide only.
    C) Pelvic radiation with cisplatin followed by additional cisplatin and etoposide.
    D) Pelvic radiation with cisplatin and etoposide followed by additional cisplatin and etoposide.

Expert Perspective: This patient is at high risk for both local and distant recurrence. For that reason, she needs both pelvic radiation therapy and systemic chemotherapy. Because the disease is limited to the pelvis, the radiation field needs to be a pelvic field. Multiple studies have shown that combination cisplatin and etoposide is tolerable with radiation therapy, and this is the regimen of choice for concurrent chemotherapy with radiation. Because patients with high-grade neuroendocrine carcinoma have improved survival if they get at least five cycles of cisplatin and etoposide (compared with those who get four cycles or less), and because patients will get only two cycles of the regimen during radiation, they will require an additional three to four cycles of the same regimen after completing pelvic radiation (Figure 42.1).

Correct Answer: D

Case Study 2

Primary Mucinous Ovarian Cancer

A 32-year-old nulliparous woman is taken to the operating room for a 22 cm left adnexal mass. Intraoperatively, the mass looks isolated to the left ovary with no gross evidence of extra-ovarian disease. The left ovary and tube are resected. Frozen section shows an invasive mucinous carcinoma of likely gynecologic origin.

4) In addition to removal of the left ovary, what other procedures should be performed?
   A) Right salpingo-oophorectomy.
   B) Hysterectomy.
   C) Omentectomy.
   D) Appendectomy.

Expert Perspective: More than 85% of patients with primary mucinous ovarian cancer will have disease limited to one ovary (stage I; Table 42.1). In the remaining 15% who will have metastatic disease, almost all will have gross evidence of metastatic disease. For premenopausal women, retention of the contralateral ovary is recommended if there is no evidence of gross disease outside the ovary. Likewise, for women who wish to retain fertility, there is no need to perform a hysterectomy if the uterus does not have any evidence of tumor involvement. In the past, appendectomy was performed in these cases to rule out an appendiceal primary, but more recent studies have shown that a normal appearing appendix is exceedingly unlikely to harbor an occult primary and therefore does not need to be resected. However, many times the appendix may be adhered to a large pelvic mass (particularly if arising from the right adnexa), so removing the appendix may be required in those cases. For patients with grossly apparent stage IA disease (i.e. disease limited to one ovary without evidence of metastatic disease), staging biopsies including omentectomy should be performed.

Correct Answer: C

5) Which of the following pathologic diagnosis is MOST likely to be found in women who present with advanced/metastatic disease (stage III or IV)?
   A) Mucinous borderline tumor.
   B) Mucinous intraepithelial carcinoma.

C) Mucinous carcinoma, expansile type.
D) Mucinous carcinoma, infiltrative type.

Table 42.1 Ovary, fallopian tube, and primary peritoneal carcinoma FIGO staging, AJCC UICC 8th edition.

Stage	Brief description
I	Tumor limited to ovaries (one or both) or fallopian tube(s)
II	Tumor involves one or both ovaries or fallopian tubes with pelvic extension below pelvic brim or primary peritoneal cancer
III	Tumor involves one or both ovaries or fallopian tubes, or primary peritoneal cancer, with microscopically confirmed peritoneal metastasis outside the pelvis and/or metastasis to the retroperitoneal (pelvic and/or para-aortic) lymph nodes
IVA	Pleural effusion with positive cytology
IVB	Liver or splenic parenchymal metastases; metastases to extra-abdominal organs (including inguinal lymph nodes and lymph nodes outside the abdominal cavity); transmural involvement of intestine

Expert Perspective: Unlike serous borderline and carcinoma, where a borderline tumor is not considered a premalignant state for high-grade serous carcinoma, mucinous borderline tumors are considered a precursor to invasive, high-grade mucinous ovarian cancer. A single ovary may have areas of benign mucinous cysts, mucinous borderline tumor, and invasive mucinous carcinoma. This progression is typically not seen in serous lesions. That said, the borderline and intraepithelial carcinomas are considered premalignant lesions and therefore unlikely to be metastatic at the time of diagnosis. There are two patterns of invasion for invasive mucinous carcinoma: expansile and infiltrative. In the expansile pattern, the glands are back-to-back with minimal or no intervening stroma. The infiltrative pattern shows haphazard glands surrounded by desmoplastic stroma. The infiltrative pattern is more aggressive than the expansile, and typically patients with metastatic disease at presentation will have the infiltrative subtype. Only 5% of women with the expansile pattern will have metastatic disease at diagnosis compared with more than 25% for those with the infiltrative pattern.

Correct Answer: D

6) **All of the following markers may be elevated in women with mucinous ovarian cancer EXCEPT:**
    A) CA19-9.
    B) CA27-29.
    C) Carcinoembryonic antigen (CEA).
    D) CA125.

Expert Perspective: Although CEA is more commonly utilized to follow patients with colon and pancreatic cancers, about one-third of patients with mucinous ovarian cancer will have an elevated CEA. CA125 may also be elevated in 10–15% of women with mucinous ovarian. This is obviously less frequent than in women with high-grade serous carcinoma, where CA125 is elevated over 85% of the time. CA19-9, which is a marker for upper gastrointestinal tumors including pancreatic, liver, and gallbladder, may also be elevated in women with mucinous ovarian cancer. CA27-29 is a serum cancer antigen that is frequently elevated in women with breast cancer. It is unlikely to be elevated in women with mucinous ovarian cancer.

Correct Answer: B

Case Study 3

Vulvovaginal Melanoma

A 72-year-old woman presents with a 1.2 cm ulcerated, pigmented lesion on the right labia majora. Biopsy reveals invasive melanoma with a tumor thickness of 2.2 mm. Metastatic workup including PET scan is negative.

7) What surgery should be recommended for this patient?
   A) Local excision with 1 cm surgical margins.
   B) Local excision with 1 cm surgical margins and sentinel lymph node biopsy.
   C) Local excision with 2 cm surgical margins.
   D) Local excision with 2 cm surgical margins and sentinel lymph node biopsy.

Expert Perspective: According to NCCN Guidelines, resection of vulvovaginal melanoma should follow those guidelines established for cutaneous melanoma. These recommendations are based on expert opinion because due to the rarity of the disease, there are no large prospective or retrospective studies guiding surgical resection. These guidelines include a surgical margin of 1 cm for invasive disease with tumor thickness ≤ 1 mm, between 1 and 2 cm for invasive disease with thickness of 1–2 mm, and 2 cm surgical margins for lesions with tumor thickness ≥ 2 mm. In addition, lymph node assessment with lymphatic mapping and sentinel lymph node biopsy should be performed. If surgeons are not trained or comfortable with sentinel lymph node biopsy, complete inguinofemoral lymphadenectomy may be considered. (Also refer to Chapter 41.)

Correct Answer: D

8) All of the following are known prognostic factors for vulvovaginal melanoma EXCEPT:
   A) Breslow thickness.
   B) Presence of ulceration.
   C) Nodal status.
   D) Surgical stage.

Expert Perspective: Breslow thickness, which is the maximum depth of invasive tumor, is probably the most important prognostic factor. The five-year disease specific survival for tumors with Breslow thickness < 1 mm is 75% compared with 33% for those with Breslow thickness > 4 mm. Women with vulvar melanoma with nodal disease at diagnosis have a five-year disease specific survival of 20–30% compared with more than 70% for those who have node negative disease. Likewise, survival was significantly shorter for women with vaginal melanoma with disease spread to regional lymph nodes. In addition to node status, surgical stage is an independent prognosticator of recurrence and death from vulvovaginal melanoma. Although ulceration is a risk factor for increased stage and nodal metastases, it has not been shown to be an independent risk factor for survival in vulvovaginal melanoma when controlling for stage and node status.

Correct Answer: B

Case Study continue: The patient does well for nine months and then is noted to have biopsy-confirmed recurrence with liver and lung metastases. The tumor is confirmed to have a *BRAF V600* activating mutation.

9) All of the following are reasonable treatment options EXCEPT:
   A) No further treatment/hospice.
   B) Dabrafenib and tremetinib.
   C) Dacarbazine.
   D) Nivolumab.

Expert Perspective: Treatment of recurrent disease follows guidelines similar to those for cutaneous melanoma. NCCN preferred regimens for first recurrence consist of immunotherapies and targeted therapies. These include anti-PD1 monotherapies with nivolumab and pembrolizumab as well as combination anti-PD1 and anti-CTLA4 agents such as nivolumab and ipilimumab. For patients with activating *BRAF V600* mutations, combination targeted therapies such as dabrafenib and tremetinib, vemurafenib and cobimetinib, and encorrafenib and binimetinib should be considered. Combinations of targeted therapies and immunotherapies also are reasonable. Patients with widely metastatic disease may opt for no further treatment, and this wish should be respected and accepted after appropriate discussion of options and prognosis. Single-agent cytotoxic chemotherapy such as dacarbazine is not recommended in the recurrent setting.

Correct Answer: C

Case Study 4

Low-grade Serous Ovarian Carcinoma

A 36-year-old woman presents with bilateral ascites, bilateral ovarian masses, and carcinomatosis in the region of the omentum on CT. Her CA125 is 240 U/mL. She undergoes primary cytoreductive surgery with the findings of stage IIIC low-grade serous ovarian cancer. No gross residual disease was present at the completion of the surgery.

10) All of the following are reasonable postoperative treatment options EXCEPT:
   A) Taxane/carboplatin with bevacizumab for six cycles followed by letrozole maintenance therapy.
   B) Taxane/carboplatin for six cycles followed by letrozole maintenance therapy.
   C) Letrozole.
   D) All of the listed options are appropriate.

Expert Perspective: All of the listed options are acceptable postoperative treatment options. NCCN guidelines for treatment of stage IIIC low-grade serous ovarian cancer include taxane/platinum chemotherapy followed by maintenance hormonal therapy as well as hormonal therapy alone. Particularly in Europe, bevacizumab is frequently combined with chemotherapy based on evidence of activity in the recurrent setting. There is an ongoing phase III trial (NCT04095364) in which women with stage II–IV low-grade serous ovarian cancer are randomized to either paclitaxel/carboplatin for six cycles followed by letrozole maintenance therapy until disease progression or letrozole monotherapy until disease progression.

Correct Answer: D

Case Study continue: The patient is treated with letrozole monotherapy. After 2.5 years, she develops a rising CA125 to 124 U/mL, and CT reveals disease progression with a mass in the perisplenic hilum and no other abnormalities on CT.

11) What is the best treatment recommendation?
   A) Paclitaxel/carboplatin for six cycles plus bevacizumab.
   B) Pegylated liposomal doxorubicin plus bevacizumab.
   C) Trametinib.
   D) Secondary cytoreductive surgery followed by systemic therapy.

Expert Perspective: With the publication of three randomized clinical trials in the study of secondary cytoreductive surgery for epithelial ovarian cancer (all subtypes), the benefit of this approach has become more controversial. However, low-grade serous ovarian cancer is known to be relatively (not completely) resistant to chemotherapy compared with high-grade serous ovarian cancer. With a solitary site of relapse, most gynecologic oncologists would recommend secondary cytoreductive surgery initially followed by some type of systemic therapy. There is no one option for systemic therapy. Furthermore, there is no standard sequencing of agents for relapse. Potential options include various chemotherapy regiments, bevacizumab with or without chemotherapy, other endocrine therapies, or targeted agents, such as MEK inhibitors.

Correct Answer: D

Case Study continue: The patient undergoes successful secondary cytoreductive surgery followed by platinum-based chemotherapy plus bevacizumab. After completion of chemotherapy and five cycles of maintenance bevacizumab, she develops a second relapse with carcinomatosis. Somatic tumor testing following secondary surgery revealed that the tumor contains a *KRAS G12V* mutation.

12) What is the recommended treatment?
   A) Pegylated liposomal doxorubicin.
   B) Tamoxifen.
   C) Trametinib.
   D) Weekly paclitaxel plus bevacizumab.

Expert Perspective: All of the options listed are acceptable, although there is no one best option based on prospective clinical trial data. Chemotherapy may have up to about a 15% probability of achieving response. Tamoxifen appears to be inferior to aromatase inhibitors in observed response rates. The most effective treatment based on available information is trametinib with overall response rates in the range of 25%. In addition, there is emerging evidence that patients whose tumors contain a mutation in the *mitogen-activated protein kinase (MAPK)* pathway have even better response rates in the range of 45–50% to mitogen-activated protein kinase inhibitor therapy.

Correct Answer: C

Case Study 5

Granulosa Cell Tumor of Ovary

A 60-year-old woman undergoes surgery for a pelvic mass and ascites. All surgical staging biopsies are negative for tumor. She is found to have stage IA granulosa cell tumor of the ovary.

13) Which of the following is the most appropriate postoperative management?
   A) Aromatase inhibitor.
   B) Paclitaxel/carboplatin for six cycles.
   C) Observation.
   D) None of the above.

Expert Perspective: For stage IA granulosa cell tumor, the appropriate management is observation. The prognosis is excellent. Only about 10% of patients will recur. The tumor type is somewhat unique in that recurrences may occur several years later.

Correct Answer: C

Case Study continue: The patient with stage IA granulosa cell tumor recurs seven years after diagnosis with pelvic and omental tumor implants. She undergoes surgery with resection of all gross disease, and final pathology confirms the diagnosis of metastatic granulosa cell tumor.

14) Which of the following would be recommended?
   A) Observation.
   B) Platinum-based chemotherapy for six cycles.
   C) Anastrozole.
   D) Bevacizumab for one year.

Expert Perspective: For metastatic granulosa cell tumor, the initial systemic therapy recommended is platinum-based chemotherapy. Historically, the most popular regimens have been either the combination of bleomycin, etoposide, and cisplatin or paclitaxel/carboplatin. Emerging evidence has suggested that paclitaxel/carboplatin is preferred related to its therapeutic index (Figure 42.2).

Correct Answer: B

15) For patients with granulosa cell tumor, which is the most reliable serum marker to follow?
   A) Alpha-fetoprotein.
   B) Inhibin.
   C) Anti-mullerian hormone (AMH).
   D) CA125.

Introduction

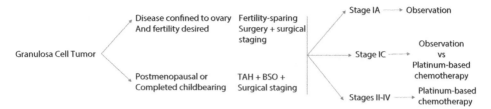

Figure 42.2 Management of newly diagnosed granulosa cell tumor of the ovary.

Expert Perspective: Serum inhibin is the most reliable serum marker for granulosa cell tumor. Serum inhibin B seems to be somewhat more predictive than inhibin A, although there are exceptions to this rule. Alpha-fetoprotein may be a marker for other sex cord-stromal tumors, such as Sertoli-Leydig cell tumors, but not for granulosa cell tumors. AMH may be a marker for granulosa cell tumor, but it does not appear to be as reliable as inhibin. CA125 may be elevated in patients with metastatic granulosa cell tumor, but it is not specific.

Correct Answer: B

Case Study 6

Clear Cell Ovarian Carcinoma

A 40-year-old woman has a 7 cm pelvic mass on ultrasound. She undergoes laparoscopic hysterectomy, bilateral salpingo-oophorectomy, and surgical staging for stage IA clear cell carcinoma of the ovary.

16) What is the most appropriate postoperative management for this patient?
 A) Observation.
 B) Pelvic radiotherapy.
 C) IV platinum-based therapy.
 D) A and C.

Expert Perspective: The optimal postoperative management of stage IA clear cell carcinoma of the ovary continues to be controversial. There are some experts who advocate observation, citing a lack of evidence of benefit of adjuvant platinum-based chemotherapy, whereas others believe that platinum-based chemotherapy is the standard. The NCCN Ovarian Cancer Guidelines actually list both as options. However, it is safe to say that the predominant view within the gynecologic cancer community favors adjuvant platinum-based chemotherapy. Part of the justification for postoperative treatment in the face of conflicting data is the extremely poor prognosis for patients with clear cell carcinoma who recur. Hopefully, future studies will provide more clarity on this important clinical management issue.

Correct Answer: D

Case Study continue: The patient with stage IA clear cell carcinoma of the ovary received adjuvant treatment with six cycles of paclitaxel/carboplatin. Two years later, she recurs with carcinomatosis, including two lesions in the liver parenchyma.

17) Which of the following options is the best choice for second-line therapy?
   A) Platinum-based chemotherapy.
   B) Platinum-based chemotherapy plus bevacizumab.
   C) Clinical trial with a targeted agent.
   D) Clinical trial with an immune checkpoint inhibitor.

Expert Perspective: The prognosis for patients with recurrent clear cell carcinoma is poor. The response rate to any standard cytotoxic chemotherapy is low, including platinum-based chemotherapy for platinum-sensitive recurrence. Anti-angiogenic agents appear to have modest activity in clear cell carcinoma. Several studies have demonstrated strong expression of Vascular endothelial growth factor (VEGF) in clear cell carcinoma, and the angiogenesis pathway appears to be very active. But whether anti-angiogenic agents are more beneficial in clear cell carcinoma than in other epithelial ovarian cancer subtypes remains unclear. In addition, several phase II trials of targeted agents in recurrent clear cell carcinoma have produced disappointing results. Importantly, there is emerging evidence that immune checkpoint inhibitors may have particular effectiveness in clear cell carcinoma compared to other subtypes, including high-grade serous carcinoma. There is preliminary evidence for support of this concept from a small number of reports, and there are several ongoing clinical trials studying immunotherapy in clear cell carcinoma of the ovary.

Correct Answer: D

Case Study 7

Uterine Serous Carcinoma

A 48-year-old woman presents with bloating, early satiety, and abdominal pain. She has had irregular menses for several years. An endometrial biopsy reveals uterine serous carcinoma. Her CA125 is elevated to 186 U/mL. CT imaging reveals peritoneal carcinomatosis and an enlarged uterus. She undergoes primary cytoreductive surgery, which achieves no gross residual disease at the completion of the case. Final pathology is consistent with stage IV uterine serous carcinoma. Molecular testing reveals that the tumor is microsatellite stable and demonstrates HER2 immunohistochemistry (IHC) 3+ staining.

18) All of the following are reasonable postoperative treatment options EXCEPT:
   A) Paclitaxel/carboplatin for six cycles.
   B) Paclitaxel/carboplatin with trastuzumab for six cycles followed by trastuzumab maintenance.
   C) Alternating megestrol acetate and tamoxifen.
   D) Paclitaxel/carboplatin with bevacizumab for six cycles followed by bevacizumab maintenance.

Expert Perspective: Based on the NCCN guidelines, all listed options are acceptable postoperative treatment options for advanced stage uterine serous carcinoma except the alternating hormonal regimen. The use of paclitaxel and carboplatin in the adjuvant setting is considered one potential standard of care. There is also an opportunity to add trastuzumab to chemotherapy in patients with HER2-positive uterine serous cancer, defined as HER overexpression (IHC 3+ expression) or HER2 amplification (on FISH analysis). In a phase II study, the addition of trastuzumab yielded improved progression free survival and overall survival (OS) in this patient population. The GOG 86P trial included serous histology and demonstrated potential for superior OS for patients treated with chemotherapy and bevacizumab. A subsequent subset analysis revealed that patients with p53 mutation derived the most benefit from bevacizumab. In general, uterine serous tumors have very low expression of estrogen receptor and progesterone receptor. Accordingly, hormonal agents, alone and in combination have not been found to have activity in uterine serous carcinoma.

Correct Answer: C

Case Study continue: The patient presents for routine evaluation during trastuzumab maintenance and is noted to have increasing abdominal pain and an elevated CA125 to 91 U/mL. Imaging reveals multifocal peritoneal recurrence.

19) What is the best treatment recommendation?
   A) Doxorubicin for 6 cycles.
   B) Pembrolizumab for 24 months.
   C) Pembrolizumab/lenvatinib for 24 months.
   D) External beam radiation therapy.

Expert Perspective: Single-agent checkpoint inhibition has not been successful in mismatch repair proficient endometrial cancer, with response rates ranging between 3 and 13%. In a phase Ib/II study, the combination of lenvatinib and pembrolizumab demonstrated a 38% response rate across patients with mismatch repair proficient endometrial cancer. This efficacy was noted across multiple histologies, including endometrioid, serous, and clear cell. This was subsequently confirmed in a randomized phase III study (KEYNOTE-775), where lenvatinib and pembrolizumab yielded improved progression-free survival and OS compared with physician's choice chemotherapy (weekly paclitaxel or doxorubicin) in mismatch repair proficient endometrial cancer. Radiation therapy is recommended for vaginal or lymph node recurrence but would not be recommended in the setting of peritoneal carcinomatosis.

Correct Answer: C

Case Study continue: After 18 months on lenvatinib and pembrolizumab, the patient is identified to have a recurrence in the lungs and peritoneum.

20) What is the recommended treatment?
   A) Weekly paclitaxel.
   B) Bevacizumab.
   C) Doxorubicin.
   D) All listed options are appropriate.

Expert Perspective: All of the options listed are acceptable and NCCN compendium listed, although there is no one best option based on prospective clinical trial data. In uterine serous carcinoma, in second-line and beyond, treatment is based on clinical trials in endometrial cancer that were not specific to uterine serous carcinoma. Across all included histologies, single-agent chemotherapy or bevacizumab have response rates of approximately 5–15% and progression-free survival of approximately three months.

Correct Answer: D

Case Study 8

Uterine Leiomyosarcoma

A 56-year-old woman undergoes surgery for enlarged uterus and pelvic pain. She undergoes a total abdominal hysterectomy and bilateral salpingo-oophorectomy. There is no evidence of disease outside of the uterus. Final pathology is consistent with a stage I leiomyosarcoma.

21) Which would the most appropriate postoperative management?
   A) Observation.
   B) Gemcitabine/docetaxel for four cycles followed by doxorubicin for four cycles.
   C) Volume-directed radiation therapy.
   D) None of the above.

Expert Perspective: There is no evidence that chemotherapy improves survival outcomes for women with stage I or II uterine leiomyosarcoma. In the GOG 277 trial, despite early closure due to slow accrual, there was no improvement in progression free survival with chemotherapy treatment (gemcitabine/docetaxel for four cycles followed by doxorubicin for four cycles) compared with active surveillance. Further, it appeared that OS was worse in the group treated with chemotherapy. Similarly, for women with early stage uterine leiomyosarcoma, adjuvant radiotherapy did not demonstrate any improvement in progression free survival or in rates of local progression in a randomized trial (Figure 42.3).

Correct Answer: A

Case Study continue: The patient notes abdominal bloating at approximately 12 months after her initial diagnosis. Imaging reveals recurrence in the lungs and peritoneal carcinomatosis.

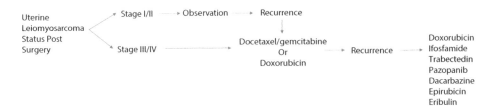

Figure 42.3 Management of uterine leiomyosarcoma.

22) Which of the following would be appropriate therapy?
   A) Doxorubicin.
   B) Paclitaxel and carboplatin for six cycles.
   C) Docetaxel and gemcitabine for six cycles.
   D) A and C.

Expert Perspective: In the treatment of metastatic or recurrent uterine leiomyosarcoma, two potential standard of care options are single agent doxorubicin or the combination of docetaxel and gemcitabine. These regimens were compared in a randomized study in sarcoma of any histology and were noted to achieve similar progression-free survival and objective response to therapy. In contrast, the combination of paclitaxel and carboplatin has not demonstrated activity in leiomyosarcoma.

Correct Answer: D

Case Study continue: The patient receives docetaxel and gemcitabine with clinical benefit for six months. Ultimately, there is progression of disease in the peritoneum.

23) What is the next best option?
- A) Trabectedin.
- B) Pazopanib.
- C) Ifosfamide.
- D) All of the above.

Expert Perspective: Each of the aforementioned options has demonstrated modest activity in recurrent uterine leiomyosarcoma in the second line or beyond. Trabectedin resulted in improved progression-free survival compared with dacarbazine. Similarly, progression-free survival was improved in patients treated with pazopanib versus placebo. Ifosfamide has been demonstrated to achieve objective response rates between 17 and 30% in women with uterine leiomyosarcoma. Thus, all are reasonable options to explore in this patient population.

Correct Answer: D

Case Study 9

Uterine Smooth Muscle Tumor of Uncertain Malignant Potential

A 36-year-old woman has a 9 cm uterine mass on ultrasound. She desires future fertility and undergoes an exploratory laparotomy with myomectomy. Final pathology is consistent with a uterine smooth muscle tumor of uncertain malignant potential (STUMP).

24) The most appropriate postoperative management for this patient is:
- A) Observation.
- B) Hysterectomy with or without oophorectomy.
- C) Doxorubicin-based chemotherapy.
- D) A and B.

Expert Perspective: Ultimately, there are no definitive guidelines for the need for hysterectomy and oophorectomy in a patient diagnosed with uterine STUMP at the time of myomectomy. Ultimately, careful review of the patient's goals and the potential for recurrence should be performed. Observation can include examination and imaging such as magnetic resonance imaging and/or transvaginal ultrasounds every 6–12 months. There are no data for the use of chemotherapy for the treatment of STUMP.

Correct Answer: D

25) What are the pathologic features that may be included in the diagnosis of a uterine STUMP?
- A) Tumor cell necrosis.
- B) High mitotic count.

C) Cytologic atypia.
D) Any one of the above in the absence of the other two is consistent with a diagnosis of STUMP tumor.

Expert Perspective: Uterine STUMP are diagnosed based on the presence of only one of the three definitive pathologic features of uterine leiomyosarcoma: (i) tumor cell necrosis, (ii) high mitotic count (≥ 10 mitoses per high power field), or (iii) moderate/severe cytologic atypia. A tumor that has two or more of these features is classified as a leiomyosarcoma.

Correct Answer: D

Case Study continue: The patient asks about her risk of recurrence.

26) Which of the following features of uterine STUMP is associated with the highest risk of recurrence?
A) High mitotic count.
B) Tumor cell necrosis.
C) Cytologic atypia.
D) There is no risk of recurrence.

Expert Perspective: Overall, the risk of recurrence of uterine STUMP is low. In small observational studies, recurrence risk appears to be associated with the pathologic feature defining diagnosis. Patients with tumor cell necrosis have the highest risk of recurrence, and tumors with high mitotic count have the lowest risk of recurrence.

Correct Answer: B

Recommended Readings

Bogani, G., Ditto, A., Lopez, S. et al. (2020). Adjuvant chemotherapy vs observation in stage I clear cell ovarian carcinoma: a systematic review and meta-analysis. *Gynecol Oncol* 157: 293–298.

Cohen, J.G., Kapp, D.S., Shin, J.Y., Urban, R., Sherman, A.E., Chen, L.M., Osann, K., and Chan, J.K. (2010 October). Small cell carcinoma of the cervix: treatment and survival outcomes of 188 patients. *Am J Obstet Gynecol* 203 (4): 347.e1–6. doi: 10.1016/j.ajog.2010.04.019. Epub 2010 Jul 1. PMID: 20579961.

Fader, A.N., Roque, D.M., Siegel, E., Buza, N., Hui, P., Abdelghany, O., Chambers, S., Secord, A.A., Havrilesky, L., O'Malley, D.M., Backes, F.J., Nevadunsky, N., Edraki, B., Pikaart, D., Lowery, W., ElSahwi, K., Celano, P., Bellone, S., Azodi, M., Litkouhi, B., Ratner, E., Silasi, D.A., Schwartz, P.E., and Santin, A.D. (2020 August 1). Randomized Phase II Trial of Carboplatin-Paclitaxel Compared with Carboplatin-Paclitaxel-Trastuzumab in Advanced (Stage III-IV) or Recurrent Uterine Serous Carcinomas that Overexpress Her2/Neu (NCT01367002): Updated Overall Survival Analysis. *Clin Cancer Res* 26 (15): 3928–3935.

Gershenson, D.M., Miller, A., Brady, W.E. et al. (2022). Trametinib versus standard of care in patients with recurrent low-grade serous ovarian cancer (GOG 281/LOGS): an international, randomized, open-label, multicentre, phase 2/3 trial. *Lancet* 399: 541–553.

Hess, V., A'Hern, R., Nasiri, N., King, D.M., Blake, P.R., Barton, D.P., Shepherd, J.H., Ind, T., Bridges, J., Harrington, K., Kaye, S.B., and Gore, M.E. (2004 March 15). Mucinous epithelial ovarian cancer: a separate entity requiring specific treatment. *J Clin Oncol* 22 (6): 1040–1044. doi: 10.1200/JCO.2004.08.078. PMID: 15020606.

Kurnit, K.C., Sinno, A.K., Fellman, B.M., Varghese, A., Stone, R., Sood, A.K., Gershenson, D.M., Schmeler, K.M., Malpica, A., Fader, A.N., and Frumovitz, M. (2019 December). Effects of gastrointestinal-type chemotherapy in women with ovarian mucinous carcinoma. *Obstet Gynecol* 134 (6): 1253–1259. doi: 10.1097/AOG.0000000000003579. PMID: 31764736; PMCID: PMC7100606.

Leslie, K.K., Filiaci, V.L., Mallen, A.R., Thiel, K.W., Devor, E.J., Moxley, K., Richardson, D., Mutch, D., Secord, A.A., Tewari, K.S., McDonald, M.E., Mathews, C., Cosgrove, C., Dewdney, S., Casablanca, Y., Jackson, A., Rose, P.G., Zhou, X., McHale, M., Lankes, H., Levine, D.A., and Aghajanian, C. (2021 April). Mutated p53 portends improvement in outcomes when bevacizumab is combined with chemotherapy in advanced/recurrent endometrial cancer: An NRG oncology study. *Gynecol Oncol* 161 (1): 113–121. doi: 10.1016/j.ygyno.2021.01.025. Epub 2021 Feb 2. PMID: 33541735.

Satoh, T., Takei, Y., Treilleux, I., Devouassoux-Shisheboran, M., Ledermann, J., Viswanathan, A.N., Mahner, S., Provencher, D.M., Mileshkin, L., Åvall-Lundqvist, E., Pautier, P., Reed, N.S., and Fujiwara, K. (2014 November). Gynecologic cancer intergroup (GCIG) consensus review for small cell carcinoma of the cervix. *Int J Gynecol Cancer* 24 (9Suppl 3): S102–8. doi: 10.1097/IGC.0000000000000262. PMID: 25341572.

Shushkevich, A., Thaker, P.H., Littell, R.D., Shah, N.A., Chiang, S., Thornton, K., Hensley, M.L., Slomovitz, B.M., Holcomb, K.M., Leitao, M.M., Toboni, M.D., Powell, M.A., Levine, D.A., Dowdy, S.C., Klopp, A., and Brown, J. (2020 October). State of the science: uterine sarcomas: from pathology to practice. *Gynecol Oncol* 159 (1): 3–7. doi: 10.1016/j.ygyno.2020.08.008. Epub 2020 Aug 21. PMID: 32839026.

Van Meurs, H.S., van Lonkhuijzen, L.R.C.W., Limpens, J. et al. (2014). Hormone therapy in ovarian granulosa cell tumors: a systematic review. *Gynecol Oncol* 134: 196–205.

WHO Classification of Tumors Online https://tumourclassification.iarc.who.int (Accessed October 13 2022).

Winer, I., Kim, C., and Gehrig, P. (2021 July). Neuroendocrine tumors of the gynecologic tract update. *Gynecol Oncol* 162 (1): 210–219. doi: 10.1016/j.ygyno.2021.04.039. Epub 2021 May 20. PMID: 34023130.

Zamarin, D., Burger, R.A., Sill, M.W. et al. (2020). Randomized phase II trial of nivolumab versus nivolumab and ipilimumab for recurrent or persistent ovarian cancer: An NRG oncology study. *J Clin Oncol* 38: 1814–1823.

Part 8

Sarcomas

43

Bone Sarcomas

Nicole Larrier, William Eward, and Richard F. Riedel

Duke University Medical Center, Durham, NC

Introduction

Bone sarcomas are rare, mesenchymal neoplasms that primarily originate in bone and account for less than 1% of all cancers. While all ages can be affected, bone sarcomas most commonly occur in children and young adults. Fewer than 4,000 new diagnoses are anticipated this year. Multimodal therapeutic approaches are key to improving outcomes for patients and treatment paradigms have been well established for both osteosarcoma and Ewing sarcoma over the years. With appropriate multidisciplinary management, the rates of long-term survival of localized osteosarcoma and Ewing sarcoma have improved from less than 20% to greater than 70%. Although the use of systemic therapy plays a critical role in the management of localized disease for osteosarcoma and Ewing sarcoma, chondrosarcoma remains particularly challenging given the lack of known effective systemic therapies. Local control for bone sarcomas can be addressed with surgery and/or radiation therapy, depending on histological subtype. An understanding of the underlying biology that leads to the pathogenesis of disease has resulted in advances, particularly in giant cell tumor of bone. Referral for genetic counseling and testing should be considered in adults suspected of carrying *TP53* mutation or *RB1* gene deletion (Chapters 45–47). However, bone sarcomas continue to remain an area of significant unmet medical need. The most common subtypes including osteosarcoma, Ewing sarcoma, and chondrosarcoma, but chordoma and giant cell tumor of bone will also be discussed in this chapter.

Case Study 1

A 17-year-old male is diagnosed with Ewing sarcoma of the left humerus diaphysis. On microscopy, there are monotonous sheets of small round blue cells that express high levels of CD99 and the nuclear transcription factor *FLI-1* (Friend leukemia integration 1 transcription factor) on immunohistochemistry. Genomic studies detect t(11;22)(q24;q12) chromosome translocations involving *FLI-1* and *EWSR1* (EWS RNA Binding Protein 1) genes. Staging studies reveal no evidence of metastatic disease. Chemotherapy with surgery and/or radiation therapy is recommended.

Cancer Consult: Expertise in Clinical Practice, Volume 1: Solid Tumors & Supportive Care,
Second Edition. Edited by Syed A. Abutalib, Maurie Markman, Al B. Benson III, and Hope S. Rugo.
© 2024 John Wiley & Sons Ltd. Published 2024 by John Wiley & Sons Ltd.

1) Is there a role for interval-compressed chemotherapy for the treatment of localized Ewing sarcoma?

Expert Perspective: Yes. The concept of interval-compressed chemotherapy was explored in a prospective, multicenter, randomized controlled trial by the Children's Oncology Group (COG). In this study, 587 patients were randomly assigned to receive chemotherapy as part of a 21- or 14-day cycle. Both treatment arms received vincristine, doxorubicin, and cyclophosphamide (VDC) alternating with ifosfamide and etoposide (IE) for a total of 14 cycles, and daily filgrastim was used for growth factor support. Across all patients, the mean cycle duration in the standard chemotherapy arm was 22.45 ± 4.87 days compared with 17.29 ± 5.40 days in the interval-compressed arm ($P < 0.001$). The five-year event-free survival was improved in the interval-compressed versus standard treatment arm, 73% versus 65%, respectively ($P = 0.048$). Five-year overall survival (OS), however, was not statistically significant between the two arms (83% vs 77%) for interval-compressed versus standard arms, respectively ($P = 0.056$). Importantly, there was no significant difference in toxicity between treatment arms. In summary, interval-compressed chemotherapy resulted in a 22% decrease in the risk of disease recurrence with no significant increase in toxicity. As a result, we would consider interval-compressed chemotherapy to be the standard of care for this patient with localized Ewing sarcoma, despite the lack of an OS benefit.

Although the COG study enrolled patients up to 50 years of age, it is important to note that patients ≥ 18 years of age represented a minority of patients enrolled (12% total) in this study. An analysis of the patients ≥ 18 years of age, reported at the American Society of Clinical Oncology (ASCO) Annual Meeting in 2008, showed no benefit for the use of interval-compressed therapy, but the total number of patients in the analysis was small (n = 67), limiting the power to detect a difference. As a result, in our opinion, the ability to draw firm conclusions on the use of interval-compressed chemotherapy in patients ≥ 18 years of age is limited. Recently, a single-institutional study reported on their experience with interval-compressed chemotherapy in patients 18 years and older. In that study, the use of interval-compressed chemotherapy was found to be feasible with no unexpected toxicity or need for significant dose reductions. In addition, the results appeared comparable with those reported in pediatric populations. Secondary malignancies, including acute leukemia, osteosarcoma, and lymphoma, occur in about 3% of survivors. Late recurrence of Ewing sarcoma, more than 5 years after initial diagnosis, occurs in 10–15% of children and adolescents, with about 25% of the late recurrences developing more than 10 years after diagnosis.

Case Study 2

A 52-year-old female presents with a one-year history of worsening back pain despite conservative treatment. Imaging reveals a 20 cm mass arising from the sacrum (Figure 43.1). Biopsy reveals a diagnosis of giant cell tumor of bone. Based on tumor size, location in the high sacrum, and anticipated surgical morbidity, the mass was deemed unresectable. The patient received a total of four embolizations over an eight-month time period with minimal improvement in symptoms. She is subsequently referred to medical oncology.

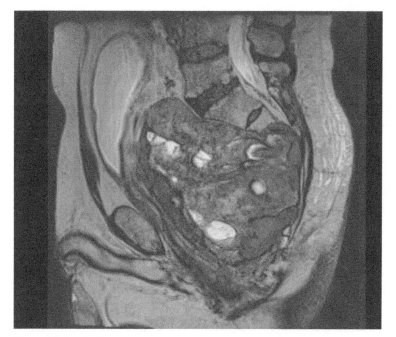

Figure 43.1 Sagittal MRI of the pelvis revealing a large sacral mass.

2) **Which of the following therapies has shown activity in giant cell tumor of bone?**
   A) Rituximab.
   B) Bevacizumab.
   C) Denosumab.
   D) Cetuximab.

Expert Perspective: Giant cell tumor of bone is a primary tumor of bone with a relatively low metastatic potential, indolent growth pattern, and high rate of local recurrence. Rarely, giant cell tumor of the bone can metastasize to the lungs. Surgery has traditionally been the preferred treatment when anticipated surgical morbidity is limited. Additional therapies such as radiation therapy and embolization have been considered as well. Studies supporting the use of systemic therapy, including chemotherapy and interferon, are of limited quality.

Denosumab is a fully human, monoclonal antibody targeting the RANK ligand, a protein with a crucial role in osteoclast differentiation and one that is expressed in the stromal cells of giant cell tumor of bone. It is currently approved by the US Food and Drug Administration for the treatment of patients with giant cell tumor of bone that is deemed unresectable or for situations where surgery would be particularly morbid. The use of denosumab in giant cell tumor of bone was initially reported in an open-label phase II study. Thirty-seven adult patients with recurrent or unresectable giant cell tumor of bone were enrolled and received monthly denosumab as a 120 mg subcutaneous injection (with additional loading doses on days 8 and 15). Patients continued denosumab until resection, disease progression, or patient desire to discontinue. Tumor response, defined as no radiographic progression up to week 25 or ≥ 90% elimination of giant cells from a pathologic specimen, was seen in 86% of patients. Treatment-related adverse events were limited. Of note, all patients in whom an on-study biopsy was performed (n = 20) exhibited a decrease of ≥ 90% giant cells with a reduction in tumor stromal cells. A recently published, multicenter, open-label, phase II study enrolled 532 subjects. The primary endpoint was safety. The most common grade 3 or more adverse events included hypophosphatemia, osteonecrosis of the jaw, extremity pain, and anemia. The majority of patients (approximately 80%) received clinical benefit, defined as improvements in pain, mobility, or function. In addition, a majority of patients had improved or stable radiographic findings.

Correct Answer: C

Case Study 3

A 54-year-old male is diagnosed with a chordoma of the sacrum involving S4–5. The patient is currently asymptomatic Staging studies reveal no evidence of metastatic disease. Surgical resection alone is recommended as the primary treatment.

3) For patients presenting with localized chordoma, are there any factors that affect morbidity and survival?

Expert Perspective: Yes. Chordomas are malignant neoplasms of purported notochordal origin that most commonly arise in the sacrum. They are typically very large by the time of diagnosis, rendering surgical resection difficult. Because conventional cytotoxic chemotherapy and radiation therapy have not been proven as effective treatment modalities, surgical resection remains the mainstay of treatment. Factors that contribute to improved local control and survival were evaluated in a large series of patients undergoing resection for sacral chordomas between 1990 and 2005. Having undergone a prior resection ($P = 0.046$) and having a high-grade tumor ($P = 0.05$) were associated with lower disease-free survival. Local recurrence ($P = 0.0001$) and metastasis ($P = 0.0001$) were associated with lower disease-free survival. Local recurrence, in turn, was more likely to occur for patients who had undergone a prior resection ($P = 0.0001$) or who underwent an intralesional resection ($P = 0.0001$). This underscores the need for a wide, margin-negative excision during the index procedure.

The issue of surgical margins was also identified as being critically important by investigators at the Rizzoli Institute. An investigation of 53 patients treated surgically for sacral chordomas found that patients with marginal or intralesional resections experienced local recurrence 63–67% of the time. Patients with wide margins or wide-contaminated margins (meaning that the tumor or its pseudocapsule was exposed intraoperatively, but further tissue was removed to achieve wide margins) were significantly less likely to experience local recurrence (22–33% of the time). Although conventional external beam radiation therapy may not have a pivotal role in treatment of this condition, it has been shown that patients with a positive margin do not have increased risk of local recurrence or death if they are treated with adjuvant radiation therapy. As a result, we recommend careful operative planning that permits wide excision of sacral chordomas at the index operation. This planning should consider the need for bowel and/or urinary diversion if the level of resection required to achieve a negative margin will interfere with sphincteric function. Patients in whom a negative margin is not achieved should undergo additional resection or receive adjuvant radiation therapy.

It is important to note that the location of sacral chordomas affects whether or not surgery is recommended as the primary treatment. As resection extends into S3 and S2, the result will be a permanent loss of bowel, bladder, and sexual function. For this reason, proton beam therapy can be considered an alternative to resection for local control of sacral chordomas, which will result in unacceptable morbidity to the patient. A study of 33 patients with sacral chordoma treated with definitive proton beam therapy found them to have disease-free survival and OS of 82% and 93%, respectively, with a median follow-up of over three years.

Case Study 4

A 61-year-old female presents with a five-month history of worsening groin and pelvic pain with weight bearing. Radiographs and an MRI reveal a 14 cm mass arising from the right acetabulum. Biopsy reveals a diagnosis of conventional chondrosarcoma. Internal hemipelvectomy with preservation of the ipsilateral lower extremity is recommended.

4) **Which of the following reconstructive options is reasonable to consider in association with hemipelvectomy?**
   A) Reconstruction using a saddle prosthesis.
   B) Reconstruction using a custom periacetabular endoprosthesis.
   C) Resection alone without reconstruction ("flail hip").
   D) All of the above.
   E) None of the above.

Expert Perspective: Chondrosarcomas are the second most common tumor of the bone and usually affect patients older than 60. There is no role for chemotherapy in the management of most chondrosarcomas, which are typically low- to intermediate-grade tumors that resemble cartilage both macroscopically and microscopically and are highly chemotherapy-resistant with the exceptions of dedifferentiated and mesenchymal chondrosarcoma. Of all tumors in or near the pelvis, those involving the acetabulum present the greatest challenge to the reconstructive surgeon. Resections involving the acetabulum, known as type II resections, disrupt the axis of weight transfer from the lower extremity to the axial skeleton. In this situation, resection of the bone does not preclude limb preservation, but it does elicit the question of how best to maximize the patient's postoperative function. The saddle prosthesis, as its name suggests, is shaped like a saddle, and the semilunar geometry articulates in a mobile way with the remnant ilium following resection. It is coupled to the femur by means of a conventional endoprosthetic replacement of the femoral neck and head. It does not require a precise anatomical fit and is therefore available on short notice. Requirements for adequate function are sufficient bone stock in the ilium to support the device and appropriate restoration of length such that the periacetabular muscles are adequately tensioned. Although the overall complication rate is high with this implant (65%), this remains a popular reconstructive option.

A semicustom periacetabular reconstruction endoprosthesis was developed in an attempt to address the high complication rate associated with the saddle prosthesis (i.e. the common occurrences of cephalad migration and instability). The periacetabular reconstruction endoprosthesis consists of a wide iliac component that is transfixed to the remnant ilium by three cross-bolts and cement. Like the saddle, the periacetabular reconstruction employs a standard femoral component and a constrained ball-and-socket joint. The functional outcomes, complication rates, and implant survivorship compare favorably relative to the saddle prosthesis. However, the iliac component of the periacetabular reconstruction requires custom fabrication based on cross-sectional imaging and takes a minimum of six weeks to acquire. In addition, its use in the United States traditionally has required a compassionate use waiver from the US Food and Drug Administration. In the last three years, there has been a relaxation of requirements for a compassionate use waiver if using a truly custom endoprosthesis if the treating clinician documents that no off-the-shelf or semicustom implant will suffice. A variety of companies will assist the surgeon in designing and fabricating a truly custom hemipelvic endoprosthesis, and outcomes have been found to be acceptable, provided that bony ingrowth of the prosthesis into the skeleton is attained.

It is important to consider whether any given patient requires an endoprosthetic reconstruction at all. Many patients do well with a "flail hip"—meaning resection of the acetabulum and preservation of the lower extremity without reconstruction of the joint itself. Although the extremity shortens significantly over time, the resultant leg length discrepancy can be corrected with shoe modification. When considering functional outcomes based on Musculoskeletal Tumour Society Scores (expressed as a percentage), the following has been shown: resection alone ("flail hip") 48–74%, saddle endoprosthesis 51–63%, and periacetabular reconstruction endoprosthesis 67%.

For these reasons, each of the three fundamental options—reconstruction with a saddle, reconstruction with a periacetabular reconstruction, and resection alone—should be under consideration for any patient undergoing a type II pelvic resection. For patients at high risk for prosthetic failure (those undergoing adjuvant radiation therapy, those with a history of infection, etc.), we favor resection alone. For those patients requiring prompt resection and who are good candidates for endoprosthetic reconstruction, we favor a saddle prosthesis. For those patients in whom surgery might be delayed (e.g. a patient receiving neoadjuvant chemotherapy for a chemotherapy sensitive disease), we have had good success with acquisition of a semicustom periacetabular reconstruction endoprosthesis.

Correct Answer: D

Case Study 5

A 20-year-old male is evaluated for unremitting left knee pain. Radiographs and magnetic resonance imaging (MRI) demonstrate a permeative bone-forming lesion in the distal left femoral metaphysis with an impending fracture. An open biopsy confirms high-grade intramedullary osteosarcoma. Staging studies reveal no evidence of metastatic disease.

Although the patient has been told that this condition is typically treated with preoperative chemotherapy, resection, and postoperative chemotherapy, attention is given to his high risk of fracture and the unlikely possibility that limb salvage could succeed following fracture through this lesion (Figure 43.2).

5) **Does neoadjuvant chemotherapy improve resectability of osteosarcoma in the extremities? If not, are there other purported benefits that would prevent immediate resection or reconstruction, with all chemotherapy deferred to the postoperative period?**

Expert Perspective: Although neoadjuvant chemotherapy has long been assumed to improve resectability of osteosarcomas, this effect has not been proven and may be an incorrect assumption. Large osteosarcomas at high risk of fracture may need to be treated with resection first.

Treatment of high-grade osteosarcoma has been repeatedly evaluated in randomized clinical trials, and the standard of care has changed little in recent decades. Purported benefits of this treatment paradigm have included delay to permit fabrication of custom implants, measurement of treatment effect on the primary tumor, and increased resectability of the tumor. Custom implants are now rarely utilized. Although measurement

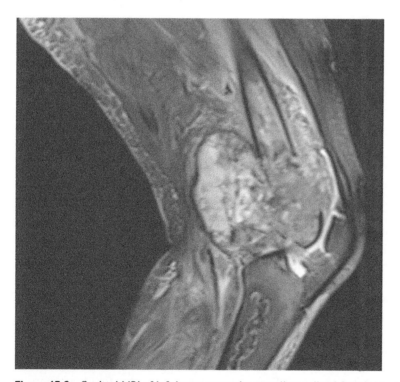

Figure 43.2 Sagittal MRI of left lower extremity revealing a distal femoral lesion with extensive soft tissue component.

of the treatment effect is prognostically valuable, changing chemotherapy protocols in response to a low rate of tumoral necrosis have shown little effect on survival. The final benefit—improved resectability of tumors due to the effect of chemotherapy—has been assumed but not demonstrated.

Recently, the perception that neoadjuvant chemotherapy renders resection of osteosarcoma easier and safer has been investigated. Twenty-four consecutive patients with distal femoral osteosarcoma with MRIs obtained before and after neoadjuvant chemotherapy were scrutinized with regard to operative planning. Four musculoskeletal oncologic surgeons and two musculoskeletal radiologists reviewed blinded and randomly ordered MRIs with regard to surgically critical anatomic details. Surgeons' expectations that chemotherapy would result in increased resectability were exposed by the fact that they believed scans in which more ablative operations were planned to be pre-chemotherapy scans. This expectation was correct only 53% of the time. In addition to this, more amputations (rather than fewer) were planned on the basis of MRIs acquired following neoadjuvant chemotherapy. We continue to keep the traditional treatment order (neoadjuvant chemotherapy, resection, and additional adjuvant chemotherapy) as our default plan. However, we acknowledge that there is no reason to delay surgery in the hopes that neoadjuvant chemotherapy will improve resectability of a large tumor. In fact, if limb salvage is threatened due to either critical tumor size or impending fracture, we recommend proceeding with prompt resection and completing all adjuvant chemotherapy postoperatively.

Case Study 6

A 15-year-old female is diagnosed with localized Ewing sarcoma of the right ilium.

6) Is it true that studies have consistently shown that pelvic Ewing sarcoma should be treated preferentially with surgery over radiation therapy for definitive local control?

Expert Perspective: Multimodality therapy with surgery, chemotherapy, and radiation is the standard of care for "Ewing sarcoma family of tumors" and results in rates of cure of greater than 50% in patients presenting with localized disease. Multi-agent chemotherapy has played a critical role in improving patient outcomes. Data have been conflicting, however, in identifying the most appropriate modality for definitive local control of pelvic Ewing sarcoma. A large institutional series from the Rizzoli Institute evaluated the role of surgery and radiation for local control of pelvic Ewing sarcoma in 129 patients. Improved local control (83% vs 67%) was observed in those patients who received surgery, with or without radiation therapy, as part of definitive local treatment as compared to radiation therapy alone. In addition, five-year event-free survival was also improved in those who received surgery (74% vs 30%; $P = 0.036$) compared with radiation therapy alone. The retrospective nature of the study, however, is a significant limitation. Furthermore, patients who received radiation therapy alone were more likely to have had larger tumor volumes at diagnosis and/or subsequent progression on chemotherapy, factors portending a poor prognosis.

An analysis of 75 patients with pelvic Ewing sarcoma treated on the Children's Oncology Group INT-0091 trial showed no difference in local control or event-free survival when comparing patients who received surgery, radiotherapy, or the combination for local control. The study, which randomized patients to two different chemotherapy regimens, did show an 11% improvement in local control for the use of a five-drug regimen (VDC–IE) compared with a standard three-drug regimen (VDC; also see Question 1).

Overall, the data emphasize the importance of aggressive multiagent chemotherapy to provide the best local control of pelvic primaries regardless of local treatment choice. With five-drug therapy, it is possible that the specific local treatment modality employed is less important. If a tumor is readily resectable with a functional reconstruction, then surgery would be the preferred modality for definitive local control. This avoids the risk of malignancy induction and possible infertility associated with radiotherapy. For those tumors where there is still a significant soft tissue mass after induction chemotherapy, and where it is felt that resolution of the residual mass would result in a margin-negative and functional resection, then radiotherapy may be employed followed by surgery. If the effect of surgery would be such that there would be gross physical dysfunction or that negative surgical margins are unattainable, then definitive radiotherapy is recommended.

Case Study 7

A healthy 60-year-old male is diagnosed with an unresectable base-of-skull conventional chondrosarcoma.

7) Which of the following are acceptable local treatment modalities?
   A) Proton therapy.
   B) Radiosurgery.
   C) Carbon ion therapy.
   D) All the above.
   E) None of the above.

Expert Perspective: Standard therapy for conventional chondrosarcoma consists of gross total resection. Tumors in the hip and pelvis can be treated with surgery with acceptable survival and reasonable morbidity. In locations such as the base of skull, however, tumors are often only partially resectable or deemed unresectable. In this scenario, radiotherapy is recommended. Even in the situation of a gross total resection, the risk of local recurrence is high, and adjuvant radiotherapy should be considered.

Historically, chondrosarcomas were considered as radioresistant. However, it is now known that doses > 70 Gy are needed to demonstrate local control of these malignancies. Conventionally delivered radiotherapy in the brain is limited to approximately 60 Gy due to the risk of damage to surrounding normal tissues such as brain and cranial nerves.

The radiotherapy modality with the longest and largest experience for treating base-of-skull lesions is proton therapy. Protons have a defined path length with rapid dose drop-off. This relatively spares the normal tissues downstream of the tumor. The largest single institution experience is from the Massachusetts General Hospital. With over 200 patients in their cohort, the local control rate at 10 years was 94%. Approximately 20% of these patients underwent only biopsy, and the majority of the remainder had a subtotal resection. The complication rate is reported as acceptable but includes a risk of blindness and other severe neurologic morbidity. Other institutions in the United States and Europe have replicated these results. Even though the number of proton therapy machines is rapidly expanding in the United States, the experience of a given center in surgery (if applicable) and in designing and executing these complex proton radiotherapy plans must be considered.

Heavy (carbon) ion therapy is currently available only in Europe and Asia. The advantage of heavy ions is similar to that of protons in the lack of exit radiation dose, and additionally in their increased biological effectiveness in treating malignancy. The number of chondrosarcoma patients treated with this promising modality is low when compared to proton therapy. The local control rate, however, appears similar to that of proton therapy. Currently, enrollment in protocols to evaluate maintaining efficacy while decreasing the risk of severe morbidity is encouraged. A randomized phase III study of carbon ion therapy versus proton therapy is ongoing in patients with low- to intermediate-grade chondrosarcoma.

Photon therapy is used to deliver most of the radiotherapy worldwide. Modern methods of treatment planning and delivery such as intensity-modulated radiotherapy (IMRT) and stereotactic radiosurgery and radiotherapy have allowed dose escalation in many sites. Recently, investigators have revisited the use of photons to treat chondrosarcoma. Doses more than 60 Gy have been delivered. In the handful of patients treated, the local control and toxicity seems to be acceptable.

In conclusion, while all options are considered acceptable local treatment options, proton therapy at an experienced center remains the gold standard for treatment of base-of-skull chondrosarcoma. Heavy ion therapy and highly conformal photon therapy show promising results, but enrollment in clinical trials to better evaluate these modalities is encouraged.

Correct Answer: A

Case Study 8

A 28-year-old female is diagnosed with a high-grade intramedullary osteosarcoma of the left distal femur. Staging studies reveal no evidence of distant metastatic disease. She receives two cycles of induction chemotherapy with methotrexate, adriamycin, cisplatin chemotherapy. Primary resection reveals a margin negative resection with evidence of 50% necrosis (<90% necrosis defined as poor responder). She is deemed to have had a poor response to chemotherapy.

8) Which of the following would be the most appropriate course of action in poor responder?
   A) Consider postoperative radiation therapy.
   B) Intensify postoperative chemotherapy to include ifosfamide/etoposide in combination with methotrexate, adriamycin, and cisplatin.
   C) Continue methotrexate, adriamycin, and cisplatin chemotherapy alone.
   D) Continue methotrexate, adriamycin, and cisplatin chemotherapy with zoledronate.
   E) Switch to an alternative systemic therapy (i.e. gemcitabine/docetaxel).

Expert Perspective: The EURAMOS-1 study was designed, in part, to investigate the role of chemotherapy intensification in patients with high-grade osteosarcoma who experienced a poor response to preoperative two cycles of methotrexate, adriamycin, and cisplatin chemotherapy. The study was a randomized, open-label, phase III study, in which patients with poor response to preoperative chemotherapy were randomized (1:1) to continuing methotrexate, adriamycin, and cisplatin chemotherapy alone or intensifying chemotherapy with the addition of ifosfamide/etoposide to methotrexate, adriamycin, and cisplatin (MAP + IE = MAPIE). Among the 618 patients enrolled who were deemed to be poor responders and randomized, the event-free survival did not differ between groups. In addition, MAPIE was associated with increased non-hematologic toxicity compared with methotrexate, adriamycin, cisplatin. As a result, current data does not support chemotherapy intensification for poor responders to methotrexate, adriamycin, and cisplatin chemotherapy. For this patient, the recommendation would be to continue methotrexate, adriamycin, and cisplatin chemotherapy. Given the margin negative resection and relative radioresistant nature of osteosarcoma, postoperative radiation therapy would not be routinely recommended. The addition of zoledronate to combination chemotherapy did not improve the event-free survival or OS rates in patients with localized (or metastatic osteosarcoma) in a randomized, open-label, phase III trial. Finally, switching to an alternative systemic therapy would not be appropriate in the absence of clear disease progression.

Correct Answer: C

Recommended Readings

Aibe, N., Demizu, Y., Sulaiman, N.S. et al. (2018). Outcomes of patients with primary sacral chordoma treated with definitive proton beam therapy. *Int J Radiat Oncol Biol Phys* 100 (4): 972–929.

Chawla, S., Blay, J.Y., Rutkowski, P. et al. (2019). Denosumab in patients with giant-cell tumour of bone: A multicentre, open-label, phase 2 study. *Lancet Oncol* 20 (12): 1719–1729.

Grier, H.E., Krailo, M.D., Tarbell, N.J. et al. (2003). Addition of ifosfamide and etoposide to standard chemotherapy for Ewing's sarcoma and primitive neuroectodermal tumor of bone. *N Engl J Med* 348 (8): 694–701.

Lu, E., Ryan, C.W., Bassale, S. et al. (2020). Feasibility of treating adults with Ewing or Ewing-like sarcoma with interval-compressed vincristine, doxorubicin, and cyclophosphamide alternating with ifosfamdie and etoposide. *Oncologist* 25 (2): 150–155.

Marina, N.M., Smelan, S., Bielack, S.S. et al. (2016). Comparison of MAPIE versus MAP in patients with a poor response to preoperative chemotherapy for newly diagnosed high-grade osteosarcoma (EURMAOS-1): An open-label, international, randomized controlled trial. *Lancet Oncol* 17 (10): 1396–1408.

National Comprehensive Cancer Network. NCCN guidelines: Bone cancer (version 1.2022). http://www.nccn.org/professionals/physician_gls/pdf/bone.pdf (accessed 3 August 2021).

Ruggieri, P., Angelini, A., Ussia, G. et al. (2010). Surgical margins and local control in resection of sacral chordomas. *Clin Orthop Relat Res* 468 (11): 2939–2947.

Thomas, D., Henshaw, R., Skubitz, K. et al. (2010). Denosumab in patients with giant-cell tumor of bone: An open-label, phase 2 study. *Lancet Oncol* 11 (3): 275–280.

Wang, J., Min, L., Lu, M. et al. (2019 November 27). Three-dimensional-printed custom-made hemipelvic endoprosthesis for primary malignancies involving acetabulu: The design solution and surgical techniques. *J Orthop Surg Res* 14 (1): 389.

Womer, R.B., West, D.C., Krailo, M.D. et al. (2012). Randomized controlled trial of interval-compressed chemotherapy for the treatment of localized Ewing sarcoma: A report from the Children's Oncology Group. *J Clin Oncol* 30 (33): 4148–4154.

44

Soft Tissue Sarcomas

Jeffrey Farma, Krisha Howell, and Margaret von Mehren

Fox Chase Cancer Center, Philadelphia, PA

Introduction

In the United States, soft tissue sarcomas (STS) have an annual incidence of 10,000–15,000 cases, leading to death in over 5,000 patients annually. STS constitute a group of mesenchymal cell tumors that can be classified based on the site of origin, such as extremity or retroperitoneal. They are rare cancers that represent <1% of all solid tumors, but unlike other solid tumors, these malignancies are seen commonly in the pediatric population. The term STS is an umbrella term for more than 70 different subtypes of malignancies that behave differently. Pathologic evaluation requires immunohistochemistry and molecular testing. Regardless of the site, most present as painless, enlarging masses. Suspected sarcomas should be confirmed with a core needle or open biopsy in the planned site of future surgical resection to minimize the risk of seeding. Surgery remains the gold standard for primary STS management when feasible, with consideration of radiation and/or systemic therapy based on location and histology. Due to the rarity of these tumors, it is imperative that they undergo sarcoma multidisciplinary team evaluation. As in many cancers, the ability to remove tumors with negative margins is one the most important prognostic factors relating to survival. Our team emphasizes the importance of upfront biopsy of tumors to determine the optimum multidisciplinary approach of initial therapy to improve outcomes, decrease the chance of local and distant recurrence, and maximize quality of life.

Case Study 1

A 38-year-old social worker noted a slowly growing lump on her right posterior upper arm. Physical exam reveals a 4 cm fatty, firm, mobile lump suggestive of a lipoma.

1) What is the next best management strategy?
   A) Needle biopsy.
   B) Resection.
   C) Incision and drainage.
   D) Obtain an ultrasound or magnetic resonance imaging (MRI) of the right upper arm.
   E) Clinical follow-up in six months.

Expert Perspective: A lipoma is a benign tumor composed of mature adipocytes that represent the most common adipocytic tumor. Imaging studies including ultrasound or MRI demonstrate a homogeneous soft tissue mass that is isodense to the subcutaneous tissue and demonstrates fat saturation. If these radiographic characteristics are confirmed, it can be followed, and biopsy would be considered unnecessary. Generally, if there is a high index of suspicion of a benign lipoma, options include surveillance or resection. Resection should be considered for pain, interval growth of the lesion, an intramuscular lipoma, masses > 5 cm in size, and/or for cosmetic reasons. Angiolipomas closely resemble lipomas, although angiolipomas are usually painful and tender; they are occasionally associated with protease inhibitor therapy in patients with HIV. Atypical lipomatous tumors/well-differentiated liposarcomas are low-grade, locally aggressive, malignant adipocytic tumors that demonstrate prominent fibrous stranding in a fatty tumor on imaging. De-differentiated liposarcomas are tumors that show evidence of a transition, either in the primary or in a recurrence, from atypical lipomatous neoplasms or well-differentiated liposarcoma to a non-lipogenic pleomorphic spindle cell sarcoma, usually of high histological grade. Radiological imaging shows the coexistence of both fatty and nonfatty solid components in the tumor. If features of malignancy are noted on imaging, a biopsy or planned resection should be done to confirm the histology.

Correct Answer: D

Case Study 2

A 60-year-old male business executive is diagnosed with a 7.3 cm high-grade pleomorphic undifferentiated sarcoma of the left distal thigh after an ultrasound-guided core needle biopsy.

2) **Which of the following should be obtained as part of his sarcoma workup?**
   A) MRI of the left thigh and computed tomography (CT) of the chest.
   B) Positron emission tomography (PET)/CT scan.
   C) MRI of the left thigh and bone scan.
   D) MRI of the thigh and MRI of the total spine.

Expert Perspective: Adequate imaging is part of the essential workup for a sarcoma and should provide details about the size of the tumor and proximity to nearby visceral structures and neurovascular landmarks. Chest imaging is imperative for initial staging, especially in high-grade extremity sarcomas, because the lung is the most common site of distant hematogenous spread. In patients with alveolar soft tissue sarcoma or angiosarcoma, central nervous system imaging should be considered. Lymph node metastases are rare in soft tissue sarcoma but can be seen in certain histologies such as small cell sarcomas, rhabdomyosarcomas, clear cell sarcoma, angiosarcoma, and epithelioid sarcomas. Myxoid/round cell liposarcomas, angiosarcomas, leiomyosarcoma, and epithelioid sarcomas can have a propensity for other soft tissue sites, and more comprehensive CT imaging of the abdomen/pelvis should be considered. Myxoid/round cell liposarcomas has increase propensity for bone metastasis. PET-CT may be beneficial in a case-by-case situation.

Correct Answer: A

Case Study 3

A 56-year-old female construction worker had a 4.5 cm tumor removed from her right lateral lower leg, with a positive medial margin adjacent to the bone. The final pathology revealed a high-grade pleomorphic sarcoma, and all other margins were negative. Postop MRI shows surgical changes, and CT chest shows no metastasis.

3) Which of the following statements is correct?
   A) She requires a below-knee amputation.
   B) Considering the tumor size is less than 5 cm, no further therapy is recommended.
   C) She should have a limb-sparing re-resection by a sarcoma surgeon.
   D) She should have adjuvant radiation therapy.

Expert Perspective: Adjuvant radiation therapy should be considered in stage II (T1 [tumor < 5 cm] and G2 or G3) or greater extremity tumors, or those cases unable to achieve an appropriate margin. Adequate margin may be defined as adequate distance between the microscopic tumor cells and resection edge of >1–2 cm or with complete removal of an enclosed organ or fascial plane. Extremity sarcomas may reside near a bone, major blood vessel, or nerve, where functional limb sparing is not feasible with re-resection. However, in the case of microscopic or close margins, the feasibility of re-resection should always be explored prior to delivery of adjuvant radiotherapy. Randomized trials and retrospective analyses support the use of preoperative or postoperative external-beam radiation therapy in appropriately selected patients with STS of extremity. The efficacy of postoperative radiation therapy was demonstrated in a prospective randomized trial comparing limb-sparing surgery with postoperative radiation therapy and limb-sparing surgery alone. Postoperative radiation therapy reduced the 10-year local recurrence rate in patients with high-grade sarcoma (no local recurrences vs 22%) as well as low-grade sarcoma (5% vs 32%). The Canadian Sarcoma group conducted a phase III randomized trial looking at preoperative radiation therapy (50 Gy in 25 fractions) versus postoperative radiation therapy (66 Gy in 33 fractions) in patients with localized primary or recurrent extremity sarcoma and showed that local control and progression-free survival rates were similar for both groups. However, preoperative radiation therapy was associated with a greater incidence of acute wound complications (35% vs 17% for postoperative radiation therapy), and late treatment-related side effects such as fibrosis, edema, and joint stiffness were more common in patients receiving postoperative radiation therapy, most likely due to the higher radiation therapy dose and larger treatment volume. Preoperative radiation therapy is preferred due to these reasons, especially if margins are expected to be close.

Correct Answer: D

Case Study 4

A young engineer in his mid-30s presents with an 11.6 cm soft tissue mass above his right elbow, which he first noted several months ago, and which has since noticeably increased in size. Biopsy is consistent with a monophasic synovial sarcoma with 30 mitoses per 10 high-power field (HPF). Immunohistochemical studies show nuclear reactivity for TLE1, weak reactivity for SMA, and patchy weak to equivocal reactivity for desmin. Fluorescence in situ hybridization (FISH) on interphase nuclei in paraffin-embedded sections reveals a clonal population of cells with rearrangement of the *SYT/SS18* locus (18q11).

4) Out of the following, what is the best recommendation for his treatment?
   A) Neoadjuvant chemotherapy, followed by radiation and then surgery in a multidisciplinary care setting.
   B) An above-elbow amputation.
   C) Limb-sparing surgery followed by adjuvant chemotherapy.
   D) Limb-sparing surgery followed by radiation therapy.

Expert Perspective: Limb-sparing surgery with or without radiation is recommended for most patients with soft tissue sarcoma of extremities to achieve local tumor control with minimal morbidity. Preoperative RT and/or neoadjuvant chemotherapy are used in certain situations to augment surgery to achieve a margin-negative resection. The benefit of adjuvant chemotherapy continues to be debated because of the challenge of performing an adequately powered randomized controlled study in a rare tumor that has tremendous heterogeneity in chemo-responsiveness of the various sarcoma subtypes. To address the problem of inadequately powered adjuvant sarcoma studies showing nonsignificant benefit in survival outcomes, the Sarcoma Meta-analysis Collaboration (SMAC) performed a meta-analysis of 14 studies, initially published in 1997. Eight of these studies used varying combinations of doxorubicin, and six studies used single-agent doxorubicin. The 10-year disease-free survival was improved (45 to 55%; $P = 0.0001$), but 10-year overall survival (OS) did not reach significance (50 to 54%; $P = 0.12$). Patients with extremity tumors appeared to have the clearest survival benefit with chemotherapy based on a subgroup analysis. An update of the SMAC analysis was published in 2008 and included four additional randomized trials. The pooled data from a total of 1,953 patients demonstrated a statistically significant improvement in local and distant recurrence with adjuvant chemotherapy. There was a statistically significant survival benefit for doxorubicin combined with ifosfamide (OR 0.56; 95% CI 0.36–0.85; $P = 0.01$) but not for doxorubicin alone (OR of 0.84; 95% CI: 0.68–1.03; $P = 0.09$). This study did not include the largest adjuvant study by the European Organization for Research and Treatment of Cancer Soft Tissue and Bone Sarcoma Group (EORTC) evaluating five cycles of adjuvant doxorubicin (75 mg/m^2) and ifosfamide (5 gm/m^2) versus observation in resected grade 2 and 3 extremity tumors. Survival in the observation arm was better than expected, leading to an interim analysis of futility. The dose of ifosfamide used in the trial was lower than what is routinely used in combination therapy for advanced disease. A separate update of the SMAC meta-analysis including this EORTC study, with a total of 2,170 patients, showed a benefit of adjuvant chemotherapy for disease-free survival and OS after 5 years, but only a nonsignificant trend toward improved survival after 10 years (OR 0.87; $P = 0.12$).

Based on retrospective analyses, the benefit of adjuvant chemotherapy appears to be much higher in patients with high-grade ≥ 5 cm tumors with certain chemosensitive histologies (i.e. myxoid or round cell liposarcomas and synovial sarcomas). Neoadjuvant chemotherapy in this setting has the advantage of response assessment to allow for a more personalized risk–benefit approach while downsizing the tumor to improve chances of

Introduction

margin-negative surgery. Multidisciplinary care in a center with expertise in sarcoma is preferred because it leads to improved outcomes.

Correct Answer: A

Case Study 5

A 42-year-old businessman in otherwise good health noted an enlarging mass on the medial lateral of his left thigh. Ultrasound revealed a 5.3 cm superficial mass (Figure 44.1). He underwent a resection by his local surgeon, and pathology revealed an intermediate grade myxoid liposarcoma with tumor extending to the resection margin. Chest X-ray shows no abnormality. MRI of the thigh shows some persistent soft tissue enhancement next to the surgical bed.

5) Which of the following would be the best option?
   A) Watchful waiting with a three-month follow-up in clinic.
   B) Adjuvant radiation therapy alone.
   C) Re-resection to obtain negative margins, and then consider postoperative radiation.
   D) Adjuvant chemotherapy with a doxorubicin-based combination.

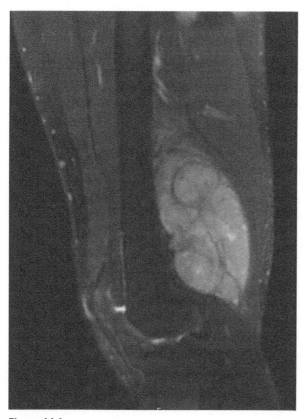

Figure 44.1

Expert Perspective: Microscopically positive surgical margins are an important adverse prognostic factor with a higher rate of local recurrence and lower rate of disease-free survival, especially in patients with extremity sarcomas. Both the surgeon and the pathologist should appropriately orientate and document surgical margins in evaluating a resected specimen. Surgical re-resection to obtain negative margins should strongly be considered if resection margins are positive on final pathology with residual disease on imaging (unless on bone, nerve, or major blood vessels). Ideally goal is to achieve an R0/R1 resection, and R2 resection should be considered for re-resection. Referral for postoperative radiation therapy should be made for high-risk patients or if the margin status is close or unclear.

Another option that can be considered for patients presenting after a total but oncologically inadequate resection of their STS is preoperative radiation followed by the planned re-resection to achieve adequate margins. A retrospective institutional review from MD Anderson Cancer Center reviewing the sequencing of radiotherapy when re-resection was planned demonstrated no evidence that the sequence influenced local control, metastatic control, disease-free survival, or disease-specific survival. Myxoid liposarcoma has been reported to be more radiosensitive then other STS histologies. In the DOREMY trial, an extensive pathological treatment response was observed in 91% of patients, meeting the primary end point, when the preoperative dose was decreased from 50 to 30 Gy.

Correct Answer: C

Case Study 6

A 39-year-old female presented with abnormal uterine bleeding. She was found to have uterine fibroids. Her gynecologist prescribed oral contraceptives. Subsequently she presented with prolonged heavy bleeding for 10 days and underwent a myomectomy that demonstrated a low-grade endometrial stromal tumor; the myomectomy specimen was removed in pieces. She then underwent a hysterectomy and bilateral salpingo-oopherectomy; no additional disease was identified. Staging studies are negative for evidence of metastatic disease. She presents for an opinion regarding additional therapy.

6) Out of the following options, what is the most appropriate?
   A) Expectant observation with imaging every three to four months.
   B) Bilateral oophorectomies.
   C) Start gemcitabine and docetaxel for four to six cycles.
   D) Start hormonal therapy.

Expert Perspective: Endometrial stromal sarcomas present either as low-grade or high-grade tumors. High-grade tumors are aggressive and managed with cytotoxic chemotherapy. Low-grade tumors are characterized by expression of estrogen and progesterone receptors.

Standard surgical resection for low-grade endometrial stromal sarcomas should include bilateral salpingo-oophorectomy, allowing for pathologic evaluation of the ovaries. In addition, a variety of retrospective series have identified a higher recurrence rate for patients whose ovaries are not resected. There are no prospective trials of the use of hormonal agents in patients following standard surgical resection. In the recurrent disease setting, aromatase inhibitors have become the preferred therapeutic approach.

Correct Answer: A

Case Study 7

A 45-year-old interior designer with a history of stage I right breast carcinoma (T1c-N0M0) six years ago now has a superficial mass in the right breast that has become more prominent over the past month, measuring around 2.5 cm, with two similar-appearing erythematous-violaceous satellite nodules on exam (Figure 44.2). She was treated with a mastectomy, reconstruction, and four cycles of TAC chemotherapy (docetaxel, doxorubicin, and cyclophosphamide) and adjuvant radiation therapy for her breast cancer. Biopsy of the main mass is consistent with an angiosarcoma. A CT of the chest, abdomen, and pelvis shows no evidence of metastasis.

7) Her treatment recommendations are likely to include which of the following?
A) Resection.
B) Resection followed by chemotherapy and radiation.
C) Systemic chemotherapy until maximal response or tolerance, followed by surgery.
D) A repeat lumpectomy followed by radiation therapy.

Expert Perspective: This patient has a radiation-induced sarcoma, which is a clinical definition based on an antecedent history of radiation exposure before the development of the sarcoma, occurrence of the sarcoma in or near the field of radiation, and pathologic confirmation of sarcoma that is histologically unique from the primary cancer. It usually presents at least three years after radiation therapy exposure, but there have been reports of these tumors presenting earlier. The most common histologic subtypes for radiation-induced sarcoma are malignant fibrous histiocytoma (undifferentiated pleomorphic sarcoma) and osteosarcoma, although other histologies (e.g. angiosarcoma, rhabdomyosarcoma, and malignant peripheral nerve sheath tumor) can occur. The prognosis for radiation-induced sarcoma is significantly worse compared with sporadic STS of the same histology. The therapy is dictated by the risk of distant metastases. High-grade tumors that are larger than 5 cm or have other high-risk features (e.g. satellite nodules or aggressive histology, like angiosarcoma) should be treated with primary chemotherapy followed by

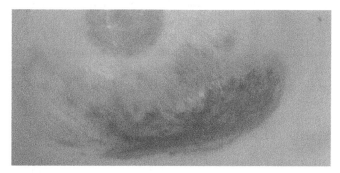

Figure 44.2

a margin-negative surgical excision of the residual disease; this frequently will include a mastectomy if they had breast conservation. Prior to surgical planning, mapping punch biopsies can be helpful to plan resection. Low-grade tumors and high-grade tumors 5 cm or smaller should be treated with a margin-negative surgical excision, and systemic chemotherapy should be considered when a negative margin is difficult.

Correct Answer: C

Case Study 8

An otherwise healthy 47-year-old female with a history of a 17 cm myxoid round cell liposarcoma of the left thigh status post complete resection and adjuvant radiation therapy presents for ongoing follow-up three years following her initial resection. On examination, she has a new palpable mass in the left breast. She is referred for biopsy that demonstrated recurrent liposarcoma. Restaging studies demonstrates an additional metastasis in the lumbar spine.

8) Which of the following therapies would be the most appropriate in the front line?
   A) Doxorubicin-based therapy.
   B) Dacarbazine.
   C) Pazopanib.
   D) Gemcitabine and docetaxel.
   E) Refer the patient for a phase I clinical trial.

Expert Perspective: Myxoid round cell liposarcoma tends to occur in the pediatric and young adult population and is characterized by a chromosomal translocation, most frequently t(12:16) (*FUS-DDIT3*) or less commonly t(12:22) (*EWSR1-DDIT3*), that is thought to play a role in tumor initiation. Most patients present with localized disease and undergo successful local therapy for their primary tumor, and 30–50% of these patients will develop metastasis and ultimately succumb to their disease. Metastases can occur in the lung, bone, and unusual soft tissue locations such that surveillance imaging should include MRI of the entire spine. The use of adjuvant or neoadjuvant chemotherapy and/or radiation therapy has improved outcomes for these patients.

Myxoid round cell liposarcoma is known for its relative sensitivity to radiotherapy and certain chemotherapeutic agents, with an approximately 50% response rate with doxorubicin and ifosfamide. The new antitumor compound trabectedin is also very effective in inducing durable responses in myxoid round cell liposarcoma patients. Dacarbazine and gemcitabine-docetaxel combination therapy are reasonable salvage options. Fixed-dose-rate gemcitabine plus docetaxel yielded higher response rates, progression-free survival, and OS compared with fixed-dose-rate, single-agent gemcitabine in a randomized trial for patients with soft tissue sarcoma who had received up to three prior regimens. The best response for the small number of myxoid round cell liposarcoma patients on this trial was stable disease. Considering this patient has not seen standard chemotherapy, a phase I trial would not be appropriate.

Correct Answer: A

Case Study 9

A 45-year-old male presents to his primary care physician with complaints of right-sided abdominal pain. Imaging of the abdomen demonstrated liver and bone metastases, as well as a mass involving the inferior vena cava. Biopsy of one of the liver metastases was performed demonstrating metastatic high-grade leiomyosarcoma.

9) What is the next best step?
   A) Referral for palliative radiation therapy.
   B) Systemic chemotherapy.
   C) Denosumab.
   D) Both B and C.

Expert Perspective: Leiomyosarcomas arise from smooth muscle cells or their precursors. Thus, they can arise from blood vessels, including the vasculature in the abdomen and pelvis. Patients presenting with primary disease of the IVC or vessels feeding the IVC will have metastases to the liver and bone more commonly than most other sarcomas where lung metastases are most common.

This patient has stage IV disease, and therefore palliative treatment including systemic chemotherapy and denosumab or other agents to decrease the risk of bone fractures is appropriate. The choice of chemotherapy should take into consideration the patient's overall status and goals of care. Treatment with a doxorubicin-based regimen or gemcitabine and docetaxel are appropriate first-line choices. A recent retrospective propensity score analysis of doxorubicin-based regimens in the treatment of leiomyosarcoma by the EORTC showed favorable overall response rate and progression-free survival with doxorubicin and dacarbazine compared with doxorubicin alone or in combination with ifosfamide.

Correct Answer: D

Case Study 10

A 28-year-old presented with lower back pain with radiation down the posterior left leg. On imaging, she was found to have a 10.5 cm expansile mass in the left psoas muscle and invading the left lateral spinal canal. Staging studies demonstrated multiple lung lesions consistent with metastases. Biopsy demonstrated alveolar soft part sarcoma.

10) Which of the following statements is accurate?
   A) Alveolar soft part sarcomas are chemotherapy sensitive, and she should be started on doxorubicin-based therapy.
   B) Alveolar soft part sarcomas do not respond to molecularly targeted therapies.
   C) Alveolar soft part sarcomas have demonstrated benefit to immunotherapy.
   D) Survival rate is poor, with one-year survival less than 10% with metastatic disease.

Expert Perspective: Alveolar soft part sarcoma is a histologically distinct, rare soft tissue sarcoma that usually presents in young patients. It has a relatively indolent course with a propensity for metastases to lung, bone, and brain; over half of patients will have metastatic disease at presentation. It is characterized by the t(X:17) (p11:25) translocation, whose fusion protein has been shown to drive *MET* signaling. The five-year survival in the reported case series at diagnosis is greater than 60%, and in patients with metastatic disease, it is around 20%. At the current time, surgery is the standard treatment, and there are no convincing data in support of conventional chemotherapy or radiation therapy. Molecularly targeted therapies (*MET* inhibitor, cediranib; *VEGFR*, sunitnib and pazopanib) have demonstrated objective responses as well as prolonged stable disease. There is also clinical trial data demonstrating the benefit of PD-1 inhibitors alone or in combination with tyrosine kinase inhibitor (TKIs). Based on the report from phase II ML39345 study, atezolizumab was approved by FDA for patients with selected unresectable or metastatic alveolar soft part sarcoma.

Correct Answer: C

Case Study 11

A 60-year-old retired accountant recently underwent resection of a 10.2 cm recurrent de-differentiated liposarcoma arising in the right retroperitoneum and pelvis (Figure 44.4). He has a history of a 19 cm retroperitoneal well-differentiated/dedifferentiated liposarcoma resected approximately four years ago with left nephrectomy. Postoperative CT scan of the abdomen and pelvis shows fat-containing areas around the surgical bed but no evidence of any residual dedifferentiated tumor.

11) What is the. next best step in his management?
   A) Follow-up imaging with CT chest/abdomen and pelvis at three-month intervals.
   B) Adjuvant chemotherapy for six cycles.
   C) Adjuvant radiation therapy.
   D) No further follow-up required.

Expert Perspective: Surgery is the mainstay of treatment for localized retroperitoneal soft tissue sarcoma. Well-differentiated and dedifferentiated liposarcomas represent the most common STS in the retroperitoneum. On a molecular level, both well-differentiated and dedifferentiated liposarcomas are characterized by amplification of chromosome 12q13–15, which includes the *MDM2* and *CDK4* genes and can be used for confirming

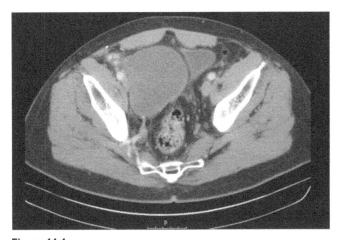

Figure 44.4

the histology. Although the clonal relationship between well-differentiated and dedifferentiated liposarcomas remains unclear, it is thought that tumor cells progressively accumulate genetic lesions as they transition to a less differentiated, nonlipogenic state. Regarding clinical outcome, the presence of de-differentiated histology is clearly associated with worse overall and recurrence-free survival and the potential for distant metastasis (e.g. to the lung); however, the frequency of metastasis is only 10–15%. For most patients with retroperitoneal, well-differentiated, and dedifferentiated liposarcomas, the burden of disease is loco-regional. Responses to chemotherapy and radiation are poor in this liposarcoma subtype, and hence adjuvant therapy is not routinely recommended. We would recommend close surveillance with imaging every three months.

Correct Answer: A

Case Study 12

A 50-year-old male presented with a one-to-two-year history of bright red per rectum, which he attributed to hemorrhoids. Flexible sigmoidoscopy examination showed a rectal mass. A transanal resection was performed and demonstrated rectal gastrointestinal stromal tumors (GISTs) with 10 mitoses/50 hpf. MRI pelvis demonstrated residual gastrointestinal stromal tumor measuring 4.2 × 4.3 × 4.2 cm, involving the proximal anal sphincter, and 3.2 cm from anal verge.

12) What would you do next?
    A) Surgery followed by adjuvant imatinib.
    B) Neoadjuvant therapy with 400 mg imatinib once daily.
    C) Neoadjuvant therapy with 400 mg of imatinib twice daily.
    D) Neoadjuvant radiation therapy.

Expert Perspective: GISTs are the most common type of gastrointestinal mesenchymal tumors, occurring throughout the GI tract but most commonly arising in the stomach or small bowel. These tumors are typically driven by mutations in the genes for *KIT* or *platelet-derived growth factor alpha (PDGFRA)* receptor protein tyrosine kinases. *KIT* (CD117) and *DOG-1* staining are present in approximately 95% of tumors. About 80–88% of these tumors have mutations in the *KIT* proto-oncogene, leading to constitutive activation of the receptor. Approximately 5% of GISTs have activating mutations in *platelet-derived growth factor alpha (PDGFRA)*.

Standard of care therapy for primary therapy is surgery. However, in this patient, resection would require an abdominal perineal resection. In situations such as this, neoadjuvant therapy is appropriate to attempt to down stage the tumor. This approach has been shown to be safe and effective. Imatinib 400 mg is the recommended dosage unless the tumor demonstrates an imatinib insensitive mutation. *KIT* exon 9 mutations in the advanced disease setting have a longer progression-free survival on higher dose imatinib, 400 mg twice a day. If the patient had a known exon 9 mutation, it would be reasonable to consider higher dose imatinib therapy, although this had not been tested prospectively.

There is no defined length of neoadjuvant therapy. Imaging to monitor response as a minimum of every three months is appropriate. Therapy should continue until response has plateaued, or at a time when surgery is feasible without excess morbidity. Collaboration with surgical oncology is important for optimal outcomes.

If surgery is accomplished, based upon the primary biopsy, the patient would be a candidate for adjuvant therapy. Risk of recurrence for patients with large (>5 cm) higher-risk GISTs is as high as 85–90%. Tumor size, mitotic index, tumor rupture, and location of the primary tumor (gastric more favorable than others) are factors impacting recurrence rates and disease-specific survival based on retrospective studies. It is important to note that the resection specimen following neoadjuvant therapy cannot be used to assess risk of recurrence as the tumor will likely demonstrate the effects of therapy.

Adjuvant therapy is recommended for at least three years based upon the Scandinavian Sarcoma Group study, SSGXVIII. This trial evaluated one year versus three years of adjuvant treatment in patients with a high risk of recurrence (tumor greater than 5 cm in size with a high mitotic rate [>5 mitoses/50 HPF] or a risk of recurrence of greater than 50%) after surgery. After 54 months of follow-up, the recurrence-free survival and OS rates were significantly higher in the 3-year group compared with those receiving one year of imatinib (five-year RFS: 65.6% vs 47.9%; HR: 0.46; 95% CI: 0.32–0.65; $P < 0.0001$; and five-year OS: 92.0% vs 81.7%; HR: 0.45; 95% CI: 0.22–0.89; $P = 0.019$). Based on the results of the SSGXVIII trial, the US Food and Drug Administration approved the use of three years of imatinib as adjuvant therapy for patients following the complete gross resection of *KIT*-positive GIST for intermediate- to high-risk patients. In patients with neoadjuvant therapy, we would recommend a total of at least three years of therapy including the time on neoadjuvant therapy.

Correct Answer: B

Case Study 13

A 69-year-old male was diagnosed with a GIST arising in the stomach with biopsy-proven liver metastasis. The gastric tumor and liver lesion are considered resectable. The tumor was sequenced and found to have a *PDGFRA D842V* mutation.

13) What would you recommend?
   A) Initiate imatinib therapy at 400 mg daily.
   B) Initiate avapritinib at 300 mg daily.
   C) Refer to a surgical oncologist for resection followed by imatinib in the adjuvant setting.
   D) Refer to a surgical oncologist for resection followed by avapritinib in the adjuvant setting.

Expert Perspective: The patient presents with metastatic disease. Although surgical resection may be feasible, the standard approach to management is systemic therapy. Randomized trials have established the efficacy and tolerability of imatinib at a starting dose of 400 mg once daily for patients with unresectable GIST. The benefit of therapy is correlated to the tumor mutation. Patients with tumors that have mutations in *KIT* exon 11 have the best overall outcome with imatinib treatment once a day. Tumors with *KIT* exon 9 mutations have a superior progression-free survival when treated with imatinib 400 mg twice a day compared with the standard dose of 400 mg daily ($P = 0.0013$). Therefore, in advanced and metastatic disease patients, it is now recommended to start with the higher dose of 400 mg twice daily when treating. Escalating the dose from the low to high over a four- to eight-week period leads to better tolerability than starting at the higher dose.

This patient's tumor has a *PDGFRA D842V* kinase domain mutation. It is resistant to imatinib. The NAVIGATOR trial, a phase I trial of avapritinib in advanced GIST, including patients with *PDGFRA D842V* GIST, demonstrated efficacy. Avapritinib therapy led to an 89% response rate in tumors with the *D842V* mutation. This resulted in FDA approval of the agent for unresectable GIST with *PDGFRA* exon 18 mutations. In general, avapritinib has similar side effects to other *KIT*-targeting TKIs. However, it has been associated with neurocognitive side effects. It is important to educate the patient and their family to monitor for changes in memory, word finding, and/or mood. Interruption of therapy and dose adjustments are recommended to mitigate against these side effects.

The benefit of surgery in patients in advanced GIST on imatinib has been the question of several trials. It has been hypothesized that with surgery, treatment with imatinib can be extended and potentially result in improved OS because tumor cells that have the potential to become resistant to imatinib are removed. Unfortunately, the trials failed to accrue, so there is no prospective data, and no trials have been done with avapritinib in this setting.

Correct Answer: B

Case Study 14

A young female in her early 30s has been experiencing increasing abdominal discomfort, early satiety, and nausea and presents to you for a second opinion. A CT of the abdomen from two months ago shows an infiltrating irregularly shaped mass approximately 11 cm involving the root of the mesentery (Figure 44.5). The biopsy is consistent with desmoid fibromatosis. She has a history of a stage III colon cancer with multiple adenomatous polyps throughout her colon consistent with Familial Adenomatous Polyposis, for which she underwent a total colectomy with ileoanal anastomosis and J-pouch more than a year ago. She completed adjuvant chemotherapy with FOLFOX six months ago. You obtain a follow-up CT that shows an increase in this mesenteric mass by 2 cm.

14) What would you recommend?
　　A) Recommend neoadjuvant systemic therapy.
　　B) Refer to radiation oncology for definitive radiation therapy.
　　C) Refer to surgery immediately.
　　D) Continue close observation.

Expert Perspective: Desmoid tumors, also known as aggressive fibromatoses, are a fibroblastic proliferation of well-circumscribed fibrous tissue that are locally invasive but do not have metastatic potential. They vary in presentation and location, from the abdominal wall of young pregnant females to intra-abdominal mesenteric masses, and to large extremity masses in older individuals. Intra-abdominal desmoids are common in patients with familial adenomatous polyposis such as Gardner's syndrome, may also arise after a surgical intervention such as a colectomy, and can lead to significant morbidity. The Wnt/beta-catenin signaling pathway is thought to be key in the molecular patho-

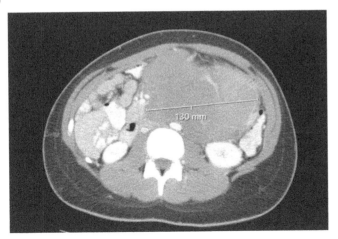

Figure 44.5

genesis of desmoid tumors. Somatic APC mutations as well as activating mutations of the beta-catenin gene are identified in the majority of sporadic desmoids (Chapter 47).

Observation is appropriate and the standard therapy for most patients with desmoid tumors, especially if they are asymptomatic and located at a site where increase in size will not alter the outcome of surgery or lead to functional limitation. Retrospective and prospective observational studies have demonstrated that desmoids can undergo spontaneous regression. For patients with large tumors causing morbidity, pain, or functional limitation, treatment choices should be based on the location of the tumor and potential morbidity of the treatment. Surgery and/or radiotherapy and/or systemic therapy are all reasonable options. Radiation is not generally recommended for retroperitoneal or intra-abdominal desmoid tumors. Because this patient's tumor involves the root of the mesentery and is likely to cause significant morbidity if untreated, systemic therapy options need to be discussed. Surgery can be very challenging in this location, and the tumor would be deemed unresectable if involving or encasing the superior mesenteric artery. Repeat resection or radiation is not offered for positive margins, and we recommend surveillance.

A variety of systemic therapy options, including nonsteroidal anti-inflammatory drugs (sulindac or celecoxib), hormonal or biological agents (tamoxifen, toremifene, or low-dose interferon), cytotoxic agents (methotrexate, vinblastine, and doxorubicin-based regimens), and TKIs (imatinib and sorafenib), have demonstrated activity in patients with advanced or unresectable desmoid tumors. Doxorubicin-based chemotherapy and the combination of methotrexate and vinblastine have shown good efficacy in patients with unresectable or recurrent tumors and are preferred if aggressive therapy is required. TKIs such as imatinib or sorafenib are less toxic options that have also demonstrated good clinical benefit (response or disease stabilization). We frequently consider a neoadjuvant approach for large symptomatic desmoid tumors.

Correct Answer: A

Recommended Readings

Gladdy, R.A., Qin, L.X., Moraco, N. et al. (2010 April 20). Do radiation-associated soft tissue sarcomas have the same prognosis as sporadic soft tissue sarcomas? *J Clin Oncol* 28 (12): 2064–2069.

Hoffman, A., Lazar, A.J., Pollock, R.E. et al. (2011 February). New frontiers in the treatment of liposarcoma, a therapeutically resistant malignant cohort. *Drug Resist Updat* 14 (1): 52–66.

Joensuu, H., Eriksson, M., Sundby Hall, K. et al. (2012). One vs three years of adjuvant imatinib for operable gastrointestinal stromal tumor: A randomized trial. *JAMA* 307 (12): 1265–1272.

Lansu, J., Bovee, J.V.M.G., Braam, P. et al. (2021). *JAMA Oncol* 7 (1): e205865.

Ogura, K., Beppu, Y., Chuman, H. et al. (2012). Alveolar soft part sarcoma: A single-center 26-patient case series and review of the literature. *Sarcoma* 2012: 907179.

Quintini, C., Ward, G., Shatnawei, A. et al. (2012 March). Mortality of intraabdominal desmoid tumors in patients with familial adeno-matous polyposis: A single center review of 154 patients. *Ann Surg* 255 (3): 511–516.

Siegel, R.L., Miller, K.D., Fuchs, H.E. et al. (2021). Cancer Statistics, 2021. *CA Cancer J Clin* 71: 7–33.

Zagars, G.K. and Ballo, M.T. (2003). Sequencing radiotherapy for soft tissue sarcoma when re-resection is planned. *Int J Radiat Onc Biol Phys* 56 (1): 21–27.

Part 9

Hereditary Cancer Syndromes and Genetic Testing

45

Hereditary Cancer Syndromes

Mary B. Daly

Fox Chase Cancer Center, Philadelphia, PA

Introduction

The past 25 years have witnessed the identification of several hereditary cancer syndromes associated with the inheritance of a germline pathogenic variant that predisposes to certain types of cancer. Characteristics of inherited cancers are early age at onset, multiple cancers in an individual, and the same cancers occurring in relatives over several generations. When a hereditary cancer syndrome is suspected, individuals are referred for genetic risk assessment and testing by a team with genetics expertise. The advantages of undergoing genetic testing include a more precise estimate of personal risk, more intense surveillance or risk-reducing surgeries, and benefit to other family members. National organizations have developed guidelines for clinical management of patients shown to have a pathogenic variant. In addition to testing tumor tissues to identify genetic variants that may guide therapy, pathology labs are now adding germline testing to tumor testing to maximize the yield of genetic information.

Case Study 1

You are treating a 53-year-old patient for a stage III uterine cancer. She mentions that her sister was just diagnosed with colon cancer at age 48. In updating her family history, you are struck by the familial pattern of cancer that you see (Figure 45.1).

1) What are the overarching concepts of hereditary cancer syndromes?

Expert Perspective: This pedigree illustrates some of the features of hereditary cancer syndromes: multiple cases of cancer in successive generations and cancers occurring at an earlier age than sporadic cancers. This pattern is suggestive of Lynch syndrome, named after Dr. Henry Lynch, who described this syndrome more than 50 years ago. Lynch syndrome is one of the hereditary cancer syndromes associated with the inheritance of a germline pathogenic variant that predisposes to certain types of cancer. Cancers seen in Lynch syndrome include colon, uterine, small bowel, gastric, ovarian, renal urinary tract, liver, and pancreatic. The genes that are responsible for Lynch syndrome, *MLH1*, *MSH2*, *MSH6*, *PMS2*, and *EPCAM*, contribute to the repair of DNA mismatch breaks. Pathogenic

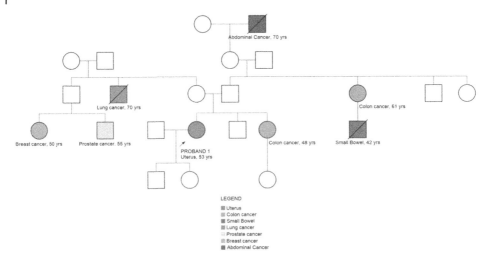

Figure 45.1 Pedigree 1.

variants in these genes disrupt the repair process and leave cells vulnerable to instability and uncontrolled growth. These changes are often illustrated by instability in the microsatellite (short, repeated sequences of DNA) in the cancer cells and have resulted in the ability to test tumors from Lynch syndrome patients for microsatellite instability (MSI) as a first step in diagnosing the syndrome. The diagnosis of Lynch syndrome, like many of the other hereditary cancer syndromes, leads to syndrome-specific screening and prevention recommendations (Chapter 47).

Most cancer-related pathogenic variants are inherited in an autosomal dominant pattern, which means the affected individual has inherited one copy of the pathogenic variant, whereas the other copy is normal. Each child of a person with a pathogenic variant has a 50% chance of inheriting it. There are some hereditary cancer syndromes inherited in an autosomal recessive condition, in which an individual has to carry two copies of an altered gene, one from each parent, to manifest the disease. When both parents are carriers of a pathogenic variant in an autosomal recessive condition, they typically do not express the trait, but there is a 25% risk of children inheriting both copies. Although ultimately all cancers are thought to be due to a lifetime accumulation of pathogenic variants in genes that regulate cellular activity, it appears that approximately 10–15% are related to the inheritance of a germline pathogenic variant. They are often unrecognized in clinical practice due to family histories that are incomplete, inaccurate, or missing altogether in the medical record.

For the most part, germline mutations associated with cancer create a predisposition to that cancer, not a certainty that it will occur. This phenomenon is called "incomplete penetrance," which means that not all carriers of a pathogenic variant in a family will develop the disease. Furthermore, those that do develop the disease will display variability in the type of cancer, the age of diagnosis, the pathologic subtype, and the degree of aggressiveness of the cancer. This variability in the expression of the pathogenic variant strongly suggests that other factors or triggers interact with the inherited genetic change to create the phenotype, or manifestation of the cancer. Loss or inactivation of the normal allele, in which case both copies of the gene are altered (called loss of heterozygosity, LOH),

Introduction

the effect of other genetic variants, epigenetic changes that can interfere with gene expression, the position of the specific variant within the gene, environmental lifestyle and hormonal factors, or other unknown factors could all contribute to the variability of risk associated with inheritance of a pathogenic variant. Several factors that can modify risk and that present opportunities for prevention have been identified in Lynch syndrome carriers, including body-mass index, diet, smoking, alcohol intake, and physical activity.

The discovery of the *BRCA1/2* genes in the mid-1990s quickly led to the availability of genetic testing in the clinical setting. As a result, healthcare providers were being approached by patients who were seeking guidance about their genetic cancer risk and their options for genetic testing. Cancer genetics risk assessment and counseling have now become an established practice in many clinical settings and indications for testing continue to expand. Refer to the American College of Medical Genetics (ACMG) (Hampel et al. 2015) for a list of the most common hereditary cancer syndromes, and see Chapters 46 and 47.

Case Study 2

You are scheduled to see a new patient recently diagnosed with invasive breast cancer at the age of 44. Her breast surgeon calls you to ask whether genetic testing for *BRCA1/2* is indicated based on her young age and her family history, because a positive test might change her surgical approach (Figure 45.2/Pedigree 2). Her family history is notable for a paternal aunt with ovarian cancer at age 54 and a paternal grandmother with breast

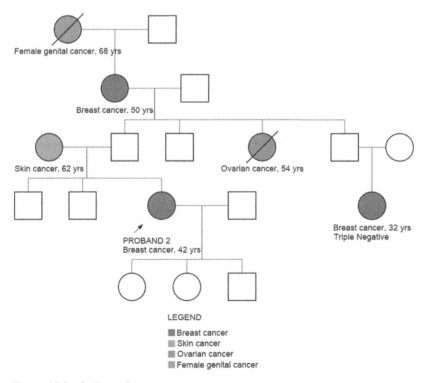

Figure 45.2 Pedigree 2.

cancer at age 50. She also has a paternal first cousin with a very young triple-negative breast cancer and a paternal great-grandmother with a history of a "female genital cancer." No one in the family has had genetic testing.

2) Who should be tested for hereditary cancer(s)?

Expert Perspective: There are several features that suggest a hereditary cancer in a patient:

- A known pathogenic variant in a family member.
- Early age of cancer onset.
- Multiple cancers in the same individual, including bilateral cancers in paired organs.
- The same cancers in close relatives occurring over several generations.
- The occurrence of rare cancers (e.g. adrenocortical carcinoma in Li Fraumeni syndrome).
- Ethnic populations known to have a high risk of hereditary cancers (known as a founder effect, in which a currently identified pathogenic variant is traced back in history to a small group of individuals isolated by geographic or sociocultural factors; e.g. increased *BRCA1/2* pathogenic variants in individuals of Ashkenazi Jewish heritage).
- Specific tumor pathology (e.g. medullary thyroid cancer seen in the MEN2 syndrome).
- Specific benign physical findings (e.g. macrocephaly seen in Cowden's syndrome, or multiple precancerous colonic polyps seen in Familial Adenomatous Polyposis Syndrome).
- Abnormal results from colon or endometrial tumor testing with microsatellite instability or immunohistochemistry, suggestive of Lynch syndrome.

Pedigree 2 displays several features of a hereditary cancer syndrome. Breast and ovarian cancer are clustering in three generations in the same lineage, with early age of onset, and with one relative with triple-negative breast cancer, which is seen more often in hereditary breast cancer syndromes. The not uncommon report of a "female genital cancer" in a relative suggests a potential diagnosis of ovarian cancer. Uncertainty about type of cancer in more distant relatives is also a common finding. The pattern in this family is consistent with hereditary breast/ovarian cancer syndrome due to a pathogenic variant in *BRCA1* or *BRCA2*. Your new patient is a good candidate for testing because she has early onset breast cancer; she is already a patient in your institution, which may minimize logistic and insurance related issues; and a positive genetic test could have immediate implications for her primary surgery.

The identification of a hereditary cancer syndrome can be hard to recognize due to a small family size, incomplete or inaccurate family history information, adoption, misattributed parentage, gender imbalance (e.g. few women in a family suspected of having hereditary breast or ovarian cancer syndrome), deaths of family members at young ages or removal of the at-risk organ before cancer would occur, or incomplete penetrance. The benefits of identifying a pathogenic variant include the ability to predict more accurate, personalized risk estimates; to define more appropriate primary and secondary prevention strategies; to inform potential risks for other family members; and increasingly for therapeutic decisions. Despite these potential benefits, some eligible individuals decide not to pursue testing for fear of discrimination, emotional distress, stigmatization, or other perceived risks. In contrast, some individuals whose personal or family history are not suggestive of a hereditary cancer syndrome elect to proceed with testing to gain a better understanding of their personal risk and for peace of mind. In both of these scenarios, patient education and counseling are valuable assets to the testing process. Several organizations, including the American Society of Oncology (ASCO), the ACMG, and the National Comprehensive Cancer Network (NCCN) have developed testing criteria for hereditary cancer syndromes.

There are several risk assessment models that, in addition to predicting the risk of cancer, may also estimate the risk of carrying a cancer-related pathogenic variant. Factors included in these models vary and may include age, family history, personal history and polygenic risk scores which are derived from the combination of several single nucleotide variants (SNV), thought to contribute to cancer risk. Model performance has been shown to differ in subgroups of individuals, and their screening potential has not been well established.

3) What does the process of genetic testing involve?

Expert Perspective: Clinical genetic testing for hereditary cancer syndromes initially started in the late 1990s in academic cancer centers and focused primarily on *BRCA1* and *BRCA2*. The counseling model developed from the early experience with high-risk families consists of in-person visits prior to and after genetic tests were performed, conducted by a genetic counseling team with expertise in genetics, oncology, and family counseling. The initial counseling session includes a risk assessment based on pedigree analysis and personal history of cancer; precursor lesions, such as multiple colonic polyps, and/or benign findings, such as the presence of café au lait spots; a review of genetic testing options based on the pattern of cancers in the family as well as insurance availability; a discussion of the possible test results; the pros and cons of testing; and a determination of the goals of the individual considering testing. An attempt is made to understand the psychosocial and cultural factors that may contribute to the impact of test results on the individual considering testing and on other family members.

The most informative person to test in the family is an affected individual whose cancer is suggestive of a hereditary cancer syndrome. However, often the best person to test may be deceased or may be unable to or uninterested in being tested. In this case, an unaffected individual may decide to pursue testing, understanding the potential uncertainty of a negative test result. Possible test results include the following:

- Positive for a known pathogenic variant.
- True negative for a known pathogenic variant in the family.
- Indeterminate, a negative test result in an individual for whom there is no known pathogenic variant in the family.
- Variant of uncertain significance (VUS), a variant whose cancer risk in unknown.

The posttest consultation includes a review of the test result; options for medical management based on best evidence, including for those in whom no pathogenic variant is identified; and implications of the test result for other family members. The counseling team attempts to understand and respond to the patient's emotional reaction to the test results. Often the counseling team will help facilitate referral to the services needed for risk management.

The introduction of next generation sequencing (NGS), discussed later in the chapter, which allows for thousands of genes to be explored at a relatively low cost, and the elimination of patent barriers has recently resulted in the availability of panels of genes that simultaneously sequence multiple genes over a wide range of hereditary cancer syndromes. Multigene panel testing can be seen as a more efficient way to explore actionable genes, particularly in families where more than one syndrome is in the differential diagnosis. It eliminates the need for sequential testing in individuals in whom the first test was negative, a situation that can cause anxiety and lead to insurance denial of additional testing. Qualifications of multigene panel testing include the possibility of finding a pathogenic variant that is discordant with the family history of cancer, the identification of pathogenic variants with low to moderate penetrance and for which medical management guidelines are not available, and an increase in the number of VUS results.

Since the first introduction of clinical genetic testing, the indications for genetic testing have expanded, and the volume of individuals seeking genetic services has increased, putting a strain on the limited genetic resources available. As a result, new counseling models have emerged, including the training of primary care and oncology practitioners and non-genetic specialists, such as nurses and other advanced practice clinicians to provide risk counseling and testing services. Genetic navigators are used in some settings to identify candidates for genetic testing, to provide basic patient education to prepare them for risk assessment, and to facilitate their referral to genetic specialists. Telehealth technologies including telephone counseling and videoconferencing, which allow for multiple family members being present for the session, are being widely adopted. Utilization of the electronic medical record to automatically identify patients appropriate for referral to genetics services has been proposed. Several online interventions to provide a scripted genetic counseling session in preparation for testing are currently being evaluated. There is limited data on the success of these newer counseling models to meet patient and provider needs, and efforts must continue to address the growing application of genetics in the oncology setting.

Case Study 3

Your resident presents to you a young patient referred to you by an endocrinologist for an early onset medullary thyroid cancer, diagnosed by ultrasound guided biopsy of a thyroid nodule. The resident has documented a family history of two additional thyroid cancers, type unknown (Figure 45.3/Pedigree 3).

4) What are the medical and surgical implications?

Expert Perspective: Although medullary thyroid cancer accounts for only 1–2% of all thyroid cancers in the general population, the lifetime incidence of medullary thyroid cancer among individuals with the MEN2A syndrome, due to a pathogenic variant in the *RET* proto-oncogene, is 20–25%. Genetic testing is indicated for anyone with this diagnosis. Other manifestations seen with pathogenic variants in MEN2A are pheochromocytoma,

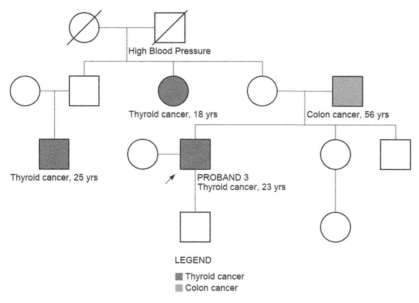

Figure 45.3 Pedigree 3.

which presents as intractable hypertension, and hyperparathyroidism. MEN2A is one of the few hereditary cancer syndromes that is seen in the pediatric setting. The typical age of onset of medullary thyroid cancer in MEN2A is between 5 and 25 years. Risk-reducing thyroidectomy is recommended by some as early as in the first year of life. Other risk-management options include routine surveillance with physical exam, thyroid ultrasound, and biochemical monitoring for elevated calcitonin levels. Screening for pheochromocytoma, which presents in early adulthood, includes regular monitoring of urine catecholamines. This case represents the potential advantages of undergoing genetic testing for a hereditary cancer syndrome, including having a more accurate estimate of personal risk with the potential to interfere in the cancer process by intensive screening to identify biomarkers or early premalignant lesions, or prophylactic surgery to remove the at-risk tissue. In addition, the potential benefits could be shared with other family members who may also be at increased risk and who could benefit from genetic testing. As more hereditary cancer syndromes are identified and characterized in terms of their genetic basis, level of penetrance, and clinical presentation, guidelines are being developed to guide clinical management options. Most of these guidelines are based on consensus of experts in the field rather than randomized controlled trials.

5) What are the risk-mitigation strategies in *BRCA1/2* carriers?

Expert Perspective: Some of the best examples of the development of risk-management strategies come from studies among *BRCA1/2* carriers (Chapters 18 and 46). Early on, clinical investigators began to pool data on the outcomes of women with *BRCA* pathogenic variants who were choosing to undergo prophylactic surgeries, to determine what impact it had on their risk of subsequent cancer. These studies showed that prophylactic removal of the breast and ovaries translated into a consistent 90–95% reduction in the risk of breast and/or ovarian cancer and to improved overall survival. The high risk of a second breast cancer in the same breast or the opposite breast among women with *BRCA* mutations who are diagnosed with a first breast cancer has led many of these women to consider bilateral mastectomy at the time of their initial surgical treatment. Unaffected women are also choosing prophylactic surgeries given the high penetrance of breast and ovarian cancer associated with *BRCA1* and *BRCA2*, the experience of cancer in their families, and the high mortality rate associated with ovarian cancer. These procedures are not without risks themselves, however. Like any surgery, prophylactic removal of the breasts poses some immediate postoperative risks. It is in most cases accompanied by breast replacement therapy, which may result in a less than optimal cosmetic result and may negatively affect body image. Prophylactic removal of the ovaries before menopause induces the onset of immediate menopause, with early and sometimes disabling menopausal symptoms. The early loss of ovarian hormones has also been linked to increases in cardiovascular disease and osteoporosis later in life.

There is a small but real chance of still developing breast or ovarian cancer despite having undergone prophylactic removal of those organs, probably as the result of microscopic amounts of residual tissue remaining after the surgery. However, with ongoing awareness of hereditary cancer syndromes among both patients and their providers, uptake of prophylactic surgeries continues to increase in developed countries among women found to carry a breast/ovarian cancer susceptibility pathogenic variant. Currently, approximately 50% of women with a *BRCA* pathogenic variant chose to undergo prophylactic mastectomy, whereas over 70% choose prophylactic removal of the ovaries. The age at which to consider prophylactic surgeries is based on our best knowledge of the expected age of incidence of cancer associated with a given syndrome but may be tailored to the ages of onset seen in a given family.

Perhaps the best evidence for heightened screening comes from studies comparing breast MRI to mammography in women with *BRCA1/2* pathogenic variants, among whom there was an alarming number of interval cancers occurring – cancers that become symptomatic or palpable in between the annual mammography screens. Several studies have reported a significantly higher detection of cancers that are smaller and less invasive among women undergoing breast MRI compared with mammography. Tumors detected by breast MRI are less likely to need chemotherapy and less likely to develop metastatic disease, which translates into reduced breast cancer mortality. The higher recall and biopsy rates seen in the early years of MRI use have decreased with improvements in technology, increased experience of radiologists, and the benefit of having consecutive MRI scans for comparison. As a result, breast MRI has emerged as an adjunct to mammography for women who are at high risk, and it is endorsed by several professional organizations, including the American Cancer Society (ACS). The current ACS guidelines recommend annual breast MRI in addition to mammography in women with a known pathogenic variant in BRCA1/2 or other genes associated with a high risk of breast cancer, women whose risk of breast cancer is predicted to exceed 20% lifetime risk by breast cancer risk models, and women who have been treated with radiation to the chest wall (e.g. for Hodgkin's lymphoma). Currently there is interest in abbreviated breast MRI that takes less time, is less costly, and would potentially increase access. The PDQ Cancer Genetics

Editorial Board (2021), which is updated on a frequent basis, provides detailed information on the clinical management of hereditary cancer syndromes.

6) What are some of the psychological implications of genetic testing in adults?

Expert Perspective: Parents who learn that they are carriers of a cancer-related pathogenic variant often express concern and even guilt about passing on their pathogenic variant to a child. Some decide not to have biologic children, whereas others may seek prenatal diagnosis, a term used to refer to a medical procedure that can determine whether a fetus is carrying a pathogenic variant. Both amniocentesis and chorionic villous sampling have been used to identify a pathogenic variant in the fetus. However, both procedures are associated with a risk of miscarriage or fetal defects, and if positive, they can lead to a difficult decision regarding pregnancy termination. More recently, preimplantation genetic testing is used to test a fertilized embryo for the known parental pathogenic variant prior to uterine implantation. Unfortunately, awareness of these reproductive options is low. Genetic testing guidelines recommend that parents considering future pregnancies be given the option of consultation with a reproductive endocrinologist.

Case Study 4

You are evaluating an African American patient with metastatic prostate cancer for a phase III clinical trial. The patient has two adult sons, three brothers, a sister, and several cousins. Other family history includes a paternal aunt with breast cancer, a paternal uncle with prostate cancer, a paternal grandmother with pancreas cancers, and a paternal cousin with breast cancer (Figure 45.4/Pedigree 4). At your encouragement, he agrees to undergo genetic testing to see whether he might be a candidate for a PARP (poly adenosine diphosphate-ribose polymerase) inhibitor trial, and he is found to have a pathogenic variant in *BRCA2*. PARP inhibitors bind the PARP enzyme to prevent it from participating in the DNA repair process. In the presence of *BRCA1/2* pathogenic variants, PARP inhibitors enhance the damage done to tumor cells and can result in cell death. Studies have shown that this class of drugs improves survival in *BRCA* carriers (Chapters 18 and 46). Although the patient has several first-, second-, and third-degree relatives who may be at risk, he is adamant that he does not want his privacy compromised by sharing this information with his family.

7) What is the standard of care for communicating genetic test information within a family?

Expert Perspective: The identification of hereditary cancer syndromes can not only provide benefit to the individuals being tested but also provide valuable information to their family members. In this case, there are several relatives who would benefit from genetic risk assessment and testing. A significant component of the genetic counseling session is devoted to a discussion of which family members would benefit from learning of the familial genetic risk, as well as information on how to communicate the information. The process of communicating genetic information within the family is referred to as "cascade testing." Cascade testing has the potential to identify those family members who would

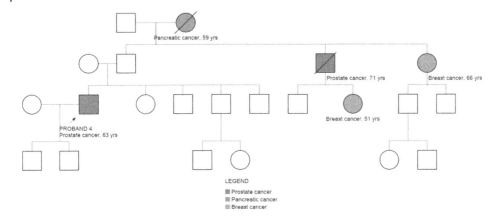

Figure 45.4 Pedigree 4.

benefit from personalized surveillance, risk-reducing strategies, or targeted therapies. In addition, relatives who are found not to carry a family pathogenic variant would be spared the more intensive interventions. Yet rates of cascade testing remain low with approximately only 30% of eligible relatives pursuing testing.

Although studies have identified the supportive role of the healthcare team as a key factor in promoting family communication about genetic risk, currently, due to concerns about privacy and confidentiality, the burden of sharing genetic testing results lies with the family member being tested, not their provider. Multiple studies have identified significant gaps in the communication of genetic test results within families. Test results are shared more often with first-degree relatives than with more distant relatives, and with female family members more than with male relatives. African American and other minority patients are less likely to share genetic test results with family members. Reasons given for not sharing test results may include lack of encouragement by their provider, limited understanding of the rationale for sharing test results, emotional distance or estrangement from family members, fear of creating worry or anxiety among relatives, feelings of guilt in possibly passing on a mutation to a child, cultural beliefs, and concerns about privacy and confidentiality. In lieu of directly sharing test results with relatives, patients may give their providers permission to contact them, which may be problematic when the family members are not part of the provider's practice. Other provider barriers include lack of sufficient training in hereditary cancer syndromes, limitations in time, and lack of institutional support. Finally, limitations at the system level include lack of access to genetic services and insurance barriers. There is ongoing debate about the provider's duty to warn at risk relatives when the patient is unwilling to share test results. Theoretic reasons to justify the provider directly contacting the family member are when there is a high likelihood of harm in the absence of disclosure, and there are proven treatments or options for prevention of the harm. In reality, it is very uncommon for a healthcare provider to violate their commitment to maintain confidentiality with their patients. Given the multiple factors which interfere with cascade testing, provision of support tools to improve cascade testing are needed, especially in populations with limited access and poor communication skills.

Case Study 5

You are caring for a patient with early stage pancreatic cancer. Recent imaging reveals a questionable new lesion in the liver, leading to a biopsy. The surgeon performing the biopsy orders genetic testing of the tumor tissue hoping to find genetic changes that may lend themselves to targeted therapy. Among the variants found in the tumor is a mutation in the *ATM* gene, which, when also found in the germline, is associated with increased rates of breast and pancreas cancer and may explain the pancreatic cancer in this patient (Figure 45.5/Pedigree 5). The family history is notable for a history of breast cancer in a first-degree relative and an abdominal cancer in a second-degree relative.

8) What is the role of tumor testing, often referred to as precision oncology?

Expert Perspective: With the availability of NGS, it is becoming increasingly common to test tumor tissues, typically in the setting of advanced disease, to identify genetic variants that may guide further therapy. Tumor DNA sequencing can detect not only acquired somatic variants, which are present only in the tumor and may have immediate targeted therapeutic implications, but also variants that are present in the germline and therefore in every cell in the body, which, if confirmed in an appropriate lab, may impact care by directing therapy choices, surgical decisions, and additional cancer screening, as well as being informative for other family members. There are challenges, however, to relying on tumor testing alone to identify germline pathogenic variants. A testing panel designed to identify somatic variants for therapeutic reasons may not include all of the genes with hereditary implications or may have reduced sensitivity. As a result, pathology labs are

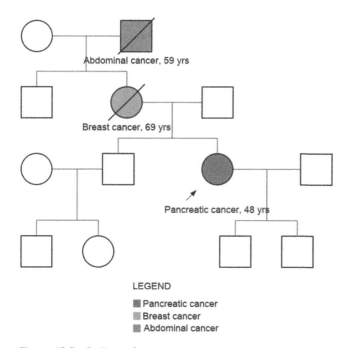

Figure 45.5 Pedigree 5.

moving away from relying on the results found in the tumor only to a newer model of routinely performing parallel tumor and germline testing, in a blood or saliva sample, to maximize the yield of genetic information. Studies have shown that simultaneous tumor/germline sequencing will identify inherited cancer predisposition variants in 3–12% of patients tested. This movement to a more comprehensive genetic analysis of both the tumor and the germline poses some unique challenges. Typically, patient consent for paired tumor/germline testing is obtained at the time of surgery without consultation with a genetic counseling team. The emphasis in this setting is on the identification of a driver mutation which may be a candidate for targeted drug therapy. The patient is mainly focused on finding an effective treatment for the advanced disease, not on learning the genetic risk for cancer. There is no consideration of family history or other indications of a hereditary cancer syndrome. In the absence of counseling, patients may be unprepared to receive germline testing results that indicate risks for additional cancers for themselves and for their families. Incidental germline findings that do not correspond with the personal or family history may be identified, leading to uncertainty regarding the clinical management of the pathogenic variant, and to the role of the pathogenic variant in the patient's tumor. Similarly, germline variants that display a low to moderate penetrance may not have corresponding evidence-based guidelines to direct preventive actions. Adding germline testing to tumor testing adds costs that are often not covered by the patient's insurance and can pose logistical problems in the coordination of obtaining the tumor and the blood sample. Despite these challenges, the potential advantages of parallel germline and tumor testing have resulted in the increasing adoption of this strategy into the mainline of oncologic care. Efforts are needed to raise public and provider awareness of the benefits of parallel genetic testing, to design alternate models for genetic counseling and informed consent in this setting, to create culturally sensitive interventions for outreach to at-risk family members, and to garner support from the health care system.

Recommended Readings

Hall, M.J., Forman, A.D., Pilarski, R. et al. (2014). Gene panel testing for inherited cancer risk. *J Natl Compr Canc Netw* 12: 1339–1346.

Hampel, H., Bennett, R.L., Buchanan, A. et al., for a Guideline Development Group of the American College of Medical Genetics and Genomics Professional Practice and Guidelines Committee and of the National Society of Genetic Counselors Practice Guidelines Committee (2015). A practice guideline from the American College of Medical Genetics and Genomics and the National Society of Genetic Counselors: Referral indications for cancer predisposition assessment. *Genet Med* 17 (1): 70–87.

Kuchenbaecker, K.B., Hopper, J.L., Barnes, D.R. et al. (2017). Risks of breast, ovarian, and contralateral breast cancer for BRCA1 and BRCA2 mutation carriers. *Jama* 317 (23): 2402–2416.

Mandelker, D. and Zhang, L. (2018). The emerging significance of secondary germline testing in cancer genomics. *J Pathol* 244: 610–615.

PDQ Cancer Genetics Editorial Board. (2021). PDQ cancer information summaries: genetics. Bethesda, MD: National Cancer Institute. Updated 8 July 2021. Available at: https://www.cancer.gov/publications/pdq/information-summaries/genetics (Accessed 23 August 2021).

Robson, M.E., Bradbury, A.R., Arun, B. et al. (2015). American Society of Clinical Oncology policy statement update: Genetic and genomic testing for cancer susceptibility. *J Clin Oncol* 33 (31): 3660–3667.

Saadatmand, S., Obdeijn, I.M., Rutgers, E.J. et al. (2015). Survival benefit in women with BRCA1 mutation of familial risk in the MRI screening study (MRISC). *Int J Cancer* 137 (7): 1729–1738.

Saslow, D., Boetes, C., Burke, W. et al. (2007). American Cancer Society guidelines for breast screening with MRI as an adjunct to mammography. *CA Cancer J Clin* 57: 75–89.

46

Hereditary Breast and Ovarian Cancer Syndromes

Kristen Whitaker and Elias Obeid

Fox Chase Cancer Center, Philadelphia, PA

Introduction

Hereditary risks underlie approximately 5–15% of all cancer diagnosis. Mutations in hereditary cancer genes cause increase cancer risks for carriers, often for a constellation of various cancers within a cancer syndrome. Hereditary breast-ovarian cancer is one of the most common cancer syndromes and is most commonly caused by mutations in *BRCA1* and *BRCA2* among others. Hereditary breast-ovarian cancer syndrome is associated with increased risks for breast, ovarian, prostate, and pancreatic cancers. Individuals with this syndrome may also be at increased risk of melanoma depending on the involved mutation. More recently there has been discovery of additional genes linked with hereditary breast-ovarian cancer syndromes. As a result of improvements in genetic testing technology (i.e. the introduction of next-generation sequencing) and decreasing costs, there is an increasing trend toward the use of multigene panel testing among individuals with a possible predisposition toward hereditary breast-ovarian cancer syndrome, rather than single- and two-gene testing that was standard practice before 2013. Although many carriers are unaware of the presence of a gene mutation increases their risk for cancer, approximately 1% of individuals have hereditary breast-ovarian cancer.

Case Study 1

During an office visit with Ms. Johnson, a 37-year-old woman with a strong family history of multiple cancers, she expresses concern about an inherited cause of cancer. She elaborates on her family history of cancer, which includes a mother with breast cancer diagnosed at age 32 and ovarian cancer at age 47, a maternal grandfather with pancreatic cancer diagnosed at age 54, two brothers with prostate cancer diagnosed at ages 41 and 56, a sister diagnosed with breast cancer at age 42, a maternal grandmother diagnosed with brain cancer at age 75, a maternal cousin diagnosed with breast cancer at age 40, a paternal grandfather diagnosed with prostate cancer at age 78, and a paternal aunt diagnosed with breast cancer at 65.

1) What genetic syndrome would be most likely present in her family?

Expert Perspective: Given the presence of breast, ovarian, pancreatic, and prostate cancers on her maternal side of the family, hereditary breast-ovarian cancer (HBOC) syndrome is the most likely genetic explanation for the cancers in her family. HBOC is characterized by an increased risk of female and male breast cancer, and ovarian cancer (includes fallopian tube and primary peritoneal cancers), as well as pancreatic and prostate cancers. Additionally, some studies have suggested a potential increased risk of melanoma, especially among *BRCA2* mutation carriers. *BRCA1* and *BRCA2* germline mutations are the most common cause of HBOC. The prevalence of *BRCA1/2* mutations in the general population is estimated at 1:400 to 1:500. Individuals of Eastern European (Ashkenazi) Jewish descent have a higher prevalence of *BRCA1/2* mutations than the general population and 1:40 individuals will carry a mutation in one of three specific mutation location in the *BRCA* genes (187delAG and 5385insC in *BRCA1* or 617delT in *BRCA2*).

Cancers in *BRCA* mutation carriers: Women with one of the *BRCA* mutations have an increased risk of developing breast cancer and often develop breast cancer at earlier ages than the general population. The lifetime risk of breast cancer in women is 46–87% in *BRCA1* mutation carriers and 38–84% in *BRCA2* mutation carriers. These women also have an elevated risk of developing second breast cancers; within 10 years this risk is 21% in *BRCA1* carriers and 10% in *BRCA2* carriers. Notably, *BRCA1* carriers have a predisposition to the aggressive triple-negative breast cancer subtype, with at least two-thirds of the breast cancers that develop in *BRCA1* carriers being triple negative. In contrast, only about a third of breast cancers in *BRCA2* carriers will be triple negative, which is similar to the proportion seen in sporadic breast cancer not associated with *BRCA* mutations. Additionally, males with *BRCA1* or *BRCA2* mutations have a 1.2% and 8–9% of developing breast cancer respectively. *BRCA1/2* carriers also have an elevated risk of ovarian cancer, estimated at 39–63% in *BRCA1* mutation carriers and 16–27% in *BRCA2* mutations carriers. Beyond elevated risks of breast and ovarian cancers, *BRCA1/2* carriers also have modestly increased risk of pancreatic and prostate cancers, and potentially melanoma (*BRCA2* carriers only). The risk of these cancers is greatest among *BRCA2* carriers.

Identification of a *BRCA* mutation in a patient with a *BRCA*-mutation related cancer (breast, pancreas, prostate, and ovarian) has important implications for the treatment of their cancer given the recent introduction of poly(adenosine diphosphate [ADP]-ribose) polymerase (PARP) inhibitors into the care of these patients with evidence from clinical trials demonstrating improved cancer outcomes when given this treatment.

Our Patient: Ms. Johnson decides to pursue genetic testing. She says that she would like to be tested for the *BRCA1/2* genes, but asks if there are any other genes that are important for testing.

2) What other genes should be considered in her situation?

Expert Perspective: Although the *BRCA1* and *BRCA2* genes are the most common cause of HBOC, there are other cancer susceptibility syndromes and/or genes that have an elevated risk of some of the cancers commonly seen in HBOC. Although often *BRCA1*- and *BRCA2*-associated HBOC can be distinguished from these other syndromes based on the constellation of tumors, it is appropriate and often advisable to consider genetic testing with a multigene panel that includes multiple cancer susceptibility. Given her family history, a multigene panel that includes at least *TP53, PTEN, CDH1, CHEK2, ATM, PALB2, STK11, RAD51C, RAD51D, MLH1, MSH2, MSH6, PMS2*, and *EPCAM* would be recommended.

Our Patient: Ms. Johnson undergoes genetic testing with a multigene panel. Her results reveal that she has a *BRCA1* mutation.

3) How should she be managed?

Expert Perspective: Because of Ms. Johnson's current age and the associated breast and ovarian cancer risks with the *BRCA1* gene, you discuss with her the immediate need to begin medical management for this gene. To manage her breast cancer risk, she has two options given her age.

1) Her first option is to implement high risk breast cancer screening, consisting of annual mammogram and breast MRI, alternated six months apart. Breast MRIs are recommended to begin at age 25, and mammograms should begin at age 30. If a breast cancer has been diagnosed before age 30 in a family with a known *BRCA* mutation, the start age should be individualized based on the family history. She should also have clinical breast exams every six months beginning at age 25. Additionally, she can consider taking chemoprevention with a medicine such as tamoxifen, which may reduce her risk of developing breast cancer although there are no data from prospective randomized trials examining chemoprevention in *BRCA1/2* mutation carriers.
2) An alternate option to intensified screening, is to consider prophylactic bilateral mastectomy. Prophylactic bilateral mastectomy reduces the risk of breast cancer by at least 90%. To manage ovarian cancer risks, all women with *BRCA* mutations are recommended to undergo risk-reducing salpingo-oophorectomies (RRSO), regardless of family history of ovarian cancer. For women with *BRCA1* mutations, risk-reducing salpingo-oophorectomy is recommended between ages 35 and 40. For women with *BRCA2* mutations, RRSO is recommended between ages 40 and 45. Oral contraceptive pills have been associated with a 14% reduction of ovarian cancer risk in women who have ever used oral contraceptive pills and 35% reduction in ovarian cancer risk among long-term users. Due to lack of effective tools to screen for ovarian cancer, completion of RRSO should be prioritized. For *BRCA1/2* mutation carriers who have not yet undergone RRSO, starting at age 35, they can consider undergoing annual transvaginal ultrasound and CA-125 blood test. However, neither screening test has been demonstrated as an effective tool for detecting early stage ovarian cancer (discussed further in Question 6).

4) Ms. Johnson with *BRCA 1* mutation understands her medical management moving forward and asks how her results impact her family member and if anyone in her family needs to be tested?

Expert Perspective: *BRCA1* and *BRCA2* hereditary breast and ovarian cancer syndrome is inherited in an autosomal dominant manner. All individuals have two copies of the *BRCA1* and *BRCA2* genes. Because *BRCA* genes have an autosomal dominant inheritance pattern, inheriting only one mutated allele even in the presence of a second normal allele is sufficient to cause hereditary breast-ovarian cancer syndrome.

Once a *BRCA* mutation has been identified within a family, the relative who first underwent genetic testing and had the *BRCA* mutation identified (i.e. the proband) should share these results with her relatives given they have risks of also carrying this mutation. At-risk relatives should receive counseling about their risk of also carrying the mutation, the availability of genetic testing to identify whether they carry this mutation, and cancer risks and medical management (discussed above) if they were found to have this mutation. First-degree relatives (siblings, children, parents) have a 50% chance of having the mutation. Second-degree relatives (nieces, nephews, aunts, uncles, grandparents, and grandchildren) have a 25% chance of having the mutation. Third-degree relatives (cousins, great-aunts, and great-uncles) have a 12.5% chance of having the mutation. If at-risk relatives undergo genetic testing and are found not to carry the familial *BRCA* mutation, they are considered to be close to general population risk for developing cancer.

Case Study 2

A 35-year-old woman presents to a genetic counseling session. She has a personal history of endometrial cancer diagnosed at age 30, thyroid cancer diagnosed at age 31, and breast cancer diagnosed at age 34. She also notes that she has a lot of skin abnormalities but is not sure what is causing them. She states that she was told by her medical oncologist that because she now has developed three cancers at an early age, she should undergo genetic testing.

5) **She asks if there is any particular inherited cancer syndrome that she should worry about.**

Expert Perspective: The constellation of breast, thyroid, and endometrial cancers in a single individual raise suspicion for a condition called Cowden syndrome, also known as *PTEN* hamartoma syndrome. Cowden syndrome is a highly variable, autosomal dominant hereditary cancer susceptibility syndrome characterized by multiple hamartomas, unusual skin and facial findings, and increased risk of multiple cancers, including breast, thyroid, and endometrial cancer. Prevalence estimates for Cowden syndrome are imprecise but currently estimated to be between 1 in 200,000 and 1 in 250,000. There appears to be a female preponderance. Individuals can present with Cowden syndrome at varying ages; this condition has been reported in individuals as young as age 13 and as old as age 65.

Cowden syndrome diagnosis is based mainly on clinical criteria as established by the International Cowden Consortium. The presence of clinical criteria aids in identifying which patients should undergo genetic testing for Cowden syndrome to determine whether they have a germline mutation in the *PTEN* gene. Eighty percent of individuals meeting clinical criteria for Cowden syndrome will have a germline mutation in the *PTEN* gene. The National Comprehensive Cancer Network (NCCN) has published Cowden syndrome testing criteria based on pathognomonic criteria and major and minor diagnostic criteria. To meet NCCN criteria for genetic testing, individuals should have three or more major criteria, but one must include macrocephaly, Lhermitte-Duclos disease (cerebellar tumors), or GI hamartomas, or two major and three minor criteria. Please see Table 46.1, which describes major and minor criteria for Cowden syndrome. Because the woman in this case presentation has breast, endometrial, and follicular thyroid cancer, she meets three major criteria for Cowden syndrome and thus qualifies for genetic testing.

In the presence of clinical criteria consistent with Cowden syndrome and/or the identification of a *PTEN* mutation, there are established recommendations for the management of cancer risks. Table 46.2 shows recommended cancer screening for individuals with Cowden syndrome.

Table 46.1 NCCN diagnostic clinical criteria for Cowden syndrome.

Major Criteria	Minor Criteria
Breast cancer	Autism spectrum disorder
Endometrial cancer(epithelial)	Colon cancer
Thyroid cancer(follicular)	Esophageal glycogenic acanthoses
GI hamartomas	Lipomas
Lhermitte-Duclos disease	Intellectual disability (i.e. IQ ≤ 75)
Macrocephaly (HC > 58 cm for females, HC > 60 cm for males)	Renal cell carcinoma
Macular pigmentation of the glans penis	Testicular lipomatosis
Multiple mucocutaneous lesions (any of the following): • Multiple trichilemmomas (≥ 3, at least one biopsy proven) • Acral keratosis • Mucutaneous neuromas • Oral papillomas(particularly on tongue or gingiva)	Vascular anomalies/malformations (including multiple intracranial developmental venous anomalies)
	Thyroid cancer (papillary or follicular variant of papillary)
	Thyroid structural lesions (e.g. adenoma, multinodular goiter)

Table 46.2 Cowden syndrome cancer risks and clinical management recommendations.

Cancer Risk	Management Recommendation
Breast	Annual mammogram and breast MRI starting at age 35 or 10 years before the earliest breast cancer diagnosis in the family
	Consider risk-reducing mastectomy
	Clinical breast exams every 6–12 months, starting at age 25 or 5–10 years before the earliest breast cancer in the family
Colon	Colonoscopy stating at age 35 or 5–10 years before the earliest colon cancer in the family if before age 40
Endometrial	Consideration of endometrial biopsy every 1 to 2 years
	Consideration of transvaginal ultrasound in postmenopausal women only
	Consideration of hysterectomy at the completion of childbearing
Kidney	Consider renal ultrasound starting at age 40, then every 1–2 years
Thyroid	Annual thyroid ultrasound starting at age 7

Case Study 3

Mrs. Brown, a 45-year-old woman with recently diagnosed high-grade epithelial ovarian cancer, states she was recommended by her oncologist to undergo germline genetic testing. She was told by her oncologist that all women with ovarian cancer are recommended to undergo germline genetic testing.

6) She asks about how commonly ovarian cancer develops due to hereditary causes and which genes might have contributed.

Expert Perspective: As noted by Mrs. Brown's oncologist, all women regardless of age and family history with epithelial ovarian cancer (including fallopian and primary peritoneal cancer) are recommended to undergo germline genetic testing as suggested by multiple medical society guidelines, such as those from the National Comprehensive Cancer Network and the American College of Obstetricians and Gynecologists (ACOG). It is estimated that up to 25% of ovarian cancer cases are caused by a heritable genetic condition. Two thirds of hereditary ovarian cancer cases are due to germline mutations in *BRCA1* or *BRCA2*. These mutations are more prevalent in those with strong family history of breast and/or ovarian cancer, a younger age at diagnosis of ovarian cancer, those with high-grade serous histology, and in certain populations, such as individuals of Ashkenazi Jewish ancestry. Women with germline *BRCA1* and *BRCA2* mutations have average cumulative risks of developing ovarian cancer by the age of 70 of about 39% (range 18–54%) and 11% (range 2.4–19%), respectively. Most of these cancers are high-grade serous cancer. Although we know that *BRCA1/2* mutations account for the vast majority of hereditary ovarian cancer, several other tumor suppressor and oncogenes have been identified and can be tested for using multigene panels to complete germline genetic testing. Mutations in the Lynch syndrome genes (*MLH1, MSH2, MSH6, PMS2*), *RAD51C, RAD51D, BRIP1, ATM,* and *PALB2* have the most well-established ovarian cancer risks. Notably, while about 15% of ovarian cancers are caused by germline mutations in *BRCA1* and *BRCA2* genes, only about 1% of ovarian cancers are caused by mutations in the mismatch repairs genes associated with Lynch syndrome. Table 46.3 shows lifetime risk of ovarian cancer in women who have mutations in established ovarian cancer susceptibility genes.

Identification of *BRCA1* or *BRCA2* mutation in a patient with ovarian cancer has been shown to be important in predicting response and susceptibility to a new class of targeted therapies called poly (ADP-ribose) polymerase (PARP) inhibitors. If Mrs. Brown did not already have ovarian cancer and underwent genetic testing and had an ovarian cancer susceptibility gene identified, strategies would be implemented aimed at reducing her future risk of developing ovarian cancer. Because screening for ovarian cancer with a Ca-125 blood test and transvaginal ultrasounds have not demonstrated efficacy in diagnosing ovarian cancer at an earlier stage, prophylactic surgery in the form of a risk-reducing salpingo-oophorectomy (RRSO) is the cornerstone of management of some women with mutations in ovarian cancer susceptibility genes. While the lifetime risk for ovarian cancer that should be used as the threshold value for recommending RRSO in women with an established hereditary cancer risk is the subject of ongoing debate, generally this has been recommended in women who have mutations in hereditary cancer susceptibility genes, which results in them having a lifetime risk of ovarian cancer that exceeds 5%. The current recommendations for RRSO in women who carry ovarian cancer susceptibility genes is shown in Table 46.3.

Given our understanding of the potential hereditary contribution to the development of a substantial portion of ovarian cancers, genetic testing should not only be performed in individuals with a personal history of epithelial ovarian cancer but also in unaffected individuals with a first- or second-degree blood relative with epithelial ovarian cancer diagnosed at any age, as well as an unaffected individual who has a probability > 5% of a *BRCA1/2* mutation based on prior probability models (such as BRCAPro).

Table 46.3 Ovarian cancer susceptibility genes and cumulative lifetimes risk of ovarian cancer.

Gene	Lifetime Risk of Ovarian Cancer	RRSO Recommendations
BRCA1	44–59%	Recommend RRSO at 35–40 years
BRCA2	11–37%	Recommend RRSO at 40–45 years
MLH1	10–20%	Consider RRSO at completion of childbearing
MSH2	17–24%	Consider RRSO at completion of childbearing
EPCAM	< 10%	Consider RRSO at completion of childbearing
PMS2	< 3%	Insufficient evidence for RRSO
MSH6	8–13%	Insufficient evidence for RRSO, manage based on family history
RAD51C	5–9%	Consider RRSO at 45–50 years
RAD51D	6–12%	Consider RRSO at 45–50 years
BRIP1	6–11%	Consider RRSO at 45–50 years
ATM	< 3%	Insufficient evidence for RRSO, manage based on family history
PALB2	3–5%	Insufficient evidence for RRSO, manage based on family history

Abbreviation: RRSO – risk-reducing salpingo-oophorectomies.

Case Study 4

Ms. McDonald, a 57-year-old woman, noted a significant family history of cancer while undergoing her annual health maintenance visit with her gynecologist. Her family history was notable for a daughter just recently diagnosed with breast cancer at age 34, two sisters with breast cancer diagnosed at age 32 and 47, a sister diagnosed with ovarian cancer at age 44, a mother with ovarian cancer diagnosed at age 51, a paternal grandfather diagnosed with pancreatic cancer at age 65 and breast cancer at age 57, a paternal uncle diagnosed with pancreatic cancer at age 83, a maternal uncle diagnosed with prostate cancer at age 75, and a maternal aunt diagnosed with breast cancer at age 79. Given her striking family history, her gynecologist sent her for a multigene panel genetic test that revealed a *PALB2* mutation.

7) She was then referred to a genetic counselor to learn more about *PALB2* mutation and its associated cancer risks and clinical management.

Expert Perspective: *PALB2* mutation was identified as breast cancer susceptibly gene in 2006. Since that time cancer risks beyond breast cancer have been identified. The estimated risks to age 80 years are 53% for female breast cancer, 5% for ovarian cancer, 2–3% for pancreatic cancer, and 1% for male breast cancer. Family history of breast cancer increases a woman's lifetime risk of breast cancer. Among women who carry a *PALB2* mutation and have a family history of breast cancer, 58% will develop breast cancer over their lifetime. Thus, in an individual with a family history including breast, pancreatic, and ovarian cancer, there should be suspicion for a *PALB2* mutation in the family.

PALB2 mutation guidelines have been established and continue to evolve to manage the cancer risks in these mutation carriers.

- To address these individuals' risk of breast cancer, they are recommended to undergo annual mammography and breast MRI beginning at age 30 or 10 years earlier than the youngest diagnosis of breast cancer in the family.
- Additionally, given cumulative lifetime risk of breast cancer that approaches that of other high-risk breast cancer genes, such as *BRCA2*, these women can also consider risk-reducing bilateral mastectomy to reduce the chance of developing a breast cancer in the future. While recent evidence does support a modest increase in risk for ovarian cancer, because this risk is lower than that which we see with other ovarian cancer predisposition genes, such as *BRCA* or *BRIP1*, there is no absolute recommendation for women to pursue RRSO to reduce future risk of ovarian cancer. Instead, decisions to pursue RRSO should be individualized and guided by the presence or absence of ovarian cancer in the family.
- For pancreatic cancer, there are currently no specific screening guidelines: at this time, no effective tool to screen for pancreatic cancer has been established. Imaging with endoscopic ultrasonography (EUS) and/or magnetic resonance cholangiopancreatography (MRCP) are being evaluated in clinical trials, but their efficacy is not established.

Case Study 5

Ms. King is a 54-year-old Caucasian female who has a history of right breast cancer diagnosed at age 30 (2003). She underwent right modified mastectomy at that time with right breast reconstruction. Her treatment consisted of chemotherapy but did not require radiation. She also received five years of antiestrogen therapy with tamoxifen. She continued to be followed closely with annual screening left mammograms and recommended routine cancer screening tests. At the time of breast cancer diagnosis, the genetic testing for the *BRCA1* and *BRCA2* genes was evidently negative for mutations.

At the age of 54 (24 years later!) she had an abnormal left mammogram. The biopsy showed ductal carcinoma *in situ* (DCIS). She decided to have left mastectomy. Ms. King has a strong family history of breast, prostate, and testicular cancer. Her father was diagnosed with metastatic prostate cancer at age 57. Her brother developed testicular cancer at age 28. Her sister developed breast cancer twice, at age 45 and again at age 56. Her maternal grandmother developed breast cancer in her 60s, and her maternal uncle was diagnosed with prostate cancer in his 60s. She presented to the genetic counselor again. A multigene panel testing was sent this time. Ms. King's multigene panel testing revealed two pathogenic mutations, one in the *ATM* gene and another in the *CHEK2* gene.

8) Can someone have more than one cancer-causing hereditary gene mutation responsible for a cancer syndrome?

Expert Perspective: Since the Supreme Court of the United States ruling that human genes cannot be patented and the availability of next-generation sequencing, multigene panel testing became widely available. With this government ruling came an increase in the yield in non-*BRCA* pathogenic variants that were previously tested through the traditional single-gene testing model, as is the case with Ms. King's test at her first cancer diagnosis in 2003. Some individuals have been found to carry more than one deleterious (cancer-causing/pathogenic) mutation; for example, a *BRCA1* and a *BRCA2* gene mutations, or a *BRCA1/2* mutation and a Lynch syndrome gene mutation. Some like Ms. King have mutations in other newly added genes to cancer risk gene panels (Table 46.4). The additional yield of multigene testing in individuals in whom a *BRCA1/BRCA2* pathogenic variant was not detected seems to be approximately 4%. Although data are limited, one

Table 46.4 Breast and ovarian cancer predisposition genes and established cancer risks.

Gene	Breast Cancer	Epithelial Ovarian Cancer	Other Cancer Risks
ATM	15–40%	< 3%	Pancreatic cancer ~5–10%
BRCA1	46–87%	39–63%	Pancreatic cancer ≤ 5% prostate cancer
BRCA2	38–84%	16–27%	Pancreatic cancer 5–10% prostate cancer
BRIP1	Uncertain*	> 10%	Unknown
CDH1	41–60%	None	Hereditary diffuse gastric cancer
CHEK2	15–40%	None	Colon cancer
NF1	15–40%	None	Malignant peripheral nerve sheath tumors GIST
PALB2	41–60%	3–5%	Pancreatic cancer 5–10%
PTEN	40–60%	None	Thyroid cancer colon cancer endometrial cancer
STK11	40–60%	None	Pancreatic cancer >15% non-epithelial ovarian cancer >10% gallbladder cancer
TP53	> 60%	None	Pancreatic cancer 5–10%
BARD1	15–40%	None	Unknown
RAD51C	15–40%	>10%	Unknown
RAD51D	15–40%	>10%	Unknown
Lynch genes (MSH2, MLH1, MSH6, PMS2, EPCAM)	Uncertain, possible increased risk with MSH6	MLH1, MSH2 >10% MSH6 ≤13% PMS2 < 3% EPCAM <10%	Pancreatic cancer 5–10% colon 46–61% endometrial 34–54% other (GI, brain, bladder, renal pelvis)

* Emerging data suggest a potential increased risk of female breast cancer, particularly triple-negative breast cancer.
Note: Estimates are only provided for well-defined cancer risks.

study has demonstrated that up to 9.5% of individuals carry clinically significant mutations in two different genes. It is important that individuals with dual gene mutations get appropriate genetic counseling, which includes attempt at discovering where the gene mutations are clustering and appropriately testing members in that branch of the family. In Ms. King's situation, both of her parents are deceased, and based on her family history alone, it is not feasible to determine or attribute which side of the family her mutations are inherited from. Testing of her cousins and descendants on both sides of her parents would be recommended until it is established which side of the family each gene (*ATM* and *CHEK2*) mutation was inherited from. While each gene could have come from different sides of her family (maternal vs paternal), it is possible that both gene mutations were inherited from one parent.

9) **How would you address her cancer risk?**

Expert Perspective: In individuals with dual gene mutations, the cancer risk is not additive. Ms. King's cancer risk is from both the *ATM* and the *CHEK2* mutation independent of one another. Therefore, her counseling would be based on what we know of risks associated with *ATM* gene mutation and *CHEK2* gene mutation.

Cancer risks with an *ATM* mutation

Ataxia-telangiectasia is an autosomal recessive disorder. The inheritance of two deleterious variants in the *ATM* gene is known to cause ataxia-telangiectasia, characterized by progressive cerebellar ataxia beginning in childhood, telangiectasias, frequent infections, and an increased risk for leukemia and lymphoma. Individuals with ataxia-telangiectasia are unusually sensitive to ionizing radiation. However, at the present time, monoallelic carriers of *ATM* gene variants are not known to be at a particularly higher risk of radiation-induced cancers. Women who carry an *ATM* gene mutation may have a 17–52% lifetime risk of developing breast cancer. Having a monoallelic mutation in the *ATM* gene increases the risk of cancer, particularly breast cancer. A statistically significant increased risk of breast cancer was found in women carriers of monoallelic (heterozygote carriers) *ATM* mutation. A meta-analysis showed the lifetime risk of breast cancer to be as high as 33%. There is also a possible increased risk for ovarian cancer for women who carry *ATM* gene mutations. However, management should be based on family history, as there is no evidence to suggest an impact from RRSO. Additionally, men who carry an *ATM* mutation have an increased risk of developing prostate cancer. At the present time, some evidence suggests a possible increased risk of pancreatic cancer as well.

Cancer risks with a *CHEK2* mutation

CHEK2 is a gene in the DDR pathway (DNA-damage response) whose mutations are considered to confer a moderately increased risk of breast cancer, and other cancers. Studies have found an approximately 1.5-fold to 3-fold increased risk of female breast cancer in women who carry the 1100delC variant in the *CHEK2* gene. The lifetime risk seems to be higher in families with a strong history of breast cancer and this variant, approaching 42%. The current information indicate women with a *CHEK2* mutation may have a 28–37% lifetime risk of developing breast cancer. Additionally, in a series of male breast cancer patients, this variant was associated with an increased risk of male breast cancer.

In a single large study, the truncating variants in *CHEK2* were not significantly associated with colorectal cancer risk; however, a specific missense pathogenic variant (I157T) was associated with a modest increased risk for colorectal cancer (odd ratio 1.5; 95% CI 1.2–3.0). Similar results were obtained in another study conducted in Poland. Therefore, individuals with *CHEK2* mutations may have an elevated risk for colorectal cancer, roughly two times higher than the general population risk. The exact risks are unclear but may approach a 10% lifetime risk.

Some studies have described a possible increased risk for a wide range of other cancers in patients with *CHEK2* mutations. A large Dutch study of 86,975 individuals reported an increased risk of cancers other than breast for carriers of the *CHEK2 1100delC* pathogenic variant including thyroid, kidney, and testicular cancer. However, these studies are not conclusive, and there are currently no medical management guidelines to address these possible risks.

In conclusion, although many different *CHEK2* mutations have been identified, estimated cancer risks for *CHEK2* gene mutations are currently based largely on studies of a single mutation (c.1100delC) that is common in patients of European ancestry. These estimates may change as ongoing research is conducted among individuals from different populations with different variants (i.e. non 1100delC).

Case Study 6

Mrs. Smith is a 58-year-old woman with a history of breast cancer diagnosed at age 30. At the time of her breast cancer diagnosis, she felt a pea-sized mass in her right breast, which soon became the size of a "golf ball." Her previous routine mammogram did not detect abnormalities. A mammogram and ultrasound led to a biopsy, which was positive for breast cancer. She had a right mastectomy and axillary node dissection with TRAM reconstruction followed by chemotherapy. She reports that she did not have radiation or hormonal therapy. Her pathology report was not available when she was seen in the cancer risk clinic. Most recently she had an abnormal left mammogram, and biopsy showed it to be a ductal carcinoma *in situ* (DCIS). She was referred by her surgeon to the genetics clinic for further evaluation given her history of breast cancer and some cancers in her family. She was contemplating lumpectomy followed by radiation versus left mastectomy.

10) Is genetic testing important in Ms. Smith's management of breast cancer and DCIS?

Expert Perspective: Mrs. Smith had early onset breast cancer, and now in her 50s she has DCIS. She is at risk of being a carrier of a genetic predisposition to breast cancer. The most common gene mutations linked to early onset and/or family history of breast cancer are *BRCA1* and *BRCA2* gene mutations, as discussed above. However, non-BRCA1/2 genes should also be considered if the tests only included these two genes in appropriate clinical context (Table 46.4). Identifying a genetic predisposition to cancer, particularly one that may carry risk for another breast cancer, such as a *BRCA1* and *BRCA2* mutations would help her in determining whether to consider mastectomy or get a lumpectomy procedure. Additionally, identifying a *TP53* gene mutation would provide valuable information to inform her surgical decision as this mutation predisposes her to radiation-induced sarcoma should she get a lumpectomy followed by radiation. Consequently, mastectomy rather than lumpectomy is typically recommended in these patients.

Mrs. Smith has a family history of breast cancer, sarcoma, and ovarian cancers. Her son who is 38 was diagnosed at age 23 with soft tissue sarcoma of the right leg. He was referred by his oncologist to a genetic counselor at that time, but he declined testing back then. Mrs. Smith was seen by a genetic counselor, and her multigene panel testing showed her to be a carrier of a pathogenic variant in the *TP53 gene*. Her son was advised to get genetic testing, and indeed, he was also found to carry the same *TP53* pathogenic variant. His sister is 34 and is healthy without a cancer diagnosis.

11) What is the spectrum of cancer diagnosis in patients with Li Fraumeni syndrome?

Expert Perspective: All types of cancers! The classical definition of the syndrome was proposed by Li and Fraumeni in 1988 and is defined below:

a) Sarcoma before age 45 years;
b) A first-degree relative with cancer before age 45 years; and
c) Another close relative (first- or second-degree relative) with either cancer before age 45 years or a sarcoma at any age.

Subsequently in 2001, Chompret et al. systematically developed clinical criteria for recommending *TP53* genetic testing, with the narrow Li Fraumeni tumor spectrum defined as sarcoma, brain tumors, breast cancer, and adrenocortical carcinoma. Those were updated in 2009 and again in 2015 by Bougerad et al. revising the criteria to include the presence of childhood anaplastic rhabdomyosarcoma and breast cancer before age 31 as an indication for testing, similar to what is recommended for choroid plexus carcinoma and adrenocortical carcinoma.

Breast cancer is also a component of the rare Li Fraumeni syndrome, in which germline variants of the *TP53* gene on chromosome 17p have been documented. Li Fraumeni syndrome is characterized by premenopausal breast cancer in combination with childhood sarcoma, brain tumors, leukemia, and adrenocortical carcinoma.

Although the most common types of cancers diagnosed in individuals with Li Fraumeni syndrome include early onset breast cancer, sarcoma, CNS tumors, and adrenocortical carcinoma, a wide spectrum of cancer types can occur. Other cancers reported with Li Fraumeni syndrome include leukemia, lymphoma, gastrointestinal (colon, gastric, pancreas), lung, ovarian, and prostate cancer, among several others.

More on Li Fraumeni syndrome: The incidence of cancer in individuals with Li Fraumeni syndrome varies depending on age. Soft tissue sarcomas (most commonly rhabdomyosarcoma) and adrenocortical carcinoma are often seen in early childhood. Bone sarcomas are frequently seen in the teenage years, and breast cancer and brain tumors are commonly seen in early adulthood. Women tend to have higher lifetime risks than men for cancer due to their significantly increased risk for breast cancer. The lifetime risk for cancer in individuals with Li Fraumeni syndrome is ≥ 70% for men and ≥ 90% for women. In one large study from France that included 415 carriers of a TP53 gene mutation from 214 families, 43% of carriers had multiple malignancies, and the mean age at first tumor onset was 24.9 years. The childhood tumor spectrum was characterized by osteosarcomas, adrenocortical carcinomas, CNS tumors, and soft tissue sarcomas (present in 23–30% collectively), whereas the adult tumor spectrum primarily encompassed breast cancer (79% of females) and soft tissue sarcomas (27% of carriers). Multiple studies have shown a link to a higher risk of having a HER2-overexpressing breast cancer in patients with *TP53*-associated breast cancers. Individuals with LFS are also at risk for developing more than one cancer; studies have shown that people with LFS have a 40–49% risk to develop a second primary cancer. In the study from France, treatment records were available for 64 carriers who received radiation therapy for treatment of their first tumor; of these, 19 (30%) developed 26 secondary tumors within a radiation field, with a latency of 2 to 26 years (mean: 10.7 years).

Recent studies, including a meta-analysis of 13 cohorts, support the use of a baseline whole-body MRI (WB-MRI) screen in all *TP53* mutation carriers in addition to the established breast cancer screening. We reviewed the family pedigree and identified family members who may be at risk for carrying the mutation. It is possible that the mutation was *de novo* (a new mutation) that started in Mrs. Smith and was not inherited from a parent. However, the breast cancer in her mother at young age raises suspicion that her mother also carried the *TP53* mutation.

Recommended Readings

Antoniou, A., Pharoah, P.D., Narod, S., Risch, H.A., Eyfjord, J.E., Hopper, J.L. et al. (2003). Average risks of breast and ovarian cancer associated with BRCA1 or BRCA2 mutations detected in case series unselected for family history: a combined analysis of 22 studies. *Am J Hum Genet* 72: 1117–1130. TsaousisG, Papadopoulos E, Apessos A, et al: Analysis of hereditary cancer syndromes by using a panel of genes: Novel and multiple pathogenic mutations. *BMC Cancer* 19:535, 201.

Antoniou, A.C., Casadei, S., Heikkinen, T., Barrowdale, D., Pylkäs, K., Roberts, J. et al. (2014). Breast-cancer risk in families with mutations in PALB2. *N Engl J Med* 371: 497–506.

Bancroft, E.K., Raghallaigh, H.N., Page, E.C., and Eeles, R.A. (2021). Updates in prostate cancer research and screening in men at genetically higher risk. *Curr Genet Med Rep* 9 (4): 47–58. doi: 10.1007/s40142-021-00202-5. Epub 2021 Oct 8. PMID: 34790437; PMCID: PMC8585808.

Chompret, A., Abel, A., Stoppa-Lyonnet, D. et al. (2001). Sensitivity and predictive value of criteria for p53 germline mutation screening. *J Med Genet* 38 (1): 43–47.

Couch, F.J., Shimelis, H., Hu, C., Hart, S.N., Polley, E.C., Na, J. et al. (2017). Associations between cancer predisposition testing panel genes and breast cancer. *JAMA Oncol* 3: 1190–1196.

Hisada, M., Garber, J.E., Fung, C.Y. et al. (1998). Multiple primary cancers in families with Li-Fraumeni syndrome. *J Natl Cancer Inst* 90: 606–611.

Kurian, A.W., Hare, E.E., Mills, M.A., Kingham, K.E., McPherson, L., Whittermore, A.S. et al. (2014). Clinical evaluation of a multiple gene sequencing panel for hereditary cancer risk assessment. *J Clin Oncol* 32: 2001–2009.

Li, S., Silvestri, V., Leslie, G. et al. (2022 January 25). Cancer risks associated with *BRCA1* and *BRCA2* pathogenic variants. *J Clin Oncol* JCO2102112. doi: 10.1200/JCO.21.02112. Epub ahead of print. PMID: 35077220.

Liede, A., Karlan, B.Y., and Narod, S.A. (2004 February 15). Cancer risks for male carriers of germline mutations in BRCA1 or BRCA2: a review of the literature. *J Clin Oncol* 22 (4): 735–742.

Näslund-Koch, C., Nordestgaard, B.G., and Bojesen, S.E. (2016 April 10). Increased risk for other cancers in addition to breast cancer for CHEK2*1100delC heterozygotes estimated from the copenhagen general population study. *J Clin Oncol* 34 (11): 1208–1216. doi: 10.1200/JCO.2015.63.3594. Epub 2016 Feb 16. PMID: 26884562.

National Comprehensive Cancer Network. (2022). NCCN clinical practice guidelines in oncology. genetic/familial high-risk assessment breast and ovarian. Version 1.

Pilarski, R., Burt, R., Kohlman, W. et al. (2013). Cowden syndrome and the PTEN hamartoma tumor syndrome: a systematic review and revised diagnostic criteria. *J Natl Cancer Inst* 105: 1607–1616.

Thompson, D., Duedal, S., Kirner, J., McGuffog, L., Last, J., Reiman, A. et al. (2005 June 1). Cancer risks and mortality in heterozygous ATM mutation carriers. *J Natl Cancer Inst* 97 (11): 813–822. doi: 10.1093/jnci/dji141. PMID: 15928302.

Tung, N., Battelli, C., Allen, B., Kaldate, R., Bhatnagar, S., Bowles, K. et al. (2015). Frequency of mutations in individuals with breast cancer referred for BRCA1 and BRCA2 testing using next-generation sequencing with a 25-gene panel. *Cancer* 121: 25–33.

Walsh, T., Casadei, S., Lee, M.K., Pennil, C.C., Nord, A.S., Thornton, A.M. et al. (2011). Mutations in 12 genes for inherited ovarian, fallopian tube, and peritoneal carcinoma identified by massively parallel sequencing. *Proc Natl Acad Sci USA* 108: 18032–18037.

Weischer, M., Bojesen, S.E., Ellervik, C., Tybjaerg-Hansen, A., and Nordestgaard, B.G. (2008 February 1). CHEK2*1100delC genotyping for clinical assessment of breast cancer risk: meta-analyses of 26,000 patient cases and 27,000 controls. *J Clin Oncol* 26 (4): 542–548. doi: 10.1200/JCO.2007.12.5922. Epub 2008 Jan 2. PMID: 18172190.

47

Hereditary Gastrointestinal and Pancreatic Cancer Syndromes

Kristen M. Shannon[1], Linda H. Rodgers-Fouche[1], and Daniel C. Chung[1,2]

[1] *Massachusetts General Hospital Cancer Center, Boston, MA*
[2] *Harvard Medical School, Boston, MA*

Introduction

Hereditary gastrointestinal (GI) and pancreatic cancer syndromes represent a phenotypically diverse group of disorders that exhibit distinct patterns of inheritance in an individual's progeny. Over the past few decades, the expansion of familial cancer registries and advancement in genomics have led to the development of clinical diagnostic criteria for specific hereditary syndromes as well as the discovery of multiple genes in which germline mutations predispose individuals to syndrome-associated neoplastic manifestations. Our chapter presents a series of case studies on genetic testing and management of hereditary gastrointestinal tumors. More specifically, we focus on genetic testing and management of hereditary gastric cancer, Lynch syndrome, familial adenomatous polyposis (FAP), attenuated familial adenomatous polyposis (AFAP), MUTYH-associated polyposis (MAP), syndrome X, constitutional mismatch repair deficiency (CMMRD), and hereditary pancreatic cancer. The topics of Peutz-Jeghers syndrome, juvenile polyposis syndrome, Cowden syndrome, and serrated (hyperplastic) polyposis syndrome are discussed elsewhere in this book in Chapters 18, 22, 23, 24, 45, and 46. The elements of informed consent that must accompany genetic evaluation as well as currently evolving genetic testing technologies are discussed in Chapter 45.

Case Study 1

A 76-year-old man undergoes hemicolectomy for colorectal adenocarcinoma. Immunohistochemistry (IHC) performed on his tumor demonstrates loss of MLH1 and PMS2 protein in the tumor sample. Genetic counseling reveals that he has no prior personal history of cancer and no family history of cancer.

1) What is the most likely reason for the absence of protein in the tumor?
   A) *MLH1* germline pathogenic variant.
   B) *PMS2* germline pathogenic variant.
   C) Hypermethylation of the *MLH1* gene promoter.
   D) *BRAF* pathogenic variant.

Cancer Consult: Expertise in Clinical Practice, Volume 1: Solid Tumors & Supportive Care,
Second Edition. Edited by Syed A. Abutalib, Maurie Markman, Al B. Benson III, and Hope S. Rugo.
© 2024 John Wiley & Sons Ltd. Published 2024 by John Wiley & Sons Ltd.

Expert Perspective: IHC to detect loss of DNA mismatch repair (MMR) protein expression is used to screen for Lynch syndrome. Lynch syndrome, or hereditary nonpolyposis colorectal cancer (HNPCC), is an inherited cancer syndrome characterized by early onset colorectal cancer as well as endometrial, urinary tract, small bowel, ovarian, gastric, pancreatic, hepatobiliary, brain, and skin tumors. Individuals with germline pathogenic variants in one of the MMR genes (*MLH1, MSH2, MSH6, PMS2*), or the *EpCAM* gene are defined as having Lynch syndrome. Nearly all colon tumors in individuals with Lynch syndrome will exhibit loss of expression of one or more of these DNA MMR genes as well as DNA microsatellite instability (MSI). The correlation between abnormal IHC and MSI results is generally good. Loss of expression of MLH1 is almost always accompanied by loss of PMS2 expression. This specific pattern can indicate the presence of a germline pathogenic variant in the *MLH1* gene but is also observed in approximately 15% of sporadic colorectal cancers due to nonheritable *MLH1* promoter hypermethylation. Thus, when *MLH1* and *PMS2* are absent on IHC, *MLH1* promoter methylation testing of the tumor sample helps to distinguish sporadic from hereditary tumors. In this case, the clinical phenotype of the patient is not suggestive of a diagnosis of Lynch syndrome (due to lack of family history of Lynch syndrome cancers and late age at diagnosis of cancer). Thus, it is more likely that his tumor is a sporadic tumor and that the loss of *MLH1* protein is due to somatic *MLH1* hypermethylation.

Correct Answer: C

Case Study 2

A 45-year-old man presents with five tubular adenomas on colonoscopy. His next colonoscopy one year later reveals an additional ten tubular adenomas. He has no family history of cancer or polyps.

2) Which genetic variants would be the most likely to explain his multiple polyps?
   A) *APC*.
   B) *MUTYH*.
   C) *MSH2, MLH1, MSH6,* and *PMS2*.
   D) Choices A and B.
   E) Choices B and C.
   F) Choices A, B, and C.

Expert Perspective: When a patient presents with multiple adenomas at an early age, one must consider the spectrum of inherited polyposis syndromes. The primary adenomatous polyposis syndromes are familial adenomatous polyposis (FAP), attenuated FAP (AFAP), or *MUTYH*-associated polyposis (MAP). FAP and AFAP are caused by pathogenic variants in the *APC* gene, and they are inherited in an autosomal dominant fashion. MUTYH-associated polyposis results from biallelic pathogenic variants in the *MUTYH* gene, and the syndrome is inherited in an autosomal recessive manner. If a patient with a suspected polyposis syndrome undergoes genetic testing and is not found to have an *APC* gene pathogenic variant, *MUTYH* gene testing should be performed to assess for MAP, as 10–20% of polyposis patients who do not have an *APC* gene pathogenic variant have biallelic *MUTYH* gene pathogenic variants. The clinical phenotype of MAP is often indistinguishable from FAP or AFAP. The typical polyp burden is usually 10–100 polyps, but sometimes more than 100 polyps can be seen. Family history often does not help to distinguish MAP from FAP. Consistent with the autosomal recessive inheritance pattern, there is often no family history of cancer in individuals with MAP. Of note, 20–25% of individuals with FAP–AFAP have the disease as the result of a *de novo* (new) *APC* gene pathogenic variant and therefore do not have a family history of the disease. Because of the inability to rely on family history for cases such as these, genetic testing for *APC* and *MUTYH* is often performed concurrently.

Correct Answer: D

Case Study 3

A 35-year-old, nulliparous woman is diagnosed with a germline pathogenic variant in the *MSH6* gene (Lynch syndrome).

3) What tumor is she most likely to develop in her lifetime?
   A) Colon cancer.
   B) Endometrial cancer.
   C) Stomach cancer.
   D) Ovarian cancer.

Expert Perspective: A germline pathogenic variant in any of the DNA mismatch repair genes (*MLH1*, *MSH2*, *MSH6*, *PMS2*, or *EpCAM*) establishes a diagnosis of Lynch syndrome, or hereditary nonpolyposis colorectal cancer (HNPCC). Individuals with Lynch syndrome are typically counseled that they have a 50–60% lifetime risk of developing colon cancer. However, colon cancer risk estimates are gene dependent and are notably lower for *MSH6* pathogenic variant carriers; the lifetime risk is estimated at 44% for males and 20% for females. Although *MSH6* pathogenic variants are associated with a lower risk for colon cancer when compared to *MLH1* or *MSH2*, females with *MSH6* pathogenic variants have a significantly increased (44%) risk for endometrial cancer (see Chapter 40). Thus, women with an *MSH6* pathogenic variant are more likely to develop endometrial cancer than colon cancer. It is essential to recognize the spectrum of extracolonic tumors that are associated with Lynch syndrome (see Chapters 45 and 46).

Correct Answer: B

Case Study 4

A 40-year-old female is diagnosed with gastric cancer. Pathologic exam reveals signet ring cells (diffuse gastric cancer). Her family history is significant for a mother with breast cancer (lobular type) diagnosed at age 45 and a father with colon cancer at age 70.

4) **Which gene would you be most concerned about?**
   A) *BRCA1/2*.
   B) Lynch syndrome.
   C) *CDH1*.
   D) *APC*.

Expert Perspective: Diffuse gastric cancers can occur in the setting of the hereditary diffuse gastric cancer (HDGC) syndrome, an autosomal dominant condition caused by an underlying germline pathogenic variant in the *CDH1* (E-cadherin) gene. The lifetime risk of diffuse gastric cancer is estimated to be as high as 70%, and women have up to a 40% lifetime risk of lobular breast cancer. Prophylactic total gastrectomy is considered the standard of care, as microscopic foci of signet ring cancer cells are identified in over 90% of gene carriers. The age at which to perform gastrectomy is not standardized, but consideration should start in the early 20s. The median age of clinically detectable gastric cancer is 38 years. *CDH1* testing identifies fewer than half of individuals with pathogenic variants who fulfil the following International Gastric Cancer Linkage Consortium (IGCLC) criteria: (i) any family with two or more documented cases of diffuse gastric cancer in first- or second-degree relatives with one case under the age of 50, or (ii) three documented diffuse gastric cancers in first- or second-degree relatives at any age. In the absence of a positive *CDH1* gene test, prophylactic gastrectomy is generally not recommended. Because conventional mammography may not be sensitive for lobular breast cancers, MRI or prophylactic mastectomy should be offered. Several other hereditary syndromes are associated with an increased risk for gastric cancer (Lynch, Li–Fraumeni, and Peutz–Jeghers), but the gastric cancers seen are typically intestinal-type cancers and not diffuse gastric cancers (see Chapters 20 and 21).

Correct Answer: C

Case Study 5

A 25-year-old woman presents with the family history shown in Figure 47.1. Her father is known to carry a pathogenic variant in the *MSH2* gene. Your patient tests negative for the familial mutation.

5) **What is the appropriate approach for her cancer screening?**
   A) Increased surveillance for colon cancer.
   B) Increased surveillance for all Lynch-associated tumors.
   C) Surveillance as if she has general-population risks for cancer.

Expert Perspective: In a family where a Lynch syndrome pathogenic variant (e.g. *MSH2* pathogenic variant) has already been identified, a negative test in a blood relative may be considered a true negative. This means that the person does not have the high risks

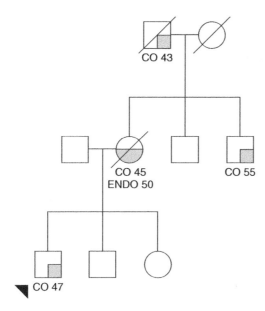

Key
squares, males
circles, females
arrowhead indicates proband
CO, colon cancer
current ages as well as ages of diagnosis of cancer are indicated
ENDO, endometrial cancer
MSH2+, positive for germline MSH2 mutation
MSH2–, negative for germline MSH2 mutation

Figure 47.1 Pedigree for Case Study 5.

for developing cancer associated with Lynch syndrome. However, since cancer is a common disease and most cancers have no known cause, a negative genetic test does not provide any assurance that a person will not develop cancer in his or her lifetime. In this case, the chances of developing cancer are like those of the average woman. It is important to note that other risk factors may become more important contributors. For that reason, she must review her personal medical history (e.g. whether she has a prior history of colon adenomas) with her physicians and be followed accordingly.

Correct Answer: C

Case Study 6

A male presents with a diagnosis of classic FAP. Genetic testing reveals a pathogenic variant in the *APC* gene. He has a seven-year-old daughter and eleven-year-old son.

6) In accordance with most other hereditary cancer syndromes, should genetic testing be deferred until his children reach adulthood?

Expert Perspective: No. Experts agree that genetic testing of children for inherited cancer syndromes needs to be considered carefully. Before testing of children can be performed, there must be some potential benefit from the testing that can be viewed as outweighing the disadvantages of testing. Since most inherited cancer predisposition syndromes are considered adult-onset diseases (i.e., predisposing to cancer in adulthood), most concede that genetic testing of minors should be deferred until adulthood. However, the classic form of FAP is an exception to this general rule.

In classic FAP, hundreds to thousands of polyps can develop in the colon. These polyps often begin to develop by the age of 12 years (range: 7–36 years). Colonoscopy to screen for colonic polyps every one to two years should begin at age 10–12 years, or 10 years before the earliest cancer diagnosis in the family, whichever is earlier. Because intervention with colonoscopy would begin at age 10, genetic testing at that age is indicated so that those children who do not have the familial *APC* pathogenic variant can avoid the costly and invasive procedure. Genetic testing in infancy may also be considered. The risk for childhood hepatoblastoma in FAP is 750 to 7,500 times higher than in the general population, although the absolute risk is estimated at less than 2%. Although no screening recommendations for hepatoblastoma have been standardized for children with FAP, screening may be considered every three months from infancy to age four or five years.

Case Study 7

A 30-year-old male presents with carpeting of adenomatous polyps in his colon. Genetic testing reveals a pathogenic variant in the *APC* gene.

7) **Which is he at higher risk for other than colon cancer?**
   A) Duodenal or ampullary cancer.
   B) Thyroid cancer.
   C) Desmoid tumors.
   D) All of the above.

Expert Perspective: The FAP syndrome results from a germline pathogenic variant in the *APC* tumor suppressor gene. This is associated with diffuse colonic polyposis and a nearly 100% risk of colon cancer without prophylactic colectomy. Following colectomy, it is important to recognize the risks of other extracolonic cancers that will require lifelong surveillance. Duodenal adenomas develop in up to 90% of FAP patients, and there is a lifetime risk of 10% of duodenal cancer. The ampulla and periampullary regions are particularly susceptible. Duodenal cancer is the second leading cause of cancer-related deaths in FAP. Papillary thyroid cancer is observed in as many as 12% of FAP families. We recommend upper endoscopy with a side-viewing examination of the duodenum at the time of colectomy or by age 30 and then at one-to-three-year intervals depending upon the findings. Thyroid ultrasound examinations should be performed every one-to-two years once the diagnosis of FAP is established. Clinically significant intra-abdominal desmoids tumors are seen in approximately 10% of FAP patients, and these typically occur postoperatively (see Chapters 4 and 44).

Correct Answer: D

Case Study 8

A 35-year-old male presents with fifty adenomatous polyps on colonoscopy. Genetic testing reveals that he has MUTYH-associated polyposis (MAP).

8) What is the risk to his siblings for also having MAP?
   A) 50%.
   B) 33%.
   C) 100%.
   D) 25%.

Expert Perspective: MUTYH-associated polyposis (MAP) is a recognized form of inherited colonic polyposis. The key distinguishing feature when compared to FAP is that MAP is inherited in an autosomal recessive manner. Consequently, an affected individual may not have a compelling family history of polyposis or colon cancer in his or her parents. Each parent is typically a heterozygous carrier of an *MUTYH* allele, and there is a 25% chance that a child will inherit a mutant *MUTYH* allele from both parents. The management mirrors that for FAP. The spectrum of extracolonic manifestations of MAP is being defined, and, like FAP, upper intestinal polyps are frequently observed. There are few reports of a higher incidence of breast cancer, but these require confirmation. The risk of colon cancer in heterozygous *MUTYH* carriers may be slightly increased (odds ratio 1.4), but this is not firmly established.

Correct Answer: D

Case Study 9

A 45-year-old female presents with adenocarcinoma of the colon. No colon polyps are seen. Her family history is depicted in the pedigree in Figure 47.2. MSI and IHC testing performed on the adenocarcinoma reveals an MSS (microsatellite stable) tumor with *MLH1, MSH2, MSH6,* and *PMS2* proteins present in the tumor.

9) What is the most likely diagnosis for this family?
   A) Lynch syndrome.
   B) *MUTYH*-associated polyposis.
   C) Syndrome X.
   D) Attenuated familial adenomatous polyposis.

Expert Perspective: A subset of families with a strong history of colon cancer in the absence of polyposis and MSI has been recognized. These families do not have Lynch syndrome or a polyposis syndrome and have been tentatively designated "syndrome X." The genetic basis of syndrome X remains elusive. A working clinical definition for syndrome X entails the fulfilment of the Amsterdam criteria with the absence of MSI. It is estimated that the colon cancer risks associated with syndrome X are not as high as with Lynch syndrome, and surveillance is recommended at three-to-five-year intervals. Exclusion of Lynch syndrome is critical in the evaluation of these families, and this can

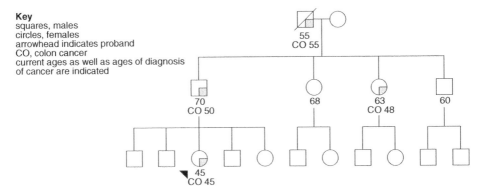

Figure 47.2 Pedigree for Case Study 9.

be accomplished by a combination of MSI testing, IHC staining for DNA mismatch repair proteins, and/or germline genetic testing. Importantly, there does not appear to be an increased risk of extracolonic malignancies as seen in Lynch syndrome. Enrollment of such families into registries is recommended.

Correct Answer: C

Case Study 10

A 13-year-old female with consanguineous parents presents with mucinous colorectal adenocarcinoma. IHC testing reveals absent *PMS2* staining on both tumor and normal tissue. Staining for *MSH2, MLH1*, and *MSH6* is preserved. There is no family history of colon cancer in either parent.

10) What is the most likely diagnosis for this patient?
   A) Li Fraumeni syndrome.
   B) Juvenile polyposis syndrome.
   C) Constitutional mismatch repair deficiency.
   D) Lynch syndrome.

Expert Perspective: Constitutional mismatch repair deficiency (CMMRD) syndrome follows an autosomal recessive inheritance pattern and is due to biallelic loss of any of the mismatch repair genes: *MLH1, MSH2, MSH6, PMS2*. CMMRD syndrome differs from Lynch syndrome, which results from heterozygous loss of an MMR gene and is autosomal dominant. CMMRD syndrome is a more aggressive cancer predisposition with younger onset and a wider spectrum of cancer risk. Individuals are at risk for hematological malignancies, brain, and other CNS tumors, as well as the gastrointestinal cancers typically observed in LS. Patients with CMMRD syndrome may also present with non-cancerous features such as café-au-lait macules (CALMs). Therefore, many patients with CMMRD have been previously misdiagnosed as having neurofibromatosis type 1. Parents of individuals with CMMRD syndrome likely have Lynch syndrome, although *de novo* cases have been reported. Affected individuals most commonly carry homozygous pathogenic variants in *PMS2*, and there is often a weak family history of cancer because of the low cancer risks in heterozygous *PMS2* carriers. Siblings of individuals with CMMRD syndrome have a 25% risk for CMMRD, a 50% risk for Lynch syndrome (if both parents have Lynch syndrome), and a 25% chance of harboring neither syndrome. Determining whether family members have CMMRD or Lynch syndrome will significantly change their medical care. For those with CMMRD, surveillance for hematological and brain tumors may begin as early as one or two years of age, and GI cancer screening may begin as early as eight to ten years of age. Relatives with Lynch syndrome typically begin screening age 20–25.

Correct Answer: C

Case Study 11

A 72-year-old male presents with adenocarcinoma of the sigmoid colon. IHC testing reveals absent MSH2 and MSH6 expression, and germline genetic testing for all Lynch syndrome genes (*MLH1, MSH2, MSH6, PMS2, and EPCAM*) is negative. The patient has no prior history of colon polyps. There is no family history of GI cancers.

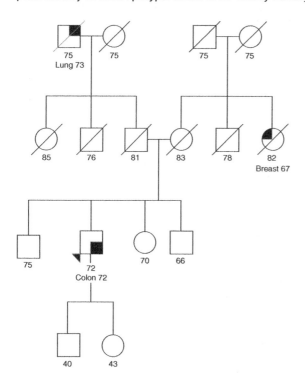

11) What is the most likely explanation for deficient mismatch repair expression?
    A) Undetectable germline *MSH2* pathogenic variant.
    B) Undetectable germline *MSH6* pathogenic variant.

C) Somatic *MSH2* pathogenic variant.
D) Somatic *MSH6* pathogenic variant.

Expert Perspective: Although it was once believed that individuals with deficient MMR tumors and negative germline genetic testing had Lynch syndrome due to an undetected germline pathogenic variant, a growing body of evidence suggests close to half of these cases are due to double somatic pathogenic variants in the MMR genes (either two sequence variants or one sequence variant with loss of heterozygosity). Individuals with double somatic MMR pathogenic variants are less likely to have the features typically observed in Lynch syndrome families (e.g. younger age at diagnosis, family history meeting Amsterdam criteria, right-sided colorectal cancers). The underlying cause of double somatic MMR pathogenic variants remains unclear. However, the cause does not appear to be heritable, and family members are not expected to be at high risk for cancer. When double somatic mutations are identified, patients and relatives' cancer surveillance and prevention recommendations should be based on the family history and not on a presumptive diagnosis of Lynch syndrome. If the personal and/or family history is suggestive of an underlying hereditary cancer syndrome, germline genetic testing for other colorectal cancer predisposition genes should be considered (e.g. *APC, MUTYH, POLE, POLD1*). Patients with MMR-deficient tumors, regardless of etiology, may still benefit from anti PD-1/PD-L1 therapies (see Chapters 22, 23, and 24).

Correct Answer: C

Case Study 12

A 67-year-old male patient presents with pancreas adenocarcinoma and seeks genetic testing. His mother was diagnosed with breast cancer at age 88, and his maternal uncle was diagnosed with melanoma at age 77. His family history is also significant for a paternal uncle with prostate cancer at age 60 and a paternal cousin with breast cancer diagnosed at age 42.

12) **What are the most appropriate germline tests to order?**
    A) Genetic testing for *BRCA1* and *BRCA2*.
    B) Genetic testing for *BRCA1*, *BRCA2*, and *CDKN2A*.
    C) Genetic testing for *BRCA2* and *CDH1*.
    D) Genetic testing panel that includes at least *APC, ATM, BRCA1, BRCA2, CDKN2A*, Lynch syndrome genes, *PALB2, STK11*, and *TP53*.

Expert Perspective: Up to 10% of pancreatic cancer cases arise due to an inherited risk. Numerous genes have been identified that increase the risk for pancreatic cancer, and some of these genes are linked to well-known hereditary cancer syndromes that increase the risk for other cancers as well. Gene panel testing is the most efficient way of determining if an individual with pancreas cancer has a hereditary cause to his/her cancer. Table 47.1 displays genes that are considered in individuals with suspected hereditary pancreatic cancer (see Chapter 28).

Correct Answer: D

Table 47.1 Hereditary pancreatic cancer genes and syndromes.

Gene(s)	Cancer(s)	Syndrome Name	Estimated Lifetime Risk of Pancreatic Cancer
APC	Colorectal, adenomatous polyps, pancreas	Familial adenomatous polyposis	2–4%
ATM	Breast, pancreas		~5–10%
BRCA1 and BRCA2	Breast, ovary, prostate, pancreas	Hereditary breast and ovarian cancer	Up to 5–10%
CDKN2A (p16)	Melanoma, pancreas	Familial atypical multiple mole melanoma	> 15%
MLH1, MSH2, MSH6, PMS2 and EPCAM	Colorectal, endometrial, ovarian, stomach, pancreas	Lynch syndrome, or hereditary non-polyposis colorectal cancer	1–6%
PALB2	Breast, pancreas		5–10%
STK11	Small bowel, breast, gastric, ovary, pancreas	Peutz-Jeghers syndrome	11–36%
TP53 (p53)	Breast, bone, brain, adrenal cortical, lung, colon, and others	Li-Fraumeni syndrome	5–10%

The risk of pancreatic cancer in the general population is about 1.6%.

Recommended Readings

Bedeir, A. and Krasinskas, A.M. (2011). Molecular diagnostics of colorectal cancer. *Arch Pathol Lab Med* 135 (5): 578–587.

Boland, C.R. and Goel, A. (2010). Microsatellite instability in colorectal cancer. *Gastroenterology* 138 (6): 2073–2087.

Boland, P.M., Yurgelun, M.B., and Boland, C.R. (2018 May). Recent progress in Lynch syndrome and other familial colorectal cancer syndromes. *CA Cancer J Clin* 68 (3): 217–231. doi: 10.3322/caac.21448. Epub 2018 Feb 27. PMID: 29485237; PMCID: PMC5980692.

Curia, M.C., Catalano, T., and Aceto, G.M. (2020 July 24). MUTYH: not just polyposis. *World J Clin Oncol* 11 (7): 428–449. doi: 10.5306/wjco.v11.i7.428. PMID: 32821650; PMCID: PMC7407923.

Engel, C., Loeffler, M., Steinke, V. et al. (2012 December 10). Risks of less common cancers in proven mutation carriers with lynch syndrome. *J Clin Oncol* 30 (35): 4409–4415.

Gamble, L.A., Heller, T., and Davis, J.L. (2021 April 1). Hereditary diffuse gastric cancer syndrome and the role of CDH1: a review. *JAMA Surg* 156 (4): 387–392. doi: 10.1001/jamasurg.2020.6155. PMID: 33404644.

Kastrinos, F. (2022 January). Inherited gastrointestinal cancers and the role of genetic evaluation and testing. *Gastrointest Endosc Clin N Am* 32 (1): xv–xvi. doi: 10.1016/j.giec.2021.10.001. PMID: 34798991.

Kaurah, P., MacMillan, A., Boyd, N. et al. (2007). Founder and recurrent CDH1 mutations in families with hereditary diffuse gastric cancer. *JAMA* 297 (21): 2360–2372.

Moreira, L., Balaguer, F., Lindor, N. et al. (2012 October 17). Identification of Lynch syndrome among patients with colorectal cancer. *JAMA* 308 (15): 1555–1565.

Wimmer, K., Kratz, C.P., Vasen, H.F. et al. (2014 June). EU-consortium care for CMMRD (C4CMMRD). diagnostic criteria for constitutional mismatch repair deficiency syndrome: suggestions of the European consortium 'care for CMMRD' (C4CMMRD). *J Med Genet* 51(6):355–365. doi: 10.1136/jmedgenet-2014-102284. Epub 2014 Apr 15.

Part 10

Special Issues in Oncology

48

Cancer of Unknown Primary

Tony Greco

The Sarah Cannon Cancer Center and Research Institute/Tennessee Oncology, Nashville, TN

Introduction

Cancer of unknown primary (CUP) is a heterogeneous, enigmatic, relatively common clinical pathological syndrome composed of many different metastatic cancer types with clinically occult primaries. Although there are biologic differences, the main clinical difference in CUP versus metastasis from known primary sites appears to be the size of the primary. In recent years it has become critical to diagnose the cancer type/tissue of origin (ToO), and this is now possible in many patients by the combined use of immunohistochemistry, molecular cancer classifier assays, and clinical features. Our understanding of CUP has evolved, and many subsets are now considered responsive/favorable and benefit from various site-specific therapies, but for most patients this depends on recognition of their ToO. Integration of comprehensive molecular profiling once the cellular context is known is important to determine the appropriate/precise therapy for the metastatic cancer each patient harbors. As therapies for many advanced metastatic carcinomas have improved, including targeted drugs and immunotherapy the accurate ToO diagnosis and subsequent site-specific treatment of CUP patients is now frequently possible. The clinical response and outcomes of CUP patients once diagnosed with a ToO and treated with site-specific therapy appear to be similar to patients with their cognate known metastatic cancers. The era of precision/molecular medicine continues to offer promise for improved diagnosis and better therapy for patients with the CUP syndrome.

Case Study 1

A 40-year-old male patient presents to your clinic with back pain. Evaluation reveals a retroperitoneal mass and several small bilateral lung lesions. Fine needle aspiration biopsy of the retroperitoneal mass revealed a poorly differentiated carcinoma. Immunohistochemistry was not possible because of too few cells. Serum alpha fetoprotein and β-hCG were normal. Core needle biopsies were then obtained from the retroperitoneal mass

Cancer Consult: Expertise in Clinical Practice, Volume 1: Solid Tumors & Supportive Care,
Second Edition. Edited by Syed A. Abutalib, Maurie Markman, Al B. Benson III, and Hope S. Rugo.
© 2024 John Wiley & Sons Ltd. Published 2024 by John Wiley & Sons Ltd.

1) Which one of the following is indicated in this patient?
A) Bilateral testicular ultrasound.
B) Immunohistochemical staining for PLAP, OCT4, and CD30.
C) In the absence of a specific ToO diagnosis other than carcinoma, begin therapy with bleomycin-etoposide-cisplatin (BEP).
D) All of the above.

Expert Perspective: This patient likely has the extragonadal germ cell cancer syndrome and is a chemotherapy-responsive or favorable CUP subset. Only half of these patients have an elevated serum AFP or beta β-hCG. Immunohistochemical (IHC) positive staining particularly with OCT4, PLAP, and CD30 would support the diagnosis. Definitive diagnosis can be made in most patients by a molecular cancer classifier assay such as the 92-gene RT-PCR assay (CancerTYPE ID) or by FISH testing for the isochromosome of 12 usually found in germ cell carcinomas. Even without a definitive diagnosis, therapy of germ cell carcinoma in these patients is appropriate in this setting and potentially curable (also refer to Chapter 35).

Several subsets of CUP patients recognized many years ago based on clinical pathological features have been defined as treatable, or favorable, subsets. These patients do not have an anatomical primary site detected, but presumed, and therapy is given based on this presumption. After administration of site-specific therapies their prognosis is similar to metastatic cancers from known primaries of the same type. These subsets include: (i) midline carcinomas usually in young man, (ii) isolated axillary adenocarcinoma in women, (iii) serous peritoneal adenocarcinoma in women, (iv) neuroendocrine tumors, (v) squamous cell carcinomas in cervical lymph or inguinal lymph nodes, (vi) a small single metastatic site, and (vii) osteoblastic bone metastasis and/or elevated serum PSA in men. More recently other CUP favorable subsets with clinical/pathologic/molecular features of colorectal, lung, and kidney adenocarcinomas have been described. All these subsets represent about 40% of all CUP and data are still limited in the remaining 60%, which can be considered an unfavorable group, but likely contain many other treatable cancers.

Correct Answer: D

Case Study 2

A 59-year-old woman is being referred for ascites and diffuse abdominal discomfort. CT scans showed multiple peritoneal nodules and ascites. Physical examination revealed moderate ascites. Core biopsy of a peritoneal nodule showed a serous adenocarcinoma. Mammography was unremarkable. Serum CEA was 100 and Ca125 350. IHC stains revealed CK7 and PAX8 positive with TTF1, CK20, CDX2, ER, and GATA3 negative. A surgical procedure was discussed, but she refused.

2) What would be your next best step to managing the care of this woman with CUP and peritoneal carcinomatosis?
A) Positron-emission tomography (PET)-CT.
B) Magnetic resonance imaging (MRI) of both breasts.
C) Upper endoscopy and colonoscopy.
D) Treatment with paclitaxel and carboplatin.

Expert Perspective: Women with this presentation, particularly with serous adenocarcinoma, fall into a subset with a more favorable prognosis (refer to Question 2) and are managed for a presumed primary from the ovary, uterine tube, or primary peritoneal carcinoma (stage III). The immunohistochemical profile of the carcinoma also fits with a gynecologic carcinoma. These tumors, like known ovarian carcinoma, are more common in those with *BRCA1/2* germline mutations, which should be tested and may help direct maintenance therapy with a PARP inhibitor. Elevated markers are relatively nonspecific, but the Ca125 can be used to monitor therpay. These patients should be evaluated and treated like stage III ovarian carcinoma, and their outcomes are similar (also refer to Chapters 38 and 39).

Correct Answer: D

3) Which of the following statements about CUP is false?
   A) CUP is a clinical pathological syndrome defined by the presence of metastatic cancer in the absence of a clinically recognized anatomical primary site.
   B) CUP represents many different types of cancers with occult primary sites but with the capacity to metastasize.
   C) In autopsy series of CUP patients a primary site was found in about 75% but is likely considerably higher since very small primary sites within solid organs can easily be missed.
   D) CUP is rare, making up less than 1% of all metastatic carcinomas.

Expert Perspective: A practical working definition for CUP is a biopsy-proven metastatic cancer with no identifiable anatomical primary site/ToO detected by history; physical examination; chest radiography; complete blood count; chemistry panel; computed tomography (CT) of chest, abdomen, and pelvis; prostate-specific antigen (PSA) in men; and mammography in women. The fact that most primary sites are found at autopsy firmly supports the many cancer types that make up this syndrome and is strong evidence regarding the natural history of this syndrome. The precise cause of the CUP syndrome remains an enigma. The mechanism of how clinically occult invasive primary cancers produce clinically detectable metastasis remains to be explained but likely is caused by acquired genetic and/or epigenetic alterations in the cancer cells. CUP is relatively common representing about 2–3% of all metastatic cancers or about 50,000–75,000 patients per year in the United States. The exact incidence is not known but likely higher than reported since many CUP patients are arbitrarily assigned a specific primary/ToO based on the physician's or pathologist's clinical opinion despite the inability to determine an anatomical primary site. These cancers are often listed as specific cancer types rather than CUP in many tumor registries.

Correct Answer: D

4) What is the frequency of adenocarcinoma histology in CUP?
   A) 65%.
   B) 25%.
   C) 5%.
   D) 3%.

Expert Perspective: Adenocarcinoma is the most common light microscopic histology. About 65% of all CUP is either well-differentiated, moderately differentiated, or poorly differentiated adenocarcinoma. About 25% are poorly differentiated carcinoma with about 5% squamous cell carcinomas and 2–3% neuroendocrine tumors and 2–3% other lineages including melanoma, sarcoma, and lymphoma. The histologic diagnosis establishes a neoplasm, and communication between the oncologist and pathologist is critical since immunohistochemical staining and molecular studies are often indicated in individual patients. Clinical features, pathology, and molecular finding are used in concert to often determine the cancer type.

Correct Answer: A

Case Study 3

A 54-year-old man presents with mid thoracic back pain, which had worsened over several months. History and physical examination otherwise unremarkable, and bone scan shows multiple bone lesions consistent with metastasis; CT scans of his chest, abdomen, and pelvis show only multiple osteoblastic lesions. A serum PSA was 650, and an MRI of his prostate was normal. Core needle biopsy of a lower lumbar vertebral body revealed adenocarcinoma with IHC stains CK7 and CK 20 negative but PSA positive.

5) What is the next best step?
 A) FDG-PET scan.
 B) EGD and colonoscopy.
 C) Multiple core biopsies of the prostate.
 D) Treat the patient.

Expert Perspective: In men with CUP and osteoblastic metastasis, prostate adenocarcinoma should be highly suspected. An elevated PSA virtually makes the diagnosis and in this setting is stage IV prostate adenocarcinoma with a clinically occult primary site. Staging by TNM should be To (undectable primary) NoM1 prostate adenocarcinoma. Documenting an anatomical primary site by biopsy of the prostate has no therapeutic implications. Additional workup in this setting is unnecessary since the therapy will not be changed, and it is appropriate to begin treatment for metastatic prostate carcinoma. Prostate adenocarcinoma presenting as CUP is relatively rare and may also include lung lesions as well as pelvic, retroperitoneal, and/or cervical adenopathy. In men with CUP, serum PSA should always be a component of the evaluation. Most of these patients also have positive PSA staining of their biopsy specimen. In some cases, gene rearrangement of *TMPRSS2::ETS* is useful and diagnostic. As a single serum or tumor marker PSA is highly reliable, which is rare with any other single stain or serum tumor marker. If feasible, germ line genetic testing for *BRCA1/2* should be obtained since a PARP inhibitor may later be a therapeutic option (also refer to chapters 34, 45, and 46).

Correct Answer: D

Case Study 4

A 75-year-old female, a smoker since age 20, presented with a chronic non-productive cough, and a chest X-ray showed left hilar adenopathy. History and physical examination otherwise unremarkable except for rather severe COPD and requirement for low-dose oxygen. ECOG performance status is 2. A PET-CT scan showed increased uptake in the left hilar lesion measuring 2 × 3 cm and a right 3 cm adrenal lesion; no lung lesions were seen. Bronchoscopy was unremarkable but a transbronchial biopsy of the left hilar lesion showed adenocarcinoma and IHC stains revealed CK7 and TTF1 positive and CK 20 negative.

6) **What additional evaluation is necessary?**
   A) Serum thyroglobulin.
   B) Next-generation sequencing (NGS) of the biopsy or liquid/blood biopsy for circulating tumor DNA (ctDNA).
   C) PD-L1 stain of biopsy.
   D) All of the above.

Expert Perspective: Useful IHC stains in the workup for this patient included cytokeratin 7 and 20 and thyroid transcription factor-1 (TTF1). CK7+ and CK20− IHC is seen in salivary gland, thyroid, breast cancer, lung cancer, mesothelioma, serous ovarian, uterine adenocarcinoma, and pancreatic cancer. TTF1 is a nuclear transcription factor and is frequently found in adenocarcinomas of the lung (about 80%; napsin A is also often positive) but TTF1 is also consistently seen in thyroid carcinoma, which would invariably have an elevated serum thyroglobulin. In this setting adenocarcinoma from an occult/undectable lung primary is the diagnosis. TNM staging as To (undetectable primary) N1M1 lung adenocarcinoma is appropriate. Genetic markers should be sought from either next-generation sequencing of the biopsy specimen or blood liquid biopsy/ctDNA. There may be important genetic alterations, which can be treated by targeted drugs or immunotherapy. A PD-L1 stain should also be obtained.

Correct Answer: D
In this patient a PD-L1 stain was reported as 90% positive, but there was no remaining biopsy specimen to obtain NGS; a blood liquid biopsy/ctDNA revealed no actionable genetic abnormalities, but a tumor mutation burden (TMB) was 42 Muts/Mb.

7) **What therapy should be offered to this patient?**
   A) Low-dose empiric pemetrexed/carboplatin or paclitaxel/carboplatin.
   B) Radiotherapy to the left hilar and the right adrenal lesions.
   C) Pembrolizumab.
   D) Pemtrexed/carboplatin for two cycles with concurrent immunotherapy with ipilimumab/nivolumab.

Expert Perspective: Some oncologists would continue to consider this patient as CUP, otherwise not specified, best treated with empiric chemotherapy. There is a lack of absolute data for targeted therapies or immunotherapies for CUP even if the available information almost certainly identifies her cancer as a metastatic adenocarcinoma from the lung. This approach for patients with CUP who have otherwise a specific highly treatable ToO is illogical and likely would provide inferior therapy.

In her setting with substantial comorbidities, a performance status of 2 with a 90% PD-L1 tumor stain and a high TMB pembrolizumab as a single agent is the preferred therapy and offers the potential for good control of her metastatic disease.

Correct Answer: C

Case Study 5

A 64-year-old man presented with pain in his left upper leg for six weeks. History and physical examination unremarkable except he had a mild limp favoring his left leg. Plain X-rays of the left hip and femur revealed a small lytic lesion in the mid shaft of the femur. CT scans of his chest/abdomen/pelvis/left femur revealed a retroperitoneal mass, paratracheal adenopathy, scattered bilateral small lung nodules, and the small lytic lesion in the left femur. All his blood work including a PSA were normal. He underwent core needle biopsies of the retroperitoneal mass revealing a poorly differentiated carcinoma with IHC CK7. CK 20, TTF1, and CDX2 negative but epithelial markers EMA, CK AE1/AE3 positive. Other than confirming a carcinoma the origin of the cancer was unknown. A 92-gene RT-PCR was performed on the biopsy specimen and revealed a 96% probability of renal cell carcinoma-clear cell type.

8) **How can this this cancer type be substantiated/confirmed?**
   A) PET scan.
   B) MRI of both kidneys.
   C) Urine cytology.
   D) IHC stains for renal cell carcinoma antigen (RCC) and PAX8 on the biopsy specimen.

Expert Perspective: This patient very likely has stage IV renal cell carcinoma with an occult primary. TNM staging as To (undetectable primary) N3M1 renal cell carcinoma is appropriate. The renal subset of CUP is now being increasingly recognized as a more favorable subset since metastatic renal cell carcinoma can often be successfully treated with several therapies including immunotherapy. IHC can often highly suggest the diagnosis, but in many instances relatively specific IHC stains for renal cell are not done initially since this diagnosis is not usually suspected and it is not possible to do an exhaustive IHC workup since there are hundreds of different stains and limited tissue. Many physicians believe that if the kidneys look normal on PET-CT or MRI, then the patient cannot have renal carcinoma. This is a common feeling about CUP from many occult primary sites but is not true since the primary site is too small to clinically detect. The 92-gene RT-PCR molecular profiling assay made a diagnosis with high probability of renal cell carcinoma. Renal cell carcinoma can be confirmed by several directed IHC stains of the biopsy specimen. There are now data showing that the renal cell subset of CUP responds similarly to known metastatic renal cell carcinoma (see Chapter 30).

Correct Answer: D

Case Study 6

A 61-year-old woman presented with right chest pain increased with deep breathing and mild shortness of breath. History and physical examination were normal other than dullness and decreased breath sounds at the right base of her lung. CT scans of chest/abdomen/pelvis revealed only a right moderate size pleural effusion. A thoracentesis and pleural biopsy were obtained revealing a poorly differentiated neoplasm felt to be a carcinoma. IHC showed CK7 positive but TTF1 negative. There was only a small amount of biopsy specimen remaining. Bronchoscopy and bilateral mammography were unremarkable.

9) Which one of the following statements is false?
   A) The cause for this pleural effusion is most likely an underlying mesothelioma.
   B) Chest tube drainage and pleurodesis may provide symptomatic relief.
   C) A molecular cancer classifier assay/ToO assay such as the 92-gene RT-PCR (CancerTYPE ID) performed on the biopsy specimen and requiring only a small number of cancer cells may be useful in determining the ToO.
   D) A battery of IHC stains done on the biopsy can often be very useful in defining the occult tumor if there is enough biopsy specimen remaining.

Expert Perspective: Isolated pleural effusions are most often adenocarcinomas with primary lung being the most common carcinoma, although mesothelioma may be difficult to differentiate. Chest tube drainage and pleurodesis may be useful for the patient. In mesothelioma IHC staining is often positive for calretinin, WT1, and CK5/6; in lung adenocarcinoma CK7, TTF-1, and napsin A are often positive. Metastasis from other occult primary sites is possible including breast—usually positive for either ER/PR/GCDFP-15 or GATA3 (Table 48.1). There

Table 48.1 Immunohistochemistry stain patterns and cancer types.[†]

Immunohistochemistry stain patterns	Possible cancer types
CK7 +/CK20 +	Mucinous ovary (can be CK20−), pancreatic (CK17+ and CDX2+), biliary, and transitional cell
CK7 +/CK20−	Adenocarcinoma lung (napsin A, mucicarmine, PAS-D+), breast (gross cystic fluid protein 15, epithelial stains+, GATA 3+, mammaglobin+), thyroid (TTF-1+ and thyroglobulin+), mesothelioma, uterine, ovary, salivary gland, embryonal, serous ovary, endocervical adenocarcinoma
CK7−/CK20 +	Colon (can be CK7+; also, CDX2+) and Merkel
CK7−/CK20−	Esophageal, small cell lung, squamous lung (desmoglein+, p40+, CK5/6+ and p63+), H&N, prostate, hepatocellular (AFP, CEA, glypican 3 and Hep par 1), adrenal, testicular (CD30, SALL4, and PLAP+) and renal (can be CK7+; CAM 5.2, Pax-8, Pan keratin, vimentin, CD 10)
HMB45, SOX10 and S100	Melanoma
Mesothelin	Mesothelioma (calretinin, D2-40, and WT1+), peritoneal (calretinin D2-40, WT1+) and ovary

[†] See text for details.

may not be enough biopsy material in this patient to obtain all the IHC, and the molecular classifier (92-gene RT-PCR assay) requires only about 300 viable cancer cells and frequently can make the correct ToO diagnosis (see Chapter 9).

Correct Answer: A

10) What is the utility of FDG-PET in evaluation of CUP?

Expert Perspective: PET-CT is not indicated in the evaluation of all CUP patients. The only direct comparison with good quality intravenous contrast CT scans of the chest/abdomen/pelvis with PET-CT showed no difference in finding a primary site, although PET was more sensitive in finding other metastasis. There are a few exceptions where PET-CT are indicated including patients who present with isolated neck or inguinal squamous cell carcinoma. In these instances, PET-CT has been shown to find the primary site rather frequently and may affect the use of definitive radiotherapy and/or surgery. In patients who present with a single small clinically isolated metastasis PET-CT may be important in finding other lesions, which would influence the choice of therapy. Occasionally in patients with predominant bone metastasis PET-CT may be superior and less expensive than the combination of CT scans and MRI to evaluate response.

11) What is the utility of tissue of origin (ToO) molecular profiling in evaluation of CUP?

Expert Perspective: CUP is not a single cancer type, and each patient has a specific cancer and therapy is indicated for their cancer type. ToO molecular profiling is useful and complements standard pathology and when combined with clinical features often accurately predicts the primary site in CUP. ToO molecular profiling appears superior to IHC in comparative studies of known cancers, but when IHC panels of stains are highly suggestive/diagnostic of a single ToO, molecular profiling to determine the cancer type/ToO is not necessary. The use of ToO molecular profiling assays on a biopsy specimen has been proven to be relatively accurate (about 85–90% of the time) when tested on patients with known cancer types. Although it is more difficult in CUP patients to validate the accuracy of ToO accuracy, there is now strong circumstantial evidence that a molecular profiling assay (92-gene RT-PCR) can usually accurately diagnose the ToO. This has become very important, particularly in the last several years, since many advanced cancers are now more treatable with improved chemotherapy regimens, targeted drugs, and immunotherapy. Data are accumulating in CUP patients of the value of NGS on biopsies or liquid biopsies when integrated into the evaluation, particularly when the cellular context/ToO is initially determined. These NGS results are expected to be similar in CUP patients once the ToO is determined. Outcomes are better for patients with cancers known to be responsive to site-specific therapies, and NGS or ctDNA is often indicated to determine optimal precision therapy.

12) What are these data with regards to outcomes of CUP patients treated with site - specific therapies based on ToO molecular profiling?

Expert Perspective: There remains debate of whether the outcome of CUP patients is improved by site specific treatment based on ToO molecular profiling. Although several prospective phase 2 and retrospective studies support an improved outcome with site specific therapy for some patients based upon the molecular diagnosis of the cancer type/ToO, only one large phase 3 randomized prospective trial is available which compared site specific therapy based on a molecular assay diagnosis verses empiric chemotherapy (gemcitabine-cisplatin). This study was designed more than a decade ago before most targeted therapies and immunotherapy were available for patients with specific cancer diagnoses. Results of this trial did not reveal any progression-free survival benefit for site specific treatment in all patients. The majority (about 75%) of patients entered in this study were molecularly diagnosed with relatively unresponsive advanced pancreaticobiliary carcinomas or metastatic squamous cell carcinomas and would not be expected to benefit from site specific treatment versus empiric chemotherapy with gemcitabine/cisplatin. However, a minority with molecular diagnoses of more treatable cancer types not expected to respond well to gemcitabine-cisplatin revealed a notable improvement in survival at 2 years compared to empiric chemotherapy (24% versus 10%) but due to the small numbers was not statistically evaluable. Additional prospective studies with the use of immunotherapies and targeted therapies particularly in sensitive tumor types are indicated.

One ongoing study (CUPISCO PHASE II) has an accrual goal of 790 CUP patients. This study requires comprehensive genetic profiling of tissue and/or blood and all patients are then treated with 3 cycles of induction empiric chemotherapy. Those who have a response or stable disease are randomly allocated 3:1 to receive targeted therapies or immunotherapy based upon their mutation profile or to continue additional cycles of induction chemotherapy. Those who have progressive disease to induction chemotherapy will have the opportunity to receive targeted therapies or immunotherapies depending on their comprehensive genetic profiling findings. This study incorporates comprehensive genetic profiling and therapy based upon the results may extend progression-free survival or overall survival for these patients. It is expected that many patients will not have a druggable target or be expected to respond to immunotherapy, thus the requirement for a large patient accrual. This study does not attempt to determine the cancer type/ToO initially which would be much more logical prior to integrating comprehensive profiling, but hopefully the results will be positive for those eventually also receiving targeted drugs or immunotherapy.

Case Study 7

A 58-year-old woman presented with right upper quadrant abdominal pain. Physical examination showed hepatomegaly. A CT scan of her abdomen and pelvis revealed multiple and diffuse liver lesions. CT scan of her chest and mammography were unremarkable. Stool was positive for occult blood. Core needle biopsies of a liver lesion revealed well-differentiated adenocarcinoma. IHC showed CK7 positive but CK 20, TTF1, CDX2, Hep-Par1, arginase1, GATA3, and ER were negative. Serum CA 19–9 and alpha fetoprotein were normal, but CEA was 100. EGD and colonoscopy were unremarkable. The pathologist felt that this was metastatic adenocarcinoma to the liver from an extrahepatic site. A 92-gene RT-PCR ToO assay performed on the biopsy specimen revealed 90% probability of cholangiocarcinoma but could not exclude gallbladder, pancreatic, or GE junction/gastric adenocarcinomas.

13) How can the diagnosis of cholangiocarcinoma be confirmed in this patient?
   A) There are no confirmatory tests.
   B) ERCP with contrast studies of the biliary tract.
   C) Albumin *in situ* hybridization of the biopsy specimen.
   D) Repeat core biopsy of a liver lesion with re-review of the histology.

Expert Perspective: Most adenocarcinoma in the liver are metastatic from an extrahepatic primary site. It is difficult to differentiate primary advanced intrahepatic cholangiocarcinoma from adenocarcinomas metastatic to the liver. Cholangiocarcinoma is frequently misdiagnosed as metastatic adenocarcinoma to the liver from an extrahepatic primary. The diagnosis in this patient is consistent with cholangiocarcinoma and the ToO profiling assay, the CK7 positivity, and the clinical features support this diagnosis. An albumin *in situ* hybridization performed on the biopsy specimen may confirm the diagnosis of cholangiocarcinoma since this is almost always positive. It is also usually positive in hepatocellular carcinoma, but the findings in this patient make this diagnosis unlikely. Hemobilia is common in cholangiocarcinoma and likely accounts for the positive occult blood in the stool. ERCP is not likely to be useful to confirm the diagnosis since intra-biliary tract lesions are usually not seen with intrahepatic cholangiocarcinoma. Only rarely is a characteristic so-called histologic cholangiolar pattern seen, and there is no need for a repeat biopsy. NGS or ctDNA may reveal treatable targets such as a FGFR2 fusion seen in 15–20% of patients with cholangiocarcinoma (refer to Chapter 27).

Correct Answer: C

Recommended Readings

Greco, F.A. (2017). Diagnosis: improved diagnosis, therapy and outcomes for patients with CUP. *Nat Rev Clin Oncol* 14 (1): 5–6.

Greco, F.A. (2014). Cancer of unknown primary site: still an entity, a biologic mystery and a metastatic model. *Nat Rev Cancer* 14 (1): 3–4. doi: 10.1038/nrc3646.

Greco, F.A. and Hainsworth, J.D. (2015). Cancer of unknown primary site. In: *Cancer: Principles and Practice of Oncology* 10the (ed. V.T. DeVita Jr, T.S. Lawrence, and S.A. Rosenberg), 1720–1737. Philadelphia: Wolters Kluwer.

Greco, F.A. and Hainsworth, J.D. (2018). Renal cell carcinoma presenting as carcinoma of unknown primary site: recognition of a treatable patient subset. *Clin. Genitourin. Cancer.* 16: e893–e898.

Hainsworth, J.D. and Greco, F.A. (2014). Gene expression profiling in patients with carcinoma of unknown primary site: from translational research to standard of care. *Virchows Arch* 464: 390–402.

Hainsworth, J.D. and Greco, F.A. (2018). Cancer of unknown primary site: new treatment paradigms in the era of precision medicine. *American Society of Clinical Oncology Education Book* 38: 20–25.

Hainswoth, J.D. Rubin M.S. Spigel D.S et al. (2013). Molecular gene expression profiling to predict the tissue of origin and direct site specific therapy in patients with carcinoma of unknown primary site: a prospective trial of the sarah cannon research institute. *J. Clin. Oncol.* 31: 217–223.

Rassy, E. Parent, P. Lefort, F. Parent, P. et al. (2020). New rising entities in cancer of unknown primary: is there real therapeutic benefit? *Crit Rev Oncol. Hematol* 147: 102882.

Rassy, E. and Pavlidis, N. (2020). Progress in refining the clinical management of cancer of unknown primaryin the molecular era. *Nat Rev Clin Oncol* 17 (9): 541–554.

Selves, J.Long-Mira, E. Mathieu, M.C. et al. (2018). Immunohistochemistry for diagnosis of metastatic carcinomas of unknown primary site. *Cancers (Basel)* 10 (4): 108. doi: 10.3390/cancers10040108.

49

Anticoagulation in Cancer

Jean Marie Connors[1,2,3]

[1] Dana-Farber Cancer Institute, Boston, MA
[2] Brigham and Women's Hospital, Boston, MA
[3] Harvard Medical School, Boston, MA

Introduction

The association between cancer and thrombosis has been recognized for over 100 years. Patients with cancer-associated thrombosis have historically had an increased risk of both reccurent venous thromboembolism (VTE) and of bleeding with conventional anticoagulants compared to those with VTE without cancer. Despite major advances in both anticoagulant treatments and in the treatment of cancers these increased risks associated with anticoagulant therapy have not diminished. Many of the advances in cancer treatments, such as targeted therapies, immunomodulatory drugs, and immunotherapies, are associated with an increased risk of VTE, with a recent national database analysis finding an increasing cumulative risk of VTE every year for the past 10 years despite no change in the population baseline risk. In this chapter commonly encountered clinical questions about the management of VTE in patients with cancer will be addressed.

Case Study 1

A 54-year-old male presents with a worsening chronic cough. Chest imaging and subsequent needle biopsy reveal the presence of metastatic lung adenocarcinoma with an *EGFR* (epidermal growth factor receptor) mutation. The patient has no prior history of venous thromboembolism (VTE), remains active, and has a normal Body Mass Index (BMI) and complete blood count (CBC). Treatment is planned with osimertinib (FDA approved treatment of patients with *EGFR T790M* mutation-positive non-small cell lung cancer [NSCLC]).

1) **Is pharmacologic VTE prophylaxis indicated for this patient? If so, what is the preferred agent?**
    A) Yes, prophylactic low-molecular-weight heparin (LMWH)
    B) Yes, prophylactic apixaban
    C) Yes, prophylactic rivaroxaban
    B) No, prophylaxis is not indicated

Expert Perspective: The use of VTE prophylaxis in ambulatory cancer patients initiating chemotherapy has demonstrated efficacy in the past with trials of LMWH; however, while the relative risk reduction in VTE was roughly 50%, the absolute risk difference in unselected ambulatory cancer patients is small. Risk assessment scores have been developed to identify those patients at increased risk who might derive greater benefit from prophylaxis. The risk for a VTE event varies among patients. Data from a prospective observational study involving approximately 2,700 cancer patients were used to derive a risk model for VTE (shown in Table 49.1).

The study authors found that the total risk score correlated with VTE risk in a separate validation cohort. The incidence of VTE was 0.3% in low-risk patients (0 points), 2% in intermediate-risk patients (1–2 points), and 6.7% in high-risk patients (≥ 3 points) over a median of 2.5 months.

The baseline risk of VTE in each patient with cancer can be estimated using this straightforward metric.

Two studies have used the Khorana risk assessment score to select patients initiating systemic cancer treatments at increased risk for VTE with a score of 2 or greater and compared the use of a DOAC at prophylactic dose with placebo to prevent VTE.

- In the AVERT trial, only 4.2% of the apixaban 2.5 mg twice daily–treated patients experienced a VTE compared to 10.2% of placebo-treated patients in the intention-to-treat analysis, with similar effect in the per-protocol population (1% vs 7.3%).
- In the CASSINI trial, participants were screened with lower extremity ultrasound prior to randomization; 4.5% were found to have a leg deep venous thrombosis (DVT), exlcuding them from the trial. Results found that 5.9% of rivaroxaban 10 mg once daily–treated patients experienced VTE compared with 8.7% in the intention-to-treat analysis; per-protocol analysis found 2.6% VTE with rivaroxaban and 6.4% with placebo.

Both trials found approximately a doubling of major bleeding with either DOAC compared with placebo, although overall rates were low, at 3.5% with apixaban vs 1.8% with placebo in the AVERT trial and 1.0% with rivaroxaban vs 2.0% with placebo in the CASSINI trial.

Table 49.1 Khorana risk assessment score.

Patient characteristic	OR (95% CI)	Risk score
Stomach or pancreas site	4.3 (1.2–15.6)	2 points
Lung, lymphoma, GYN, bladder, or testicular site	1.5 (0.9–2.7)	1 point
Platelet count ≥ 350,000 per µL	1.8 (1.1–3.2)	1 point
Hemoglobin < 10 g/dL	2.4 (1.4–4.2)	1 point
WBC count > 11,000 per µL	2.2 (1.2–4)	1 point
BMI ≥ 35 kg/mg^2	2.5 (1.3–4.7)	1 point

BMI: Body Mass Index; CI: confidence interval; GYN: gynecological; OR: overall response; VTE: venous thromboembolism; WBC: white blood cell.
Source: Connors JM, "Venous Thromboembolism Prophylaxis in Ambulatory Cancer Patients." *New Engl J Med*. At Press. Copyright 2014 Massachusetts Medical Society. Reproduced with permission of the Massachusetts Medical Society.

Current NCCN, ASCO, ITAC, ASH and ESMO guidelines overall suggest the use of prophylaxis in patients with multiple myeloma on immunomodulatory drug therapy and suggest considering prophylaxis in those with other cancers and a Khorana risk score of 2 or greater starting a new chemotherapy regimen. We also use empiric prophylaxis for ambulatory patients treated with a history of prior unprovoked or life-threatening VTE or strong inherited thrombophilias (such as homozygous factor V Leiden).

The patient in this case has no past history of thrombosis and no other VTE risks. His Khorana risk score is 1 (intermediate risk), with a VTE incidence rate of 2%. Additional studies are needed to identify ambulatory cancer patients better prospectively at high risk for VTE who may benefit from such prophylactic anticoagulation.

Of importance, the efficacy and safety of prophylactic anticoagulation in the hospitalized cancer patient and in patients undergoing oncology surgery, who have a higher risk of postop VTE than non-oncology patients, have been clearly demonstrated. We have not covered these indications in this chapter. As in all situations where anticoagulation treatment is considered, the risks and benefits need to be carefully evaluated and understood for each individual patient.

Correct Answer: D

Case Study continued: After three months of treatment, restaging computed tomography (CT) scan is performed. Incidental pulmonary embolus is found in a right lower lobe segmental artery. Although the patient is fatigued and has an infrequent nonproductive cough, his heart rate is 85 beats per minute, his blood pressure is 128/72, and room air oxygen saturation is 96%. Brain natriuretic peptide is within normal limits, and there is no evidence of right heart strain on physical exam. CT also suggests a response to therapy, and plans are to continue with the current treatment regimen.

2) **Which of the following agents would be preferred for initial treatment of asymptomatic right lower lobe segmental artery thrombosis in a cancer patient?**
   A) Warfarin
   B) Intravenous (IV) unfractionated heparin (UFH)
   C) Dalteparin
   D) Any oral Xa inhibitor

Expert Perspective: This patient presents with an apparently asymptomatic pulmonary embolism (PE). In a retrospective study, however, 75% of cancer patients who were diagnosed with unexpected PE did in fact have symptoms, including fatigue and dyspnea, that had been previously attributed to the cancer or its treatment. Clinicians need to have a high index of suspicion for VTE in the evaluation of new symptoms in the cancer patient. Treatment of incidental VTE is warranted. A study comparing recurrent VTE, bleeding, and mortality rates in oncology patients with incidentally detected versus symptomatic PE found no difference in outcome for either group, suggesting that the incidental PE group had just as high a risk of adverse events associated with VTE as symptomatic patients. Regardless of symptoms, the presence of thrombus serves as an indicator for true hypercoagulable state. In our experience, when patients with asymptomatic VTE are observed and reimaged, there is a high rate of extension or development of new thrombus in other locations.

Initial treatment of acute VTE requires the use of rapid-acting agents to prevent clot propagation. Use of warfarin alone is associated with an unacceptably high rate of thrombus extension and is not appropriate initial therapy in this patient or any patient with acute VTE. Intravenous UFH, LMWH, fondaparinux, and the oral Xa inhibitors apixaban, edoxaban, and rivaroxaban have all been demonstrated to have good efficacy and safety in the initial treatment of VTE in the general population and in patients with cancer. LMWH has many pharmacokinetic advantages over UFH, including fixed weight-based dosing with no need for monitoring. LWMH was determined to be the first-line agent for treatment of cancer-associated VTE based on the CLOT trial, in which approximately 700 patients who were actively receiving chemotherapy were randomized to treatment with dalteparin 200 units/kg/day for one month followed by a decrease in dose to 150 units/kg/day for five months, or initial dalteparin for 5–7 days followed by warfarin for six months. The probability of recurrent VTE was 9% for those treated with dalteparin alone versus 17% for warfarin ($P = 0.002$). There was no difference in risk of bleeding.

3) Should this patient be hospitalized?

Expert Perspective: There would be no reason to hospitalize this ambulatory patient for treatment with UFH. Although the current standard of care of PE in many institutions is to admit patients for treatment and observation, we have found that many reliable patients who have an unexpected finding of PE can be treated in the outpatient setting. Clinical judgment incorporating an assessment of clot burden, degree of symptoms, oxygen saturation and hemodynamic function, and risk of bleeding can be used to determine the need for hospitalization. A meta-analysis of 13 studies with a total of 2,458 patients supports outpatient treatment in low-risk patients. Despite the use of different risk stratification schemes, the risk of recurrent VTE, fatal PE, and major bleeding was low.

4) How about a DOAC in this patient compared to LMWH?

Expert Perspective: Although LMWH has been the standard of care for initial treatment of cancer-associated VTE in ambulatory patients, recent studies of DOACs in cancer patients have resulted in guideline changes that now recommend apixaban, edoxaban, and rivaroxaban as first-line treatment as well as LMWH given the non-inferiority findings for the prevention of recurrent VTE with edoxaban, rivaroxaban, and apixaban in the large randomized clinical trials.

Edoxaban must be used following an initial five-day treatment of LMWH. Major bleeding was found to be higher with edoxaban and rivaroxaban compared to dalteparin, with subanalyses revealing that the increased risk is seen primarily in patients with GI tract cancers. Apixaban had no increased risk of major bleeding compared to daletparin. As this patient does not have a GI tract malignancy, any of the Xa inhibitor DOACs can be used. Drug-drug interactions with the use of these Xa inhibitor DOACs in patients with cancer need to be considered as certain antibiotics, antifungals, antivirals, and seizure medications can affect plasma concentrations of these oral anticoagulants. These interactions occur via p-glycoprotein transport in the case of edoxaban, or both p-glycoprotein and CYP3A4 for rivaroxaban and apixaban.

Guidelines from the American Society of Clinical Oncology (ASCO), National Comprehensive Cancer Network (NCCN), European Society for Medical Oncology (ESMO), and American College of Chest Physicians (ACCP) endorse the use of LMWH or the Xa inhibitor DOACs as monotherapy for six months in this population.

5) What are additional caveats using warfarin in cancer patients?

Expert Perspective: While oncology patients have sometimes had recurrent VTE on warfarin, warfarin management itself in this population is difficult due to drug–drug interactions, hepatotoxicity from chemotherapy, and absorption issues due to the significant gastrointestinal impact of chemotherapy. It should be noted that the CLOT trial had a warfarin time in therapeutic range (TTR) of only 46%, reflecting the management difficulty in this population. Most of the recurrent events occurred during the first month of anticoagulation treatment, when optimal warfarin dose is being defined. Almost half of the recurrent events in the warfarin arm occurred when the international normalized ratio (INR) was < 2.0, which may account for some of the differences seen between the treatment arms. For certain patients, however, transitioning to warfarin after initial therapy with LMWH may be appropriate or unavoidable.

The cost of LMWH and a DOAC can be prohibitive for many patients, and for those with creatinine clearance less than 30 mL/min, both LMWH and a DOAC should be used with caution.

Correct Answer: D

Case Study continued: After six months of treatment, this patient is hospitalized with acute kidney injury related to volume depletion and ibuprofen use. Recent restaging scans showed partial recanalization of segmental pulmonary emboli. Metastatic NSCLC remains at present, stable. Osimertinib is currently on hold for several months. Initial labs show a creatinine clearance of 15 mL/min, with normal platelet count.

6) What is the next best management strategy?
   A) Switch to enoxaparin 1 mg/kg once daily and monitor anti-Xa level
   B) Discontinue Xa inhibitor DOAC, and transition to warfarin
   C) Change to dabigatran
   D) Continue Xa inhibitor DOAC at therapeutic dose

Expert Perspective: Indefinite anticoagulation is indicated given the prior pulmonary embolus and chronic hypercoagulable state in the setting of metastatic malignancy. Discontinuing anticoagulation at this point has been shown to result in high recurrence rates. This patient may have a short-term increased risk of VTE given concurrent hospitalization.

The Xa inhibitor DOACs were evaluated in patients with creatinine clearance greater than or equal to 30 mL/min. All have some degree of renal clearance, and although apixaban has the least renal clearance, how to adjust the dose for renal insufficiency for the treatment of VTE is not known. LMWH is almost exclusively cleared by the kidneys, but there is guidance for monitoring with established anti-Xa levels. In this patient, there are two approaches that can be employed.

- One is to use LMWH at a decreased dose, with close monitoring and dose adjustment based on anti-Xa levels. The current creatinine clearance is borderline for this approach. (Choice A)
- Alternatively, one could transition to warfarin. This is the less preferred option since the patient is hospitalized. (Choice B)

While Xa inhibitor DOAC or LMWH are preferred for initial treatment of VTE in cancer patients, superiority for long-term treatment after six months has not been evaluated. Given this patient's impaired renal function and lack of ongoing chemotherapy, warfarin is also a valid option. Transitioning directly to warfarin can be accomplished without the need to continue a parenteral agent until therapeutic INR is reached, since the current goal in this patient of anticoagulation is secondary prevention of a new VTE event, not prevention of clot propagation. If the patient remains hospitalized, which increases his thrombotic risk, intravenous UFH bridge can be initiated.

Correct Answer: A

Case Study continued: The patient recovers but is readmitted two months later to the intensive care unit with persistent hemoptysis. INR on warfarin is 2.1. Anticoagulation is stopped and reversed. Lower-extremity Doppler ultrasound shows no evidence of DVT, and there is no new PE on chest CT.

7) **Is an inferior vena cava (IVC) filter indicated for secondary prophylaxis of pulmonary embolism?**

Expert Perspective: Unfortunately, this challenging scenario is commonly encountered in clinical practice. The patient has now developed a contraindication to anticoagulation but remains at risk of recurrent VTE. Improvements in IVC filter technology (such as the development of retrievable filters) make them more attractive, but data regarding efficacy are lacking. Only one randomized controlled trial of IVC filter use has been performed in any patient population, and patients in this study were also given full-intensity anticoagulation. Although there was a lower incidence of PE during the first 12 days following filter placement (1.1% vs 4.8%), there was a twofold increase in the rate of lower-extremity DVT in patients with filters at two years. After eight years, the filter group still demonstrated increased DVT rates and decreased PE rates, but there was no difference in mortality.

Studies of IVC filters in cancer patients are limited to retrospective case-control studies. Their use does not obviate the need for anticoagulation as the filter itself does not address the underlying hypercoagulable state. Overall, there are often increased complications, including increased rates of lower extremity DVT, with no demonstrated improvement in survival in oncology patients.

Case Study continued: In this patient, who has no lower extremity DVT, we would strongly advise against the use of an IVC filter as there is no evidence to support clinical benefit.

8) **When should IVC filter be considered in cancer patients?**

Expert Perspective: We reserve the use of IVC filters for those with acute DVT of the lower extremity in a large proximal thigh vein who have an absolute contraindication to anticoagulation, such as large untreated brain metastases or primary central nervous system (CNS) tumor, or for those with severely limited cardiac or pulmonary function in whom a new PE would truly be life-threatening. Other situations include perioperative retrievable filter placement in those patients with similar absolute contraindications to anticoagulation. Patients need to be continually reassessed for their ability to tolerate anticoagulation. Anticoagulation should be started as soon as practical to prevent development of lower-extremity DVT or filter thrombosis. Given lack of lower extremity DVT and no new PE, the use of prophylactic dose anticoagulation in this patient with hemoptysis can be considered to prevent VTE while minimizing risk of bleeding as he has already received months of therapeutic dose anticoagulation, although data for this approach are lacking. When anticoagulation is restarted, the IVC filter should also be removed. Retrieval of IVC filters has often been overlooked, with studies demonstrating at best an 8.5–18% retrieval rate. As the use of IVC filters has not been shown to improve survival and is in fact often associated with increased morbidity, the life expectancy of the cancer patient must also be considered before filter placement. For those with advanced-stage disease and short life expectancy, IVC filter placement may be an unnecessary intervention with a higher risk of harm than benefit.

Case Study 2

A 42-year-old woman is diagnosed with squamous cell carcinoma of the head and neck. Treatment is planned with combined radiation and chemotherapy with cisplatin. A port-a-cath is placed in the right internal jugular vein for venous access due to small peripheral veins. She presents one week later with right arm swelling. There is no evidence of compartment syndrome. Ultrasound demonstrates an occlusive right axillary vein thrombus.

9) Which of the following is the most appropriate next step in management?
   A) Start enoxaparin 1 mg/kg twice a day
   B) Remove port-a-cath immediately
   C) Start therapeutic Xa inhibitor DOAC
   D) A or C

Expert Perspective: Catheter-associated thrombosis is a known complication of central venous access devices. One prospective trial of approximately 440 oncology patients showed that 4.3% of patients with central lines developed catheter-associated thrombosis. Upon diagnosis of DVT, the first step is to reevaluate the indication for the line. In this case, the patient requires access for necessary chemotherapy. She has no known contraindication to anticoagulation. There is no clear evidence that early catheter removal in the absence of severe symptoms affects outcome. In one study of 74 patients with catheter-associated thrombosis, investigators were able to treat with anticoagulation and leave the line in place with low risk of line failure or of recurrence or extension of upper-extremity DVT.

Thus, in this case, we would favor initiation of anticoagulation with therapeutic LMWH or Xa inhibitor DOAC and would keep the line in place. In this patient consideration of ability to swallow oral medications needs to be considered, as many patients with head and neck cancer receiving concurrent chemotherapy and radiation therapy often require a PEG tube for feeding; in this case LMWH may be preferable, even though both apixaban and rivaroxaban can be crushed for administration through feeding tubes. If symptoms fail to improve within one to two weeks, then line removal can be considered. NCCN guidelines recommend anticoagulation for as long as the catheter is in place, with a minimum total of three months of therapy. Over time, patients with chronic central access catheters that are not routinely being used and are not on anticoagulation are at risk for superior vena cava syndrome due to thrombus or stenosis.

10) What is the role of central access catheter prophylaxis?

Expert Perspective: The question of routine central access catheter prophylaxis has been addressed in several studies, often with low-dose anticoagulation. Two meta-analyses have found conflicting results. Many individual studies were small, and different agents were used—including UFH, LMWH, and fixed low-dose warfarin. A randomized, placebo-controlled trial of dose-adjusted warfarin with target INR 1.5–2.0 in 174 patients found no evidence of efficacy.

At present, routine central access catheter thromboprophylaxis is not recommended for all patients. We reserve its use for patients with a history of significant thrombosis or strong inherited thrombophilia. Intensity (prophylaxis versus full intensity) is determined after assessment of the patient's baseline VTE and bleeding risks.

Correct Answer: D

Case Study continued: The patient begins therapeutic enoxaparin 1 mg/kg twice daily, and her arm swelling improves. However, after two weeks she refuses injections due to abdominal skin bruising and pain.

11) What recommendation should be made?
   A) Change to once daily fondaparinux
   B) Change to a Xa inhibitor DOAC
   C) Discontinue anticoagulation
   D) A or B

Expert Perspective: Subcutaneous hemorrhage and pain at injection sites are sometimes encountered in patients on LMWH. Patients should be taught proper injection technique, encouraged to use ice packs on the site after injection, and advised not to wipe the site with alcohol after the injection to minimize bruising. Other sites beside the abdomen can be used for injection, including the upper thigh, buttocks, and triceps areas. Patients can be instructed to insert just the tip of the needle into the skin, past the beveled edge but not to the hub of the syringe, to minimize trauma with injections.

Often, the above instructions combined with reassurance and counseling on the benefits of parenteral anticoagulation are sufficient for many patients to continue with LMWH. If these measures are unsuccessful, a change in therapy may be required. In our experience, fondaparinux is associated with less burning upon injection. The FDA approved once-daily administration of fondaparinux or dalteparin can often be better tolerated than the twice-daily dosing of enoxaparin. While enoxaparin 1.5 mg/kg daily is widely used in other settings, it has not been evaluated in the oncology population.

Xa inhibitor DOAC can be considered if not initially started, although patients with head and neck cancers have been underrepresented in the large phase III randomized control trials of DOAC in patients with cancer-associated VTE. Warfarin would not be the first choice given possible drug interactions with cisplatin and expected variations in nutritional status and the potential need for enteral support on this highly emetogenic chemotherapy regimen. Anticoagulation is required while the catheter remains in place.

Correct Answer: D

Case Study continued: The port-a-cath was removed after completing chemotherapy. Restaging scans at six months show no evidence of disease. An upper-extremity ultrasound shows continued right subclavian vein occlusion with collateral flow. Symptoms have resolved, and arm swelling is no longer present. D-dimer is < 500. The patient expresses a preference to stop anticoagulation if possible.

12) What recommendation should be made?
- A) Stop anticoagulation
- B) Continue anticoagulation indefinitely
- C) Data to support A or B choices are lacking

Expert Perspective: The patient appears to have developed chronic organized thrombus in the right subclavian vein despite six months of anticoagulation. The line has been removed, and planned cancer treatment is complete. The decision regarding cessation of anticoagulation should be made based on individual considerations of risk versus benefit, while incorporating patient preferences. In this case, the indication for extended anticoagulation is not definite. The provoking factors of cancer, chemotherapy, and central access catheter use are no longer present, and the patient has received adequate duration of anticoagulation therapy for the initial clot. There is no evidence of post-thrombotic syndrome, which might indicate a need for continued anticoagulation to prevent recurrent thrombus in the same arm. Stopping anticoagulation can be safely considered provided the patient is educated to contact a provider immediately for any new symptoms. Data to support either approach are lacking.

D-dimer measurement is not specifically validated for cancer patients with provoked VTE. Thus, treatment decisions should not be made based on the D-dimer value alone until prospectively validated in an oncology-specific population.

Correct Answer: C

Case Study 3

A 63-year-old woman with a history of metastatic pancreatic adenocarcinoma is found to have new occlusive right portal vein thrombosis on restaging scans at six weeks. Right upper quadrant ultrasound confirms the presence of thrombus with markedly decreased Doppler flow in the right portal vein. There is no evidence of cavernous transformation. She is currently on cycle 4 of weekly gemcitabine, and the tumor burden is stable. Recent mild transaminitis and right upper quadrant discomfort were previously attributed to chemotherapy. Platelet count is 90,000 per µL, and prothrombin time (PT) and activated PTT values are normal.

13) **What step should be taken next?**
    A) Start aspirin 325 mg daily
    B) Start apixaban 10 mg twice a day for seven days followed by 5 mg twice a day
    C) Start dalteparin 200 units/kg daily for one month followed by a decrease in dose to 150 units/kg/day for five months
    D) No treatment is required for an incidental portal vein clot

Expert Perspective: Patients with cirrhosis or underlying malignancy are at increased risk of portal vein thrombosis. The risk is further increased in the presence of inherited thrombophilias and myeloproliferative disorders (including *JAK2* mutations). Complete portal vein occlusion reduces the liver blood flow by up to two-thirds and is associated with hepatocyte apoptosis in animal models. Anticoagulation is indicated for the treatment of acute portal vein thrombosis to prevent clot extension and facilitate recanalization. In cancer patients, we view the development of any thrombosis as demonstration of a hypercoagulable state. With persistent malignancy and ongoing chemotherapy, this patient is at increased risk for extension of thrombus. Anticoagulation in this patient should prevent progression to complete thrombosis of the right portal vein and extension to the main portal vein and other splanchnic vessels.

The role of anticoagulation for management of chronic portal vein thrombosis is more controversial, particularly in patients with increased bleeding risk due to cirrhosis and esophageal varices; this is the patient population from which most of the data are derived. There is still controversy about the role of anticoagulation in this setting. We do not recommend anticoagulation for the cancer patient with clearly old thrombus and good collateral circulation.

In this patient, treatment with apixaban following the VTE treatment dose strategy can be used. Although pancreatic cancer is a GI tract malignancy, the Xa inhibitor DOAC can be considered for use if there is no intra-luminal GI tract tumor. Alternatively, use of therapeutic-dose dalteparin would also be acceptable.

Patients with a platelet count of 90,000 per µL can be safely anticoagulated unless there are other major contraindications to anticoagulation. The platlet thereshold for eligibility was 75,000 per µL for the phase III randomized control trials DOAC trials in patients with cancer-associated VTE. Generally accepted practice endorsed by ASCO, NCCN, ITAC, ASH and ACCP is to hold anticoagulation for platelet counts lower than 50,000 per µL; however, individual patient assessments have allowed us to continue anticoagulation with platelet counts down to 30,000 per µL. The severity and age of thrombus determine the importance of anticoagulation. In patients with severe persistent thrombocytopenia and new acute clot such as main pulmonary artery PE, platelet transfusion support may be necessary to allow anticoagulation treatment.

Correct Answer: B or C (While apixaban may be better tolerated, there is no difference in efficacy and major bleeding between apixaban and dalteparin as shown in the Caravaggio trial. Insurance cost may affect anticoagulation choice)

Case Study continued: The patient is started on therapeutic apixaban. Six weeks later, she develops right lower extremity swelling and pain. Lower extremity Doppler ultrasound reveals occlusive right femoral vein thrombosis. Neurologic exam remains normal.

14) **What step should be taken next?**
    A) Change to warfarin
    B) Add antiplatelet agent

C) Switch to LMWH at therapeutic dose
D) Place IVC filter

Expert Perspective: Oncology patients remain at increased risk of recurrent VTE, even while receiving effective anticoagulation. In the CLOT trial, this risk was 9% for the group treated with dalteparin over six months. There is no single optimal approach to management of recurrent VTE while on therapy. Patient compliance and effectiveness of medication administration need to be assessed. In patients who have recurrent VTE on a DOAC, difficulty with absorption, such as in the setting of nausea and vomiting, or drug-drug interactions that might decrease DOAC plasma concentration also needs to be considered.

Switching to LMWH is a reasonable next step after a recurrent VTE with DOAC treatment. If recurrent events occur while on therapeutic-dose LMWH, the next step would be dose escalation of LMWH as this has been evaluated in a small series. One retrospective cohort study examined the outcomes of 70 oncology patients with recurrent, symptomatic VTE. The majority of patients had metastatic disease. The dose of LMWH was increased by 20–25% for those already on therapeutic dosing. During a three-month follow-up period, 8.6% of patients had a second, recurrent VTE, while 4.3% had bleeding complications. Larger trials are needed to fully evaluate the efficacy and safety of this approach. Dose escalation may not be appropriate for patients with known CNS metastases, significant thrombocytopenia (platelet count below 50,000 per μL), or other significant bleeding risk factors.

IVC filter placement is also an option for this patient given the proximal DVT. However, the risk of recurrent DVT is as high as 35% over eight years following IVC filter placement (see Case Study 1, Question 4). The filter itself may serve as a nidus for further thrombus formation in the setting of a hypercoagulable state. For this patient, we would favor switching to LMWH as the initial approach.

Correct Answer: C

Recommended Readings

Agnelli, G., Becattini, C., Meyer, G., Muñoz, A., Huisman, M.V., Connors, J.M. et al. (2020 April 23). Caravaggio investigators. Apixaban for the treatment of venous thromboembolism associated with cancer. *N Engl J Med* 382 (17): 1599–1607. doi: 10.1056/NEJMoa1915103. Epub 2020 Mar 29. PMID: 32223112.

Al-Samkari, H. and Connors, J.M. (2019 December 6). Managing the competing risks of thrombosis, bleeding, and anticoagulation in patients with malignancy. *Hematol Am Soc Hematol Educ Program* 2019 (1): 71–79. doi: 10.1182/hematology.2019000369. PMID: 31808892; PMCID: PMC6913483.

Blom, J.W., Doggen, C.J.M., Osanto, S. et al. (2005). Malignancies, prothrombotic mutations, and the risk of venous thrombosis. *Jama* 293: 715–722.

Carrier, M., Abou-Nassar, K., Mallick, R., Tagalakis, V., Shivakumar, S., Schattner, A. et al. (2019 February 21). AVERT investigators. Apixaban to prevent venous thromboembolism in patients with cancer. *N Engl J Med* 380 (8): 711–719. doi: 10.1056/NEJMoa1814468. Epub 2018 Dec 4. PMID: 30511879.

den Exter, P.L., Hooijer, J., Dekkers, O.M. et al. (2011). Risk of recurrent venous thromboembolism and mortality in patients with cancer incidentally diagnosed with pulmonary embolism: a comparison with symptomatic patients. *J Clin Oncol* 29: 2405–2409.

Khorana, A.A., Soff, G.A., Kakkar, A.K., Vadhan-Raj, S., Riess, H., Wun, T. et al. (2019 February 21). CASSINI investigators. Rivaroxaban for thromboprophylaxis in high-risk ambulatory patients with cancer. *N Engl J Med* 380 (8): 720–728. doi: 10.1056/NEJMoa1814630. PMID: 30786186.

Kraaijpoel, N., Bleker, S.M., Meyer, G., Mahé, I., Muñoz, A., Bertoletti, L. et al. (2019 July 10). UPE investigators. Treatment and long-term clinical outcomes of incidental pulmonary embolism in patients with cancer: an international prospective cohort study. *J Clin Oncol* 37 (20): 1713–1720. doi: 10.1200/JCO.18.01977. Epub 2019 May 22. PMID: 31116676.

Lee, A.Y.Y., Levine, M.N., Baker, R.I. et al. (2003). Low-molecular-weight heparin versus a coumarin for the prevention of recurrent venous thromboembolism in patients with cancer. *N Engl J Med* 349: 146–153.

Mulder, F.I., Horváth-Puhó, E., van Es, N., van Laarhoven, H.W.M., Pedersen, L., Moik, F. et al. (2021 April 8). Venous thromboembolism in cancer patients: a population-based cohort study. *Blood* 137 (14): 1959–1969. doi: 10.1182/blood.2020007338. PMID: 33171494.

Raskob, G.E., van Es, N., Verhamme, P., Carrier, M., Di Nisio, M., Garcia, D. et al. (2018 February 15). Hokusai VTE cancer investigators. Edoxaban for the treatment of cancer-associated venous thromboembolism. *N Engl J Med* 378 (7): 615–624. doi: 10.1056/NEJMoa1711948. Epub 2017 Dec 12. PMID: 29231094.

Schrag. D., Uno, H., Rosovsky, R., et al. (2023 Jun 13). CANVAS investigators. direct oral anticoagulants vs low-molecular-weight heparin and recurrent VTE in patients with cancer: a randomized clinical trial. *JAMA* 329: 1924–1933. doi: 10.1001/jama.2023.7843. PMID: 37266947; PMCID: PMC10265290.

Young, A.M., Marshall, A., Thirlwall, J., Chapman, O., Lokare, A., Hill, C. et al. (2018 July 10). Comparison of an oral factor Xa inhibitor with low molecular weight heparin in patients with cancer with venous thromboembolism: results of a randomized trial (SELECT-D). *J Clin Oncol* 36 (20): 2017–2023. doi: 10.1200/JCO.2018.78.8034. Epub 2018 May 10. PMID: 29746227.

50

Identification and Management of Immunotherapy-Related Adverse Events in Oncology

Ozge Gumusay[1], Laura A. Huppert[2], Dame Idossa[3,4], and Hope S. Rugo[2]

[1] Acibadem University, School of Medicine, Department of Medical Oncology, Istanbul, Turkey
[2] UCSF Helen Diller Family Comprehensive Cancer Center, San Francisco, CA
[3] Division of Hematology, Oncology, and Transplantation, University of Minnesota, Minneapolis, MN
[4] Masonic Comprehensive Cancer Center, Minneapolis, MN

Introduction

Immune checkpoint inhibitors (ICIs) have revolutionized the treatment of cancer in the last decade. They include anti-cytotoxic T lymphocyte antigen 4 (anti-CTLA-4), anti-programmed cell death 1 (anti-PD-1), and anti-programmed cell death 1 ligand 1 (anti-PD-L1) antibodies, which are efficacious in multiple cancer types and have demonstrated unprecedented survival in some cases. However, while manipulating the immune system to induce antitumor response, ICIs can also cause immune-related adverse events, which differ from standard chemotherapy toxicities. Immune-related adverse events typically present are usually delayed in onset with prolonged duration. These adverse events most commonly involve the skin, endocrine glands, gastrointestinal system, and liver but can affect almost any organ system. Less frequently, immune-related adverse events can also affect the cardiovascular, pulmonary, musculoskeletal, ocular, and central nervous system, leading to severe and sometimes fatal outcomes. The toxicities due to ICIs require early recognition and optimal management.

Case Study

A 58-year-old woman was diagnosed with *de novo* metastatic estrogen receptor (ER)-positive, progesterone receptor (PR)-positive, human epidermal growth factor receptor 2 (HER2)-negative invasive ductal breast cancer six years ago. She received multiple lines of endocrine therapy and one line of chemotherapy for metastatic breast cancer to lung, liver, and bone. She then received pembrolizumab (anti-PD-1) combined with endocrine therapy for three months in a clinical trial. She presented to the emergency department three months after her last cycle of pembrolizumab with nausea, vomiting, and diarrhea. She reported eight episodes of diarrhea per day for the last 14 days, which she described as liquid, bloody, and mucinous. EGD demonstrated esophagitis, and colonoscopy showed severe circumferential diffuse inflammation throughout the entire examined colon. Biopsy

Cancer Consult: Expertise in Clinical Practice, Volume 1: Solid Tumors & Supportive Care,
Second Edition. Edited by Syed A. Abutalib, Maurie Markman, Al B. Benson III, and Hope S. Rugo.
© 2024 John Wiley & Sons Ltd. Published 2024 by John Wiley & Sons Ltd.

was consistent with ileitis and colitis due to pembrolizumab. She started 1 mg/kg/day of steroid therapy. Her symptoms did not improve initially but resolved with 2 mg/kg/day of steroids and the initiation of infliximab.

1) What are immune checkpoint inhibitors?

Expert Perspective: Monoclonal antibody–based ICI reinvigorate antitumor immune responses by interrupting co-inhibitory signaling pathways and enhancing the function of antitumor T lymphocytes. Ipilimumab, which targets cytotoxic T-lymphocyte associated protein 4 (CTLA-4), was the first approved ICI for the treatment of patients with advanced melanoma (see Chapter 36). Subsequently, several monoclonal antibodies to programmed cell death protein 1 (PD-1) and programmed death-ligand 1 (PD-L1) have been developed. The depiction of T cell activation and inhibition, and the role of ICIs to promote antitumor activity is displayed in Figure 50.1.

2) Why do immune-related adverse events occur?

Expert Perspective: The exact pathophysiology underlying the occurrence of specific or unique immune-related adverse events is not clear. Translational studies have proposed that immune-related adverse events develop through a combination of pathways involving autoreactive T cells, autoantibodies, and cytokines. T-cell activation contributes to the development of immune-related adverse events by leading to the production of inflammatory cytokines and B cell–mediated autoantibodies. There are differences in organ-specific toxicities in patients treated with anti-CTLA-4 therapy or anti-PD-1 therapy. Colitis and hypophysitis occur more frequently with anti-CTLA-4 therapy,

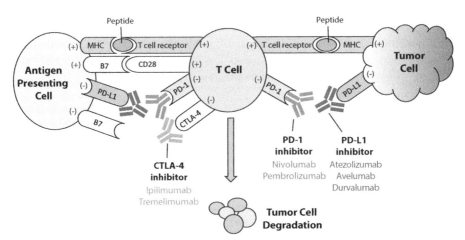

Figure 50.1 T-cell activation and inhibition and the role of immune checkpoint inhibitors: T-cell activation is mediated by the interaction of the T-cell receptor and the CD28 receptor on the T cell with the major histocompatibility complex (MHC) and the CD28 receptor on the antigen-presenting cell. T-cell inhibition is mediated by the PD-1 and CTLA-4 receptors on the T cell and the PD-L1 on the APCs. When effector T cells are active, they can recognize and destroy the tumor cells. However, when they are inactivated this tumor degradation does not occur. Immune checkpoint inhibitors (ICIs) work by inhibiting the PD-1, PD-L1, or CTLA-4 receptors, thus effectively blocking the breaks so that the T cells can remain active and more effectively promote tumor cell degradation.

whereas pneumonitis and thyroiditis are more common with anti-PD-1 therapy. Patients who develop thyroid disorders while on anti-PD-1 therapy may have antithyroid antibodies, which sometimes are present at baseline and other times are only detectable after treatment initiation. In addition to T cell–mediated immunity, anti-PD-1 and anti-PD-L1 treatments modulate humoral immunity and thereby enhance preexisting antithyroid antibodies. Studies have demonstrated that immune-related adverse events may also develop through cross-reactive tumoral antigenicity, where the targeted T-cell antigens are present in both tumor and normal tissue. Cytokines may have a role in the pathophysiology of immune-related adverse events. In previous trials, interleukin-17 (IL-17) elevations were reported in patients with ipilimumab-induced colitis and IL-17 elevations were observed in preclinical models of colitis.

3) Why do immune-related adverse events occur in some patients and not in others?

Expert Perspective: There are some variations in the risk of immune-related adverse events, and it is unclear why some patients do not develop adverse events after ICI therapy, whereas other patients develop serious immune-related adverse events. One hypothesis is that certain individuals have a predisposition to autoimmunity. In one study of 453 patients with melanoma who received ipilimumab, no association was identified between one specific genotype (HLA-A status) and the risk of immune-related adverse events. However, larger genome-wide studies may be needed to investigate the relationship between genetic factors and the risk of immune-related adverse events. Several studies have investigated the potential risk factors of immune-related adverse events, including history of autoimmune disease, age, ethnicity, increased body mass index, genetic factors, and variations in the microbiologic composition of patients' gastrointestinal flora. Age does not appear to be a risk factor, as elderly patients tolerate ICIs much like younger patients. Further studies are needed to confirm whether other epidemiologic factors contribute to the likelihood of developing immune-related adverse events.

4) What is the timing of immune-related adverse event(s)?

Expert Perspective: In general, immune-related adverse events can occur at any time during the treatment course with immunotherapy, including after treatment discontinuation. Dermatologic toxicities are usually the first to appear, typically within the first two to three weeks after treatment initiation. The exception to this is vitiligo, which usually occurs months after treatment initiation. Gastrointestinal symptoms typically occur within six weeks from treatment initiation, and hepatic toxicities usually occur within 8–12 weeks from treatment initiation. Endocrinopathies usually occur within nine weeks of ICI initiation. Renal, cardiac, pulmonary, CNS, vascular, and rheumatologic toxicities are rarer and can occur at any point during the treatment course.

5) What is the incidence of immune-related adverse events in single-agent anti-PD-1 vs anti-PD-1 or anti-PD-L1 plus anti-CTLA-4 agents?

Expert Perspective: The incidence of immune-related adverse events is variable and dependent on the organ specific toxicity, type of ICI used, and tumor type. In a meta-analysis of 36 phase II/III trials, the pooled incidence of any grade immune-related adverse events with monotherapy ICI ranged between 54% and 76%. In another meta-analysis of seventeen trials, the incidence of immune-related adverse events was higher in combination ICI therapy and were 88% (95% CI 84–92%) compared to 41% (95% CI 35–47%) with single-agent ICI therapy.

6) What are the most common immune-related adverse events?

Expert Perspective: Dermatologic toxicities are the most common immune-related adverse event, occurring in up to 40% of patients receiving anti-CTLA-4 inhibitors and in 20% of those receiving PD-1/PD-L1 inhibitors. Endocrinopathies such as hypothyroidism are also common. Less common immune-related adverse events include ophthalmologic, renal, pancreatic, neurologic, cardiac, and hematologic toxicities.

Non-endocrine Toxicities

7) How is the immune-related adverse event colitis typically diagnosed?

Expert Perspective: Colitis is diagnosed with direct visualization and biopsy. For grade II symptoms, lactoferrin (markers of inflammatory diarrhea) can be used to stratify the patients who need more urgent endoscopy. For patients with grade III/IV colitis, urgent endoscopy is warranted. Infectious causes of diarrhea should be ruled out in all patients with colitis. Screening laboratory tests including HIV, hepatitis A and B, and quantiferon, which should be checked in the event patients need to be started on infliximab. There should be a low threshold to consider repeat endoscopy in patients who are not responding to immunosuppressive treatment (also see Question 21, Question 25, and Table 50.1).

8) What are the most common dermatologic immune-related adverse events?

Expert Perspective: The most common dermatologic toxicities are pruritis, morbilliform exanthems, vitiligo, and lichenoid dermatitis. Pruritis can occur in 11–18% of patients treated with PD-1 inhibitors and up to 30% of patients treated with anti-CTLA-4 or dual checkpoint inhibition. Though it is not associated with an underlying rash, secondary dermatologic findings such as excoriations and lichenization can be present. At times, pruritis can be a prodrome to other dermatologic toxicities such as bullous pemphigoid, so it is important to clinically follow intense or refractory pruritis very closely. On the other hand, morbilliform exanthems are transient and coalescing pink macules and papules. These can occur in 11% of patients treated with PD-1 monotherapy and in about 25% of patients receiving anti-CTLA-4 or combination ICI therapy. Vitiligo can be seen in up to 25% of patients treated with ICI for melanoma but are rarely seen in patients treated for other malignancies. Lichenoid dermatitis is characterized as pruritis, violaceous papules/plaques, which can at times involve the mucosal surface. It is seen in approximately 20% of patients receiving anti-PD-1 and anti-PD-L1 therapy and occurs less frequently in those being treated with anti-CTLA-4 therapy (refer also to Chapter 36).

9) How should immune-related hepatitis be diagnosed? Is a liver biopsy necessary to diagnose immune-related hepatitis?

Expert Perspective: It depends on the level of injury. Prior to use of ICI, all patients should be screened for hepatitis B, and those with evidence of chronic hepatitis B infection should be placed on prophylactic antivirals. For all patients receiving immunotherapy, aspartate aminotransferase (AST), alanine transaminase (ALT), and bilirubin should be monitored before each dose. If elevated transaminases are noted, repeat viral testing should be pursed. Careful medication reconciliation should also be completed including over the counter, complementary, and herbal supplements to assess for associations with hepatotoxicity. For grade II or higher transaminase elevations (between 2.5 and 5 times upper limit of normal), imaging should be obtained to evaluate for possible hepatic metastasis and/or biliary obstruction. Radiographic findings are not typical but can at times show hepatomegaly, periportal edema, and lymphadenopathy. If no other etiology has been identified, then patients should be promptly started on glucocorticoids for presumed immune-related hepatitis. Biopsy is not necessary for diagnosis; however, if there is grade IV hepatic toxicity (> 20 times upper limit of normal), a liver biopsy can be considered if there are no contraindications (see also Question 21, Question 25, and Table 50.1).

10) How should immune-related pneumonitis be diagnosed?

Expert Perspective: Pneumonitis associated with ICI is rare and presents as interstitial lung disease. Symptoms can include dry cough, shortness of breath, fever, chest pain, and hypoxia. It can present as organizing pneumonia, nonspecific interstitial pneumonia, hypersensitivity pneumonitis, and diffuse alveolar damage. Pneumonitis is diagnosed on CT scan by demonstrating the presence of focal or diffuse inflammation of the lung parenchyma. For grade II symptoms, treatment with ICI should be held and patients should have extensive infectious evaluation. Patient should be placed on empiric broad spectrum antibiotics until infectious etiologies have been fully excluded. Patients should also be treated with immune suppression. If there is no symptom improvement within 48–72 hours, patients should be admitted and managed as grade III toxicity with inpatient management, and prolonged immunosuppression. Patients with grade 3 or higher pulmonary toxicity require permanent discontinuation of ICI (see also Question 21, Question 25, and Table 50.1).

Endocrine Toxicities

11) How should the immune-related adverse event thyroiditis be diagnosed?

Expert Perspective: Autoimmune thyroid disease is a common immune-related adverse event, which can be caused by either hypothyroidism or hyperthyroidism. Thyroid disorders often present with fatigue and other non-specific complaints, so it is important to keep thyroid disorders on the differential diagnosis and monitor for it with lab tests routinely while patients are on ICI therapy. Thyroid function should be monitored with each ICI infusion, or at least every four to six weeks.

For the diagnosis of hypothyroidism, a high thyroid stimulating hormone (TSH) and a low free thyroxine (T4) indicates primary hypothyroidism, whereas a low TSH and low free T4 suggests hypophysitis. In a meta-analysis of 38 randomized clinical trials evaluating the use of ICIs in advanced solid tumor malignancy by Barroso-Sousa et al. (2018), the incidence of hypothyroidism ranged from 3.8% to 7.0% for single-agent PD-1, PD-L1, or CTLA-4 inhibitors to 13.2% for combination PD-1/CTLA-4 inhibitors. Patients with asymptomatic and subclinical hypothyroidism who have elevated TSH with normal free T4 can proceed with ICI but should be monitored closely. Patients who develop hypothyroidism

Table 50.1 Monitoring, presentation, diagnosis, management of common immune-related adverse events.

irAEs	Presentation	Diagnosis	Management
Dermatologic	Rash, pruritus, bullous dermatitis Dermatomyositis Dermal hypersensitivity reaction Sweet syndrome Pyoderma gangrenosum DRESS SJS/TEN	Rule out alternative etiology of skin problem (e.g. infection, other drug rash, skin lesion linked to another systemic disorder). Complete skin examination and determination of lesion type. Consider skin biopsy	Grade 1: Emollients, topical corticosteroids and/or oral or topical anti-histamines. Avoid skin irritants, avoid sun exposure. Proceed with ICI treatment. Grade 2: High potency topical corticosteroids, and/or oral steroids. Proceed with ICI. Grade 3-4: Withhold ICI. Treat with systemic 1–2 mg/kg/d steroids and dermatology consultation. Treat until symptoms improve to grade ≤ 1 then taper over 4-6 weeks. • Consider IVIG or rituximab for grade ≥ 3 bullous dermatitis • Permanently discontinue ICI treatment if grade 4 or SJS/TEN Consider gabapentin/pregabalin for grade ≥ 3 pruritus
Diarrhea or colitis	Diarrhea Urgency Abdominal pain and/or cramping Fever	Evaluate baseline bowel habits CBC, Comprehensive metabolic panel, ESR, TSH, CRP. Rule out infection: stool culture, Clostridium difficile, CMV DNA PCR, stool ova and parasites. Consider lactoferrin/calprotectin CT Abdomen/pelvis. Consider GI consultation for EGD/colonoscopy with biopsy	Grade 1: Symptomatic management: oral fluids, loperamide, avoid high fiber/lactose diet. Grade ≥ 2: Hold ICI until recovery to grade ≤ 1; evaluate for infection; start 1–2 mg/kg/d steroids; gastroenterology consult. If no response within 3–5 d, consider adding infliximab. In refractory cases or cases with a contraindication to infliximab, vedolizumab can be used; earlier initiation of biologic therapy may lead to improved outcomes. Grade 3: Discontinue ICI; consider resuming anti-PD-1 or anti-PD-L1 after resolution of toxicity. Grade 4: Permanently discontinue ICI
Hepatitis	Elevation of AST/ALT Fulminant hepatitis	Comprehensive metabolic panel. Rule out infectious causes: viral studies. Rule out drug-induced hepatitis, including alcohol ANA, ANCA, ASMA if autoimmune hepatitis suspected. Rule out NASH and thrombosis. Abdomen CT to evaluate liver metastases Consider liver biopsy	Grade 1: Continue ICI treatment with increased frequency of LFT monitoring. Grade 2: Hold ICI until recovery to grade ≤ 1; start systemic 0.5-1mg/kg/d if no improvement. Grade 3-4: Hold ICI; monitor liver enzymes, hepatology consult; start 1–2 mg/kg/d steroids. Grade 4: Permanently discontinue ICI; start 1–2 mg/kg/d steroids Grade > 1 transaminitis with elevated bilirubin;-Bilirubin 1–2xULN: hold ICI, initiate 1–2 mg/kg/d steroids - Bilirubin 3-4X ULN: permanently discontinue ICI; initiate 1–2 mg/kg/d steroids. For steroid-refractory cases, or if no improvement after 3 days, consider mycophenolate mofetil

	Symptoms	Workup	Management
Pneumonitis	Cough, chest pain, wheezing, shortness of breath, new hypoxia, fatigue, respiratory failure	Consider CT Chest. Consider infectious work up: nasal swab, sputum culture. Consider bronchoscopy with BAL and consider transbronchial lung biopsy. Imaging findings are variable and include cryptogenic organizing pneumonia, nonspecific interstitial pneumonitis, hypersensitivity pneumonitis, or usual interstitial pneumonitis/pulmonary fibrosis	Grade 1: Consider holding ICI, reassess in 1–2 weeks, consider CT Chest. Grade 2: Hold ICI; consider pulmonary consultation; consider empiric antibiotics; initiate 1-2 mg/kg/d steroids. If no improvement after 48–72 hours of steroids, treat as grade 3 Grade 3–4: Permanently discontinue ICI; pulmonary and infectious disease consultation; consider empiric antibiotics; initiate 1–2 mg/kg/d steroids; assess steroid response within 48 hours and plan taper over 6 weeks or longer. If no improvement after 48 hours, consider adding infliximab, IVIG or mycophenolate mofetil
Thyroid Disorders	Hypothyroidism Hyperthyroidism Myxedema Thyroid storm	TSH, free T4 Morning cortisol level for concurrent adrenal insufficiency TSH receptor antibodies if Graves' disease is suspected	Asymptomatic hypothyroidism: Thyroid hormone replacement if TSH > 10 mIU/L Symptomatic hypothyroidism: Thyroid hormone replacement Hyperthyroidism: If symptomatic, consider endocrine consultation and propranolol for symptom control ICI can be continued in the setting of hypothyroidism or thyrotoxicosis
Adrenal Insufficiency	Hypophysitis Dysfunction of thyroid, adrenal or gonadal axis Symptoms: Headache, dizziness, nausea/emesis, anorexia, fatigue	Lab: Evaluate morning cortisol and ACTH TSH, free T4 LH, FSH, testosterone (men), estradiol (women) Imaging: MRI of sella Secondary adrenal insufficiency: Low ACTH, low	Endocrine consultation. Hold ICI until acute symptoms resolve, and hormone replacements are initiated Treat with hormone replacement as indicated:- Secondary adrenal insufficiency: steroid replacement (physiologic steroid replacement hydrocortisone 20mg AM, 10mg PM). Acutely symptomatic or hospitalized patients may require stress doss hydrocortisone (e.g. 50mg every 6–8 hours) - Central hypothyroidism: Thyroid hormone replacement and follow free T4 level for dose titration

ACTH: adrenocorticotropic hormone; ALT: alanine transaminase; ANA: antinuclear antibodies; ANCA: anti-neutrophil cytoplasmic antibody; ASMA: anti-smooth muscle antibody; AST: aspartate transaminase; BAL: bronchoalveolar lavage; CMV: cytomegalovirus; CRP: C-reactive protein; CT: computed tomography; d: day; ICI: immune checkpoint inhibitor; DRESS: drug rash with eosinophilia and systemic symptoms; EGD: esophagogastroduodenoscopy; ESR: erythrocyte sedimentation rate; FSH: follicle-stimulating hormone; GI: gastrointestinal; ICI: immune checkpoint inhibitor; irAEs: immune-related adverse events; IVIG: intravenous immunoglobulin; LFT: liver function test; LH: luteinizing hormone; MRI: magnetic resonance imaging; NASH: non-alcoholic steatohepatitis; PCR: polymerase chain reaction; SJS/TEN: Stevens-Johnson syndrome or toxic epidermal necrolysis; T4: thyroxine; TSH: thyroid-stimulating hormone; ULN: upper limit of normal.

should be treated with the thyroid hormone replacement, levothyroxine. Levothyroxine can be initiated for TSH levels above 10 mIU/L. After thyroid replacement is started, TSH and free T4 levels should be evaluated six to eight weeks later.

For the diagnosis of hyperthyroidism, the patient will have a low TSH and a high free T4. In the meta-analysis described above by Barroso-Sousa et al., the incidence of hyperthyroidism ranged from 0.6% to 3.2% for single-agent PD-1, PD-L1, or CTLA-4 inhibition to 8.0% for combination PD-1/CTLA-4 inhibition. Thyroiditis is a self-limiting process and leads to permanent hypothyroidism after one month after the thyrotoxic phase and two months from initiation of immunotherapy. Conservative treatment during the thyrotoxic phase of thyroiditis is recommended. Symptomatic patients can be treated with beta blockers, preferably with alpha-receptor blocking capacity. Thyroid hormone levels should be repeated every two to three weeks.

12) What does autoimmune hypophysitis entails?

Expert Perspective: Hypophysitis is a term used to describe inflammation of the pituitary gland or pituitary stalk, typically affecting the production of one or more pituitary hormones. Symptoms include headache, fatigue, nausea, vomiting, polyuria, and polydipsia. When the diagnosis of hypophysitis is suspected, it can be established by detecting low levels of pituitary hormones such as low TSH, adrenocorticotropic hormone (ACTH), luteinizing hormone (LH), follicle-stimulating hormone (FSH), prolactin, and/or growth hormone (GH). MRI of the pituitary can demonstrate pituitary enhancement or swelling. In the meta-analysis by Barroso-Sousa et al., the incidence of autoimmune hypophysitis ranged from < 0.1% to 3.2% for single-agent PD-1, PD-L1, or CTLA-4 inhibition to 6.4% for combination PD-1/CTLA-4 inhibition. Management of autoimmune hypophysitis involves high-dose glucocorticoids (e.g. 1 mg/kg prednisone daily) as soon as possible to try to reduce the inflammation and prevent the need for long-term hormone replacement therapy. Often, supplementation with levothyroxine and hydrocortisone is required.

13) How do patients with adrenal insufficiency typically present, and how are they treated?

Expert Perspective: Adrenal insufficiency is a life-threatening condition that can present with fatigue, hypotension, and electrolyte imbalances (hyponatremia, hyperkalemia). Labs are notable for a low serum cortisol. If adrenal crisis is suspected, the patient should be referred for immediate hospitalization to receive intravenous glucocorticoids, fluids, and evaluation for sepsis. In a case series of over 50,000 patients with ICI adverse drug reactions, 451 cases of primary adrenal insufficiency (0.9%) were identified. ICI-associated primary adrenal insufficiency was associated with significant morbidity (> 90%) as well as mortality (7.3%).

14) Does new-onset diabetes mellitus occur after ICI therapy?

Expert Perspective: Yes. ICI therapy can also lead to the development of acute-onset type 1 diabetes mellitus (DM1) due to autoimmune destruction of the pancreatic beta cells. Patients typically present with elevated serum glucose and may develop diabetic ketoacidosis (DKA). Patients should be treated with insulin therapy and typically require hospitalization for DKA management. Unlike the management of other immune-related adverse events, the use of steroids and immunosuppression are not effective for reversal of DM1. The development of DM1 is rare, occurring in < 1% of patients on ICI therapy in most case series.

Rare Immune-related Adverse Events

15) Which neurologic toxicities occur with ICI therapy?

Expert Perspective: ICI therapy can cause a variety of neurologic side effects. Common neurologic immune-related adverse events include headache and peripheral neuropathy. Rarely, neurologic immune-related adverse events may include myasthenia gravis, acute inflammatory demyelinating polyneuropathy (AIDP), posterior reversible encephalopathy syndrome (PRES), aseptic meningitis, transverse myelitis, cerebellar inflammation, and cranial neuropathies. In a retrospective observational study including patients with advanced melanoma on nivolumab +/- ipilimumab enrolled in 12 clinical trials, 35 of 3,763 (0.93%) patients developed serious neurologic immune-related adverse events, including neuropathy (n = 22), encephalitis (n = 6), aseptic meningitis (n = 5), neuromuscular disorder (n = 3), and non-specific neurologic events (n = 7). The median onset was 45 days after ICI initiation, but the timing ranged from 1 day to 170 days. Treatment includes initiation of high-dose steroids for most conditions and may also require additional immunosuppressive agents in some cases. Most neurologic immune-related adverse events resolved with appropriate treatment, but the median time to resolution was 32 days. Permanent discontinuation of ICI therapy is recommended in cases of severe neurologic immune-related adverse events.

16) Which immune-related cardiovascular toxicity has been reported with ICI treatment?

Expert Perspective: Cardiovascular toxicity is also possible with ICI therapy. Immune-related myocarditis is a rare but serious side effect that can cause inflammation of the heart muscle. Symptoms may include chest pain, shortness of breast, palpitations, or fatigue. Serum troponin is elevated. It is important to first rule out acute coronary syndrome (ACS) and other cardiac pathologies. Prompt recognition and initiation of immunosuppression are essential to try to reduce the inflammation and damage. Management requires inpatient admission, cardiology consult, initiation of high-dose steroids, and consideration of additional immunosuppressive agents if steroids are not sufficient, such as mycophenolate, infliximab, intravenous immunoglobulin (IVIG), and/or abatacept. Permanent discontinuation of ICI therapy is recommended in most cases of cardiac immune-related adverse events.

17) What rheumatologic immune-related adverse events have been observed?

Expert Perspective: Rheumatologic immune-related adverse events are also observed with ICI therapy, including myositis, sicca syndrome, inflammatory arthritis, vasculitis, and lupus nephritis. Arthralgias and myalgias are also well described. In a systematic review that contained data from 52 studies, arthralgia prevalence ranged from 1% to 43%, and myalgia was reported in 2–20%. Five studies reported arthritis, and two reported vasculitis. Management of these conditions is often performed in conjunction with rheumatology consultation and may warrant steroids or additional immunosuppression if symptoms are severe.

18) Should ICI be considered in new renal dysfunction?

Expert Perspective: Yes, and it usually happens months after start or after discontinuation of ICI therapy. ICI-associated acute kidney injury (ICI-AKI) is a rare complication of ICI therapy. The most common pathology is acute tubulointerstitial nephritis (ATN), but thrombotic microangiopathy and immune complex glomerulonephritis can also occur. There are no clinical features that reliably distinguish ICI-AKI from other etiologies of AKI. Interestingly, the latency period between starting ICI therapy and the development of ICI-AKI is often longer than other immune-related adverse events, so ICI-AKI should be considered even months after discontinuation of ICI therapy. In a combined analysis of 3,695 patients, the overall incidence of ICI-AKI was 3%, with a higher incidence (5%) among patients receiving combination ICI therapy. The incidence of severe AKI, defined as an increase in serum creatinine more than threefold above baseline, an increase in serum Cr to > 4.0 mg/dl, or the need for renal replacement therapy, was 0.6%.

19) What types of ocular toxicities have been reported with ICI treatment?

Expert Perspective: ICI treatment can cause inflammation of the eye, causing episcleritis, uveitis, conjunctivitis, or orbital inflammation. Symptoms may include eye pain, photophobia, blurred vision, or dryness of the eye. If an ophthalmologic immune-related adverse events is suspected, ophthalmology consultation is recommended, and treatment with topic glucocorticoids may be used. Oral glucocorticoids are sometimes required for severe or refractory cases.

20) How are immune-related adverse events graded?

Expert Perspective: Immune-related adverse events are graded according to the Common Terminology Criteria for Adverse Events (CTCAE) from the US National Cancer Institute, which categorizes toxicity on a scale of 1 to 5, in ascending order of severity. The grading of immune-related adverse events may be difficult due to subtle distinctions between grade 2 and 3 toxicities, such as the number of stools in a day, which is often affected by recall bias. Therefore, using clinical judgment is important in these cases.

21) How are immune-related adverse events treated?

Expert Perspective: Most immune-related adverse events are treated by inducing temporary immunosuppression with oral corticoids, high-dose steroid therapy (oral prednisolone 1–2 mg/kg/day or IV equivalent), or additional immunosuppressants in more severe cases. The management of immunotherapy toxicities depends on the grade of severity, type of immune-related adverse events, and number of adverse events. The patient's medical history, comorbidities, underlying disease status, and ability to tolerate corticosteroids must be incorporated into decisions about optimal treatment strategies. The management of common immune-related adverse events is summarized in Table 50.1. We have outlined general principles of the management of immune-related adverse events below.

- For grade 1 immune-related adverse events, ICI treatment can be continued with close monitoring, with the exception of some neurologic, hematologic, and cardiac toxicities.
- For grade 2 immune-related adverse events, steroid treatment with 0.5–1 mg/kg prednisone/equivalent is recommended, and ICI therapy should be held until toxicity resolves to grade ≤ 1. ICI should be stopped permanently in grade 2 immune-related adverse events lasting for six weeks or longer except in endocrinopathies.
- For grade 3 or 4 immune-related adverse events, ICI treatment should be held, and dose adjustment is not recommended. Cautious re-treatment with ICIs can be considered when immune-related adverse events revert to grade ≤ 1. Patients should be treated with-high dose steroids (oral prednisolone 1–2 mg/kg/day or IV equivalent) until resolution to ≤ grade 1, at which point steroid treatment should taper slowly over four to six weeks. In some cases, longer steroid tapers (six to eight weeks or more) may be required to prevent recurrent irAEs, especially with pneumonitis and hepatitis.
- If there is no improvement with steroids in one to three days, other immunosuppressant and immunomodulatory agents can be considered.
- For grade 4 toxicities, ICI should be stopped permanently except in endocrinopathies controlled on hormone replacement.
- ICI should be stopped permanently if there is an inability to reduce glucocorticoids dose to 7.5 mg/day prednisone or equivalent for patients treated with anti-CTLA-4 antibodies and less than 10 mg/day within 12 weeks for anti-PD-1 antibodies.

22) What prophylaxis should be considered when patients are on steroids to control immune-related adverse events?

Expert Perspective: When patients are on prolonged high-dose steroids, it is important to consider prophylaxis for steroid-induced complications. Proton pump inhibitors or H2 blockers should be considered for GI prophylaxis. For patients receiving at least 20 mg prednisone or equivalent/day for three weeks or more, the addition of prophylactic antibiotics for pneumocystis pneumonia (PCP) can be considered. Prophylaxis against fungal infections (e.g. fluconazole) should be considered in patients receiving prednisone ≥ 20 mg daily for six to eight weeks or more.

23) What are the treatment options for the management of steroid-refractory cases?

Expert Perspective: For steroid-refractory patients including patients with severe immune-related adverse events that are not responsive to steroids within 48–72 hours, early initiation of additional immunosuppressive agents, monoclonal antibodies, IVIG, or plasmapheresis should be considered.

- **Additional immunosuppressive agents:** Mycophenolate mofetil can be used for the management of steroid-refractory immune-related adverse events, particularly for immune-related hepatitis, nephritis, pancreatitis, and uveitis. Other immunosuppressive agents including tacrolimus, cyclosporine, and sulfasalazine have been less commonly used for steroid-refractory immune-related adverse events.

- **IVIG and plasma exchange:** IVIG is used as a second-line therapy for neurological and hematological immune-related adverse events. Plasma exchange can be used in immune-related adverse events caused directly by autoantibodies, such as some hematological or neuromuscular immune-related adverse events, which can remove autoantibodies from the circulation and is effective in severe cases of myasthenia gravis or Guillain-Barre syndrome.
- **Monoclonal antibodies:** Infliximab has shown efficacy in patients with moderate-to-severe colitis and inflammatory arthritis induced by ICI. In most patients, infliximab 5 mg/kg should be repeated after two weeks for persistent symptoms. Vedolizumab, a monoclonal antibody to the integrin $\alpha 4\beta 7$ that inhibits the migration of T cells into inflamed gastrointestinal mucosa, can be used for immune-related colitis. Tocilizumab (an anti-IL-6 antibody) has been used for the management of a few steroid-refractory immune-related adverse events, such as pneumonitis, cerebritis, and polyarthritis. Rituximab has shown efficacy for the treatment of steroid-refractory patients with severe encephalitis, autoimmune cytopenias, or severe bullous skin disease.

24) Should endocrine replacement therapy be given permanently, for the rest of the patient's life?

Expert Perspective: Treatment for most immune-related adverse events is typically limited to a few months, but management of thyroid disorders and adrenal insufficiency with hormone replacement therapy is required for the remainder of the patient's life. If adrenal insufficiency and hypothyroidism are both present, steroids should be started before thyroid hormone replacement to prevent adrenal crisis. Patients with adrenal insufficiency should be educated about the potential life-threatening nature of adrenal crisis and stress doses of hydrocortisone should be provided in case of infection, trauma, or illness.

25) Is it safe to re-treat patients with immunotherapy after an immune-related toxicity?

Expert Perspective: One of the most important questions in clinical practice is the safety of re-treatment with immunotherapy following immune-related adverse events. In clinical trials, ICI therapy is permanently discontinued if a serious immune-related adverse event occurs due to a study therapy. When restarting ICI treatment, clinicians must consider the severity of the prior event, the availability of alternative treatment options, the overall status of the cancer, and the goals/preferences of the patient. Re-treatment with ICI is contraindicated if there is a life-threatening toxicity, particularly cardiac, pulmonary, or neurologic toxicity. The type of toxicity is also an important consideration in making re-treatment decisions. In cases of thyroid, adrenal, and pituitary disorders, for instance, patients can be re-treated with ICI after hormone repletion and resolution of acute symptoms. Given the complexity of re-treatment decisions, multidisciplinary and collaborative management approaches are required to decide whether re-treatment with ICI should be pursued following immune-related adverse events.

Conclusion

With the increased use of ICIs, clinicians have observed common and also rare immune-related adverse events. It is important to understand these toxicities, which can help lead to early recognition and optimal management. Further studies are needed to characterize the pathophysiology leading to toxicity, better understand which patients are at highest risk for immune-related adverse events, improve preventive treatment approaches, and to optimize treatment strategies for these complications.

Recommended Readings

Barroso-Sousa, R., Barry, W.T., Garrido-Castro, A.C. et al. (2018). Incidence of endocrine dysfunction following the use of different immune checkpoint inhibitor regimens: a systematic review and meta-analysis. *JAMA Oncol* 4 (2): 173.

Cappelli, L.C., Gutierrez, A.K., Bingham, C.O. et al. (2017). Rheumatic and musculoskeletal immune-related adverse events due to immune checkpoint inhibitors: a systematic review of the literature. *Arthritis Care Res (Hoboken)* 69 (11): 1751–1763. doi: 10.1002/acr.23177.

Eigentler, T.K., Hassel, J.C., Berking, C. et al. (2016). Diagnosis, monitoring and management of immune-related adverse drug reactions of anti-PD-1 antibody therapy. *Cancer Treatment Reviews* 45: 7–18. doi: 10.1016/j.ctrv.2016.02.003.

Kennedy, L.B. and Salama, A.K. (2020). A review of cancer immunotherapy toxicity. *CA: Cancer J Clin* 70 (2): 86–104.

Martins, F., Sofiya, L., Sykiotis, G.P. et al. (2019). Adverse effects of immune-checkpoint inhibitors: epidemiology, management and surveillance. *Nat Rev Clin Oncol* 16 (9): 563–580.

NCCN Clinical Practice Guidelines in Oncology (NCCN Guidelines). (2022). Management of immunotherapy-related toxicities. Version1.2022-February 28.

Postow, M.A., Sidlow, R., and Hellmann, M.D. (2018). Immune-related adverse events associated with immune checkpoint blockade. Longo DL, ed. *N Engl J Med* 378 (2): 158–168. doi: 10.1056/NEJMra1703481.

Puzanov, I., Diab, A., Abdallah, K. et al. (2017). Managing toxicities associated with immune checkpoint inhibitors: consensus recommendations from the Society for Immunotherapy of Cancer (SITC) toxicity management working group. *J Immunother Cancer* 5 (1): 1–28.

Ramos-Casals, M., Brahmer, J.R., Callahan, M.K. et al. (2020). Immune-related adverse events of checkpoint inhibitors. *Nat Rev Dis Primers* 6 (1): 1–21.

51

Geriatric Oncology

Sukeshi Patel Arora[1] and Efrat Dotan[2]

[1] Mays Cancer Center, University of Texas Health, San Antonio, TX
[2] Fox Chase Cancer Center, Temple Health, Philadelphia, PA

Introduction

Age is perhaps the most significant risk factor for cancer incidence. With increased longevity of the population, early detection, and more effective therapies, the number of older cancer patients and survivors will continue to rise. Due to the variability in aging, chronological age and performance status alone are inadequate to assess the health span of an individual. On the other hand, a multi-domain assessment of geriatric syndromes by comprehensive geriatric assessment (CGA) can predict functional decline, morbidity, and mortality in older adults receiving anticancer therapy. The CGA has also been shown to be predictive of chemotherapy-related toxicity and prognosis. Thus, a CGA should be routinely incorporated into the evaluation and care of older adults with cancer before the start of treatment. This will better determine their functional and global health status as well as reduce their morbidity and mortality, as recommended by multiple guidelines, including National Comprehensive Cancer Network (NCCN) and American Society of Clinical Oncology (ASCO). However, CGA is still underutilized due to the challenges of its incorporation into routine clinical care. Furthermore, older patients with cancer are underrepresented in clinical trials, resulting in a lack of data to guide therapy in this population. Here, we review geriatric oncology principles that every clinician caring for older adults with cancer should know and implement in their clinical practice to enhance and personalize care for this vulnerable group of patients.

1) What geriatric syndromes should we assess in older adults with cancer?

Expert Perspective: Traditional tools, such as chronological age and the Eastern Cooperative Oncology Group (ECOG) or Karnofsky performance status (KPS), do not evaluate physiological reserve and have poor predictive value for clinical outcomes in older adults with cancer. Frailty is a biological geriatric syndrome of decreased reserve and resistance to stressors, resulting in vulnerability to adverse outcomes. Patients who are frail are at increased risk of falls, disability, hospitalization, and death. Further, frailty in older adults with cancer is correlated with poor tolerance of chemotherapy, increased hospitalization, falls, disability, decreased activities of daily living (ADLs), and death. The CGA is the gold standard tool for assessment of frailty by evaluation for the presence of known geriatric syndromes, such as constipation, dementia, delirium, depression, failure to thrive, falls, incontinence (fecal and/or urinary), neglect and abuse, osteoporosis or spontaneous fractures, pressure ulcers, and sarcopenia.

2) What is a comprehensive geriatric assessment (CGA)?

Expert Perspective: The CGA is a multidisciplinary, objective evaluation of a patient that assesses geriatric domains that can affect prognosis, treatment decisions, and outcomes in older adults. This type of assessment carries even more significance when caring for older adults with cancer and personalizing anticancer therapies for this population. CGA scores are strongly correlated to both prognosis and treatment-related toxicity. The domains covered by CGA include functional status, comorbidity, cognition, mental health, social support, nutrition, and geriatric syndromes. ASCO and NCCN guidelines, recommend conducting a CGA before treatment initiation to evaluate the functional and global health status of older adults with cancer and personalize therapy based on these findings. This approach will allow for reduction in morbidity and mortality. Further, repeating CGA during treatment may identify new deficits in geriatric domains that were not present at baseline and guide further adjustment to therapy or the referrals to supportive care services.

Table 51.1 highlights the domains that should be evaluated in a CGA, with examples of assessment tools that have been validated in older adults with cancer in each of these areas. Providers can select the individual tools from this list that fit their practice for assessment of each of these domains. In addition to these domains, clinicians should screen for geriatric syndromes (i.e. dementia, delirium, falls, neglect and abuse, fecal and/or urinary incontinence, osteoporosis, failure to thrive, constipation, pressure ulcers, and sarcopenia).

3) What is a geriatric screening tool, and how do you use it?

Expert Perspective: Despite the data supporting the benefit of conducting a CGA, its incorporation into clinical practice is challenging due to time constraints and lack of personnel. As a result, geriatric screening tools can be used to identify patients at risk who may benefit from a more comprehensive evaluation with CGA. There are several geriatric screening tools that have been validated in older adults with cancer and can be administered quickly in a busy practice.

The screening tools, however, do not evaluate all domains, specifically lacking assessment of cognition, psychosocial status, and nutrition, areas that are commonly affected by cancer diagnosis in older adults. Therefore, in concerning cases a follow-up with a CGA is necessary to ensure assessment of all aspects of the patient's overall health and ensure comprehensive support during therapy. The best geriatric screening tool is the one that can be consistently implemented into your clinical practice. Two tools frequently used in the geriatric literature are the G8 questionnaire and the Vulnerable Elders Survey (VES-13). These screening tools take a few minutes to complete, are available in several languages, and have a self–reported version available, which can facilitate implementation in clinical practice.

The G8 is a validated screening tool in older adults with cancer. The G8 contains questions on eight items: age, appetite changes, weight loss, mobility, neuropsychological problems, body mass index, medication, and self-rated health questions. A cutoff value of 14 for the G8 tool had a good sensitivity estimate (85%) without deteriorating the specificity

Table 51.1 Domains of a comprehensive geriatric assessment (CGA).

Domain	Performed by patient vs provider	Examples of Assessment Tools
Function and mobility	Self-reported by patient	Activities of Daily Living (ADLs) Independent Activities of Daily Living (IADLs) falls
	Provider	Timed "up and go" (TUG) timed 10-meter walk test short physical performance battery (SPPB)
Comorbidity	Provider	Charlson Comorbidity Index (CCI) Cumulative Illness Rating Scale-Geriatric (CIRS-G)
Social functioning and support	Self-reported by patient	MOS Social Support Survey RAND Health Care Social Support Survey Instrument
Cognition	Provider	Mini-Cog Mini-Mental State Examination (MMSE) Blessed Orientation Memory Concentration Test (BOMC)
Psychological	Self-reported by patient	Geriatric Depression Scale (GDS) Mental Health Inventory (MHI-17) Distress thermometer (NCCN)
Pharmacy	Provider	Number of medications Prescription and over-the-counter medication list Beers criteria Medication Appropriateness Index (MAI) Screening Tool to Alert Doctors to Right Treatment (START) Screening Tool of Older Persons' Prescriptions (STOPP)
Nutrition	Provider and self-reported by patient	Body Mass Index (BMI) Percent unintentional weight loss in the last 6 months Mini-nutritional assessment (MNA)

excessively (65%). A G8 score ≤ 14 is associated with increased mortality and quality of life (QOL) and warrants referral for a full CGA. A limitation of this tool is related to the items of the G8, which may correlate with symptoms resulting from the patient's cancer diagnosis rather than geriatric syndromes, which a CGA would identify.

In recent years, the ELCAPA study group developed a modified G8 screening tool, using only six items, which showed better diagnostic performance with greater uniformity across cancer types. The six independent predictors for abnormal CGA are weight loss, cognition/mood, performance status, self-rated health status, polypharmacy (six or more medications per day), and history of heart failure/coronary heart disease. The modified G8 demonstrated a sensitivity of 89.2%, specificity of 79.0%, and area under the receiver-operating curve (AUROC) of 91.6%, with higher AUROC values for all tumor sites and stable properties on the validation set when compared to the original G8. Thus, the modified G8 screening tool helps identify older adults with cancer who need a CGA with more specificity than the original G8. If the score is 6 or higher, then CGA is recommended.

The Vulnerable Elders Survey (VES-13) is a simple function-based tool to identify older adults at risk of health deterioration. VES-13 defines vulnerable older adults as those who are age 65 and older and who are at increased risk of functional decline or death over the next two years. The 13-item questionnaire includes age, self-rated health, limitations in physical function, and disability. A score of 3 or more identifies individuals as vulnerable, and this vulnerable group had 4.2 times the risk of death or functional decline over two years, compared to those who scored < 3. Of note, patients > 85 years of age automatically receive 3 points, which makes this tool less useful in the oldest of the old. This is a function-based screening tool, which relies on patient self-reporting, and thus, can be easily incorporated into clinical settings. A limitation is that the self-report format may underestimate the prevalence of underdiagnosed conditions.

The ONCODAGE prospective multicohort study evaluated the diagnostic accuracy of G8 and VES-13 as a predictive screening tool to identify older adults with cancer who would benefit from a CGA. This study showed the G8 was more sensitive (76.5% vs 68.7%; $P = 0.0046$), and the VES-13 was more specific (74.3% vs 64.4%; $P < 0.0001$).

These three tools are summarized in the Table 51.2 below.

Table 51.2 Geriatric screening tools: G8, modified G8, and VES-13 Questionnaires.

Questionnaire	G8	Modified G8	VES-13
Items evaluated	1) Decline in food intake 2) Weight loss 3) Mobility 4) Neuropsychological problems 5) BMI 6) 3+ medications per day 7) Self-related health 8) Age	1) Weight loss 2) Cognition/mood 3) Performance status 4) Self-rated health status 5) Polypharmacy (≥ 6 per day), 6) History of heart failure/coronary heart disease	1) Age 2) Self-rated health 3) Difficulty with stooping, lifting, reaching, handling small objects, walking quarter of a mile, heavy housework 4) Difficulty with shopping, managing money, walking, light housework, bathing
Score	0 (worst) – 17 (best) Score $\leq 14 \rightarrow$ CGA	0–35 Score $\geq 6 \rightarrow$ CGA	0 (best) – 10 (worst) Score $\geq 3 \rightarrow$ CGA
Sensitivity for abnormal CGA	77–92%	89.2%	69–88%
Specificity for abnormal CGA	40–75%	79%	62–86%

4) What are chemotherapy toxicity prediction tools, and how do I use them in clinical practice?

Expert Perspective: Chemotherapy toxicity tools are helpful to predict risk of grade 3 or higher toxicity from chemotherapy in older adults with cancer. These tools can be used to inform decision-making for chemotherapy intensification/de-intensification and determine the need for early interventions and closer monitoring during treatment. Chemotherapy toxicity tools are less time consuming and easier to interpret than the CGA, thereby making them accessible to oncologists in communities with limited resources. Three validated chemotherapy toxicity tools (Table 51.3) are as follows:

Table 51.3 Chemotherapy toxicity prediction tools in older adults with cancer.

Characteristics	CRASH	CARG	CARG-BC
Study inclusion criteria	• Age ≥ 70 years • Diagnosis of cancer • Scheduled to receive a new chemotherapy regimen (1st–4th line) • No diagnosis of dementia • No concomitant radiotherapy	• Age ≥ 65 years • Diagnosis of cancer • Scheduled to receive a new chemotherapy regimen	• Age ≥ 65 years • Diagnosis of stage I–III breast cancer • Scheduled to receive adjuvant or neoadjuvant chemotherapy
Factors included in the scoring model			
Geriatric assessments (cutoff/score)	IADL: • < 26 = 1 • ≥ 26 = 0 ECOG PS: • 1–2 = 1 • 3–4 = 2 Mini Mental State Examination: • < 30 = 2 • ≥ 30 = 0 Mini Nutritional Assessment: • < 28 = 2 • ≥ 28 = 0	Hearing: • Excellent/good = 0 • Fair/poor/totally deaf = 2 Falls during last 6 months: • 0 = 0 • ≥1 = 3 IADL: taking medications: • Without help = 0 • With some help/completely unable = 1 Walking limitations one block: • Not limited at all = 0 • Limited a little/a lot = 2 Decreased social activity: • None/a little of the time = 0 • Some/most/all the time = 1	Falls during last 6 months: • 0 = 0 • ≥1 = 4 Walking limitations ≥ 1 mile: • Not limited at all = 0 • Somewhat/very limited = 3 Availability of someone to provide advice about a crisis: • Most/all the time = 0 • None/little/some of the time = 3
Patient characteristics	-	Age: • < 72 years = 0 • ≥ 72 years = 2	-

(Continued)

Table 51.3 (Continued)

Characteristics	CRASH	CARG	CARG-BC
Clinical parameters	Diastolic blood pressure: > 72 mmHg = 1	-	-
Laboratory parameters	LDH: > 459 U/L = 1	Hemoglobin: • ≥ 11 g/dL (male) or ≥ 10 g/dL (female) = 0 • < 11 g/dL (male) or < 10 g/dL (female) = 3 Creatinine clearance (Jeliffe formula): • ≥ 34mL/min = 0 • < 34mL/min = 3	Hemoglobin: • >13 g/dL (male) or > 12 g/dL (female) = 0 • ≤ 13 g/dL (male) or ≤ 12 g/dL (female) = 3 Liver function tests: • normal = 0 • Outside normal reference range = 3
Disease characteristics	-	Cancer type: • Other = 0 • GI/GU = 2	Breast cancer stage: • I = 0 • II-III = 2
Treatment features	Chemotoxicity toxicity score based on regimen (assigned by the study team): • 0–0.44 = 0 • 0.45–0.57 = 1 • > 0.57 = 2	Chemotherapy dose: • Reduced = 0 • Standard = 2 Number of chemotherapy agents: • Mono-chemotherapy = 0 • Polychemotherapy = 2	Anthracycline use: • No = 0 • Yes = 1 Planned chemotherapy duration • ≤ 3 months = 0 • > 3 months = 4
Outcomes	Grade 4 hematological toxicity Grade 3–4 non-hematological toxicity Combined toxicity	Grade 3–5 toxicity	Grade 3–5 toxicity
Risk groups	Low: 50% Medium-low: 58% Medium-high: 77% High risk: 79%	Low (0–5 points): 30% Intermediate (6–9 points): 52% High risk (10–19 points): 83%	Low: 27% Intermediate: 45% High: 76%

- The Chemotherapy Risk Assessment Scale for High-Age Patients (CRASH) score combines laboratory values and some geriatric assessment variables to predict the risks associated with a proposed therapy. The study that led to the validation of CRASH score included patients who were 70 years of age or older, had histologically proven cancer, and were initiating a new first-line to fourth-line chemotherapy. This prediction model includes the specific chemotherapy regimen considered, laboratory values (creatinine, albumin, hemoglobin, lactate dehydrogenase [LDH], liver function tests), and geriatric assessments variables (function, cognition, and nutrition). The combined hematologic and non-hematologic risk categories identified patients at low risk (50%), medium-low risk (58%), medium-high risk (77%), and high risk (79%) for experiencing adverse events.
- The Cancer and Aging Research Group (CARG) chemotoxicity assessment tool uses elements of the CGA to help risk-stratify elderly patients. The validation study included patients age ≥ 65 years with various malignancies undergoing chemotherapy treatments. These patients completed a pre-chemotherapy assessment that included demographics, tumor/treatment variables, laboratory results, and geriatric assessment variables (function, comorbidity, cognition, psychological state, social activity/support, and nutritional status). This tool was compiled based on these factors identifying a few simple questions that the patient can answer without the need for a full CGA to be performed. It assesses the likelihood of older cancer patients developing grade 3–5 toxicity from systemic chemotherapy. The following variables are captured: age, type of malignancy, the chemotherapy regimen under consideration (single- vs multi-agent treatment), hemoglobin, creatinine clearance, hearing, ability to take medications, physical activity, and social activity. The score ranged from 0 to 19, and the median risk score was 7. The risk score predicted incidence of grade 3–5 toxicity as follows: low (0–5 points, 30%), intermediate (6–9 points, 52%), or high risk (10–19 points, 83%) of chemotherapy toxicity ($P < .001$). One limitation is that patients with gastrointestinal and genitourinary cancers score higher for cancer type, which makes this tool less useful in these patient cohorts.
- The CARG-BC score is the newest validated tool and first disease-specific tool that was derived from the original CARG chemotherapy assessment tool. This eight-item weight risk tool was developed for older patients with early stage breast cancer (stage I–III) receiving neoadjuvant or adjuvant chemotherapy to predict chemotherapy-related grade 3–5 toxicity in this setting. This model includes breast cancer stage, chemotherapy regimen and its duration, along with liver function tests, hemoglobin, falls, limited mobility, and social support. In the validation cohort, the rates of grade 3–5 toxicity were 27%, 45%, and 76% in patients with low, medium, and high-risk scores, respectively. These categories also correlated with hospitalization rate and reduced chemotherapy dose intensity. This tool is an example of how different variables are important for each disease type and the need for further research to develop disease-specific toxicity tools.

These tools are highly useful in a busy clinical practice to assess the risk associated with systemic chemotherapy. However, they do carry a few limitations, mainly related to the fact that they were developed for patients receiving chemotherapy, and so, the utility in newer agents, such as targeted therapy or immunotherapy, is unclear. Further, independent validation studies are needed in diverse populations, different malignancies, and across different geographical locations.

5) How do we evaluate function in older adults: Performance status versus functional status?

Expert Perspective: Traditionally, ECOG or KPS have been used to determine eligibility for systemic therapy for all patients with cancer regardless of physiologic age; however, the utility of these scores to predict toxicity, QOL, and survival in older adults has been understudied. Traditional performance status scores are subjective and lack sensitivity to predict toxicity from therapies. In addition, these scores do not account for diversity of health status in these patients, which can be evaluated by comprehensive assessment of functional status. Functional status can be measured with objective and subjective tools (Figure 51.1).

Performance measures objectively assess the inability or restriction to perform an action, whereas self-reported measures subjectively reflect the inability or limitation to perform socially defined activities or roles. Self-reported measures include the individual's ability to complete ADLs and IADLs. ADLs are basic self-care skills needed for an individual to be independent at home. IADLs include complex skills that are needed for an individual to be independent in the community. Dependence in IADLs has been associated with decreased chemotherapy tolerance as well as lower survival in older adults with cancer. Performance-based measures are used to assess functional status and include gait speed (or walking speed) and Timed Up and Go (TUG). Gait speed predicts survival in older adults with cancer, with studies showing that a decline in gait speed correlates with mortality. Therefore, gait speed can identify patients who may benefit from preventive interventions. The Timed Up and Go, or TUG, test is a quick screening tool to evaluate mobility and motor function in older adults. The TUG test score of 13 seconds or greater can identify patients who are at higher risk of falls. In such patients, a more comprehensive functional assessment should be done. Ideally, the global functional status should be evaluated to help identify which patients are at higher risk for functional decline and toxicity so that early interventions may be implemented. Physical therapy (PT) or occupational therapy (OT) along with interventions to improve safety at home should be considered in any patient who is found to

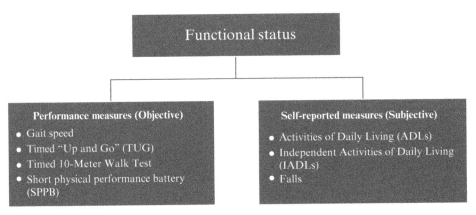

Figure 51.1 Functional status: Performance and self-reported measures.

Introduction

have or is at risk for functional decline. Incorporating social workers and home-based health workers into patient care teams will help identify patients who are at higher risk and who would benefit from such interventions.

6) What are the types of geriatric oncology models of care?

Expert Perspective: There are several models of care for older adults with cancer (See Figure 51.2). Given limited access to geriatricians and geriatric oncologists, models have developed over time to adapt to the different clinical environments.

The gold standard has traditionally been a comprehensive multidisciplinary clinic in which the patient meets with the geriatrician and geriatric oncologist in the same setting for a CGA and oncologic treatment plan. During this visit, the patient also sees support services, such as dietician, pharmacist, physical/occupational therapist, and social worker, thus avoiding extra clinic visits. In this model, the same assessment will continue longitudinally during the patient's treatment course to address any changes or challenges that arise during therapy. As needed, additional supportive services, such as palliative care and social services, can be added to the treatment team. Although this model is ideal for providing patients with the most comprehensive care, its main limitation is the significant resources that are required for its execution. Furthermore, with the shortage in geriatric oncologists and the limited access to support services in remote centers, implementation of this model can occur only in few select centers with high resources and expertise.

An alternative model is one in which the patient is co-managed by a geriatrician and an oncologist. In this shared model, patients see the geriatrician and oncologist in different clinics, possibly on a different day. The CGA is completed by the geriatrician, while the oncologic assessment is carried out by the oncologist. After seeing the patient, the care team meets and discusses the patients during an interdisciplinary team meeting to develop a comprehensive plan for care for the patient. The plan must include evaluation and referral to other support services, such as physical therapy, nutrition, and social work, as needed. The individual specialists continue to follow the patient during their treatment in their respective clinics. This model is more appealing and feasible in a moderate resource setting; however, it carries the burden of multiple appointments and visits required of the patient and caregivers.

A model that maybe more feasible in centers with limited resources is the consultative model. Under this model, a geriatric screening is done in by the oncologist to identify higher-risk patients who would benefit from a CGA by a geriatrician or geriatric oncologist. Only

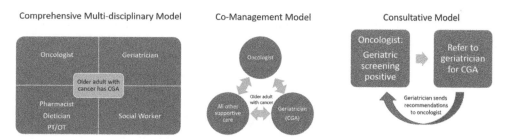

Figure 51.2 Three common geriatric oncology models of care.

those patients are referred to the specialized team for evaluation, and the summary recommendations are given back to the treating oncologist to inform the treatment plan. In this model, the oncology team carries the burden of conducting a geriatric screening tool repeatedly during the treatment course and ensuring the appropriate patient is referred. Furthermore, the lag between these visits may affect treatment initiation and ultimately outcome.

7) How can we improve inclusion of older adults with cancer in clinical trials?

Expert Perspective: Despite the increasing number of older adults with cancer that are seen in oncology clinics, data is still lacking to guide treatment approach in this vulnerable patient population. This is in part due to underrepresentation of older adults in clinical trials. Patients of the age ≥ 70 years are 42% of the overall cancer population. However, only 24% of participants in registration trials with the US Food and Drug Administration (FDA) are aged ≥ 70 years. Also, < 10% of older adults with cancer participated in National Cancer Institute (NCI)-sponsored clinical trials. A study by Ludmir et al. evaluated phase III clinical trials over two decades for age disparities. They found that enrollment criteria restrictions based on performance status or age cutoffs were associated with age disparities. They also found that industry-funded trials were not more likely to use these enrollment restrictions than non-industry-funded trials. Additionally, age disparities were larger among trials evaluating targeted systemic therapy and among lung cancer trials.

As a result, treatment decisions for older patients with cancer are based on data from studies conducted on younger patients. Therefore, the impact of these therapies on the QOL and functional independence of the older patient is unclear. As a community, we must realize the importance of including real-world older patients on clinical trials. As oncologists, we should remove the bias of age alone when considering patients for clinical trials. Furthermore, investigators must design clinical trials that will provide useful information for all patients. Table 51.4 outlines the efforts that could help increase the accrual of older adults to clinical trial by the clinical investigator and the treating oncologist.

8) If a deficit in a geriatric domain is found, what is the intervention?

Expert Perspective: Geriatric assessment should be repeated along the continuum of care for it may elucidate findings and needs that may change over time. Inclusion of a multidisciplinary team in the care of the patient is critical to address any challenges that arise during therapy. If a deficit in a geriatric domain is uncovered, interventions should be done to decrease morbidity and improve QOL during treatment.

The "Older Adult Oncology" NCCN guidelines as well as the ASCO guidelines provide comprehensive examples for interventions for oncologists to consider when identifying a deficit in a domain. In addition, comanagement with a geriatrician and/or primary care physician (PCP) can aide in delivery of interventions. Table 51.5 adapts recommendations from the above guidelines.

9) What are special considerations in the approach to decision-making for older adults with cancer that may be unique from younger patients?

Table 51.4 Efforts to increase enrollment of older adults onto cancer clinical trials.

Efforts by clinical investigator	Efforts by treating oncologist / oncology community
Development of elderly-specific clinical trials with inclusion of CGA. • Development of sub-cohort of older adults to take part in large studies. • Ensuring a minimum number of older patients enrolled on trials to fit the percent of older patient with each cancer in the population. • Reporting of data that is of significance for older adults, beyond survival (i.e. QOL, functional independence). • Avoid restrictive eligibility criteria. • Participate in real-world prospective database of older adults with cancers, which include CGA focused on survival, toxicity, geriatric outcomes, and QOL.	Avoid age bias and consider all older adults for clinical trials. • Ensure accessibility to clinical trials in the community, where most older adults are treated. • Improve how we communicate with older adults and create materials and messages that match their health literacy skills. (e.g. provide research materials in large font). • Learn how to be a better advocate for older adults in clinical trials and join organizations that serve them.

Expert Perspective: For an oncologist, there are unique considerations that must be weighed when caring for an older adult with cancer beyond stage, cancer biology, performance status, and patient preferences that affect decision-making. Chronological age is measured in years, but biological age is assessed by a person's physical and mental functions. Life expectancy calculators, such as ePrognosis, can estimate a patient's prognosis based on comorbidities, and therefore, can be helpful during shared decision-making with patients. Additionally, morbidity, including treatment-related toxicities, should be discussed with patients in the setting of curative- versus palliative-intent approaches. For example, in the palliative setting, agents with high risk of causing neuropathy may be omitted from chemotherapy regimens to avoid significant increased risk of falls and effect on independence. Further, functional independence and caregiver support should be considered at baseline and through the treatment trajectory. An older adult who is living functionally independent is still at increased risk for toxicities compared to younger counterparts. Further, the patient's goals (i.e. palliation), values (i.e. QOL), and decision-making capacity may carry more weight than survival (i.e. extending life at any cost).

Case Study 1

Early breast cancer

A 75-year-old female presents with a 1-centimeter ER-positive, Her2-negative breast cancer. She had a lumpectomy showing pT1N0 breast adenocarcinoma. She meets with you after surgery to discuss adjuvant treatment options, including recommendations regarding radiation therapy.

10) What do you recommend?

Table 51.5 Deficits in geriatric domains and suggested interventions.

Deficit in domain	Intervention
Physical function	Referral to physical medicine and rehabilitation PT/OT referral Home safety evaluation Promote physical activity / exercise
Comorbidity	Optimize medical condition prior to treatment Coordinate with subspecialists and PCP Evaluation of life expectancy
Cognition	Involve caregiver Assess inappropriate medications that can be stopped or changed Delirium prevention Evaluate capacity Advanced care planning Cognitive testing with referral to neuropsychologist or geriatrician
Psychological	Complimentary non-pharmacological modalities (e.g. meditation) Referral to psychology/psychiatry Treat anxiety/depression Support programs, spiritual care
Nutrition	Nutrition consult Oral care Supplemental nutrition Occupational therapy for assistive devices Speech therapy and swallowing assessment Dental evaluation for dentures Evaluate food insecurity
Polypharmacy	Medicine reconciliation Discontinue inappropriate medications Evaluate for drug-drug and drug-disease interactions

Expert Perspective: Radiation is an important part of adjuvant therapy in early breast cancer after breast conservation surgery. There are some clinical situations where adjuvant radiation may not be warranted. For example, patients 70 years and older with low-risk early stage breast cancer (i.e. luminal A, tumor size T1–T2, and node negative) who underwent breast conservation surgery have a < 3% chance of relapse. Stueber et al. found that such low-risk patients who received adjuvant radiation did not have significant differences in recurrence-free survival when compared to those who did not receive radiation. Additionally, total mastectomy in low-risk patients with the goal of sparing radiation is, therefore, not necessary. Thus, patients 70 years and older with early stage breast cancer can be treated with breast conservation surgery without adjuvant radiation and referred for oncologic discussion for systemic adjuvant therapy (Chapter 11).

Case Study 2

Metastatic colorectal cancer

A 77-year-old man has a new diagnosis of metastatic colorectal cancer to the liver, *RAS* wild type, *BRAF* wild type, Her2 negative, microsatellite stable. His past medical history is significant for controlled hypertension, diabetes mellitus type 2, and coronary artery disease. A geriatric assessment is conducted. He reports history of two falls last month, and he requires help with meals preparation, finances, laundry, and bathing. He uses a rollator walker for mobility. His daughter is his primary caregiver. He has good kidney function and no history of bleeding.

11) What treatment options would you discuss with him?

Expert Perspective: Based on the case above, the patient has multiple medical problems, including falls, and is dependent in 1 of 6 ADLs and 3 of 8 of IADLs. He has limited mobility and uses a walker. He is frail and not a candidate for standard combination chemotherapy for first-line treatment of metastatic colorectal cancer. However, he may be a candidate for the combination of capecitabine and bevacizumab. This is based on the AVEX study led by Cunningham et al., which randomized patients 70 years and older with previously untreated metastatic colorectal cancer, who were not candidates for oxaliplatin-based or irinotecan-based chemotherapy regimens, to capecitabine (1000 mg/m^2 orally twice a day on days 1–14) alone or with bevacizumab (7.5 mg/kg intravenously on day 1), given every three weeks. Patients were treated until disease progression, unacceptable toxic effects, or withdrawal of consent. Progression-free survival was longer with bevacizumab and capecitabine than with capecitabine alone (median 9.1 months vs 5.1 months; HR 0.53; $P < 0.0001$). Treatment-related adverse events of grade 3 or worse were in 40% patients in the combination group versus 22% in the capecitabine group, and treatment-related serious adverse events in 14% and 8% patients, respectively. The most common grade 3 or worse adverse events of special interest were hand-foot syndrome 16% versus 7%, diarrhea 7% versus 7%, and venous thromboembolic events 8% versus 4%, respectively. The most common any-grade adverse event of special interest for bevacizumab was hemorrhage 25% versus 7%. Thus, bevacizumab and capecitabine is an effective and well-tolerated regimen for older adults with metastatic colorectal cancer who are not candidates for standard front-line combination chemotherapy. This could be discussed with the patient and his family to consider as a treatment option (see Chapter 24).

Case Study 3

Metastatic lung adenocarcinoma

An 81-year-old man has a new diagnosis of metastatic lung adenocarcinoma, *EGFR* negative, PDL1 0%, no other targetable mutations (including *ALK, KRAS, ROS1, BRAF, NTRK 1/2/3,*

MET, RET). Imaging does not show brain metastases. He has ECOG performance status 1. His past medical history is significant for hypertension, hyperlipidemia, and chronic obstructive pulmonary disease (COPD). He has rheumatoid arthritis for which immunotherapy is contraindicated. He is independent in ADLs and IADLs, taking his medications without help, and has good hearing. He has had no falls in the last six months. He has dyspnea on exertion at less than one block. His physical health or emotional problems interfere with his social activities a little. Hemoglobin is 11.6 g/dL and creatinine clearance is 47. He is interested in treatment options, but he wants to know the risk of chemotherapy as his QOL and spending time with his family is very important to him in the palliative setting.

12) How do you proceed to counsel him?

Expert Perspective: Based on the case above, the treating oncologist can use the CARG chemotherapy toxicity tool to review risks of grade 3–5 toxicity from systemic chemotherapy with the patient. For patients with non-small cell lung cancer that does not have targetable mutations and for patients with contraindications to immunotherapy, palliative chemotherapy is typically recommended. Doublet chemotherapy (i.e. carboplatin/paclitaxel) versus single-agent chemotherapy (i.e. paclitaxel) are discussed with the patient. Based on the CARG chemotherapy toxicity tool, the risk of grade 3–5 chemotherapy-related toxicity with doublet chemotherapy is predicted to be 59% at standard doses versus 44% with a dose reduction. The risk of chemotherapy toxicity with single-agent chemotherapy is predicted to be 44% at standard dose versus 30% with a dose reduction. After discussion of risks and benefits of doublet versus single-agent chemotherapy, shared decision-making results with the plan to start with dose-reduced doublet chemotherapy with growth factor support to prevent complications from neutropenia. His goal is to continue chemotherapy if he can so that he can spend time with his grandchildren as long as he has an acceptable QOL. This case illustrates how chemotherapy toxicity prediction tools are superior to performance status in predicting toxicity and how these tools can be are necessary for shared decision-making regarding risks/benefits for chemotherapy (see Chapter 7).

Recommended Readings

Chapman, A.E., Elias, R., Plotkin, E., Lowenstein, L.M., and Swartz, K. (2021). Models of care in geriatric oncology. *J Clin Oncol* 39 (19): 2195–2204.

Cunningham, D., Lang, I., Marcuello, E., Lorusso, V., Ocvirk, J., Shin, D.B. et al. (2013 October). AVEX study investigators. Bevacizumab plus capecitabine versus capecitabine alone in elderly patients with previously untreated metastatic colorectal cancer (AVEX): an open-label, randomised phase 3 trial. *Lancet Oncol* 14 (11): 1077–1085. doi:10.1016/S1470-2045(13)70154-2. Epub 2013 Sep 10. PMID: 24028813.

Extermann, M., Boler, I., Reich, R.R., Lyman, G.H., Brown, R.H., DeFelice, J., Levine, R.M. et al. (2012). Predicting the risk of chemotherapy toxicity in older patients: the chemotherapy risk assessment scale for high-age patients (CRASH) score. *Cancer* 118: 3377–3386.

Hurria, A., Mohile, S., Gajra, A., Klepin, H., Muss, H., Chapman, A. et al. (2016 July 10). Validation of a prediction tool for chemotherapy toxicity in older adults with cancer. *J Clin Oncol* 34 (20): 2366–2371. doi: 10.1200/JCO.2015.65.4327. Epub 2016 May 16. PMID: 27185838; PMCID: PMC5321104.

Li D, Sun CL, Kim H, Soto-Perez-de-Celis E, Chung V, Koczywas M, Fakih M, Chao J, Cabrera Chien L, Charles K, Hughes SFDS, Katheria V, Trent M, Roberts E, Jayani R, Moreno J, Kelly C, Sedrak MS, Dale W. Geriatric Assessment-Driven Intervention (GAIN) on Chemotherapy-Related Toxic Effects in Older Adults With Cancer: A Randomized Clinical Trial. *JAMA Oncol.* 2021Nov 1;7(11):e214158. doi: 10.1001/jamaoncol.2021.4158. Epub 2021 Nov 18. PMID: 34591080; PMCID: PMC8485211.

Mohile, S.G., Dale, W., Somerfield, M.R., Schonberg, M.A., Boyd, C.M., Burhenn, P.S. et al. (2018 August 1). Practical assessment and management of vulnerabilities in older patients receiving chemotherapy: ASCO guideline for geriatric oncology. *J Clin Oncol* 36 (22): 2326–2347. doi: 10.1200/JCO.2018.78.8687. Epub 2018 May 21. PMID: 29782209; PMCID: PMC6063790.

Mohile SG, Mohamed MR, Xu H, Culakova E, Loh KP, Magnuson A, Flannery MA, Obrecht S, Gilmore N, Ramsdale E, Dunne RF, Wildes T, Plumb S, Patil A, Wells M, Lowenstein L, Janelsins M, Mustian K, Hopkins JO, Berenberg J, Anthony N, Dale W. Evaluation of geriatric assessment and management on the toxic effects of cancer treatment (GAP70+): a cluster-randomised study. *Lancet.* 2021 Nov 20;398(10314):1894–1904. doi: 10.1016/S0140-6736(21)01789-X. Epub 2021 Nov 3. PMID: 34741815; PMCID: PMC8647163.

Older adult oncology NCCN guidelines. Version 2.2022. https://www.nccn.org/professionals/physician_gls/pdf/senior.pdf

Owusu, C., Koroukian, S.M., Schluchter, M., Bakaki, P., and Berger, N.A. (2011 April). Screening older cancer patients for a comprehensive geriatric assessment: a comparison of three instruments. *J Geriatr Oncol* 2 (2): 121–129. doi: 10.1016/j.jgo.2010.12.002. PMID: 21927633; PMCID: PMC3173499.

Sattar, S., Alibhai, S.M., Wildiers, H., and Puts, M.T. (2014 October). How to implement a geriatric assessment in your clinical practice. *Oncol* 19 (10): 1056–1068. doi: 10.1634/theoncologist.2014-0180. Epub 2014 Sep 3. PMID: 25187477; PMCID: PMC4200997.

Stueber, T.N., Diessner, J., Bartmann, C., Leinert, E., Janni, W., Herr, D. et al. (2020 May 20). Effect of adjuvant radiotherapy in elderly patients with breast cancer. *PLoS One* 15 (5): e0229518. doi: 10.1371/journal.pone.0229518. PMID: 32434215; PMCID: PMC7239665.

Wildiers, H., Heeren, P., Puts, M., Topinkova, E., Janssen-Heijnen, M.L., Extermann, M. et al. (2014 August 20). International society of geriatric oncology consensus on geriatric assessment in older patients with cancer. *J Clin Oncol* 32 (24): 2595–2603. doi: 10.1200/JCO.2013.54.8347. PMID: 25071125; PMCID: PMC4876338.

52

Palliative Medicine for Curable and Terminal Cancers

Isabelle Blanchard, Kavitha Jennifer Ramachandran, and Divya Gupta

Stanford University, San Francisco, CA

Introduction

With the development and use of novel therapeutic agents, patients with curable and terminal cancers are living longer and requiring further palliation or supportive care of their symptoms, be it from their underlying disease or from side effects of therapies. As a result, there is a growing need for input from palliative care specialists to appropriately manage symptoms, especially in the context of which stage of disease a patient is in and their goals of care. Although there is a wide variety of treatment options for symptom management, individualizing therapy is critical and becoming increasingly complex, especially when patients have various comorbidities, intolerances/allergies, personal preferences, or are taking other medications where there is a possibility for drug-drug interactions. Ultimately, palliative care has become a vital component of the overall care of cancer patients.

Case Study 1

A 53-year-old woman presents with metastatic colon cancer involving the liver, abdominal pleura and lymph nodes, thoracic spine, and brain. Palliative care consultation was placed for symptoms of vertigo and nausea with projectile vomiting.

Initial treatment included a right-sided hemicolectomy for an obstructing adenocarcinoma of the cecum. She has since received multiple regimens of systemic chemotherapy including phase I treatment, as well as undergone craniotomy, stereotactic radiosurgery for brain metastases, and radiation therapy to the thoracic spine. Currently, she is not a candidate for any further chemotherapy and was recently informed of a poor prognosis of four to six weeks to live.

The patient is now admitted with a two-to-three-day history of nausea, vomiting, vertigo, and headache. She attributes her nausea to the administration of opioids and has a history of akathisia with metoclopramide. For nausea, she finds ondansetron to be ineffective and prefers to take lorazepam 0.25–0.5 mg as needed.

Her Edmonton Symptom Assessment Scale is: Pain 5, fatigue 6, nausea 7, depression 0, anxiety 0, drowsiness 2, appetite 2, feeling of well-being 1, shortness of breath 0, sleep 0.

Her symptoms are significant for left-sided, constant, frontal headache, which is worse in the morning hours and non-radiating intermittent chronic mid- to low-back pain. Headache has persisted for the past three days, and she rates the intensity as 5 of 10. She achieves some pain relief with acetaminophen. In addition, she reports vertigo with any type of movement or with standing. Otherwise, the remainder of the review of systems is negative.

Vital signs include afebrile temperature, pulse 56, respiration rate 17, BP 121/90, and O_2 saturation was 94% on room air. Physical examination is notable for a chronically ill-appearing woman who is somewhat anxious and talks openly about her concerns. Laboratory values are within normal limits.

1) **Which of the following factors may be contributing to the patient's nausea?**
   A) Gastroparesis.
   B) Increased intracranial pressure.
   C) Anxiety.
   D) Vestibular dysfunction.
   E) All of the above.

Expert Perspective: Nausea with or without symptoms of vomiting is not uncommon in patients with advanced cancer. A stepwise, thoughtful approach is needed for the workup of nausea including a detailed history and physical examination. Once an underlying mechanism is identified, therapy can be tailored to each unique clinical scenario. However, as in this case, multiple factors may play a role requiring more than one intervention in order to block multiple pathways resulting in emesis.

The first step in the evaluation of nausea includes a thorough history characterizing the symptom with attention for clues to the underlying etiology. Early satiety may indicate gastroparesis, nausea and vomiting in the morning hours with symptoms of head discomfort suggest increased intracranial pressure, nausea relieved by infrequent, large emesis may indicate a bowel obstruction, and a temporal pattern of nausea associated with emotional reaction suggests underlying anxiety. Cancer that has metastasized to the liver, peritoneum, or brain is often associated with nausea.

A complete review of medications is extremely critical. Research indicates common factors resulting in nausea and vomiting include medications (i.e. opioids, chemotherapy, antibiotics) and constipation. Other factors associated with nausea in cancer patients include infections, metabolic abnormalities, gastroparesis secondary to autonomic dysfunction, radiation especially to the abdomen and pelvis, and bowel obstruction.

Physical examination may provide additional clues regarding the underlying etiology for nausea and vomiting. Loss of heart rate variability or orthostatic hypotension suggests autonomic dysfunction, evidence of mucositis or thrush may result in oropharyngeal or esophageal irritation, abdominal distention or masses provide evidence of abdominal cancer or malignant ascites, and rectal examination may reveal impaction suggesting constipation.

Nausea and vomiting are the result of stimulation of the following pathways:
a) Chemoreceptor trigger zone with its porous blood-brain barrier is localized to the area postrema in the floor of the fourth ventricle where chemosensitive nerve cell projections are bathed by cerebrospinal fluid that is in equilibrium with blood in the fenestrated local capillaries;
b) Cortex with input from the senses;

c) Peripheral pathways via mechanoreceptors in the upper gastrointestinal tract, vagal and splanchnic nerves, glossopharyngeal nerves, and sympathetic ganglia;
d) Vestibular system.

In cancer patients, common causes of nausea include opioid use, chemotherapy, autonomic dysfunction, and bowel obstruction. Opioid treatment results in nausea and vomiting in 40% of patients by stimulation of the chemoreceptor trigger zone, gastroparesis, constipation, and alterations in vestibular function. In advanced cancer patients with chronic nausea, autonomic dysfunction may result in gastroparesis and constipation. Autonomic failure affects the majority of patients with advanced cancer and is associated with decreased survival.

Autonomic dysfunction in cancer patients has a multifactorial etiology including cachexia, medications including chemotherapy, direct tumor invasion of nerves or paraneoplastic syndrome, and comorbidities such as diabetes or heart failure.

Measures to prevent constipation and avoid medications that may exacerbate autonomic dysfunction should be implemented.

Correct Answer: E

2) To control the patient's intractable nausea with vomiting, which medication would you initiate?
  A) Metoclopramide.
  B) Dexamethasone.
  C) Haloperidol.
  D) Diphenhydramine.
  E) Ondansetron.

Expert Perspective: Two approaches to the management of nausea and vomiting have been proposed. One approach involves treatment based on the underlying mechanism and found to be effective in up to 90% of patients with advanced disease. Others have proposed initiation of an empirical anti-emetic regimen, usually a dopamine antagonist, irrespective of the underlying etiology. No head-to-head comparison of the two strategies has been studied to date.

In clinical practice, patients with advanced cancer often have symptoms of nausea and vomiting due to multiple underlying factors. All potential reversible etiologies must be assessed and treated while simultaneously administering an antiemetic to control symptoms. A dopamine antagonist such as metoclopramide or haloperidol would be a sensible empiric treatment for nausea.

In the case presentation, the patient has a history of akathisia to metoclopramide. Her history of head discomfort and early morning nausea with MRI revealing progression of brain metastasis would argue to initiate dexamethasone as first-line therapy. With the above change in treatment, the patient has less projectile vomiting but continues to be symptomatic despite a trial of several anti-emetic medications.

Case Study continued: In the next 48 hours, the patient develops increased confusion with periods of agitation at night resulting in distress to the patient, family, and nursing staff. Family at bedside observes that agitation has a temporal relationship with the administration of lorazepam which causes brief sedation followed by agitation and confusion. Memorial delirium assessment scale was conducted by palliative care fellow at beside and found to be 10/30.

Correct Answer: B

3) Which of the following treatments is the first-line therapy to control agitation secondary to underlying delirium?
   A) Repeat dose of lorazepam.
   B) Haloperidol.
   C) Chlorpromazine.
   D) Diphenhydramine.
   E) Physical restraints.

Expert Perspective: Delirium is a common symptom at the end of life and results in distress not only for patients but also for their family and health care providers. Delirium is characterized by a disturbance in consciousness with an inability to focus, shifts in attention, and perceptual disturbances, which fluctuate over time. The majority of patients have a good recollection of their experience while delirious, resulting in distress. Appropriate interventions are needed to treat underlying precipitation factors including infections, dehydration, electrolyte abnormalities such as hypercalcemia and hyponatremia, organ failure, medications such as opioids and benzodiazepines, intracranial disease, as well as a number of other factors and must be initiated rapidly. In cancer patients, delirium is frequently underdiagnosed resulting in undertreatment. Several clinical tools to assess for delirium exist, but only the Memorial Delirium Assessment Scale (MDAS) and the brief observational Nursing Delirium Screening Scale (NuDESC) are both diagnostic and able to quantify the severity of delirium, allowing patients to be monitored over time.

Limited research exists examining pharmacological treatment of delirium. In hospitalized patients with AIDS, Breitbart et al. performed a seminal double-blind, randomized comparison trial of haloperidol, chlorpromazine, and lorazepam. Both haloperidol and chlorpromazine were effective; however, chlorpromazine was associated with a significant decline in cognitive function. The arm receiving lorazepam was stopped early secondary to side effects including excessive sedation, worsening mentation and disinhibition, and ataxia. The combination of haloperidol with lorazepam has been proposed for the treatment of agitated, delirious patients in order to minimize extrapyramidal side effects but more studies are needed. In addition, atypical antipsychotic medications secondary to decreased risk of extrapyramidal adverse effects are being evaluated in the treatment of delirium; however, high-quality randomized controlled trials are lacking.

Correct Answer: B

Case Study continued: The same day, the patient's primary oncologist visits the patient, who is agitated and distressed. He recommends transfer to an inpatient palliative care unit and consideration for palliative sedation.

4) For which of the following conditions is palliative sedation clearly indicated?
   A) Chronic nausea.
   B) Anxiety and depression.

C) Terminal delirium with agitation.
D) Transient respite care.
E) Existential pain.

Expert Perspective: Patient is transferred to the acute palliative care unit, and reversible causes of delirium were worked up and treated by an interdisciplinary team. Patient remained agitated despite administration of haloperidol (>10 mg/day), and a trial of chlorpromazine was initiated and found to be ineffective in controlling symptoms. No reversible etiology was noted, and the patient was diagnosed with terminal delirium.

Correct Answer: C

Case Study continued: Discussions with the patient's family caregivers about palliative sedation to control symptoms at the end of life were deliberated and agreed upon.

5) **Which of the following medications titrated to control symptoms would be appropriate for palliative sedation?**
   A) Intermittent lorazepam as needed for agitation.
   B) Continuous midazolam titrated to control symptoms.
   C) Continuous morphine drip titrated to control symptoms.
   D) Scheduled haloperidol every four hours.
   E) Scheduled haloperidol every four hours with intermittent lorazepam as needed for agitation.

Expert Perspective: Palliative sedation is a treatment of last resort for refractory symptoms in patients with cancer. Symptoms are refractory when they are inadequately controlled despite aggressive treatment that does not compromise consciousness. An interdisciplinary team with specialists in pain and symptom management should ideally be involved in assessment and treatment of symptoms before categorizing them as refractory.

A potential for misunderstanding exists regarding palliative sedation, which may result in distress for a patient's family and health care providers as well as loss of reputability of the physicians involved and institutions, resulting in potential litigation.

The European Association of Palliative Care has outlined four "problem practices":

i) Abuse of palliative sedation with the goal of hastening death.
ii) Injudicious use of palliative sedation when health care providers inadequately assess or treat symptoms, resort to sedation out of frustration or burnout, or use of palliative sedation upon request of a distressed family member.
iii) Injudicious withholding of palliative sedation when avoidance of difficult discussions or concerns about hastening death result in providing ineffective treatments.
iv) Substandard implementation of palliative sedation including inadequate consultations with all parties involved regarding indications for sedation, goals of care, outcomes and risks; inadequate monitoring of symptoms while providing sedation; escalation of sedatives when not required; use of inappropriate medications (e.g. opioids); or inadequate emotional and spiritual support is provided for a patient's family.

Indications for palliative sedation vary widely between groups and settings and consensus is often lacking. Emergency situations where palliative sedation for patients with advanced cancer is clearly indicated include intractable convulsions, massive hemorrhage, asphyxiation, terminal dyspnea or delirium refractory to medical therapy. At our institution, the most common indications were delirium (82%), dyspnea (6%), and other symptoms (6%) including bleeding and seizures. In terminal patients, indications with no clear consensus for palliative sedation include refractory depression, anxiety, or existential distress.

No evidence exists for a first-line treatment for palliative sedation, but benzodiazepines are the most commonly used sedative. Of the benzodiazepines, midazolam is the most frequently used and is typically administered parenterally. Because of its short half-life, midazolam is easily titrated to control symptoms and possesses anxiolytic and anticonvulsant properties, which make it desirable for palliative sedation. Barbiturates, such as phenobarbital and propofol, are also occasionally used for palliative sedation. Opioids such as morphine are not useful agents for palliative sedation since they provide sedation only at toxic doses, and their use is associated with side-effects including worsening delirium, myoclonus, and respiratory sedation. However, if patients are on chronic opioid therapy for the management of pain, they should be continued.

Correct Answer: C

Case Study 2

A 36-year-old premenopausal female presents with newly diagnosed stage III invasive ductal carcinoma of the right breast. She was just started on ovarian suppression with monthly goserelin injections and is about to start standard chemotherapy.

Her social history is notable for a remote history of methamphetamine abuse and cigarette smoking. She lives at home with her supportive husband and does not have any children currently though may be interested in having children in the future. She does not align herself with a particular faith but does consider herself to be a spiritual person. Moreover, she works as an ad executive, and her appearance and confidence are very important to her. She is currently worried about hair loss and neuropathy associated with chemotherapy. She is referred to palliative care to discuss symptom relief and alternatives to typical medications for her treatment.

Physical examination is unremarkable with stable vital signs. Weight 63.4 kg, height 66 inches, BMI = 22.6. Laboratory values are within normal limits.

She does not endorse any pain currently but is interested in understanding more about non-opioid pain control, especially tetrahydrocannabinol (THC)/cannabidiol (CBD)-based.

6) Which of the following is NOT an example of a coanalgesic?
  A) Glucocorticoids.
  B) Opioids.
  C) Cannabis and cannabinoids.
  D) Anticonvulsants.

Expert Perspective: Coanalgesics or adjuvant analgesics describe a class of medications with a major clinical use other than pain control that can be used as an analgesic. Examples include glucocorticoids and anticonvulsants. There is growing interest in the use of cannabinoids as a coanalgesic though unfortunately there is limited data regarding its efficacy especially in patients with cancer-related pain. In the US, there are two synthetic cannabinoids (dronabinol and nabilone) that are approved for treatment of chemotherapy-induced nausea and vomiting as well as appetite stimulation in wasting illnesses. An oromucosal spray containing THC and CBD called Nabiximols is available in other countries for use as an adjunctive treatment for opioid-refractory pain. Results of placebo-controlled clinical trials of Nabiximols in chronic cancer-related pain, however, were equivocal but did not identify new safety concerns or evidence of tolerance during extended use. Other published randomized trials have demonstrated short-term benefit for smoked or vaporized cannabis in patients with neuropathic pain, though none of the trials included patients with cancer-related pain. Opioids is NOT an example of coanalgesic.

Correct Answer: B

7) Which of the following statements regarding alopecia due to systemic chemotherapy is false:
   A) Alopecia is a transient and usually reversible consequence of systemic chemotherapy.
   B) Systemic chemotherapy-associated alopecia can be emotionally traumatic for patients and cause them to delay necessary therapy.
   C) There are currently no FDA approved therapies for the prevention of chemotherapy associated alopecia.
   D) None of the above are false statements.

Expert Perspective: Alopecia is a common, transient, and usually reversible side effect of cytotoxic chemotherapy that can be emotionally traumatic for patients and cause them to delay therapy. Scalp hypothermia has been increasingly used to prevent chemotherapy-associated alopecia. It induces local vasoconstriction of scalp blood vessels to reduce the delivery of chemotherapy to the scalp, decreases the metabolic rate of hair follicle cells, and reduces cellular drug uptake. There are two automated scalp cooling devices (DigniCap and Paxman) that have been cleared by the FDA for use in the US based on two clinical trials involving patients receiving neoadjuvant chemotherapy for breast cancer. The efficacy of scalp hypothermia, however, is variable and dependent on the type and intensity of planned chemotherapy. For instance, there is significantly less hair preservation in patients receiving anthracyclines compared with non-anthracycline-based regimens. Adverse events associated with scalp hypothermia include cold intolerance, headaches, and lightheadedness. Despite this, it is currently listed as an option for alopecia prevention in the breast cancer NCCN guidelines. Patients should be counseled on the high costs associated with treatment and that insurance companies may not cover the full cost.

Correct Answer: C

Case Study continued: As the patient begins chemotherapy, her husband becomes her primary caretaker. Her husband presents with her to palliative care clinic and asks for resources for caregiver support.

8) Which of the following statements regarding caregiver support is true?
   A) On average, caregivers provide care for cancer patients for ~10 hours per week.
   B) Caregiver well-being can have direct and indirect effects on the quality of cancer care for patients.
   C) There are no adverse outcomes associated with caregiving for caregivers.

Expert Perspective: Cancer caregiving is a major source of stress for caregivers and can have a negative impact on their health and quality of life. Some of the tasks caregivers perform include attending appointments, keeping track of side effects, managing or controlling symptoms, administering medicine, and other medical/nursing tasks (administering IV infusions, managing ventilators, providing tube feeding). They typically provide an average of 35 hours of care to cancer patients per week. Multiple studies have demonstrated that caregiving can be associated with worsening physical health, insomnia, and poor mental health. Moreover, caregiver well-being has direct and indirect effects on the quality of cancer care, including care from the health care team, the caregiver themselves, and the patient regarding their own self-management. As a result, supporting caregivers has tangible consequences with regards to the quality of care patients receive. There has been support for technology-driven interventions for informal caregivers, including those that help assess the burden of caregiving, facilitate further integration of caregivers into formal health care settings, and provide content regarding symptom management and coping.

Caregivers have a multitude of coping strategies, of which the most common is turning to their spirituality. Spiritual care, which includes the religious and existential aspects of care, is one of the domains endorsed by the National Consensus Project (NCP) for Quality Palliative Care. Spiritual distress is a significant aspect of overall distress, and health care providers should be trained to perform spiritual screening and document a patient's spirituality/religious preferences in the patient record. Care plans should include a referral to trained spiritual care providers as appropriate, the development of spiritual goals, and interventions to address those goals.

Correct Answer: B

Case Study continued: After initiating chemotherapy, the patient develops significant neutropenia, putting her at risk for infections and neutropenic fever. As a result, she gets started on filgrastim, a G-CSF (granulocyte colony-stimulating factor) injection, to decrease the duration of neutropenia with each cycle of chemotherapy. Unfortunately, shortly after starting G-CSF therapy, she develops severe bone pain, one of the most common side effects associated with G-CSF.

9) How best to treat bone pain related to G-CSF?

Expert Perspective: The etiology of G-CSF-associated pain is uncertain but is thought to be related to the expansion of granulocyte progenitor cells in the bone marrow that occurs as a result of the drug. NSAIDs have only been modestly effective at reducing the severity of bone pain. On the other hand, antihistamines, loratadine in particular, have been reported to be very effective in relieving bone pain from G-CSF therapy. The patient is started on the antihistamine, loratadine, and her bone pain significantly improves.

Case Study 3

A 63-year-old man with a diagnosis of non-small cell lung cancer was initially treated with four cycles of neoadjuvant chemotherapy including carboplatin and paclitaxel. He had a significant clinical response and underwent a left-sided pneumonectomy. Despite treatment, he developed recurrence of his cancer in his kidney and subsequently received docetaxel plus amplimexon with continued progression of his underlying disease. He presents to an outpatient palliative care clinic with complaints of decreased appetite, weight loss, and severe fatigue. Despite his symptom burden, he continues to work. Patient also describes syncopal episodes after getting up from a seated position. His past medical history is significant for renal vein thrombosis. Medications include megestrol acetate, prescribed for anorexia by his oncologist and lovenox.

His Edmonton Symptom Assessment Scale is: Pain 0, fatigue 9, nausea 0, depression 0, anxiety 0, drowsiness 3, shortness of breath 2, appetite 2, sleep 2, feeling of well-being 7.

Physical examination is unremarkable with stable vital signs. Weight 81.2 kg, height 193 cm, BMI = 21.8, laboratory values are significant for a hemoglobin of 10.8.

10) **Which of the following are known complications of megesterol acetate?**
    A) Edema.
    B) Adrenal insufficiency.
    C) Thromboembolism.
    D) Hypogonadism in male patients.
    E) All of the above.

Expert Perspective: Megestrol acetate is an appetite stimulant with predominantly progestational and anti-gonadotropic effects. Side effects of megestrol include edema, adrenal insufficiency, thromboembolism, and hypogonadism in male patients. Systematic reviews have concluded that megestrol has a beneficial effect on appetite and overall weight; however, no effect was reported on lean body mass and overall quality of life. To reduce the risk of side effects, it is recommended to start at the lowest effective dose and titrate to a maximum of 800 mg/day.

Correct Answer: E

Case Study continued: For symptoms of anorexia, the patient has noticed a significant improvement since initiating megestrol. In view of his symptom improvement, he was suggested to consider decreasing his dose to 400 mg to continue at the lowest effective dose. In addition, a testosterone, morning cortisol, and thyroid panel were ordered. For his fatigue, he was recommended to resume exercising as tolerated twice a week and offered a trial of methylphenidate, which he declined in favor of a non-pharmacological approach. At the one-month follow-up visit his labs were: thyroid stimulating hormone 1.67, cortisol 1.9, total testosterone 31, and albumin of 3.4. His symptom burden was unchanged. He was discontinued on megestrol and supplemented with steroids, dexamethasone 4 mg in the morning, with instructions to taper. The following month, he rated fatigue a 1/10 and was compliant with recommendations to exercise and his appetite remained good while he was on steroids.

11) **Which of the following is the best assessment of weight in cancer patients with cachexia?**
    A) Body Mass Index (BMI).
    B) Dual-energy X-ray absorptiometry (DEXA).
    C) Bioelectrical impedance analysis (BIA).
    D) Computed tomography.

Expert Perspective: Body mass index is easily calculated with a patient's weight and height. In general, BMI <20 has been used as a marker for nutritional deficiency and cachexia. However, the accuracy of BMI has been shown to be limited and does not factor a patient's age, gender, or proportion of bone, lean body mass, and fat content. Chronically ill patients despite having a normal BMI may have decreased fat-free mass and increased fat mass.

DEXA scans are a highly accurate measure of weight and can differentiate body composition but are mainly used in the research setting. Computed tomography and magnetic resonance imaging may also be useful, but due to the high cost, their use in clinical practice is limited. Bioelectrical impedance analysis is a low-cost assessment of weight and can distinguish fat-free mass and fat mass. But in patients with cancer, bioelectrical impedance analysis underestimates fat-free mass compared to DEXA, and edema may affect the accuracy of the recordings.

Correct Answer: B

Case Study continued: The patient continues to lose weight and is distressed about his weight loss. He is counseled in the clinic by a nutritionist and requests another pharmacological intervention to treat his weight loss.

12) Which of the following pharmacological interventions has shown promising results in the treatment of cancer cachexia?
    A) Dronabinol.
    B) L-carnitine (4 g/day) and celecoxib.
    C) L-carnitine (4 g/day), celecoxib, and megestrol acetate.
    D) Cyproheptadine.

Expert Perspective: Alterations in body image as a result of cachexia often result in distress for both cancer patients and their family. Cachexia is an ominous sign of impending death and psychosocial support for patients and family is critical. With regards to cachexia, the social benefits of eating at the dinner table and the pleasure of tasting food should be emphasized over the exact amount of total caloric intake. Often, patients and family have to be counseled that decreasing appetite and oral intake resulting in cachexia is not an uncommon symptom but a part of the natural process that occurs with advancing illness.

There are several treatments undergoing research for the treatment of cancer cachexia. Initial pilot studies of dronabinol, a cannabinoid, showed promise for the treatment of anorexia; however, a double-blind, placebo-controlled study failed to show a beneficial effect. Cyproheptadine, a histamine antagonist with anti-serotonergic properties, in a small pilot study reported a small improvement in appetite but no significant effect on weight. The tetracyclic antidepressant mirtazapine induces weight gain and increases food intake at standard doses, and a phase II trial did demonstrate weight gain and improved appetite for non-depressed patients who took mirtazapine.

Interventions that appear to be promising for the treatment of cancer cachexia include L-carnitine and NSAIDs. L-carnitine is a quaternary ammonium compound required for the transport of fatty acids to the mitochondria where they are utilized to generate metabolic energy. In cancer patients, decreased caloric intake and diminished endogenous synthesis results in low levels of L-carnitine. A recent well-designed placebo-controlled clinical trial reported that L-carnitine supplementation increased BMI and quality of life in patients with pancreatic cancer. NSAIDs such as celecoxib have been shown to increase weight in cancer patients either as a single agent or in combination with megestrol acetate.

Other interventions that may be promising in the treatment of cancer cachexia is omega-3 fatty acids, eicosapentaenoic acid, and docosahexaenoic acid, which are found in fish oil and known to reduce inflammation. Initial studies have been inconclusive; however, recent studies have been more encouraging. The recent positive results have been attributed to efforts to improve compliance with fish oil supplementation and provide interventions earlier in the disease trajectory.

Since the underlying mechanism of anorexia-cachexia syndrome is complex, researchers have argued that a single therapeutic agent would be ineffective in reversing weight loss and that a better approach would be to incorporate multimodal therapy targeting simultaneously multiple underlying physiological processes that result in weight loss. One study examined the combination of L-carnitine (4 g/day) and celecoxib (300 mg/day) with or without megestrol acetate and found identical responses.

Up to four different agents for the treatment of cancer cachexia have been studied, and more research is needed to delineate the right combination of medications that provide benefit without side effects. For this patient, a combination of L-carnitine and celecoxib may be reasonable to initiate.

Correct Answer: B

Case Study 4

A 56-year-old woman with metastatic non-small lung cancer, has been referred by her oncologist for the management of fatigue. She has complications of a malignant pleural effusion, which has required a thoracentesis. Recently, she has received chemotherapy with carboplatin, pemetrexed, and bevacizumab, which was followed by maintenance pemetrexed and bevacizumab. She is maintaining her weight and her Zubrod performance status is 1. The patient has significant pain at the site of pleurodesis, which is described as aching, intermittent. She also has a history of chronic neck and low-back pain and describes the pain as intermittent, sharp, and worse with activity. Hydrocodone with acetaminophen (10/325 mg) was prescribed for pain, which she takes up to 12 tablets a day.

Past medical history is notable for thyroid follicular cancer treated with total thyroidectomy followed by iodine treatment. She is married with two teenaged children. Social history is otherwise unremarkable.

Her Edmonton Symptom Assessment Scale is: Pain 8, fatigue 8, nausea 6, depression 8, anxiety 3, drowsiness 8, shortness of breath 3, appetite 8, feeling of well-being 8, sleep 3.

Review of systems is significant for the following: The patient requires frequent napping, which does not relieve symptoms of fatigue. She also had a history of fleeting thoughts of hurting herself but denies having a plan in place. She denies symptoms of anhedonia, feelings of hopelessness, worthlessness, or guilt. In the past, the patient has been prescribed bupropion and mirtazapine for symptoms of clinical depression, which she discontinued because she "didn't like the way the medications made her feel." She occasionally takes lorazepam to assist with falling asleep, which she recently has been taking on a nightly basis.

Other medications include rosuvastatin, dexamethasone with chemotherapy, furosemide as needed for lower extremity edema, thyroid supplementation, and two blood pressure medications, losartan and amlodipine.

Laboratory values are notable for hemoglobin of 10.9 g/dL; otherwise, complete blood count and electrolyte panel are normal. PET-CT scan revealed stable residual nodule in left upper lobe consistent with treated malignancy.

For pain, the patient has been previously prescribed morphine, which caused itching, rash, hives, and difficulty breathing. She is reluctant to use any strong opioids at this time. She feels that hydrocodone is controlling her pain and was instructed to continue hydrocodone but not exceed eight tablets per day.

Vital signs: Temperature 36.5, pulse 94, respiratory rate 18, blood pressure 109/59, O_2 saturation 95%, weight 76.8 kg. Physical examination is otherwise normal with the exception of dry oral mucosa and flat affect.

13) **Which of the following statements regarding the role of lorazepam for the treatment of sleep disturbances in patients with advanced cancer is correct?**
    A) When used for a short term it reduces the time of sleep onset and improves sleep efficacy.
    B) Prolonged use may result in fragmented sleep, tolerance, and/or dependence.
    C) It may cause daytime delirium, sedation, and fatigue in older adults.
    D) It may exacerbate respiratory suppression when are used in combination with opioids.
    E) All of the above.

Expert Perspective: Benzodiazepines are used because of their sedative properties to reduce the time to sleep onset and to improve sleep efficiency. Unfortunately, tolerance to these medications occurs rapidly, and their prolonged use can cause sleep disturbances, such as fragmented sleep and dependence on medication for sleep onset. In addition, several side effects have been observed with benzodiazepines, such as daytime sedation, delirium, and fatigue. Benzodiazepine dose has also been associated with increased falls particularly in adults with cancer.

Correct Answer: E

14) **With regards to the patient's cancer-related fatigue, which of the following would NOT help improve her symptoms?**
    A) Trial of methylphenidate.
    B) Weaning lorazepam and discontinue diuretic if not clearly indicated.
    C) Dexamethasone.
    D) Modafinil.
    E) Antidepressants.

Expert Perspective: Pharmacological treatments for fatigue are limited, and a paucity of randomized controlled trials exists for patients with advanced cancer. Glucocorticoids, including dexamethasone (8 mg/day for 14 days), has been shown to improve fatigue in patients with advanced cancer. Long-term use of glucocorticoids is limited by side effects including increased infections, insomnia, elevation of blood glucose, myalgia, mood swings, edema, poor wound healing, and gastritis. Cancer patients at the last stages of life may derive the most benefit from glucocorticoids.

Psychostimulants including methylphenidate (5 mg at breakfast and lunch time titrated to a maximum of 40 mg/day) and modafinil (200 mg in the morning) have been shown to be helpful in the management of fatigue in cancer patients; however, the data from randomized controlled trials are mixed. Caution should be applied in cancer patients with heart disease and cognitive dysfunction.

Correct Answer: E

Case Study continued: In this patient's case lorazepam was weaned off, and furosemide was discontinued. She presented with no clear signs of major depression; however, she was closely monitored over the next three months. For symptoms of fatigue, a trial of methylphenidate was initiated and titrated to 10 mg in the morning and mid-day. Her symptoms of fatigue and her mood have improved. On follow-up visit, the patient's oncologist recommends that acetaminophen should not be used on a continuous basis. Workup of her back pain revealed underlying metastasis to his seventh thoracic vertebra.

15) **Which opioid would you recommend for her chronic back pain?**
    A) Morphine.
    B) Codeine.
    C) Oxycodone.
    D) Fentanyl.

Expert Perspective: True allergy to morphine results in hives or difficulty breathing. Often, nausea and itching as a result of morphine administration is confused with an allergic reaction. The patient appears to have a true allergy to morphine. Morphine as well as codeine, hydrocodone, hydromorphone, oxycodone, and oxymorphone belong in the same class of phenanthrenes and it is advisable to try an opioid in another class such as fentanyl (phenylpiperidines) or methadone (phenylheptylamines).

Correct Answer: D

Case Study continued: Her fentanyl dose has been increased to 125 mcg every 72 hours, and she was using hydromorphone 4 mg for breakthrough pain. The patient's husband called the clinic regarding poorly controlled pain and confusion, and she was admitted to the hospital for further workup. MRI reveals no evidence of brain metastasis. Workup revealed no sources for infection, no electrolyte abnormalities, or reversible etiologies that would result in confusion.

16) **The switching of one opioid to another opioid using an equianalgesic table is known as opioid rotation. Which of the following are indications to rotate opioids?**
    A) Neurotoxicity from opioids such as hallucinations, myoclonus, and confusion.
    B) Uncontrolled pain despite opioid titration and addition of adjuvants.
    C) Financial burden of the cost of an opioid.
    D) Opioid-related nausea despite adequate medical management.
    E) All of the above.

Expert Perspective: Opioid rotation is recommended for the development of adverse effects including opioid-induced neurotoxicity such as confusion, myoclonus, and hallucinations as well as uncontrolled pain despite the adjustment of dose. Other practical concerns that might result in opioid rotation include minimizing the number of pills or cost of the medication, better compliance (e.g. rotation to a transdermal delivery system in a patient unable to tolerate an oral regimen), and in cases of organ failure (e.g. rotation to methadone in the setting of renal failure).

Correct Answer: E

17) **Which opioid would be the best to control his pain?**
    A) Increase fentanyl patch to 150 mcg every 72 hours with hydromorphone 4 mg as needed for breakthrough pain.
    B) Change to methadone 10 mg every 12 hours with oxycodone 5 mg every four hours as needed for breakthrough pain.
    C) Change opioids to oxycodone extended release 20 mg every 12 hours with oxycodone 5 mg every four hours as needed for breakthrough pain.
    D) Change to morphine extended release 100 mg every 12 hours with morphine 15 mg every four hours as needed for breakthrough pain.

Expert Perspective: The reason why opioid rotation is successful is unclear. Incomplete cross-tolerance to the analgesic effects of opioids being greater than the cross-tolerance to adverse effects may play a role. Opioid rotation to methadone is difficult secondary to the lack of reliable equianalgesic conversion ratios, large inter-individual variability in pharmacokinetics, and pharmacological interactions of methadone with other drugs. Rotation to methadone is best performed by a specialist in palliative care or pain management and requires strict monitoring.

The patient presents with delirium most likely secondary to opioid escalation resulting in neurotoxicity. Opioid rotation would be indicated, and methadone would be a reasonable second-line strong-opioid under close supervision. Compared to other strong opioids, methadone has a number of potential advantages including no known active metabolites and no significant elimination by the kidneys. In addition, methadone is a relatively potent N-methyl-D-aspartate (NMDA) receptor antagonist. NMDA as well as other excitatory amino acids have been implicated in the development of neuropathic pain and opioid tolerance. The use of methadone as a first-line strong-opioid for the treatment of cancer pain is unclear, and more research is needed. After rotating her opioids, the patient's delirium improved.

Correct Answer: B

Recommended Readings

Breitbart, W. and Alici, Y. (2008). Agitation and delirium at the end of life: "We couldn't manage him". *JAMA* 300 (24): 2898–2910.

Fearon, K., Strasser, F., Anker, S.D. et al. (2011). Definition and classification of cancer cachexia: an international consensus. *Lancet Oncol* 12: 489–495.

Litzelman, K. (2019 August). Caregiver well-being and the quality of cancer care. *Semin Oncol Nurs* 35 (4): 348–353.

Ripamonti, C.I., Giuntoli, F., Gonella, S., and Miccinesi, G. (2018 July). Spiritual care in cancer patients: a need or an option? *Curr Opin Oncol* 30 (4): 212–218.

Silva, G.B., Ciccolini, K., Donati, A., and Hurk, C.V.D. (2020 September-October). Scalp cooling to prevent chemotherapy-induced alopecia. *An Bras Dermatol* 95 (5): 631–637.

Weeks, J.C., Catalano, P.J., Cronin, A. et al. (2012). Patients' expectations about effects of chemotherapy for advanced cancer. *N Engl J Med* 367: 1616–1625.

Wood, G.J., Shega, J.W., Lynch, B. et al. (2007). Management of intractable nausea and vomiting in patients at the end of life "I was feeling nauseous all of the time ... nothing was working". *JAMA* 298 (10): 1196–1207.

Index

Locators followed by 'f' and 't' refer to figures and tables respectively.

a

ABC-06 trial   323–324
abdominal/abdomen:
  cavity   502
  cryptorchidism   438
  distention, initial treatment for   499–501
  pain   587
  perineal resection   589
  skin bruising   658
abemaciclib   140, 141t
abiraterone/prednisone   426, 432–433
abnormal uterine bleeding   584
ACCORD 03 trial   343, 351
ACCORD 16 trial   356
acetaminophen   703
ACOG. See American College of Obstetricians and Gynecologists (ACOG)
ACS. See American Cancer Society (ACS)
ACTICCA-1 trial (NCT02170090)   321
ACTION. See Adjuvant Clinical Trial in Ovarian Neoplasms (ACTION)
acute kidney injury   655
acute myeloid leukemia (AML)   184
acute palliative care unit   697
adagrasib, NSCLC patients   90
ADAURA trial   67, 68
ADC. See antibody drug conjugate (ADC)
adenocarcinoma   541, 643
  of colon   629–630
  histology in CUP   641–642
  in liver   647–648
  metastatic lung   651
  of sigmoid colon   633
adenomatous polyps in colon   630
adenosarcomas   531–532
adenosquamous cervical cancer   541
adjuvant chemoradiotherapy,
    gastroesophageal cancer   237
adjuvant chemotherapy   501, 507–509
  benefit of   321
  bladder cancer   382–383
  colon cancer   258, 260–261
  endometrial cancer   528–529
  gastroesophageal cancer   237
  male breast cancer   216
  NSCLC:
    stage I-III   65t
    stage II-III   64, 66
  SCLC   100
Adjuvant Clinical Trial in Ovarian Neoplasms (ACTION)   507
ADJUVANT-CTONG 1104 trial   67
Adjuvant Lapatinib and Trastuzumab Treatment Optimization (ALTTO) trial   161
adjuvant radiation therapy   482–483
  DCIS   120–123
  SCLC   100
adjuvant systemic therapy, breast cancer   129–130
adjuvant temozolomide   8
adjuvant therapy:
  breast cancer   136–137
  extended, HER2-positive breast cancer   158–161
  in gastric adenocarcinoma:
    with nodal disease   243–244
    without nodal disease   244

Cancer Consult: Expertise in Clinical Practice, Volume 1: Solid Tumors & Supportive Care,
Second Edition. Edited by Syed A. Abutalib, Maurie Markman, Al B. Benson III, and Hope S. Rugo.
© 2024 John Wiley & Sons Ltd. Published 2024 by John Wiley & Sons Ltd.

adrenal insufficiency 670
adriamycin 577
ADT. *See* androgen deprivation therapy (ADT)
adults:
   genetic testing in 605
   malignant tumors 4
advanced/metastatic disease 551–552
AFAP. *See* attenuated FAP (AFAP)
AFP. *See* alpha fetoprotein (AFP)
aggressive fibromatoses 591
agitation 695–696
AJCC8 staging system 481–482
alanine transaminase (ALT) 666–667
alcohol abuse 309
alopecia 699
alpelisib 146, 148
alpha fetoprotein (AFP) 310, 557
ALT. *See* alanine transaminase (ALT)
alveolar soft part sarcoma 587–588
amenorrhea, chemotherapy-induced 226–227, 226t
American Association for the Study of Liver diseases (AASLD) 310
American Brachytherapy Society 408
American Cancer Society (ACS) 604
American College of Obstetricians and Gynecologists (ACOG) 616
American Joint Committee on Cancer (AJCC) staging system 411
   mesothelioma 108, 109–110t
American Society for Radiation Oncology 119
American Society of Clinical Oncology (ASCO) 59, 119, 136, 177, 181, 390, 568, 601, 677
American Society of Oncology 27
American Thyroid Association (ATA) 40
AML. *See* acute myeloid leukemia (AML)
anal cancer:
   anal canal 347
   anal margin 347
   anticipated trials 355–356
   biomarkers in 347
   case study 345
   chemoradiation in 352–353
   chemotherapy agents 354
   desciprion of 343–345
   5-FU-based chemoradiotherapy in 353–354
   HPV:
      infection 345–346
      vaccines 346

   involvement of lymph nodes 349–350
   macroscopic disease 352
   microscopic disease 352
   palliative chemotherapy in metastatic disease 356–357
   planning target volumes in 350
   radical chemoradiation therapy 354–355
   radical chemoradiotherapy for 350–352
   rectum 347
   sentinel lymph node biopsy in staging 347–348
   squamous cell carcinoma 346
   surgical margins 348–349
   surgical procedure of 350
anaplastic thyroid cancer 39
   BRAF V600E mutation 47
   management algorithm 48f
   metastatic 47–48
   stages 47
   systemic therapies 47–48
anastrozole, DCIS 124, 125t
androgen deprivation therapy (ADT) 406, 410–411
   metastatic prostate cancer 427
   monotherapy 424
   radiation therapy 413–414
androgen receptor signaling inhibitors 425, 427–428
angiosarcoma 585
anorexia-cachexia syndrome 703
anorexia, symptoms of 701
anthracycline 157
anthracycline-taxane-based chemotherapy, TNBC 182–183
antibody drug conjugate (ADC) 197
anticoagulation in cancer:
   cessation of 659
   description of 651
   initiation of 657–658
   stopping 659
anticonvulsants 698–699
antihistamine loratadine 700
antihormonal therapy, DCIS 123–124
antineoplastic agents 512–513
APC gene 630
apixaban, CYP3A4 for 654
apparent diffusion coefficient (ADC) map 400
ARASENS trial 417
aromatase inhibitors 555–556
aromatase inhibitor therapy, breast cancer 132, 133

asbestos-induced mesothelioma 105–106
ASCO. *See* American Society of Clinical Oncology (ASCO)
aspartate aminotransferase (AST) 666–667
ASSURE trial 363–364
astrocytoma 3, 7–8
  grade 3, 8–9
  grade II 9, 10*f*
asymptomatic right lower lobe segmental artery thrombosis 653
asymptomatic tumors 7
ATA. *See* American Thyroid Association (ATA)
ATEMPT trial, phase II 154
atezolizumab 315, 364, 383
ATLAS trial 133–134*f*
ATM mutation 620
ATRX mutation 7
attenuated familial adenomatous polyposis (AFAP) 625
attenuated FAP (AFAP) 626–627
aTTom trial 133–134*f*
autoimmune hypophysitis 670
autosomal recessive manner 631

b

Barcelona Clinic Liver Cancer (BCLC) staging system 311–312, 312*f*
Barret's esophagus 235, 245–246
basal cell carcinoma:
  AJCC 8 and BWH T-staging systems for 488*t*
  high risk of metastasis 488–489
  low- and high-risk criteria for 488–489
  primary 488
  quadriceps femoris muscle 489–490
  risk factors of patients 488–489
base-of-skull conventional chondrosarcoma 575
BCIRG-006 study. *See* Breast Cancer International Research Group 006 (BCIRG-006) study
BCSS. *See* breast cancer-specific survival (BCSS)
BEACON study, phase III 286
benign mucinous cysts 552
benign tumors 3
benzodiazepines 704
betel nut chewing, oral cavity squamous cell carcinoma 19
bevacizumab 315, 501–502, 505, 516, 537, 539
  addition of 520

anti-VEGF 315
  benefit from 539–540, 559
  chemotherapy with 520
  documented benefits of 519
  in epithelial ovarian cancer 519
  inadvisability of employing 519
  in neuro-oncology 11
  in platinum-resistant ovarian cancer 520
  side effects of 11
  single agent 537
  therapy, maintenance 503
  treatment with 11, 502
bilateral ascites 554
bilateral ovarian masses 554
bilateral pelvic lymphadenectomy 413
bilateral salpingo-oophorectomy 530, 584
bile duct cancer 319
biliary tract cancers 319–320
bilirubin 666–667
biochemical recurrence 423
  conventional imaging in 395–396
bladder cancer 375, 383–385
  adjuvant chemotherapy 382–383
  advanced/metastatic 386
  cisplatin-based regimens 385
  lymph node dissection 379–380
  maintenance therapy 385–386
  neoadjuvant chemotherapy 379, 380–382
  and preferred management 377*t*
  therapy 376–379, 386–387
  TNM staging AJCC UICC 8th edition 376*t*
bladder neck margins 394
bladder-sparing 378
bladder wall, asymmetric thickening of 378
bleomycin 447, 448, 556
blood-based testing 92
Bloom Syndrome 107
body mass index 701–702
bone:
  health, treatment for 428–429, 429*t*
  metastases 336, 337–338
  strengthening agents 429–430
bone sarcomas:
  description of 567
  multimodal therapeutic approaches of 567
  therapies 569
bowel:
  involvement with tumor 519
  obstruction, history of 506
  perforation, risk of 519

brachytherapy 407
BRAF and MEK inhibitors (BRAF/MEKi) 458
BRAF mutations 46, 47, 355, 469–470, 554
brain cancers 3
brain metastases 449–450, 471
BRCA:
  mutations 513
  pathogenic variant 604
BRCA1/2 genes 599, 603–605
BRCA1/2 mutations 147, 193–194
BRCA2 mutations 503, 604, 605, 612–613, 616, 621
BRCA pathogenic variants 228
breast cancer 130, 508–509, 599, 618, 687.
    See also HER2-positive breast cancer; HER2-positive metastatic breast cancer; inflammatory breast cancer (IBC); male breast cancer; metastatic breast cancer (MBC)
  adjuvant systemic therapy 129–130
  adjuvant therapy 136–137
  ATLAS and aTTom trials 133–134*f*
  axillary node-negative 136
  CDK 4/6 inhibitor 133
  early stage, HER2-negative 135
  EBCTCG analysis 132*f*
  endocrine therapy 132–133, 133*f*, 134*f*
  history of 621
  Mammaprint™ 130
  metastatic triple-positive 174–175
  monarchE trial 133–135*f*
  OLYMPIA trial 135, 135*f*, 136
  Oncotype Dx™ 130, 599, 618, 687
  poly (ADP-ribose) polymerase inhibitors 134–136
  predisposition genes 619*t*
  pregnancy and fertility 225–232
  RxPONDER study 130–132
  screening 613
  TAILORx trial 136
  triple-negative, early-stage 179–189
Breast Cancer International Research Group 006 (BCIRG-006) study 152
breast cancer-specific survival (BCSS) 154
breast-conserving therapy 118–119, 216
Breslow thickness 553–554
bullous pemphigoid eruptions 459
bupropion 703
BWH, alternative staging system 480–481, 481*t*

C

cabazitaxel 433
cabozantinib 44, 369
cachexia:
  cancer patients with 701–702
  malignant pleural mesothelioma 107
  treatment of 702–703
CALGB trial. *See* Cancer and Leukemia Group B (CALGB) trial 9633
caloric intake 702–703
Canadian Sarcoma group 581
cancer. *See also specific types*
  risk with ATM mutation 620
  risk with CHEK2 mutation 620–621
  screening, approach for 628
  syndrome, mutation responsible for 618–619
Cancer and Aging Research Group (CARG) chemotoxicity assessment tool 683
Cancer and Leukemia Group B (CALGB) trial 9633 56–57, 64
cancer cachexia, treatment of 703
cancer of unknown primary (CUP) 639, 641
  adenocarcinoma histology in 641–642
  clinical response and outcomes of patients 639
  definition for 641
  FDG-PET in evaluation of 646
  and peritoneal carcinomatosis 640–641
  renal subset of 644
  subsets of patients 640
  tissue of origin (ToO) molecular profiling in evaluation of 646
  treatment of 639
cancer-related pathogenic variants 598
CAO/ARO/AIO-12 trial 272
capecitabine 321, 336–337, 340
  HER2-positive breast cancer, metastatic 172–173
  TNBC 185
CapeOX adjuvant chemotherapy, colon cancer 261–262
CAPTEM regimen (capecitabine combined with temozolomide) 337
carboplatin 384, 537, 558–559
  cycles of 507
  hypersensitivity 517
  NSCLC 66
  plus gemcitabine 520
  SCLC 101

carboplatin–paclitaxel chemotherapy   512
carcinoembryonic antigen (CEA)   49, 283, 552–553
carcinoma, immunohistochemical profile of   641
carcinomatosis   554
carcinosarcomas   530–532
caregiver support   699–700
CARMENA trial   365
Carney complex   40
catheter-associated thrombosis   657
catheter prophylaxis   658
catheter thromboprophylaxis   658
CCRT. *See* concurrent chemoradiotherapy (CCRT)
CCTC. *See* China Clinical Trials Consortium (CCTC)
CDK4/6 inhibitor (CDK4/6i)   140–141, 141*t*, 142
CDKN2A mutation   457
CDNK2A/B homozygous deletion   8
CEA. *See* carcinoembryonic antigen (CEA)
CECILIA   537–538
CELESTIAL trial   315
cemiplimab   486–487, 541
central nervous system tumors:
    bevacizumab in neuro-oncology   11
    brain tumors   3–4, 6
    diagnosis in   3–4
    genetic conditions   5, 5*t*
    glioblastoma treatment   9–10
    grade 3 IDH mutant astrocytoma   8–9
    grade 1 meningioma   6–7
    oligodendroglioma, care treatment of   7–8
    primary brain cancers   4–6
    pseudo-progression and necrosis   10–11
    tumors in adults   4, 4*t*
cervical adenocarcinoma   538
cervical cancer   533
    advanced   536–537
    bevacizumab use in   539
    checkpoint inhibitor therapy   541
    cisplatin-based chemotherapy   533–534
    definitive chemoradiation   536
    GOG study   537
    IB1   534
    international multicenter study   535
    KEYNOTE-826 trial   540
    Moore criteria   540
    prospective trials   534
    screening   546–547
    stage IIIC1   536
    survival outcomes   536
    treatment of   533–534
cervical intraepithelial neoplasia (CIN)   533
cervix, high-grade neuroendocrine carcinoma of   549–551, 550*f*
cervix uteri, FIGO staging of cancer of   534, 534*t*
cetuximab   22, 355–356
CGA. *See* comprehensive geriatric assessment (CGA)
CHAARTED trial   416–417
CheckMate-9LA trial   85, 88, 90, 91*f*
CheckMate 141 trial   36
CheckMate 274 trial   382
Checkmate-577 trial   240
CheckMate 816 trial   72
CHEK2 mutation   620–621
chemotherapy:
    amenorrhea, chemotherapy-induced   226–227, 226*t*
    with bevacizumab   520
    cisplatin-based   382–383, 543
    concomitant   8
    cytotoxic   370, 371, 508–509, 558
    empiric   643–644
    induction   575
    metastatic esophagogastric cancer   251–252
    pregnancy   226, 229–231
    TNBC   181–184, 191, 192
Chemotherapy Risk Assessment Scale for High-Age Patients (CRASH) score   683
chest wall debulking   114
childbearing   509
Children's Oncology Group INT-0091 trial   574–575
China Clinical Trials Consortium (CCTC)   59
cholangiocarcinoma   319–320, 648
chondrosarcomas   571, 575
chordomas, localized   570–571
chromosomal translocation   586
chronic back pain   705
chronic portal vein thrombosis   660
chronological age   687
CIN. *See* cervical intraepithelial neoplasia (CIN)
circulating-tumor DNA (ctDNA)   92, 188, 196, 264, 383
circumferential peripheral and deep margin assessment (CCPDMA)   482

cirrhosis   312–313, 317t, 660
cisplatin   322, 381, 384, 449–450, 534,
    550–551, 556
  chemotherapy   577
  and gemcitabine combination,
    nasopharyngeal carcinoma   25
  laryngeal cancer   21
  oropharyngeal cancer, HPV-related   23
  SCLC, limited-stage   98, 99
  superiority of   517
  systemic chemotherapy with   549–550
cisplatin-based chemotherapy   382–383, 543
ClarIDHy trial   324
CLARINET study   336, 339
clear cell carcinomas   369, 558
clear cell ovarian carcinoma   557–558
  cytotoxic chemotherapy   558
  NCCN Ovarian Cancer Guidelines   557
  postoperative management   557
  second-line therapy   558
  stage IA   557
CLEOPATRA trial   164–165, 164f
CLOT trial   655
CMMRD syndrome. See constitutional
    mismatch repair deficiency (CMMRD)
    syndrome
coanalgesics   698–699
COBRA trial phase II/III   264
CodeBreaK-100 trial   89, 90
colitis   666
colon cancer:
  adjuvant chemotherapy   258, 260–263
  anti-EGFR therapy   263
  ATOMIC trial   261
  AVANT trial   263
  biological agents, adjuvant chemotherapy
    regimen   263
  chemotherapy duration   258
  ctDNA evaluation   264
  family history of   631
  history of   631
  management options   257–259
  MOSAIC trial   258
  MSI-H   256, 258–259
  NSABP C-08 phase III trial   263
  oxaliplatin with 5FU-based therapy   258, 260
  PETACC-8 phase III trial   263–264
  polyp   265
  QUASAR2 phase III trial   263
  stage II   256–259
  stage III   259–264

colorectal adenocarcinoma   625–626
colorectal cancer. See also rectal cancer
  AJCC staging   269t
  incidence and death rates   255
  recurrent and metastatic   283–288
  survival   255
Common Terminology Criteria for Adverse
    Events (CTCAE)   672
compartment syndrome   657
completion hysterectomy   538
completion oophorectomy   509
comprehensive geriatric assessment (CGA)
    677
  definition of   678
  domains of   679t
  screening tool   678, 680t
concomitant chemotherapy   8
concurrent chemoradiotherapy (CCRT)   19–20
CONKO-001 trial   304
constitutional mismatch repair deficiency
    (CMMRD) syndrome   625, 632
contralateral ovary   551
conventional chondrosarcoma   571, 575
Cowden syndrome   40, 614
  cancer risks and clinical management
    recommendations   615t
  diagnosis   614
  NCCN diagnostic clinical criteria for   615t
creatinine clearance   655
cryopreservation   185–186, 229
ctDNA. See circulating-tumor DNA
CUP. See cancer of unknown primary (CUP)
curable and terminal cancers, palliative
    medicine for:
  description of   693
  patient's nausea   694
cutaneous squamous cell carcinoma
    477–483
  AJCC8 staging system and   480, 481t
  high-risk   480
  histopathological evaluation   485–486
  Mohs micrographic surgery   484–485
  preferred management option   483–484
  and risk groups   479t
cyclin-dependent kinase 4/6 (CDK 4/6)   133
cyclin-dependent kinase inhibitors (CDKIs)
    197
cyclophosphamide   226, 231
cystectomy   378–379
  and neoadjuvant chemotherapy   382
  trimodality approach   379

cystic mass 507
cystoscopy/transurethral resection of a bladder tumor (TURBT) 376
cytologic atypia 562
cytoreduction 339–340, 505
cytoreductive nephrectomy 364–366
cytotoxic chemotherapy 370, 371, 508–509, 520

d
dalteparin 658
DCIS. *See* ductal carcinoma in situ (DCIS)
ddMVAC. *See* dose-dense version of MVAC (ddMVAC)
Decipher test 406
de-escalation therapy, HER2-positive breast cancer 154
definitive brachytherapy 408
delirium, agitation secondary to underlying 696
denosumab 430, 569
de novo HER2-positive metastatic breast cancer:
　CLEOPATRA trial 164–165, 164f
　CT scans 163
　first-line treatment 164–165
　SystHERs 164
dermatofibrosarcoma protuberans:
　extensive subcutaneous extension 491
　medical history of 490
　radiological workup for patient with 490–491
dermatologic immune-related adverse events 666
dermoscopy 457
desmoid tumors 591, 630
DESTINY-Breast03 trial 166–168, 169f, 221
DESTINY-Breast09 trial 165
DESTINY-Gastric01 study 252
dexamethasone 11
DEXA scans 702
diabetes mellitus 303
diabetic ketoacidosis (DKA) 670–671
differentiated neuroendocrine carcinoma 340
differentiated thyroid carcinoma:
　biomarkers 41–42
　BRAF V600E mutation 46
　distant metastases 43–44
　dynamic risk stratification 41
　EBRT 42

locoregional recurrence 43
patient risk categories 41
poorly differentiated 46
RAI refractory 44–45, 45f
RAI therapy 40–41
surgical options 40
systemic therapy 44–45
thyroid lobectomy 40
total thyroidectomy 40, 43
TSH suppressive therapy 42, 42t
diffusion weight imaging (DWI) 400
digital rectal examination (DRE) 391
distal femoral lesion 573, 573f
DKA. *See* diabetic ketoacidosis (DKA)
DNA repair 506, 514, 627
docetaxel 432–433, 530, 561
dopamine antagonist 695
dose-dense version of MVAC (ddMVAC) 381
doxorubicin 143, 145, 592
DRE. *See* digital rectal examination (DRE)
ductal carcinoma in situ (DCIS) 621
　accelerated partial breast irradiation 123
　active surveillance 126
　adjuvant radiation therapy 120–123
　antihormonal therapy 123–124
　breast cancer and 621
　breast-conserving therapy 118–119
　clinical trials, comparison of 120, 121t
　DCISionRT scoring 126
　DCIS Score 126
　grade 2 estrogen receptor positive 118
　ipsilateral axilla 118
　margin width, appropriate 119
　nipple-sparing mastectomy and reconstruction 119–120
　randomized clinical trials, radiation 120, 122t
　risk-prediction models 124, 126
　tamoxifen therapy 123–124, 124t
　treatment guidelines 118f
Dukes B colon cancer 257
duodenal adenomas 630
duodenal cancer 630
DWI. *See* diffusion weight imaging (DWI)
dynamic intravenous contrast–enhanced (DCE) imaging 400
dynamic risk stratification 41
dysphagia 27, 32, 34, 99, 236, 238
dyspnea 79

e

Early Breast Cancer Trialists' Collaborative Group (EBCTCG) 151, 187
Eastern Cooperative Oncology Group (ECOG) 33, 37, 677
EBCTCG. *See* Early Breast Cancer Trialists' Collaborative Group (EBCTCG)
EBRT. *See* external beam radiation therapy (EBRT)
EBV. *See* Epstein-Barr virus (EBV)
ECOG. *See* Eastern Cooperative Oncology Group (ECOG) score
ectopic Cushing syndrome 97
Edmonton Symptom Assessment Scale 693, 701, 703
EGD. *See* esophagogastroduodenoscopy (EGD)
ELCAPA study 679
embryo cryopreservation 185–186, 229
embryonal carcinoma 441
empiric chemotherapy 643–644
encephalomyelitis 97
endocrine syndromes 97
endocrine therapy:
　breast cancer 132–133
　HR+ MBC 139, 140
　male breast cancer 218, 219
endocrine toxicities 667
endometrial adenocarcinoma 527
　cytotoxic agent in 527
　metastatic 529
endometrial cancer:
　abdominal radiation 527
　adenocarcinoma of endometrium 524
　adjuvant chemotherapy 528–529
　adjuvant therapy in 528*f*
　of chemotherapy and hormonal therapy in 524
　cisplatin-doxorubicin-paclitaxel regimen 526–527
　combination chemotherapy 526
　cytotoxic chemotherapy 524–525
　description of 523
　dMMR 525–526
　doxorubicin plus cisplatin 526
　hormonal therapy 524
　intermediate-risk 530–531
　metastatic 527
　papillary serous carcinoma of 528
　randomized phase III study 525
　stage I 528
　stage III 527
　stage IV 526
　use of pembrolizumab 525
　women with Lynch syndrome 526
endometrial carcinoma 529, 531
endometrial sarcoma 530, 531
endometrial stromal sarcomas 530, 531–532, 584
endoprosthetic reconstruction 572
endoscopic ultrasound (EUS), pancreatic adenocarcinoma 292, 293, 300, 305, 306
EORTC 26101 study 11
EORTC 30994 trial 382
epidermal growth factor receptor (EGFR) mutations 355
epithelial ovarian cancer 512–513, 519, 615–617
　asymptomatic female with 514
　cytoreductive surgery 514
　paclitaxel delivery 518
　platinum-associated toxicities 515
　platinum-based chemotherapy 513, 515
　primary chemotherapy 513, 514
　secondary cytoreduction in 514, 555
　second-line carboplatin-based chemotherapy 515
　second-line therapy of 518
　single-agent pegylated liposomal doxorubicin 518
Epstein-Barr virus (EBV) 25, 32
ER. *See* estrogen receptor (ER)
erdafitinib 387
erionite 106
esophageal cancer 235, 237, 240, 241, 354. *See also* gastroesophageal cancer
esophageal dysplasia 245–246
esophagectomy 111, 236, 237, 239, 240
esophagogastroduodenoscopy (EGD) 21, 236, 238–245, 333, 334, 647, 663
estrogen receptor (ER) 663
etoposide 550–551, 556
　SCLC, limited-stage 98, 99, 101
　systemic chemotherapy with 549–550
European Association of Palliative Care 697
European Organization for Research and Treatment of Cancer Soft Tissue and Bone Sarcoma Group (EORTC) 582
European Randomized Study of Screening of Prostate Cancer (ERSPC) trial 390, 401
EV-302 study 387
Ewing sarcoma 567

interval-compressed chemotherapy for
treatment of 568
of left humerus diaphysis 567
pelvic 574
of right ilium 574
excisional biopsy, LCIS 127
extended adjuvant therapy, HER2-positive
breast cancer 158–161
external beam radiotherapy (EBRT)
techniques 42, 46, 407
extracolonic malignancies 632
extragonadal germ cell cancer
syndrome 640
extrahepatic distal cholangiocarcinoma
322
extrapleural pneumonectomy 111
extremity sarcomas 581

f

FALCON phase III trial 141
false-positive results 53–54
familial adenomatous polyposis (FAP) 40,
267, 591, 625–627
cancer-related deaths in 630
hepatoblastoma in 630
syndrome 630
familial medullary thyroid carcinoma 40
familial melanoma 456–457
family cancer history 4–5
fam-trastuzumab deruxtecan-nxki (Enhertu)
197
FAP. See familial adenomatous polyposis (FAP)
fatigue 704–705
management of 703
symptoms of 703
febrile neutropenia 157–158, 162, 250, 450
Federal Drug Administration (FDA) 325
femoral neck 571–572
fertility:
preservation 508–509
sparing surgery 509
systemic breast cancer therapies on
185–186
fibroblast growth factor receptor (FGFR)
signaling 253, 324, 387
filter thrombosis 657
fine-needle aspiration (FNA) biopsy 33
FISH. See fluorescence in situ hybridization
(FISH)
fluorescence in situ hybridization
(FISH) 581–582

fluoropyrimidine-platinum doublet,
metastatic esophagogastric cancer
250–251
fluoropyrimidines 260
fluorouracil group 534
FNCLCC ACCORD phase 3 trial 243
FOLFIRINOX, pancreatic adenocarcinoma
299
fondaparinux 658
futibatinib 325

g

gallbladder:
adenocarcinoma 320–322
cancer 319–320
ischemia 313–314
Gardner syndrome 40
gastric cancer 628
gastroenterology 21
gastroesophageal cancer, early-stage:
adjuvant chemoradiotherapy 237
adjuvant chemotherapy 237
adjuvant therapy 243–244
Barret's esophagus 235, 245–246
definitive chemoradiation 238
diagnosis 236
esophageal dysplasia 245–246
incidence 235
management strategy 237, 242–243
neoadjuvant chemoradiotherapy 241
neoadjuvant therapy 238, 242
nodal disease 243–244
perioperative chemotherapy 241
residual disease 239–240
risk factors 235
surgery, after neoadjuvant
chemoradiation 238–239
surveillance 237
targeted therapy 245
TNM staging 236t
gastroesophageal reflux disease (GERD)
235, 245
gastrointestinal fistula, rate of 539
gastrointestinal mesenchymal tumors 589
gastrointestinal stromal tumors (GISTs)
589–590
abdominal discomfort 591
benefit of surgery in patients 591
G-CSF. See granulocyte colony-stimulating
factor (G-CSF)
gemcitabine 25, 321, 322, 381, 530, 561

gemcitabine-cisplatin, chemotherapy with 323
gemcitabine plus oxaliplatin (GEMOX) 322
genetic testing in adults 605
GERD. *See* gastroesophageal reflux disease (GERD)
geriatric domains, deficits in 686–688*t*
geriatric oncology 677, 685–686, 685*f*
germ cell tumor 447
  advanced stage disease 447–451
  chemotherapy for 450
  description of 437–438
  serum tumor 438–439, 439*t*
  stage I disease 439–444
  stage II disease 444–447
germline mutations 598
germline testing 180, 607–608, 633
giant cell tumor of bone 568, 569
GISTs. *See* gastrointestinal stromal tumors (GISTs)
Gleason score of radical prostatectomy specimen 394
glioblastoma 3, 4, 8–11
glioma 6
glucocorticoids 698–699
GnRH agonists. *See* gonadotropin-releasing hormone (GnRH) agonists
gonadotropin-releasing hormone (GnRH) agonists 145, 186, 218, 229
Goteborg trial 390–391
granulocyte colony-stimulating factor (G-CSF) 700
granulosa cell tumor of ovary 556–557
  management of newly diagnosed 556, 557*f*
  postoperative management 556
  serum marker 556–557
  stage IA 556
groin pain 571
Guardant RevealTM ctDNA test 264
gynecologic cancer community 557
Gynecologic Oncology Group 529, 530–531, 533–534

h

hand-foot syndrome 185
HDGC syndrome. *See* hereditary diffuse gastric cancer (HDGC) syndrome
head and neck cancer. *See also* recurrent/metastatic HNSCC
  CCRT 19–20
  HNSCC 15, 16, 23
  HPV 16, 19
  hypopharynx 18*t*, 27
  larynx cancer 19–21
  mucosal lip and oral cavity TNM staging 16*t*–17*t*
  nasopharyngeal carcinoma 25
  oropharyngeal cancer 17*t*–18*t*, 19, 23, 26
  paranasal sinuses 15
  partial glossectomy 23
  PET-CT 22
  prognosis 31
  radiation therapy, concurrent cisplatin 23–24
  risk factors 15
  salivary gland cancers 15, 28
  total laryngectomy 20
  TSH evaluation 27
  upper aerodigestive tract 15, 16*t*–17*t*
head and neck squamous cell carcinoma (HNSCC) 15. *See also* recurrent/metastatic HNSCC
  HPV 16, 23, 32
  primary 33
  risk factors 32
  tobacco use 32
heavy (carbon) ion therapy 575
Hellenic Oncology Research Group (HORG) study 153
hematologic syndromes 97
hematuria 376
hemicolectomy 693
hemipelvectomy, association with 571
hepatitis B virus (HBV) 309
hepatitis C virus (HCV) 309
hepatocellular cancer:
  diagnostic approaches 311
  risk factors for 309, 310*t*
  screening methods for hepatocellular carcinoma 310
  staging and initial workup 311–312
  treatment 312–317
hepatocellular carcinoma (HCC) 310
  diagnostic for 311
  screening methods for 310
  staging system 311–312, 312*f*
  treatment for 316*t*
  treatment of 313–314
HER2. *See* human epidermal growth factor receptor 2 (HER2)
HER2CLIMB-02 trial 168

hereditary breast-ovarian cancer (HBOC)
    syndrome   611, 612
hereditary cancer syndromes:
    cascade testing   605–606
    features   600–601
    genetic testing for   601–602, 639–630
    identification of   597, 600–601, 605
    multigene panel testing   602
    next generation sequencing (NGS)   602
    overarching concepts of   597–599
    posttest consultation   601–602
    precision oncology   607–608
    telehealth technologies   602
    training in   606
hereditary diffuse gastric cancer (HDGC)
    syndrome   628
hereditary gastrointestinal (GI) and
    pancreatic cancer syndromes   625
hereditary melanoma   456–457
hereditary nonpolyposis colorectal cancer
    (HNPCC)   267, 626
hereditary pancreatic cancer   625, 635t
HER2-positive breast cancer:
    ALTTO trial   161
    anthracycline with trastuzumab   152
    ATEMPT trial, phase II   154
    congestive heart failure and acute
        leukemia   152
    de-escalation therapy   154
    extended adjuvant therapy   158–161
    future trials   161t
    KAITLIN randomized phase III trial   154
    neoadjuvant therapy   155–158
    NeoALTTO study, phase III   160
    PERSEPHONE trial, phase III   153–154
    pertuzumab   155–157
    post-neoadjuvant therapy   158
    T-DM   1, 154–155
    trastuzumab   151–154
    treatment algorithm, early stage   160f
HER2-positive metastatic breast
        cancer   166–167
    CNS metastases   170
    de novo   163–165
    DESTINY-Breast03 trial   166–167
    DESTINY-Breast09 trial   165
    HER2CLIMB regimen   174
    HER2-low   177
    novel therapies   177
    recurrent   165–167
    trastuzumab deruxtecan   170–171

trastuzumab emtansine   167–168,
    173–175
treatment:
    first-line   164–165, 167–168
    second-line   168–169
    third-line   171–173, 173f
    tucatinib   172–173
high-power field (HPF)   581–582
high-risk disease   411–413
HIMALAYA trial   315
HIPEC. *See* hyperthermic intraperitoneal
    chemotherapy (HIPEC)
HNPCC. *See* hereditary nonpolyposis
    colorectal cancer (HNPCC)
HNSCC. *See* head and neck squamous cell
    carcinoma (HNSCC)
Hodgkin's lymphoma   508–509
homologous recombination deficiency (HRD)
    tumors   195
homologous recombination repair (HRR)
    genes   180
HORG study. *See* Hellenic Oncology
    Research Group (HORG) study
hormonal syndrome   332–333
hormone receptor positive (HR+) MBC:
    BRCA1/2 mutation   147
    CDK4/6i   140–141, 141t
    chemotherapy choice   142–143
    CNS metastasis   143–144
    ECOG 2108 trial   144
    endocrine therapy   139, 140
    first-line treatment   140–142, 145
    locoregional treatment   144
    PARP inhibitor, somatic BRCA hormone
        receptor positive (HR+) MBC
        mutation   147
    PIK3CA mutation   146
    PI3K inhibitor, PIK3CA mutant   146
    second-line treatment   142
    systemic treatment   139
    TBCRC048 phase II trial   147
    treatment approach   148f
    visceral crisis   142–143
hormone-sensitive prostate cancer
    415–416
HPF. *See* high-power field (HPF)
HPV. *See* human papillomavirus (HPV)
HRD tumors. *See* homologous recombination
    deficiency (HRD) tumors
HRR genes. *See* homologous recombination
    repair (HRR) genes

human epidermal growth factor receptor 2 (HER2) 663
human papillomavirus (HPV) 16, 533
　infection 345–346
　　positive and negative cancers 346
　　related cancers 549
Hurthle cell thyroid cancer 39
hydrocodone 703, 704
hyperparathyroidism 602–603
hyperthermic intraperitoneal chemotherapy (HIPEC) 502
hypocalcemia 430
hypopharyngeal cancer 18t, 27
hypophosphatemia 570
hysterectomy 584

i

IALT. See International Adjuvant Lung Trial (IALT)
IASLC. See International Association for the Study of Lung Cancer (IASLC)
IBC. See inflammatory breast cancer (IBC)
IBD. See inflammatory bowel disease (IBD)
ICIs. See immune checkpoint inhibitors (ICIs)
IDEA. See International Duration Evaluation of Adjuvant Therapy (IDEA)
iDFS. See invasive disease-free survival (iDFS)
IDH1 gene 9
IDH2 gene 9
IDH mutant astrocytoma 3, 8–9
ifosfamide 529–530
IGCLC criteria. See International Gastric Cancer Linkage Consortium (IGCLC) criteria
IGRT. See image-guided radiotherapy (IGRT)
IHC. See immunohistochemistry (IHC)
image-guided radiotherapy (IGRT) 407
imatinib, efficacy and tolerability of 590–591
IMDC. See International Metastatic RCC Database Consortium (IMDC)
IMIG. See Mesothelioma Interest Group (IMIG)
immediate cytoreductive nephrectomy 365
immune checkpoint inhibitors (ICIs) 459, 663, 664
　adverse events 664
　immune-related adverse events 665
　T-cell activation and inhibition 664, 664f
immune-related adverse events 185, 671–672
　immune-related cardiovascular toxicity 671
　management of 672–674
　　monitoring, presentation, diagnosis, management of 668–669t
　neurologic toxicities 671
　renal dysfunction 672
　rheumatologic 671–672
　steroid-refractory cases 673–674
　steroids to control 673
　treatment for 674
immune-related hepatitis 666–667
immune-related pneumonitis 667
immune-related toxicity, immunotherapy after 674
immunohistochemistry (IHC) 625–626, 645, 645t
immunosuppressive agents 673
immunotherapy:
　metastatic esophagogastric cancer 252
　NSCLC, recurrent and metastatic 79–81, 83, 87t, 89–94
　recurrent/metastatic HNSCC 34
　SCLC 101
　thyroid cancer 45
　TNBC 192–193
　use of 647
IMpassion130 phase III trial 222
IMpassion131 phase III trial 222, 223
IMRT. See intensity modulated radiation therapy (IMRT)
induction chemotherapy 575
inferior vena cava (IVC) filter 656–657, 661
inflammatory bowel disease (IBD) 278–279
inflammatory breast cancer (IBC)
　clinical trials 208, 209t
　definition 201
　diagnostic criteria 202–203, 203f
　genes, altered 205
　HER2 positive 205–206
　histopathological findings 204
　hormone receptor positive 206
　metastatic 207–208
　molecular profile 204–205
　predisposing factors 202
　prognosis 202
　prospective research 208, 209t
　radiation treatment 207
　radiographic findings of 203–204
　stage III 202, 205–206
　surgical treatment 206–207
　treatment 205–208
　triple negative 206
　TRYPHAENA study 205

inguinal cryptorchidism   438
inherited cancer syndromes   614, 615t, 629
inherited thrombophilias   660
INR. *See* international normalized ratio (INR)
intensity-modulated radiotherapy (IMRT)   112, 356, 407, 575
intermediate-risk disease   405
internal hemipelvectomy   571
International Adjuvant Lung Trial (IALT)   56
International Association for the Study of Lung Cancer (IASLC)   108
International Classification of Disease (ICD) classification   319
International Collaborative Neoplasm Studies (ICON1) trial   507
International Duration Evaluation of Adjuvant Therapy (IDEA)   261, 262
International Gastric Cancer Linkage Consortium (IGCLC) criteria   628
International Germ Cell Consensus (IGCC) Classification   448, 449t
International Metastatic RCC Database Consortium (IMDC)   361–362
international normalized ratio (INR)   655
interstitial lung disease   170–171
interval-compressed chemotherapy   568
interval cytoreductive surgery   502
intractable hypertension   602–603
intrahepatic cholangiocarcinoma   320, 324
intramedullary osteosarcoma   572–573
invasive disease-free survival (iDFS)   131
invasive ductal carcinoma (IDC)   215, 698
invasive lobular carcinoma (ILC)   215
invasive mucinous carcinoma   551, 552
invasive tumor   437
ipilimumab   113, 341
ipsilateral lower extremity   571
irAEs. *See* immune-related adverse events (irAEs)
isocitrate dehydrogenase gene (IDH mutation)   7
isolated pleural effusions   645
isolated tumor cells   545
isolated tumormetastasis (ITC)   544

j
JBR.10 trial   64

k
KAITLIN randomized phase III trial   154
Karnofsky performance status (KPS)   677
KATHERINE trial   167
Kattan preoperative nomogram   393–394
Khorana risk assessment score   652–653, 652t
kidney cancer. *See* renal cancer
KPS. *See* Karnofsky performance status (KPS)
KRAS G12C mutation   89–90
KRAS mutations   355

l
LACE. *See* Life after Cancer Epidemiology (LACE); Lung Adjuvant Cisplatin Evaluation (LACE)
Lambert-Eaton myasthenic syndrome   97
laparoscopic hysterectomy   557
lapatinib, HER2-positive breast cancer   159–161
large cell neuroendocrine carcinoma (LCNEC)   335
larynx cancer:
    CCRT   19–20
    stage I and II   19
L-carnitine   702–703
LCIS. *See* lobular carcinoma in situ (LCIS)
LDCT. *See* low-dose computed tomography (LDCT) imaging
left inguinofemoral node dissection   543
left knee pain   572–573
left ovary, removal of   551
left sentinel lymph node   544
leiomyosarcomas   531–532, 562, 587
lenvatinib   559
letrozole monotherapy   555
Life after Cancer Epidemiology (LACE)   188
Li Fraumeni syndrome   622–623
limb-sparing surgery   581–582
limited-stage SCLC:
    cisplatin and etoposide   98, 99
    concurrent chemoradiation   98–99
lipoma   579–580
lipomatous neoplasms   580
lipomatous tumors/well-differentiated liposarcomas   580
liposarcomas   586, 589
liposomal doxorubicin   506
liquid biopsy   92, 93, 196
liver:
    biopsy   666–667
    cancer   309–310
    lesion, biopsy of   366
    metastases, treatment approach for   336
    transplantation   313

LMWH. *See* low-molecular-weight heparin (LMWH)
lobular breast cancer 628
lobular carcinoma in situ (LCIS)
  excisional biopsy 127
  pleomorphic (nonclassic) 127
  risk reduction 127
  treatment guidelines 118*f*
locoregional recurrence, differentiated thyroid cancer 43
lorazepam 703–705
low-dose computed tomography (LDCT) imaging 52–54, 60
low-grade serous ovarian carcinoma 554–556
  letrozole monotherapy 555
  postoperative treatment options 554–555
  secondary cytoreductive surgery 555
  stage IIIC 554–555
  stage II–IV 555
  systemic therapy 555
  taxane/platinum chemotherapy 554–555
low-molecular-weight heparin (LMWH) 651–652, 654, 656
  initial five-day treatment of 654
  switching to 661
low-risk disease, definitive treatment of 403–404
lumbar spine, metastasis in 586
Lung Adjuvant Cisplatin Evaluation (LACE) 57, 64
lung cancer. *See also* non-small cell lung cancer; small cell lung cancer
  adjuvant chemotherapy 56–60
  chest radiographs 52
  early stage 51
  false-positive results 53–54
  LDCT imaging 52, 53
  mortality 51, 53
  NELSON trial 53
  NLST 52–53
  NSCLC 56–60
  PET imaging 54
  randomized controlled trials, screening 52–53
  staging, AJCC 8th edition 64*t*
lung NETs 338
lymph node 349–350
  adjuvant therapies 550–551
  assessment 550
  dissection 379–380, 447, 535, 536
  metastases 580
  status 535–536
lymphoscintigraphy 231
lymphovascular invasion 441, 530
Lynch syndrome 5, 267, 319, 597–598, 625, 626
  developing cancer associated with 629
  family history of 626
  genes 632
  pathogenic variant 628
  presumptive diagnosis of 634

m

macroscopic disease 352
male breast cancer:
  adjuvant endocrine therapy 218, 219
  adjuvant/neoadjuvant chemotherapy 216
  bone-modifying agents 219
  diagnosis 215
  HER2, 220–221
  hormone receptor positive 219–220
  incidence and prevalence 213–214
  Oncotype and Mammaprint 216–218
  prognosis 215–216
  radiation therapy 216
  receptor subtype 215
  risk factors 214–215, 214*t*
  surgical management 216
  surveillance 220
  survivorship 223
  targeted therapies 219
  treatment, metastatic setting 221
  triple-negative 221–223
malignant bowel obstruction 506
malignant cancers 3
malignant fibrous histiocytoma 585
malignant pleural mesothelioma 108
  diagnosis 107–108
  extrapleural pneumonectomy 111
  locoregional 110–112
  markers 107
  MARS randomized trial 110
  nivolumab and ipilimumab 113
  pathogenesis 105–107
  pleurectomy decortication 111, 112
  second-line therapy 113–114
  staging 108–110
  surgery 112
  targeted molecular agents 113
  treatments 110–113
  VATS 108

mammalian target of rapamycin (mTOR) inhibitors 45, 369
Mammaprint™ 130
MammaPrint molecular assays 216–217
margetuximab, HER2-positive metastatic breast cancer 172, 173
mastectomy:
  IBC 206
  male breast cancer 216, 220
  nipple-sparing 119–120
MBC. *See* metastatic breast cancer (MBC)
MDAS. *See* Memorial Delirium Assessment Scale (MDAS)
MDS. *See* myelodysplastic syndrome (MDS)
mediastinal germ cell tumors 438
medullary thyroid cancer 602
medullary thyroid carcinoma 39, 48
  familial 40
  metastatic 49
  total thyroidectomy 49
megesterol acetate, complications of 701
melanoma 545
  adjuvant and neoadjuvant therapy 460–464
  advanced 464–466
  AJCC 8th edition for 459–462*t*
  biosynthetic pathway 456
  BRAF V600E/K mutation 469–470
  CDKN2A mutation 457
  curative therapy 464
  desccription of 455
  diagnosis of 457–458
  family history of 455–456
  genetic counselor 456–457
  management of 470
  with metastases to brain 470–473
  neoadjuvant immunotherapy, non-metastatic bulky nodal disease with 468–469
  optimal therapy 468–470
  parameters used to select adjuvant therapy 466–467
  potential increased risk of 612
  stage IV 458
  staging 459–460
Memorial Delirium Assessment Scale (MDAS) 695–696
Memorial Kettering-Integrated Mutation Profiling of Actionable Cancer Targets (MSK-IMPACT) 196

Memorial Sloan Kettering Cancer Center (MSKCC) 124, 279, 361–362
MEN2A 602–603
  pathogenic variants in 602–603
  syndrome 602–603
meningiomas 3, 6
  grade1 6–7
  grade2 6–7
  grade3 4
  molecular sequencing of 7
Merkel cell carcinoma 492
  treatment approach for patient and tumor 492, 492*f*
  workup and tumor surveillance 493–495
mesenchymal neoplasms 567
mesothelioma. *See also* malignant pleural mesothelioma
  asbestos-induced 105–106
  environmental exposures 105–107
  genetics 106–107
  pathogenesis 105–107
  staging 108–110
  SV40, 106
Mesothelioma Interest Group (IMIG) 108
metabolic syndrome 309
metastatectomy, TNBC 197
metastatic adenocarcinoma 647
metastatic breast cancer (MBC). *See also* HER2-positive metastatic breast cancer
  HR+ MBC 139–148
  initial treatment 140–142
  locoregional treatment 144
  male patient 145
  second-line treatment 142
  triple-negative 191–197
  triple-positive 174–175
  visceral crisis 142–143
metastatic cancer 416, 640
metastatic castrate-resistant prostate cancer, PSMA-based therapies in 434
metastatic cervical cancer 537, 540, 541
metastatic colon cancer 693
metastatic colorectal cancer 689
  diagnosis of 689
  treatment options 689
metastatic disease 356–357, 364, 551–552, 567, 570
metastatic endometrial adenocarcinoma 529
metastatic endometrial cancer 527

metastatic endometrial sarcomas, high-dose chemotherapy in 530
metastatic esophagogastric cancer:
  chemotherapy 251–252
  first-line regimen 249–250
  fluoropyrimidine-platinum doublet, third drug to 250–251
  immunotherapy 252
  targeted therapies 252–253
metastatic granulosa cell tumor 556
metastatic lesions 3
metastatic lung adenocarcinoma 651
  diagnosis of 689–690
  proceed to counsel 690
metastatic neuroendocrine carcinoma 340–341
metastatic pancreatic adenocarcinoma 659–660
metastatic prostate cancer 421, 422f
  ADT 427
  androgen receptor signaling inhibitor 427–428
  bone health, treatment for 428–429, 429t
  bone strengthening agents 429
  castrate-sensitive 426t
  germline testing and molecular phenotyping 430–431
  high-volume 425
  management strategy 423–425
  optimal sequencing 432
  PARP inhibitors in 431
  PET-based imaging 423
  phase III trials in 426t, 429t
  radical prostatectomy 424–429
  treatment options 421, 422t, 426–427
metastatic urothelial carcinoma 383
MGMT methylated glioblastoma 9
microsatellite instability high (MSI-H) phenotype 256, 258–259
microsatellite-instable (MSI) disease 506, 598
microscopic disease 352
microwave ablation (MWA) 312–313
Milan criteria 313
mirtazapine 703
mismatch repair (MMR) 279, 632–633
mitogen-activated protein kinase (MAPK) pathway 556
mixed adenocarcinoid tumors 329
MLH1 gene 626
MMR. *See* mismatch repair (MMR)
Mohs micrographic surgery 483f, 484–485

molecular biomarkers, use of 4
molecularly targeted therapies (MET) 588
molecular testing 80, 90, 92, 294–295
monoclonal antibodies 674
monophasic synovial sarcoma 581–582
MSH6 gene 627
MSH2 gene, pathogenic variant in 628
MSI disease. *See* microsatellite-instable (MSI) disease
MSI-H. *See* microsatellite instability high (MSI-H) phenotype
MSKCC. *See* Memorial Sloan Kettering Cancer Center (MSKCC)
MSK-IMPACT. *See* Memorial Kettering-Integrated Mutation Profiling of Actionable Cancer Targets (MSK-IMPACT)
mTOR inhibitors. *See* mammalian target of rapamycin (mTOR) inhibitors
mucinous colorectal adenocarcinoma 632
mucinous ovarian cancer 552
multiple endocrine neoplasia type 2A 40
multiple lung lesions 587
multiple polyps 626–627
muscle-invasive bladder cancer 380
MUTYH-associated polyposis (MAP) 625–627, 631
MVAC regimen 383–384
myelodysplastic syndrome (MDS) 184
myeloproliferative disorders 660
myometrium 530
myxoid round cell liposarcoma 586

n
Nabiximols 699
nasopharyngeal carcinoma 25, 32
National Cancer Database (NCDB) study 70, 221, 534
National Cancer Institute (NCI) 40
National Comprehensive Cancer Network (NCCN) 40, 118, 123, 132, 136, 139, 165, 172–173, 180, 181, 187, 215, 237, 240, 242, 244, 250, 256, 258, 478, 501, 538–539, 601, 614, 616, 677
National Lung Screening Trial (NLST) 52–53, 100
National Thyroid Cancer Treatment Cooperative Study Group 40
nausea:
  causes of 694
  evaluation of 694

management of 695
and vomiting 694, 695
NAVIGATOR trial 591
NCCN. *See* National Comprehensive Cancer Network (NCCN)
NCDB study 538–539
NCI. *See* National Cancer Institute (NCI)
necrosis 10–11
NELSON trial 53
neoadjuvant chemoradiotherapy, gastroesophageal cancer 241
neoadjuvant chemotherapy:
 benefit of 381
 with carboplatin/paclitaxel 504
 cycles of 700–701
 male breast cancer 216
 ovarian cancer 502–503
 for patients with muscle-invasive disease 382–383
 TNBC 181–182
neoadjuvant immunotherapy, nonmetastatic bulky nodal disease with 468–469
neoadjuvant therapy:
 criteria for 501
 gastroesophageal cancer 238, 242
 HER2-positive breast cancer 155–158
 NSCLC 71–73
 rectal cancer 271–272
 results for 501
NeoALTTO study 160
NEOCRTEC5010 study 238
nephrectomy 363, 364
neratinib:
 HER2-positive breast cancer 158–159
 HER2-positive metastatic breast cancer 172
 IBC 206
neuroendocrine carcinoma 334–335
neuroendocrine cervical cancers 549
neuroendocrine tumors (NETs)
 adjuvant treatment 330
 description of 327
 ENET 328, 328f, 331t
 evaluation 330, 334
 grade3, 335–336
 incidental rectal 330
 lung 338
 management 328
 metastatic pancreatic 339
 pancreatic 340
 peptide receptor radiotherapy in 337

staging 329t, 331
treatment of incidental appendix 327
type 1 gastric 333–334, 334t
neurologic syndromes 97
neuro-oncology, bevacizumab in 11
next generation sequencing (NGS)
 IBC 204
 TNBC 196
NGS. *See* next generation sequencing (NGS)
nivolumab 113, 341
NLST. *See* National Lung Screening Trial (NLST)
N-methyl-D-aspartate (NMDA) receptor antagonist 706
nodal disease 243–244
non-malignant brain tumors 6
nonmelanoma skin cancers 477
 AJCC8 and BWH systems 480–482, 481t, 488t
 cutaneous squamous cell carcinoma 477–483
 high-risk factors 478–480
 therapy for 482–483
non-metastatic castrate-resistant prostate cancer 427
nonseminomas 445–446, 448
 stage I 442
 surveillance schedule of 443t
 testicular germ cell, stage II 445t
 treatment 449
nonseminomatous germ cell tumors 440
nonsentinel lymph node involvement 542, 542t
non-small cell lung cancer (NSCLC). *See also* recurrent and metastatic NSCLC
 ADAURA trial 60
 adjuvant clinical trials and meta-analyses 57, 58t
 CALGB trial9633 56–57
 first-line therapy 80–83
 IALT 56
 squamous cell 90–91
 stage III 73–75
 stage I-III, adjuvant chemotherapy 65t
 stage II-III 64, 66
  adjuvant chemotherapy 64, 66
  adjuvant immunotherapy 68–69
  adjuvant radiotherapy 69–70
  adjuvant targeted therapy 66–68
  carboplatin 66
  chemotherapy regimen, choice of 66
  neoadjuvant therapy 71–73

stage IV   80
surgical resection   63
TNM staging system   57, 58t
trial data   82t
tumor size and redefining T scoring   57–60
novel therapeutic agents   693
NSABP C-08 phase III trial   263
NSCLC. *See* non-small cell lung cancer (NSCLC)
Nursing Delirium Screening Scale (NuDESC)   696

O

OFS. *See* ovarian function suppression (OFS)
olaparib   431
monotherapy, TNBC   194
pancreatic adenocarcinoma   299–300
TNBC   181, 185
older adults:
adjuvant therapy   688
approach to decision-making for   686–687
with cancer in clinical trials   686, 687t
chemotherapy toxicity prediction tools in   681–682t
geriatric assessment   686
geriatric syndromes in   677–678
performance *vs.* functional status   684–685, 684t
oligodendroglioma   3
classification of   7–8
grade2, 7–8
grade3, 7–8
pathology   7–8
radiation treatment   8
standard of care treatment of   7–8
treatment of   7–8
oligometastatic disease   49, 415
oligometastatic prostate cancer, SBRT in management of   415–416
OlympiaD trial   147
OLYMPIA trial   135, 135f, 136
ONCODAGE prospective multicohort study   680
oncological outcomes, benefits in   404–405
Oncotype DX™   130, 256–257
Oncotype 21-gene assay recurrence score   216–217
opioid rotation   705–706
optimal cytoreduction   501
orchiectomy   443

oropharyngeal cancer:
betel nut chewing   19
HPV associated   32
HPV-related   16, 17t, 23, 26
p16 negative   17t
recurrent   36
risk factors   32
T2N3bM0, 21,T1N1M0   22–23
tobacco use   32
osimertinib   93, 94
osteoblastic metastasis   642
osteoclast inhibitors   429
osteonecrosis   570
osteopontin   107
osteosarcoma   585
EURAMOS-1 study   576–577
of left distal femur   576
neoadjuvant chemotherapy   573, 574
resectability of   573
treatment of   573
ovarian cancer   520, 599–600, 604, 611–612, 616
abdominal distention, initial treatment for   499–501
abdominal pain   516
chemotherapy in   501–502, 507–508
conservative therapy for   508–509
description of   499
DESKTOP III trial   504
epithelial   512–513
fertility preservation   508–509
FIGO staging criteria for   499, 500t
future management   516
germline testing   512
GOG-0213 trial   504
high-dose chemotherapy   516
hyperthermic intraperitoneal chemotherapy   502–503
intraperitoneal (IP) chemotherapy   502
management strategies   512
NCCN guidelines is for women   508
non-platinum-based strategy   512
NOVA study   505
optimal cytoreduction   501
PARP inhibitor maintenance therapy   503–504
patient experiences   516
platinum program   516
platinum-sensitive   504–505, 517
predisposition genes   619t
primary chemotherapy   517

primary platinum-based therapy 511
secondary cytoreduction 515
second-line:
   management of 515
   therapy of 513, 516, 518–519
   treatment strategies 511–520
single-cytotoxic-agent treatment 516
SOC-1 trial 505
substantial portion of 616–617
susceptibility genes and cumulative lifetimes risk 617t
treatment of 502
ovarian function suppression (OFS) 137
ovarian tissue cryopreservation 229

p

paclitaxel/carboplatin 506, 529–530, 537, 557, 558–559
   cycles of 507
Paget's disease 533
PALB2 mutation 617–618
palbociclib 140, 141t, 145
palliative care 506
palliative chemotherapy in metastatic disease 356–357
palliative sedation 696–697
   control symptoms 697
   indications for 697–698
   treatment for 698
pancreas adenocarcinoma 644
pancreatic adenocarcinoma:
   adjuvant FOLFIRINOX 301, 304
   anticoagulation management 294
   cross-sectional abdominal imaging 292–293
   diabetes mellitus and 303
   endoscopic biliary decompression 294
   EUS 292, 293, 300, 305, 306
   EUS-directed FNA 293
   FOLFIRINOX 299
   gemcitabine/cisplatin 299
   germline genetic testing 295
   molecular testing 294–295
   multidisciplinary consultation 297–298
   neoadjuvant chemotherapy 302
   neoadjuvant FOLFIRINOX 300–301
   olaparib 299–300
   pain control 306–307
   PREOPANC-1 trial 302
   screening 305–306
   second-line treatment 296–297
   somatic tumor molecular profiling 295
   surgical resection 302
   systemic treatment 295–296
pancreatic cancer 607
PAOLA-1 trial 503
papillary thyroid cancer 46, 630
para-aortic lymph nodes 536
paraganglioma 330–332
   peptide receptor radiotherapy in 332
   systemic therapy 332
parenteral anticoagulation, benefits of 658
PARPi. *See* poly (ADP-ribose) polymerase inhibitor (PARPi)
PARP inhibitors. *See* poly adenosine diphosphate-ribose polymerase (PARP) inhibitors
PCI. *See* prophylactic cranial irradiation (PCI)
PDGFRA D842V kinase domain mutation 590, 591
PD-1/PD-L1 inhibitor therapy 387
pegylated liposomal doxorubicin (PLD) 517, 518–519
pelvic lymph node dissection 380
pelvic mass 556
pelvic pain 571
pelvic radiation therapy 531
pembrolizumab 26, 185, 377, 381, 386, 540, 541, 559
   enfortumab vedotin with 386
   HNSCC, recurrent/metastatic 33–34
   IBC 206
   NSCLC, recurrent and metastatic 84
   TNBC 183–184, 193
peptide receptor radiotherapy 332–333, 337
percutaneous ethanol injection (PEI) 312–313
perineural invasion 394, 478
peripheral neuropathy 386–387
peripheral sensorimotor neuropathy 541
peritoneal cavity 502
pertuzumab:
   HER2-positive breast cancer 155
   neoadjuvant therapy, HER2-positive breast cancer 156–157
PETACC-8 phase III trial 263–264
pheochromocytoma 330–331, 603
PIK3CA mutations 146
plasma exchange 674
platelet-derived growth factor alpha (PDGFRA) receptor 589

platinum-based chemotherapy   503, 520
platinumbased therapy   505
platinum-resistant disease   506–507
platinum-resistant neuroendocrine
    carcinoma   341
platinum-resistant ovarian cancer,
    management of   518–519
platinum-sensitive recurrent ovarian cancer:
  secondary cytoreduction in   504–505
  standard treatment of   505
  treatment options   506–507
PLD. *See* pegylated liposomal doxorubicin
    (PLD)
pleomorphic (nonclassic) LCIS   127
pleural effusion   645
pleurectomy decortication   111, 112
Pleurx catheter   506–507
PMS2, 626
pneumonitis   667
poly adenosine diphosphate-ribose
    polymerase (PARP) inhibitors   431,
    503–504, 511, 513
  as "maintenance therapy," 520
  use of   505
polyp   265
polypharmacy   679
poly(ADP-ribose) polymerase (PARP)   9
poly (ADP-ribose) polymerase inhibitor
    (PARPi)
  HR+/HER2-negative breast
    cancer   134–136
  non-metastatic IBC   207
  TNBC   194–195
polyposis, absence of   631
polyps, history of   626
positron emission tomography (PET)
  IBC   203–204, 204f
  NLST   54
Post-Operative Radiation Therapy in
    Endometrial Cancer (PORTEC-2)
    trial   531
pregnancy and fertility, breast cancer patients:
  adjuvant chemotherapy   228–229
  anti-HER2 treatment   230–231
  BRCA pathogenic variant   228
  chemotherapy-induced amenorrhea
    225–227
  delivery, optimal timing of   230–231
  elective abortion   230
  ER status   227
  fetal/infant risk of malformations   228

systemic therapy   231–232
taxanes   232
PREOPANC-1 trial   302
primary brain tumors   3
primary mucinous ovarian cancer   551–553,
    552t
primary vaginal carcinoma   545
PRIMA trial   503
procarbazine, lomustine, and vincristine
    (PCV)   8
PRODIGE23, 268
progesterone receptor (PR)   663
PRONET group   335
prophylactic bilateral mastectomy   613
prophylactic brain irradiation   549
prophylactic cranial irradiation
    (PCI)   101–102
prophylactic mastectomy   628
prostate adenocarcinoma   406–407, 424–425,
    642
prostate biopsy tissue   406
prostate cancer   389, 421
  active surveillance, radical prostatectomy,
    and radiation therapy   392–393, 404,
    405t
  adjuvant radiotherapy   409
  ADT   414
  androgen deprivation therapy
    (ADT)   410–411
  biomarkers   395
  brachytherapy   407
  clinically node-positive   415
  definitive brachytherapy   408
  description of   389
  diagnosis of   402–403
  disease-free survival rate   393–395
  early and locally advance   399
  external beam radiotherapy (EBRT)   407
  high-risk disease   411–413
  high-volume metastatic   416–418
  intermediate-risk   405, 407–409
  invasive therapies for   395
  local radiotherapy   395–396
  low- and very low-risk disease   403–404
  low volume metastatic   415–416
  management options   406
  multi-parametric MRI   399–401, 400t
  NCCN risk stratification for   405t
  negative biopsies   403
  patient qualify for active surveillance
    392–393

PI-RADS score system 400t
predict oncologic outcomes 406
prostatectomy 407
prostatic bed 411
PSA screening 390-392
radiation therapy 410, 413
risk of 402
screening 401-418
treatment options 407
Prostate Cancer Intervention Versus Observation trial (PIVOT) 404
prostate health index 402-403
prostate specific antigen (PSA) 389, 399
Prostate Testing for Cancer Treatment trial (ProtecT) 404
prostatic adenocarcinoma 405-406
ProtecT. *See* Prostate Testing for Cancer Treatment trial (ProtecT)
proton therapy 575
PRRT in PGGL 333t
pseudocapsule 570
pseudo-progression, diagnosis of 10-11
psychostimulants 705
PTEN mutation 614
pulmonary embolism (PE) 653, 656-657

q
quadrant abdominal pain 647
quadriceps femoris muscle 489-490
quality of life (QOL) 679
QUASAR2 phase III trial 263

r
radiation exposure 6
radiation-induced cancer:
  LDCT 54
  lungs 54-55, 55t
  NSCLC 56-60
radiation-induced necrosis 11
radiation-induced sarcoma 585
radiation therapy, male breast cancer 216
radiation treatment:
  cumulative dose and fractionation of 11
  IBC 207
radical chemoradiotherapy 350-352, 354-355
radical cystectomy 379, 381, 383
radical hysterectomy 550
radical prostatectomy 406, 423, 424-429
RADICALS trial 410
radioactive iodine (RAI) therapy:

refractory differentiated thyroid cancer 44-45, 45f
thyroid cancer 40-41
radiofrequency ablation (RFA) 312-313
radiotherapy 314
RAI. *See* radioactive iodine (RAI) therapy
RAINBOW study 252
RAPIDO trial 268
RAVES trial 410
RECIST. *See* Response Evaluation Criteria in Solid Tumors (RECIST)
rectal cancer, early-stage:
  adjuvant FOLFOX chemotherapy 274-275
  capecitabine 272-273
  5-FU continuous infusion 272-273
  IBD patients 278-279
  initial management 268-271
  MMR 279-280
  PRODIGE23, 268
  RAPIDO trial 268
  risk factors 267
  surveillance 275
  total mesorectal excision 273-274, 276-277
  total neoadjuvant therapy 270, 270t-271t
  treatment, neoadjuvant therapy 271-272
recurrent and metastatic colorectal cancer:
  capecitabine + bevacizumab 284
  chemotherapy combination 284
  encorafenib + cetuximab 286
  FOLFIRI and bevacizumab 285, 287
  pembrolizumab 285-286
  surgical resecton 287
  trastuzumab and pertuzumab 288
recurrent and metastatic NSCLC 84-85, 86t, 87f, 87t
  dual immunotherapy 82-84
  first-line therapy 80-83, 90-91
  ipilimumab plus nivolumab 85
  KRAS G12C mutation 89-90
  liquid biopsy 92, 93
  molecular testing 80, 90, 92
  single-agent immunotherapy, high PD-L1 patients 84
  smoking status, treatment 88-89
  systemic treatment, PD-L1 negative 85, 87, 89f
  tissue-based testing 92
  tissue biopsy 94
recurrent/metastatic HNSCC:
  biomarkers 33-34

CPS 33, 34
FNA biopsy 33
immunotherapy 34, 36
PD-L1 combined positive score 33–34
recurrent laryngeal SCC 34–35
risk factors 32
single-agent chemotherapy 36
systemic treatment 35–36
recurrent ovarian cancer:
 maintenance strategy in 520
 treatment of 512–513
renal cancer 361
 adjuvant therapy 363–364
 management 371–372
 nephrectomy in treatment plan 364–366
 patients predictive of shortened survival 362–363t
 patients treated with systemic therapy 361–363
 therapy 366–367, 370–371
 TNM staging 366t
 treatment option 367–369
renal cell carcinoma (RCC) 361, 364, 367, 644
 description of 368
 immunotherapy therapy 368
 kidney transplant 368–369
renal medullary carcinoma 371, 372
Response Evaluation Criteria in Solid Tumors (RECIST) 195
retroperitoneal mass 639
retrospective analyses 514
rhabdoid de-differentiation 370, 371
ribociclib 140, 141t
right breast carcinoma, stage I 585
right hemicolectomy 329
risk-reducing salpingo-oophorectomy (RRSO) 616
rivaroxaban, CYP3A4 for 654
Rizzoli Institute 570
RTOG90-1, 534
RTOG pilot study 351
rucaparib 431, 505
RxPONDER trial:
 iDFS 131, 132
 outcomes, premenopausal and postmenopausal patients 130, 131

S
sacituzumab govitecan 388
 TNBC 191, 197
 triple-negative IBC 208

sacral chordomas, location of 571
sacral mass, pelvis revealing 568, 569f
sacrum, chordoma of 570
salivary gland cancer 15, 28
salvage laryngectomy 20
salvage radiation therapy 396
Sarcoma Meta-analysis Collaboration (SMAC) 582
sarcomas 545
 extremity 581
sarcomatoid 370, 371
 de-differentiation 370
SCC. See squamous cell carcinoma (SCC)
SEER. See Surveillance, Epidemiology, and End Results (SEER)
semicustom periacetabular reconstruction endoprosthesis 572
seminal vesicle involvement by tumor 394
seminomas 439–440
 stage I 442, 444
 stage II 445t
 treatment 448
sentinel lymph node 347–348, 542, 543
sentinel lymph node biopsy (SLNB) 118, 119, 129
Sertoli-Leydig cell tumors 557
serum alpha fetoprotein 639
serum inhibin 556–557
serum thyroglobulin, differentiated thyroid cancer marker 41–42
SIADH. See syndrome of inappropriate antidiuretic hormone secretion (SIADH)
Siewert types, gastroesophageal junction adenocarcinoma 240–241
sigmoid colon, adenocarcinoma of 633
SignateraTM test 264
Simian virus 40 (SV40) 106
simultaneous integrated boost (SIB) 356
single-agent checkpoint inhibition 559
single-agent pegylated liposomal doxorubicin 518
single nucleotide variants (SNV) 601
skin punch biopsy 204
sleep disturbances, treatment of 704
SLNB. See sentinel lymph node biopsy (SLNB)
small cell lung cancer (SCLC) 549
 adjuvant chemotherapy 100
 adjuvant radiation therapy 100
 carboplatin 101
 with CNS metastases 102
 diagnosis of 97

extensive-stage 101
hematogenous metastases 99
immunotherapy 101
limited-stage 98–99
PCI 101–102
risk factors 99
screening tests 100
second-line therapies 102
staging system 100
surgery 100
symptoms 99
SMARCB1 gene 371
SMART. *See* Surgery for Mesothelioma After Radiation Therapy (SMART)
Society of Surgical Oncology 119
soft tissue sarcomas (STS) 586
  adjuvant radiation therapy 581
  adjuvant therapy 590
  chemotherapy 587
  description of 579
  management strategy 579–580
  multidisciplinary care 582–583
  neoadjuvant therapy 589–590
  oncologically inadequate resection of 584
  positive surgical margins 584
  primary biopsy 590
  recommendation for treatment 582
  retrospective analyses 582–583
  stage IV disease 587
  workup 580
somatic tumor testing 430–431
somatostatin receptor imaging 336–337
sonidegib 489–490
sorafenib 44, 366–367
sotorasib, NSCLC patients 89
spinal cord tumors 3–4
squamous cell cancer 343
squamous cell carcinoma (SCC) 346, 533
  anal cancer 346
  of cervix 533, 535
  of head and neck 657
  laryngeal, recurrent 34, 35
  management 657
  metastatic 33, 37
  oropharyngeal, recurrent 31, 36–37
  treatment of 537
squamous cell vaginal cancer, risk factors for 545
SRS. *See* stereotactic radiosurgery (SRS)
stereotactic body radiotherapy (SBRT) 407–408
stereotactic radiosurgery (SRS)

breast cancer 170
SCLC 100
steroid therapy 672–673
subcutaneous hemorrhage 658
subtotal glandular therapy 407
sunitinib 365, 366–367
supraclavicular lymph node 371
Surgery for Mesothelioma After Radiation Therapy (SMART) 112
surgical lymph node 536
SURTIME trial 365
Surveillance, Epidemiology, and End Results (SEER) 40, 70, 118, 127, 144, 214, 216
SV40. *See* Simian virus 40 (SV40)
SWENOTECA group 440
SWOG S1 609, 341
SWOG 1500 study 369
SWOG 8814 trial 130
syndrome of inappropriate antidiuretic hormone secretion (SIADH) 97
syndrome X 625, 631
systemic chemotherapy 322, 699
systemic therapeutic(s) 323
Systemic Therapies for HER2-Positive Metastatic Breast Cancer Study (SystHERs) 164
SystHERs. *See* Systemic Therapies for HER2-Positive Metastatic Breast Cancer Study (SystHERs)

t

tacrolimus, liver transplant on 544
TAILORx trial 136
talazoparib, TNBC 194
tamoxifen:
  vs. anastrozole, DCIS 124, 125*t*
  DCIS 123–124, 124*t*
targeted therapies, use of 647
taxanes 184–185, 232
TBCRC 048 trial 147, 195
T4bN0M0 laryngeal squamous cell carcinoma 20–21
TCH. *See* trastuzumab (TCH)
T-DM1. *See* trastuzumab emtansine (T-DM1)
temozolomide 8, 9, 340
testicular cancer, stage II 444–445
thoracentesis 91, 108, 645, 703
thoracic back pain 642
thyroid cancer 602
  anaplastic 39, 46–48
  differentiated 40–46

histologic types 39–40
Hurthle cell 39
medical and surgical implications 602–603
medullary 48–49
papillary 46
radiation exposure 39
thyroiditis 667
thyroid lobectomy 40
thyroid-stimulating hormone (TSH)
evaluation, head and neck cancer 27
suppressive therapy, thyroid cancer 42, 42t
tisotumab vedotin-tftv 541
tissue-based testing 92
tissue of origin (ToO)
empiric chemotherapy 647
genetic profiling 647
molecular profiling 646–647
TMB. *See* tumor mutational burden (TMB)
TME. *See* total mesorectal excision (TME)
TNBC. *See* triple-negative breast cancer (TNBC)
T2N3bM0 oropharyngeal squamous cell carcinomas 21
TNM clinical staging:
colorectal cancer 269t
esophagus and gastroesophageal junction cancers 236t
hypopharyngeal cancer 18t
lung cancer 64t
NSCLC 57, 58t
oropharyngeal cancer, HPV-related 17t
oropharyngeal cancer, p16 negative 17t–18t
SCLC 100
T1N1M0 oropharyngeal squamous cell carcinomas 22–23
topotecan 506
total abdominal hysterectomy 530
total mesorectal excision (TME) 267, 268, 273–277
total neoadjuvant therapy, rectal cancer 270, 270t–271t
total thyroidectomy:
differentiated thyroid cancer 40, 43
medullary thyroid carcinoma 49
RAI therapy 40–41
toxicity 384
transarterial chemoembolization (TACE) 313–314
transarterial embolization (TAE) 314

transarterial treatments 314
transrectal biopsy, risks associated with 403
transurethral resection of a bladder tumor (TURBT) 378
trastuzumab (TCH)
duration, breast cancer 152–154
gastroesophageal cancer 245
HER2-positive breast cancer 151–152
neoadjuvant therapy, HER2-positive breast cancer 156
pregnancy 230
trastuzumab deruxtecan (T-Dxd)
interstitial lung disease 170–171
metastatic esophagogastric cancer 252
metastatic IBC, HER2 positive 208
toxicity, HER2-positive metastatic breast cancer 170–171
trastuzumab emtansine (T-DM1)
HER2-positive breast cancer 154–155
HER2-positive metastatic breast cancer 167–168
IBC 206, 207
neoadjuvant therapy, HER2-positive breast cancer 158
toxicity 174
trastuzumab maintenance 559
treatment-related (radiation) necrosis 11
triple-negative breast cancer (TNBC)
BRCA1/2 mutations 193–194
CDKIs 197
chemotherapy 181–183, 191, 192
CNS involvement 196–197
definition 179
Enhertu 197
fertility 185–186
future areas of development 189
genetic counseling 194
germline testing 180
immune checkpoint inhibition 183–184
immunotherapy 192–193
lifestyle recommendations 188–189
metastatectomy 197
metastatic pattern, spread 196
neoadjuvant chemotherapy 181–182
NGS 196
novel therapies 197
PARP inhibitors 194–195
pathogenic germline variant 180–181
postsurgical findings, disease management 186–187
prognostic markers 179–180

recurrence monitor 187–188
sacituzumab govitecan 191, 197
somatic BRCA mutations 195
systemic therapy 181
systemic treatment, side effects of 184–185
TBCRC 048 trial 195
Trousseau syndrome 97
TRYPHAENA study 205
TSH. *See* thyroid-stimulating hormone (TSH)
tubular adenomas on colonoscopy 626
tucatinib:
  HER2-positive metastatic breast cancer 172–173
  IBC 207
tumor:
  absence of protein in 625–626
  cell death of 10
  differentiation and proliferation rate 327
  response, definition of 570
tumor mutational burden (TMB) 29, 192, 356, 644
tunica albuginea 440–441
TURBT. *See* cystoscopy/transurethral resection of a bladder tumor (TURBT)
Turin criteria, poorly differentiated cancer 46
tyrosine kinase inhibitor (TKIs) 588

u

ultrasound guided biopsy 231
uncommon gynecologic cancers, description of 549
unfractionated heparin (UFH), ambulatory patient for treatment with 654
United Kingdom National Anal Cancer Trial (ACT II) 343–344
United States Preventative Task Force (USPTF) 53
University of California, San Francisco (UCSF) criteria 313
urinary tract infections (UTIs) 375
urothelial bladder cancer 375
urothelial carcinoma 375
US Preventive Services Task Force (USPSTF) 390
USPTF. *See* United States Preventative Task Force (USPTF)
uterine cancer, stage III 597
uterine leiomyosarcoma 560–561
  aforementioned options 561

appropriate therapy 560
management of 560, 560f
postoperative management 560
stage I or II 560
treatment of 560–561
uterine sarcomas 531–532, 562
uterine serous carcinoma 558–559
  NCCN guidelines 558–559
  postoperative treatment options 558
  treatment recommendation 559
uterine smooth muscle tumor of uncertain malignant potential (STUMP) 561–562
  diagnosis of 561–562
  features of 562
  pathologic features 561
  postoperative management 561
  risk of recurrence 562

v

vaginal brachytherapy 531
vaginal cancer 533
  histologies of 545
  radiation therapy for 546
  risk factors for 545
  stage II 546
vaginal intraepithelial neoplasia (VAIN) 533
vaginal melanoma 553–554
valrubicin 377
Van Nuys Prognostic Index (VNPI) 124
variant of uncertain significance (VUS) 195
vascular endothelial growth factor (VEGF) 362, 365, 501–502, 558
VATS. *See* video-assisted thoracoscopic surgery (VATS)
venous thromboembolism (VTE) 651
  AVERT trial 652
  baseline risk of 652
  CASSINI trial 652
  initial treatment of acute 654
  management strategy 655–656
  pharmacologic prophylaxis 651–653
  prophylaxis in ambulatory cancer patients 651–652
  treatment of incidental 653
video-assisted thoracoscopic surgery (VATS)
vincristine, doxorubicin, and cyclophosphamide (VDC) 568
viral infections 310
VISION trial 418
vismodegib 489–490

VNPI. *See* Van Nuys Prognostic Index (VNPI)
volumetric modulated arc therapy (VMAT)   356
vomiting, management of   695
Vulnerable Elders Survey (VES-13)   678, 680
vulvar cancer   533
   with palpable left inguinal adenopathy   543
   radiation therapy   544–545
vulvar intraepithelial neoplasia:
   treatment   544
   on vulvar biopsy   544
vulvar intraepithelial neoplasia (VIN)   533
vulvar melanoma   545
vulvar squamous cell carcinoma:
   description of   542
   GROINSS-V   542
   NCCN guidelines   543

vulvovaginal melanoma   553–554
   biopsy   553
   NCCN guidelines   553
   prognostic factors for   553
   recurrence and death from   553–554

W

warfarin   655, 659
WBRT. *See* whole brain radiation therapy (WBRT)
West-German Study Group phase II ADAPT trial   157
WHO Classification of Tumors of the Digestive System   327
whole brain radiation therapy (WBRT)   102, 170
Wnt/beta-catenin signaling pathway   592
World Health Organization (WHO) classification system   3

Printed and bound by CPI Group (UK) Ltd, Croydon, CR0 4YY
14/11/2023

08188336-0001